Prosthetics & Orthotics
in Clinical Practice

A Case Study Approach

Prosthetics & Orthotics
in Clinical Practice

A Case Study Approach

Bella J. May, EdD, PT, CEEAA, FAPTA
Professor Emerita Georgia Health Science University,
    Augusta, Georgia;
President, BJM Enterprises, Dublin, California;
Adjunct Professor, Department of Physical Therapy,
    California State University–Sacramento, Sacramento,
    California

Margery A. Lockard, PT, PhD
Associate Clinical Professor
Department of Health Sciences and Health Administration
Drexel University, Philadelphia, Pennsylvania

F.A. Davis Company • Philadelphia

F. A. Davis Company
1915 Arch Street
Philadelphia, Pennsylvania 19103
www.fadavis.com

Printed in the United States of America

Last digit indicates print number: 10 9 8 7 6 5 4 3 2 1

Acquisitions Editor/Publisher: Margaret M. Biblis
Manager of Content Development: George W. Lang
Developmental Editor: Peg Waltner
Art and Design Manager: Carolyn O'Brien

As new scientific information becomes available through basic and clinical research, recommended treatments and drug therapies undergo changes. The author(s) and publisher have done everything possible to make this book accurate, up to date, and in accord with accepted standards at the time of publication. The author(s), editors, and publisher are not responsible for errors or omissions or for consequences from application of the book, and make no warranty, expressed or implied, in regard to the contents of the book. Any practice described in this book should be applied by the reader in accordance with professional standards of care used in regard to the unique circumstances that may apply in each situation. The reader is advised always to check product information (package inserts) for changes and new information regarding dose and contraindications before administering any drug. Caution is especially urged when using new or infrequently ordered drugs.

Library of Congress Cataloging-in-Publication Data

May, Bella J.
  Prosthetics & orthotics in clinical practice : a case study approach / Bella J. May, Margery A. Lockard.
    p. ; cm.
  Includes bibliographical references and index.
  ISBN-13: 978-0-8036-2257-9
  ISBN-10: 0-8036-2257-0
  1. Prosthesis—Case studies. 2. Orthopedic apparatus—Case studies. 3. Orthopedic apparatus—Case studies. 4. Physical therapy. 5. Physical therapy assistants. I. Lockard, Margery A. II. Title.
  [DNLM: 1. Prostheses and Implants—Case Reports. 2. Amputation—rehabilitation—Case Reports. 3. Amputees—psychology—Case Reports. 4. Orthotic Devices—Case Reports. 5. Physical Therapy Modalities—Case Reports. WE 172]
  RD755.M365 2011
  617'.9—dc22

                                                                2010033098

To all who "do not follow where the path leads, rather go where there is no path and leave a trail" (author unknown) as they facilitate each person's return to a meaningful life.

BJM

To my husband who took care of everything else, without complaining, so I could sit behind the computer for hours on end!

MAL

In the last decade, many changes have taken place in the field of physical therapy and in the care of individuals who need prostheses and orthoses. Improved technology, major developments in computerized components and robotics, as well as new materials have enabled many disabled individuals to return to useful and functional lives. Military personnel who have lost limbs or lost the use of parts of limbs are now able to remain in the military and fulfill all required duties.

In the same decade, the expectations of physical therapists and physical therapist assistants have also changed dramatically. Physical therapists are now educated at the doctoral level and expected to make diagnoses, establish treatment plans, implement or supervise the implementation of complex interventions, as well as participate in research to further the knowledge base of the profession. As its cousin *Amputation and Prosthetics: A Case Study Text,* this book is designed to assist the physical therapy student become an effective clinical decision maker when working with individuals in need of prostheses and orthoses. It is also designed to help the physical therapist assistant student gain the knowledge and skills necessary to be an effective member of the physical therapy team. Although written primarily as a text, this book can also serve as an excellent reference for the practitioner who may not be current in these areas.

The case studies found in each chapter and the accompanying activities facilitate an active learning process. Whether individually or in small groups, working through the stimulus questions enables the student to apply the information provided to actual situations. The decision-making process of the physical therapist is emphasized in the student activities; the role of the physical therapist assistant is also considered in the specifically designed physical therapist assistant activities. Even though the book contains information and concepts beyond the practice of the physical therapist assistant, understanding each other's scope of practice continues to be important for effective teamwork. The online faculty manual is a guide for the faculty—particularly faculty who do not have a strong background in these areas.

Whether working with only one or two patients in need of appliances or in a facility where similar patients are treated frequently, this book can be a resource for all practitioners and improve their ability to provide the most up-to-date care for all individuals in need of prostheses or orthoses.

BELLA J. MAY, EdD, PT, CEEAA, FAPTA

CONTRIBUTOR

Robert S. Gailey, PhD, PT
Associate Professor
University of Miami Miller School of Medicine
Department of Physical Therapy
Coral Gables, Florida
Director
Functional Outcomes Research and Evaluation Center
Miami Veterans Affairs Healthcare System
Miami, Florida

REVIEWERS

Elaine L. Bukowski, PT, DPT, MS (D)ABDA
Professor of Physical Therapy, Associate Director of
    Post-Professional DPT Program
Richard Stockton College of New Jersey
Pomona, New Jersey

Deborah A. Edmondson, PT, EdD
Associate Professor, Academic Coordinator of Clinical
    Education
Tennessee State University
Department of Physical Therapy
Nashville, Tennessee

Cheryl Ford-Smith, PT, DPT, MS, NCS
Associate Professor
Virginia Commonwealth University
Department of Physical Therapy
Richmond, Virginia

Robert H. Fuchs, PT, MA, ATP, CSCS
Associate Professor, Physical Therapist
University of Nebraska Medical Center
Division of Physical Therapy Education
Omaha, Nebraska

Natalie R. N. Housel, PT, EdD
Associate Professor
Tennessee State University
Department of Physical Therapy
Nashville, Tennessee

ACKNOWLEDGMENTS

While writing a book appears to be a solitary endeavor, it is not. There are many individuals who contribute to a book directly or indirectly. Throughout my career, my patients have helped me learn how to be a more effective practitioner and to consider each as an individual and not to make assumptions about goals based on age or disability. To all my patients over the years, I owe a debt of gratitude, and much that I have learned from them is part of this book.

My students have also taught me a great deal and, in their evaluations of my courses and previous texts, have helped me make this text as readable and "user friendly" as I can. Students in the California State University Sacramento physical therapy classes of 2008 and 2009 actually reviewed many of the prosthetic chapters in development and provided good feedback on what was helpful and what was confusing.

Many of the photographs were freely donated by component manufacturers; their prompt responses, explanations, and materials enabled us to include the most current and clear photographs and descriptions. Over the years, my patients have willingly let me photograph them to enhance both publications and teaching. Special thanks go to Lindsay M. Morehead who willingly endured numerous photo shoots during the past 2 years.

Thanks also to my coauthor Margery A. Lockard, who has made the complex field of orthotics clinically available to students and practitioners. Most especially, I thank the editors who kept the book moving even when I despaired of it reaching publication. Margaret M. Biblis initially proposed combining prosthetics and orthotics and, through the years of development and production, was a patient listener to my complaints and an enabler of the whole process. Margaret "Peg" Waltner carefully edited each chapter, tried hard to keep us on time, and made sure every "t" was crossed and "i" was dotted. Without the hard work and support of these individuals and others in the artistic and production staff of F. A. Davis, this book would never have seen the light of day.

BELLA J. MAY

Having used the earlier editions of this textbook, *Amputations and Prosthetics: A Case Study Approach,* to support courses in Prosthetics and Orthotics that I have taught over the years, I was honored to be invited by Bella J. May to help her update and expand the book to include orthotic devices. I was particularly excited about this project because it provided the opportunity to present this material as I had tried to teach it for many years: not as two separate bodies of information that just happened to be fused together in one course, but in a way that helps students see the similarities among prosthetic and orthotic devices: how they work biomechanically; how they are selected or prescribed; and how to train individuals to use their devices to achieve their functional goals. I thank Bella for this extraordinary and rewarding opportunity.

Another focus of the book that has been exciting for me is that it not only presents the necessary information about the devices, their componentry, and what types of patients typically use them, but also graphically shows students the processes involved in making the clinical decisions about device selection and prescription, how to train patients in their use, and how to diagnose problems when they arise. The development of many of the graphics that illustrate these decision-making processes are a direct result of years of student questions that guided me to organize, outline, and clarify how to apply knowledge and examination findings to get to the decision that was needed. I owe a huge debt to all the persistent students from Hahnemann, Arcadia, Temple, and Drexel universities who kept asking "why and how."

Prosthetics and orthotics is not a subject matter that can be described with just a "sea of words." Students must see and ultimately touch and move the devices to understand how they work and can help clients. Thus, I am thankful to the editors who supported our efforts to ensure that all the major concepts in the text are presented visually in the many photographs and drawings throughout the text. I would like to thank all the friends and clients who were willing to share their devices with you, the reader, and paused or adjusted their schedules for the camera. These include Carol Chew, Rocco DiSimone, Bob Dyer, Jeff Emrey, Father Greg Hickey, Michael Kennedy, Beth Lockard, Rita McClerkin, Christopher Nowak, Brian Smithman, and Liz Thompson. I would also like to thank photographer Jason Torres for his extraordinary skill and willingness to "keep snapping" until the picture was right.

I also need to thank the prosthetic and orthotic professionals who helped me to find examples of all the devices and materials that I wanted to show. Jack LaWall, CPO, and Tim Rayer, CP, were very supportive to me in this project, always took my calls with a smile, and always came up with the materials I needed. Thanks also go to Jane Fedorczyk, PT, PhD, CHT, ACT, director of the Hand and Upper Quarter Rehabilitation Programs in the Department of Physical Therapy at Drexel University, who provided most of the upper limb orthoses and splints.

Thanks also go to the extensive and creative team at F. A. Davis who provided technical and managerial support and guided this textbook from an idea to reality. We are fortunate to have Publisher Margaret Biblis working with us, whose vision, energy, and experience kept us focused, and development editor Peg Waltner, whose patience, persistence, and positivity were a constant in keeping this project moving forward.

Finally, I could never have completed this project without the unfaltering support of my husband, children, and friends, who gave up countless hours of time and attention, smilingly "covered the bases," and never asked, "how can she still be working on that book"!

MARGERY A. LOCKARD

CONTENTS

Foundation for Prosthetics/Orthotic Practice

Introduction to Prosthetics and Orthotics

OBJECTIVES

At the end of this chapter, all students are expected to:

1. Discuss the key milestones in the history of prosthetics and orthotics.
2. Discuss the rationale for learning about prosthetics and orthotics.
3. Discuss the role and function of members of a clinic team.

People have used external devices to help them function throughout the history of humankind. Shoes and foot inserts made of animal hair were early orthoses as innkeepers recognized their client's painful feet and provided padding from animal hair gathered in the barns. There is evidence of the use of splints to support broken or injured limbs since the early dawn of civilization. A 45,000-year-old skull in the Smithsonian Institution gives evidence from teeth alignment that he may have been missing one arm. More evidence of amputations, prostheses, and bracing can be found in the records of the early Greek, Roman, and Egyptian civilizations with more emphasis on science and medicine.[1] An early recorded amputation was performed by Hegesistratus, who, in 484 BCE escaped from the stocks by cutting off one of his feet; he is reported to have carved himself a wooden foot to compensate.[2]

The history of developments in prosthetics and orthotics is interesting as part of the study of human civilization development. Such a study indicates the effects of both scientific and creative endeavors directed to improve human function. As one studies historical developments in health care, the influence of wars becomes evident. Wars have always created large numbers of young people with disabilities, and governments have long believed they had an obligation to those who have been injured in their cause. The study of history further illustrates the role of research and the interrelationship between increased knowledge in human anatomy and physiology and improved methods of rehabilitation and care.

PHYSICAL THERAPY

The focus of this book is the use of prostheses and orthoses to improve human function. Physical therapists (PTs) examine patients/clients, evaluate data to make clinical judgments, diagnose to determine the impact of the problems on function, and then select and implement appropriate interventions.[3] Determining the need for prostheses or orthoses, working closely with **prosthetists** and **orthotists** in selecting appropriate components, and teaching patients and families the proper use and care of the devices are integral parts of these functions. Physical therapists' assistants (PTAs) work with the physical therapists in carrying out selected interventions and must also understand the fit and function of such devices. To fulfill these functions, the student must learn the different types of devices, their biomechanical principles, how they should be properly fitted, and how to teach clients the proper use and care of all devices. Today's growing technological advances have led to a great variety of currently available simple and complex devices, and continued research and development lead to new components and capabilities. To aid in the development of clinical judgment and clinical decision making both at the professional and assistant levels, this book incorporates patient cases, study questions, and clinical problems.

Diagnosis

Diagnosis by and in physical therapy practice is a topic of increasing interest within the profession. Throughout the book, physical therapy students will be asked to develop an appropriate diagnosis from the evaluative data. It is imperative that PTs make diagnoses to guide the prognosis, plan of care, and interventions.[3] There is a working definition of diagnosis: "Diagnosis is both a process and a descriptor. The diagnostic process includes integrating and evaluating the data that are obtained during the examination for the purpose of guiding the prognosis, the plan of care, and intervention strategies. Physical therapists assign diagnostic descriptors that identify a condition or syndrome at the level of the system, especially the human movement system, and at the level of the whole person."[3]

Patients who need a **prosthesis** or **orthosis** to improve function have movement dysfunctions. An individual who has just undergone an amputation and is referred for postsurgical physical therapy could be diagnosed as having gait and balance instability associated with a transtibial amputation for a diabetic ulcer. The diagnosis helps to organize and classify related syndromes to guide assessment and intervention. There may be one or more than one diagnosis for any given patient depending on the complexity of the condition. The reader is referred to several issues of *Physical Therapy* in 2009 for more in-depth information.[4,5] However, as a guide for students using the diagnostic process to work through cases presented in this book, **Box 1.1** outlines the current criteria and guidelines.[6] Physical therapists have been making diagnoses for many years although not using that designation. The process of clinical decision making is discussed in more detail in Chapter 20.

BOX 1.1 | Criteria and Guidelines for Diagnostic Descriptors

1. Use recognized anatomical, physiological, or movement-related terms to describe the condition or syndrome of the human movement system.
2. Include, if deemed necessary for clarity, the name of the pathology, disease, disorder, or symptom that is associated with the diagnosis.
3. Be as short as possible to improve clinical usefulness.

From Norton B: Diagnosis dialogues presentation at DxPT, APTA Annual Conference, San Antonio, TX, June 2008.

Activity

1. Review the historical developments presented in this chapter. In study groups, discuss the changes that have occurred and impetus for the changes and become familiar with some of the terminology. What do you think are the important concepts to understand to be effective as a physical therapist or physical therapist assistant?
2. If available, look and feel different prostheses and orthoses to gain a better understanding of the effects of technological advances.
3. Review the *Guide to Physical Therapist Practice,* second edition, and identify practice patterns related to the use of orthotics and prosthetics in practice.[7]
4. Review the World Health Organizations' International Classification of Functioning, Disability, and Health[8] to use as appropriate with the patient situations presented in this text.[9]

AMPUTATION SURGERY THROUGH THE AGES

Early **amputations** were only performed because of trauma or gangrene. Hippocrates (450–377 BCE) advocated performing amputation because of gangrene and cutting through "dead" tissue. Bleeding was controlled with **cauterization**. The emphasis was on surgical speed rather than shaping the residual limb. Many did not survive the shock of the amputation or the postoperative infections that frequently followed. Over the next decades, surgical techniques continued to improve and amputations were performed for chronic ulcers, tumors, and congenital deformities.[10]

Ambroise Pare[10] (1510–1590), a French army surgeon, reintroduced the use of ligatures, originally set forth by Hippocrates. This technique was more successful than crushing the amputation limb, dipping it in boiling oil, or other means of cautery that had been used during the Dark Ages to stop bleeding. Pare was the first to describe phantom sensation. General improvements and development in surgical techniques which continued through the centuries contributed to improvements in amputations, survival, and eventually residual limb preparation.

The relationship between the residual limb and the prosthetic socket is critically important in the person's eventual ability to functionally use a prosthetic device. With improved control of bleeding followed by the introduction of anesthesia, surgeons could begin to look at other surgical techniques rather than the standard cutting of the limb at one level, usually above the knee. James Syme[10] of Edinburgh performed the first successful amputation at the ankle joint in 1842; the procedure carries his name. He also advocated thigh amputations through the cortical bone of the condyles or the trochanters. In 1867, Joseph Lister[10] published his principles of antiseptic surgery that markedly reduced mortality during and after surgery. Lister also experimented with catgut as a ligature (1880) rather than silk or hemp that were not absorbed by body tissues and often caused inflammation and hemorrhage. These developments were all precursors to the improved surgical approaches to amputation that came in the 20th century.

The 20th Century

In the early 1900s, surgeons attempted to build bone bridges at the ends of transtibial (below-knee) amputations to allow for greater end bearing and to reduce breakdowns at the end of the residual limb. Traditionally, severed muscles were allowed to retract, and eventually, bone ends pushing against the distal skin of the residual limb in the open-ended sockets of the times caused pain and ulcerations. World War I with its 4200 U.S. amputations and almost 100,000 amputations in all armies led to improved skin flaps and greater consideration for levels of amputation. It was generally agreed that the middle third of the lower leg and lower to middle third of the thigh were the most ideal length for a residual limb.[10]

World War II led to further improvements in surgical techniques and greater consideration for the shape of the residual limb. Myoplasty, the suturing of the ends of severed muscles over the end of the bone, was first advocated in 1949[2] but did not gain in popularity until the 1950s when it was adopted by Dederich[11] and popularized by Burgess.[12] Myodesis, the suturing of severed muscles to distal bone, was advocated by Weiss[13] in the 1960s. Both myodesis and myoplasty are designed to provide muscle fixation for improved function and shape of the residual limb. In 1958, Michael Berlemont, in France, demonstrated immediate postsurgical fitting of prostheses.[10] The technique that involves placing the residual limb in a rigid postsurgical dressing fabricated using prosthetic principles was also advocated by Weiss[13] and was brought to the United States by Sarmiento[14] and Burgess.[12]

In the l960s and 1970s, a number of factors combined to lead surgeons to reconsider the transfemoral amputation as the level of choice for severely ischemic limbs. Immediate postoperative fitting reduced postoperative edema, allowing healing at transtibial levels, even for individuals with severe ischemia. Improved circulatory evaluation techniques provided accurate information on the presence of collateral circulation. The use of the long posterior flap with its increased blood supply also contributed to the healing capabilities of transtibial amputations.[15] All of these factors contributed to a reversal in the number of transtibial and transfemoral amputations performed for severe limb ischemia and concomitantly increased the number of individuals becoming successful prosthetic ambulators.

The Development of Prostheses Through the Ages

Early prostheses were usually made by local artisans or the individual who had sustained the loss. Most lower extremity limbs employed a simple peg with some straps for suspension. Upper extremity limbs were fabricated to hold a weapon or shield. Prostheses were made of wood or metal as dictated by availability and the preference of the fabricator.

In 1561, Pare designed an artificial limb of iron that employed an articulated joint for the first time (**Fig. 1.1**).[2] In 1696, Pieter Andriannszoon Verfuyn (Verduin'),[2] a Dutch surgeon, introduced the first known transtibial prosthesis with an unlocked knee joint. In concept, it resembled the thigh-corset prosthesis used in more recent times. A thigh cuff bore part of the weight and was connected by external hinges to a leg piece whose socket was made of copper and lined with leather. The leg piece terminated in a wooden foot. In 1843, James Potts[2] of London introduced a transfemoral (above-knee) prosthesis with a wooden shank and socket, a steel knee joint, and an articulated foot with leather thongs connecting the knee to the ankle. This enabled dorsiflexion (toe lift) whenever the wearer flexed the knee. The device was known as the "Anglesey (Anglesea) leg" because it was used by the Marquis of Anglesey following the loss of his leg in the Battle of Waterloo (**Fig. 1.2**).

During the American Civil War (1861–1865), interest in artificial limbs and amputation surgery increased because of the number of individuals surviving amputations (30,000 in the Union army) and the commitment of federal and state governments to

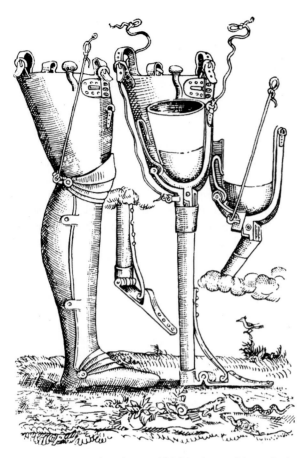

FIGURE 1.1. An above-knee artificial leg invented by Ambroise Paré (mid-16th century). *(From Paré A: Oeuvres Complétes, Paris, 1840, with permission from the National Library of Medicine.)*

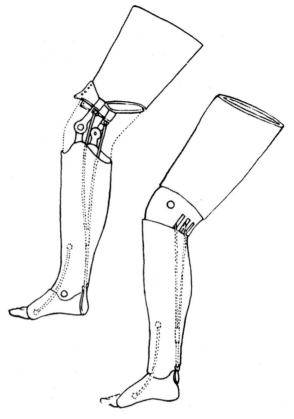

FIGURE 1.2. The Anglesey (Anglesea) leg (1816) with articulated knee, ankle, and foot. (Left) Below knee. (Right) Above knee. *(From Bigg HH: Orthopraxy: the mechanical treatment of deformities, debilities and deficiencies of the human frame, ed. 3. J & A Churchill, London, 1877, with permission.)*

pay for artificial limbs for veterans. J. E. Hanger,[2] who lost a leg during the Civil War, replaced the cords of his prosthesis with rubber bumpers at the ankle to control plantar flexion and dorsiflexion. The J. E. Hanger Company opened in Richmond, Virginia, in 1861, and in 1862 the first law providing free prostheses to people who lost limbs in warfare was enacted by the U.S. Congress.[2]

In 1863, the suction socket (**Fig. 1.3**) that employed the concept of using pressure to suspend an artificial limb was patented by an American, Dubois D. Parmelee,[16] who also invented a polycentric knee unit and a multiarticulated foot. In 1870 Congress passed a law that not only supplied artificial limbs to all honorably discharged persons from the military or naval service who had lost a limb while in the U.S. service, but also entitled them to receive one every 5 years.

THE WORLD WARS

Fewer Americans (4403) lost a limb during World War I (1914–1918) compared to the British (42,000) or to the total number of amputations (approximately 100,000) in all of the armies of Europe. However, the war was an impetus for improvements in artificial limb developments.[16] Collaboration between prosthetists and surgeons in the care of veterans with amputations led to the formation of the Artificial Limb Manufacturers Association in 1917. Little progress was made in the field of prosthetics and amputation surgery in the period between the two wars, but World War II again spurred developments. The American Orthotic and Prosthetic Association (AOPA) was established in 1949 and developed educational criteria and examinations to certify prosthetists and orthotists.[2]

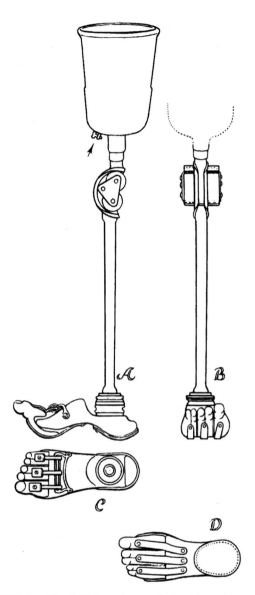

FIGURE 1.3. The D. D. Parmelee prosthesis with suction socket, patented in 1863. *(From Historical development of artificial limbs. In Orthopaedic appliances atlas, Vol 2, Artificial limbs. JW Edwards, Ann Arbor, MI, 1960, p. 11, with permission.)*

Committee on Prosthetic Research and Development (CPRD), and the Committee on Prosthetic-Orthotic Education (CPOE) influenced the development of modern prosthetics and orthotics.[2] Plastics replaced wood as the material of choice, socket designs followed physiological principles of function, lighter weight components were developed, and more cosmetic alternatives were fabricated. Most modern prosthetic principles had their inception in the work of these committees.[2]

Since the 1970s, prosthetic developments have grown at an exponential rate. Computer-assisted socket designs, new materials spawned by the space age, better research into human function, miniaturization, and computer chips all have contributed to vastly improve general and specialized prosthetic components. Prosthetics and orthotics have emerged as sciences as well as art. The consumer is also making greater demands on the prosthesis, seeking limbs that will enable him or her to participate in all aspects of life, including sports and leisure activities. The Iraq and Afghanistan wars have brought many young people into the world of the amputee; they seek prostheses that will enable them to stay in the military if desired and perform all the physical activities needed for their jobs. Flexible intimate fit sockets suspended by suction were developed for transfemoral and transtibial amputations. Gel-filled liners provide a shock-absorbing interface between the residual limb and the hard socket. Gel liners insure an intimate fit suspending the prosthesis with virtually no pistoning, making the artificial limb an integral part of the lower extremity. There are a wide variety of prosthetic feet designed to respond dynamically and incorporating multiple axes of motion similar to the human foot. Research highlighted the importance of swing phase as well as stance phase in normal walking, leading to multiaxis and computer-assisted knee mechanisms. Initial development of prototype active feet and knee components are currently in use and close to reaching the marketplace. Researchers are attempting to find a method to bring sensation into the prosthetic limb.

The upper extremity has always posed a major challenge for prosthetists. The great complexity of hand function is difficult to duplicate mechanically. The loss of sensation limits the function of the hand or hook, and researchers have yet to develop replacement for sensory function. Research in this area is continuing. Developments in external power and virtual reality are probably the highlight of modern upper extremity prostheses. Myoelectric controls are

In 1945, in response to the demands of veterans for more functional prostheses, the National Academy of Sciences (NAS) initiated a study to develop design criteria for artificial limbs that would improve function.[2] The Committee on Artificial Limbs (CAL) contracted with universities, industrial laboratories, health providers, and others to spearhead major changes in all facets of prosthetics and orthotics. From 1947 to 1976 under NAS sponsorship and Veterans Administration (VA) support, the CAL, the now used fairly routinely for transhumeral and transradial amputations. Virtual reality is increasingly used as part of both upper and lower extremity training and will be discussed further in appropriate chapters.

HISTORY OF ORTHOTICS

People have been wearing shoes for many centuries. Early shoe designs dating back thousands of years suggest that appearance has always been as important as comfort; in early times, wearing shoes was a status symbol as only the rich could afford them. As materials and artisans became more plentiful and shoes became more affordable, people started to consider comfort as well as style. Early innkeepers provided travelers with matted animal hair for foot covering, and eventually, artisans began to specialize in making shoes. These early cobblers added leather and felt. Responding to customers' need for adaptations, they began to make pads and inserts to provide more comfort. Early arch supports were made by laminating layers of leather strips together, molding them to shoe lasts, and then shaping the arch support by hand for wearing inside shoes. A variety of shoes and shoe adaptations followed with the advent of electricity and new equipment. New materials were developed and universal lasts for different sizes became available for mass production. Cobblers continued to be in demand to make adaptations for comfort and accommodation of deformities.[15]

Concomitant with the development of more sophisticated and adapted shoes came the development of splints and braces to support damaged limbs. Skilled metal workers, not only made prosthetic devices for those who had lost a limb but also made supportive devices for people with fractures and other injuries. Brace makers eventually became the orthotists of today.

In the 18th century, the French physician Nicolas Andry suggested that a body's misshape did not have to be permanent, particularly in children. He suggested that, much like a gardener who ties a misshapen tree to correct the shape, devices could be developed to correct a misshapen spine or limb so that, with growth, the deformity could be corrected.[15]

As in prosthetics, the greatest improvements in the orthotics came in the 20th century after both world wars and the polio epidemics of the late 1940s and early 1950s. Manufacturers, orthotists, orthopedists, and others involved in the rehabilitation of the severely disabled began to use and adapt the now wide array of prefabricated parts into functional orthoses for specific purposes. Initially somewhat heavy and cumbersome, orthoses became increasingly functional and usable with new knowledge of human function and new lighter and more malleable materials.

THE 21ST CENTURY

The 21st century is bringing many changes in the field of prosthetics and orthotics and in the care of individuals in need of prostheses and orthoses. Robotics are moving from the realm of science fiction to practical applications. Fairley[16] reported on the development of a lower extremity exoskeleton suit developed at the University of California Berkeley. The suit weighs about 31 lbs with a battery pack, and a computer allows the wearer to perform activities such as carrying a heavy weight without feeling the weight or tiring. Another suit developed in Japan allows the disabled wearer to perform activities of daily living the person cannot otherwise perform. This suit detects biosignals generated on the surface of the skin when the person attempts to make selected movements. Robotic developments in prosthetics seek to create active rather than responsive movements.

The 21st century will likely bring changes in surgery and reconstruction. Work being done on nerve transplants is already beginning to salvage limbs that otherwise would be nonfunctional and often require amputation. Virtual reality is increasingly being used for both upper and lower extremity rehabilitation. Some of these areas will be explored in a bit more detail in relevant chapters.

Prosthetists and Orthotists

Prosthetists and orthotists today, unlike their earlier counterparts who learned their trade as apprentices, are educated through university-based programs, must complete an internship, and must pass national licensing boards. Completion of an accredited educational program and passing the licensing examination entitles one to use the initials "CP" or "CO," indicating a Certified Prosthetist or Certified Orthotist after his or her name. Prosthetists and orthotists guide research and publish findings in professional journals. National and international prosthetic manufacturers strive to develop lighter and more functional components. Prosthetic and orthotic designs are based on increasing knowledge of human physiology and functional needs, and specialized devices are developed for individuals with particular needs.

National and international meetings provide opportunities for continuing education. Prosthetists and orthotists are the most knowledgeable people about their ever-more broad and complex fields. Even though many practitioners are certified both as prosthetists and orthotist "CPOs," many more are specializing in one or the other field. As in physical therapy, there is further specialization within each area.

In almost every area of practice, you as a physical therapist or physical therapist assistant will encounter patients who need a prosthetic or an orthotic device. Working closely with your local prosthetist or orthotist on the selection and fit of the device will greatly improve your patient care. Even prefabricated devices that anyone can buy over the counter can benefit from proper fitting to the individual. In some settings, you may be working as part of a rehabilitation team where a group of experts work together with the patient to determine and execute the plan of care. Prosthetists and orthotists need to be integral members of that team.

A number of clinical centers throughout the country hold regular amputee clinics with all patients reviewed on a regular basis.[17] The clinic team plans and implements comprehensive rehabilitation programs designed to meet the physical, psychological, and economical needs of the client. Most clinic teams are located in rehabilitation facilities, university health centers, or Department of Veteran's Affairs medical centers. The team generally includes a physician, physical therapist, occupational therapist, prosthetist, social worker, and vocational counselor. Other health professionals who contribute to the team are a nurse, dietitian, psychologist, and possibly, administrative coordinator. Clinic meeting frequency is dictated by the caseload; clients are seen regularly and decisions are made using input from all team members. A screening session held by the physical and occupational therapists prior to the actual clinic allows for the careful evaluation of each person and improves the effectiveness of the clinic.[17] In centers without a clinic, close communication between the client, surgeon, and physical therapists, with the later addition of the prosthetist, is important to insure an optimum outcome.

Unfortunately, amputee clinics are not the norm, and in many places, patients are referred directly to a prosthetist, sometimes many months after amputation, and without intervention by physical therapists. This can lead to complications and limited outcomes and will be discussed further in later chapters.

SUMMARY

Knowing something of the history and development of a field is helpful in understanding the rationale for change and new concepts. Advanced knowledge of human function, as well as new and lighter materials, improved computers, and even smaller chips that contain greater amounts of information have led to much more functional appliances that help those with movement dysfunctions achieve greater levels of independence. All physical therapists and physical therapist assistants need to have a basic knowledge of prosthetics and orthotics to guide the rehabilitation of individuals with movement dysfunctions. Often, the physical therapists will discern the need for an appliance or a modification and are instrumental in obtaining the most appropriate appliance for each person. Physical therapists and physical therapist assistants need to stay up to date on changes in technology, component availability, and management. A good resource that opens the door to many areas of the prosthetic and orthotic world is www.oandp.com.

KEYWORDS FOR LITERATURE SEARCH

Amputation
Amputee
Amputee rehabilitation
Orthoses
Orthotist
Prosthesis
Prosthetist
War amputee

REFERENCES

1. History of the study of locomotion. University of Vienna Web site. http://www.univie.ac.at/ (accessed March 2009).
2. Wilson, AB Jr: History of amputation surgery and prosthetics. In Bowker JH and Michael JW (eds): Atlas of Limb Prosthetics: Surgical and Prosthetic Principles. Mosby Year Book, St. Louis, 1992.
3. Norton BJ: Harnessing our collective professional power: diagnosis dialogue. Phys Ther 87(6, June): 635–638, 2007.
4. Coffin-Zadai CA: Disabling our diagnostic dilemmas. PTJ 87:641–653, 2007.
5. Norton BJ: Diagnosis dialogues: progress report. PTJ 87:1270–1273, 2007.
6. Norton BJ (moderator): Dx diagnosis. Session held at the annual conference of the American Physical Therapy Association. San Antonio, TX, June 2008.

7. APTA. Guide to Physical Therapist Practice, 2nd ed. Alexandria, VA, 2001.

8. World Health Organization/United Nations Economic and Social Commission for Asia and the South Pacific: Training manual on disability statistics, Chapter 2: the ICF framework. www.unescap.org/stat/disability/manual/Training-Manual-Disability-Statistics.pdf

9. Jette A: Towards a common language for function, disability and health. Phys Ther 86:726–724, 2005.

10. Bowker JH, Pritham CH: The history of amputation surgery. In Smith DG, Michaelk JW, and Bowker JH (eds): Atlas of Amputations and Limb Deficiencies, 3rd ed. American Academy of Orthopaedic Surgeons, Rosemont, IL, 2004, pp 3–19.

11. Dederich R: Technique of myoplastic amputations. Ann R Coll Surg Engl 40:222–227, 1967.

12. Burgess E, Traub JE, and Wilson AB Jr: Immediate postsurgical prosthetics in the management of lower extremity amputees. Veterans Administration TR 10-5, Washington, DC, 1967.

13. Weiss M: Myoplastic amputation, immediate prosthesis and early ambulation. U.S. Department of Health Education and Welfare, U.S. Government Printing Office, Washington, DC (no date given).

14. Talbott JH: A Biographical History of Medicine: Excerpts and Essays on the Men and Their Work. Grune & Stratton, New York, 1970.

15. Bunch WH: Introduction to orthotics. In American Academy of Orthopaedic Surgeons (ed): Atlas of orthotics: Biomechanical Principles and Application, 2nd ed. C. V. Mosby, St. Louis, 1985.

16. Fairley MI: Robot: robotic technology adds a new dimension to orthotics. O and P Edge, March 2009, pp 22–26. (www.oandp.com/edge)

17. May BJ: A statewide amputee rehabilitation programme. Prosthet Orthot Int 2:24–26, 1978.

Biomechanical Principles in Prosthetics and Orthotics

OBJECTIVES

At the end of this chapter, all students are expected to:

1. Describe the goals of prosthetic and orthotic devices.
2. Describe the types of forces applied by prosthetic and orthotic devices.
3. Describe the gait cycle and the phases of gait.
4. Describe the distance and temporal characteristics of gait.
5. Describe the typical changes in gait that are associated with aging.
6. Discuss the biomechanical effects of limb loss and use of a prosthetic or orthotic device on balance.

Physical Therapy students are expected to:

1. Explain the biomechanical methods by which prosthetic and orthotic devices accomplish their goals.
2. Discuss the biomechanical issues of the interface between the device and the user's anatomy.
3. Discuss the kinematics and kinetics of gait, including internal and external moments during each phase of gait.
4. Discuss muscle activity and function during gait.

CASE STUDY

Harry Green is a 67-year-old African American widow who suffered a thrombotic cerebral vascular accident (stroke) with right hemiparesis 3 weeks ago. Although he has type 2 diabetes (without peripheral neuropathy) and hypertension, he is medically stable with his current medications. Prior to his stroke, Mr. Green lived independently and was active at home and in the community. He is an inpatient in a rehabilitation hospital. Although sensation, cognition, and communication are intact, he has moderate weakness in both his right upper and lower extremities, with the greater weakness distally. He also has difficulty dissociating volitional movements in his right extremities; thus, when he tries to flex his right hip, he is compelled to flex all three joints in the extremity in the same direction at the same time. For example, when he walks, taking a step on the right is difficult because when he flexes his right hip to take a step, he is unable to extend his knee. He is, however, able to walk with assistance using a four-point cane, but his gait is slow, inefficient, and not always safe. He has little voluntary muscle activity in the right foot and ankle, which produces a right foot drop during gait, making right step initiation and swing more difficult. He exhibits varus positioning of his right ankle at initial foot contact as well as knee instability during right stance phase. For example, sometimes his right knee buckles causing balance difficulty, although he has had no falls to date. In his upper extremity, he has some voluntary muscle activity, which is greater in flexor muscles than extensors. He has some voluntary grasp and release in his right hand and can hold onto an object if placed in his hand. Using his upper extremity requires much effort and he does not use it functionally at present.

Case Study Activities

All Students:

1. Identify and discuss Mr. Green's gait abnormalities and provide biomechanical explanations for his loss of balance and potential for falls.
2. Discuss how Mr. Green's age may affect his gait and interact with his newly acquired gait impairments resulting from his stroke.
3. Identify the gait deficits and problems that Mr. Green presents in each of the phases of gait.

FORCES AND PROSTHETIC AND ORTHOTIC DEVICES

The prosthetic and orthotic devices discussed in this text are devices or appliances applied externally to the user's body to replace a missing body part (**prosthesis**) or to replace a missing function (**orthosis**). Ultimately, the goal of the appliance is to improve the user's mobility and ability to perform daily functional activities. In order to accomplish their goals, prosthetic and orthotic devices apply forces to the user's anatomy, following the rules of mechanics. Thus, practitioners, who identify the need for appliances and then select or prescribe, fit, and train clients with them, must understand the biomechanics of how the devices apply forces as well as the biomechanical behavior of the user/appliance unit during functional activities and mobility. This chapter reviews selected relevant biomechanical principles and demonstrates their applications in prosthetic and orthotic devices. In addition, the chapter reviews common methods of assessing gait and functional mobility, including examples of how practitioners can use these assessments in clinical decision making with clients who wear prosthetic or orthotic devices. The chapter is not intended to provide a comprehensive discussion of the science of biomechanics or gait and functional analysis. Readers are encouraged to access other dedicated biomechanics texts for more complete and in-depth presentations of these topics.

Terminology and Definitions of Forces

The purpose of this section is to review the terminology used to describe forces and how they behave. This terminology is used in subsequent sections of this chapter that present the methods by which prosthetic and orthotic devices apply or manipulate forces to accomplish their goals.

A **force** is a push or a pull exerted by one object on another. It is described as a vector by its magnitude, direction, and point of application. When a force is applied to an object, it can affect that object by moving, accelerating or decelerating it. Thus, a force is also described by the acceleration of the body to which it has been applied and is proportional to the mass of the object.

When forces are applied to a body producing a movement, the resulting motion is described by the plane or planes in which it occurs and the type of resultant displacement. A *sagittal* plane divides a body into right and left parts. A *frontal* or coronal plane divides a body into anterior and posterior parts, and a *transverse* plane is usually a horizontal plane. Displacement is described as translation, rotation, or curvilinear movement. *Translation* is linear displacement of a moving segment. *Rotation* or rotatory motion is angular displacement around a fixed axis or center of rotation (CoR). Axes of rotation are always perpendicular to the plane of the movement. Thus, flexion and extension occur in the sagittal plane around a medial–lateral (ML) axis; abduction and adduction occur in the frontal plane around an anterior–posterior (AP) axis; internal (medial) and external (lateral) rotations occur in the transverse plane around a vertical (longitudinal or long) axis. Translation and rotation can and often do occur together as shown in **Figure 2.1A**. Although combined, the movements in this example occur in one plane—the sagittal plane. Many functional movements, however, occur simultaneously in more than one plane, which allows for a greater range of movement as well as a greater variety of movement patterns. *Curvilinear* motion is a combination of translation and rotation of a body segment. When this type of motion occurs, the axis about which the segment moves is not fixed, but moves in space as the object moves (**Fig. 2.1B**). In the example shown, in order to place the foot on the opposite thigh, as one might do to put on a sock or tie a shoe, the knee flexes while the leg segment rotates about the sagittal plane (vertical) axis at the hip. The result is that the leg segment moves through a three-dimensional curvilinear path.

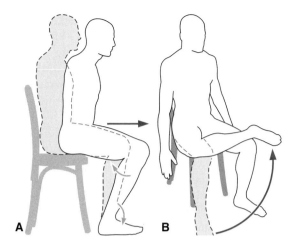

FIGURE 2.1. Translation, rotation, and curvilinear movement. A, As the buttocks translate forward with the feet remaining fixed, rotation of the knees and ankles occurs simultaneously. B, The leg segment traces a curvilinear path as the knee flexes, while the leg rotates about a sagittal axis at the hip. Start positions are shaded; end positions are clear.

When a prosthetic or orthotic device with mechanical joints is worn over an anatomical joint, the two must move together either in cardinal plane movements or more complex three-dimensional curvilinear movement. In either case, the anatomical and mechanical axes must closely align with one another for efficient and pain-free movement to occur. Misalignment

between anatomical and mechanical axes during movement results in migration of the appliance on the wearer's body, producing pain, excessive pressure, or even deforming forces. Thus, prosthetic and orthotic practitioners must be able to estimate the locations of anatomical axes of rotation on their clients and monitor their alignment with moving mechanical joints. **Table 2.1** provides estimates for the locations of the anatomical axes that can be found on a patient and guidelines for alignment with mechanical axes.

Forces acting on the joints of the human body produce or restrain joint movement and are classified as external or internal forces. **External forces** are pushes or pulls from sources outside of the body. *Gravity*, the attraction of the earth's mass to all other masses, is an important external force that affects the body during all activities. The *weight* of an object, including the human body and its parts (or limb segments), is a quantity equivalent to the mass of the object multiplied by the pull of gravity on the object's mass, the acceleration of gravity (9.8 m/sec^2). Thus, the weight of the body is a force that can produce joint movement. The **line of gravity**, or "weight line" as it is sometimes called, is a line from the object's center of mass (CoM) to the center of the earth. For the human body, the CoM is located just anterior to the second

TABLE 2.1	Guidelines for Alignment of Prosthetic/Orthotic Mechanical Axes With the Anatomical Joints in the Lower Limb		
Axis	**Hip Joint**	**Knee Joint**	**Ankle Joint**
Mechanical ML axis (for motion in the sagittal plane)	Height: 1 inch superior to apex of greater trochanter AP: ½ inch anterior to apex of greater trochanter	Height: ~¾ inch proximal to tibial plateau (joint line); ~ through the femoral epicondyles AP: ~half the AP diameter of the knee, not including the patella	Height: at the distal tip of the medial malleolus AP: on medial side, at center of medial malleolus; on lateral side, at center of lateral malleolus
Orientation of the mechanical ML axis in the transverse plane	Neither internally nor externally rotated; parallel to the axis at the knee	Perpendicular to the plane of motion of the leg/shank	Rotated to coincide with the anatomical tibial torsion, typically ~ 10° to 20° external rotation in relation to the knee axis
Orientation of the mechanical ML axis in the frontal plane	Parallel to the floor or perpendicular to the midsagittal line	Parallel to the floor or perpendicular to the midsagittal line	Parallel to the floor or perpendicular to the midsagittal line

AP, anterior–posterior; ML, medial–lateral.

sacral vertebral body. The location of the line of gravity with respect to the axis of rotation at an anatomical joint can produce or limit movement at the joint. For example, when a person leans backwards causing the line of gravity to fall posterior to the hip joint axis, gravity will cause an extension moment (force) at the hip (**Fig. 2.2**). If the same person leans forward, the line of gravity will fall anterior to the hip and knee causing hip flexion and knee extension moments.

Another important external force is the ground reaction force (GRF). Whenever the body contacts the ground, the ground pushes back on the body. This force of the ground on the foot is called the **ground reaction force vector** (GRFV). It is a composite or resultant force vector that represents the magnitude and direction of the force applied to the foot during weight-bearing and can be visualized as the line connecting the body's CoM and the point of contact of the foot with the ground, called the center of pressure (CoP). This composite force vector is composed of component vertical, AP, and ML forces and is measured by force plates in the ground. The location of the GRFV with respect to the joints or anatomical axes of rotation in the limb affects joint movement. For example, if a person takes a step and shifts weight onto the leg with the knee flexed, the GRFV will pass posterior to the knee and anterior to the hip, causing external hip and knee flexion moments (**Fig. 2.3**). The forces applied by prosthetic and orthotic devices are also external forces. Prosthetic and orthotic devices may be designed to manipulate the location of the line of gravity or the GRFV to produce or control joint motion.

Internal forces are produced by sources within the body, such as muscle contraction and the viscoelastic nature of connective tissues, including joint capsules and ligaments. Internal forces produce joint movements but also function to counteract the external forces that act on the body (**Fig. 2.4**). Internal force vectors or moments at a joint are expressed as composites of all the internal forces acting on a joint at a point in time.

Most of the forces (internal or external) that produce joint motion in humans act at some distance from the joint's center or axis of rotation. Thus, the resulting joint motion is primarily rotation (often with a smaller amount of concomitant translation). The result of this force application at a distance from the rotation center is called a **moment** and is measured as *torque* or angular motion. Moments are named by the direction of the resultant joint movement. In Figure 2.4, the line of gravity produces an external ankle dorsiflexion moment that is countered or

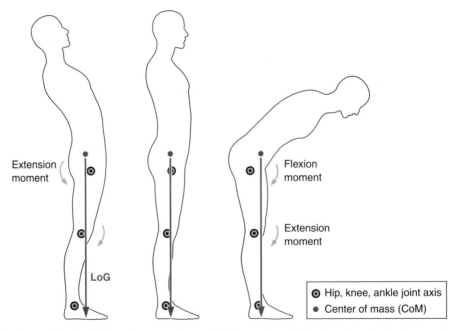

FIGURE 2.2. The body weight, localized as the center of mass (CoM), acts through the line of gravity (LoG) to produce external forces that affect the joints. In a neutral erect position, the LoG is close to the joint axes of rotation and has little effect. (O, joint axis of rotation; ●, location of center of mass.)

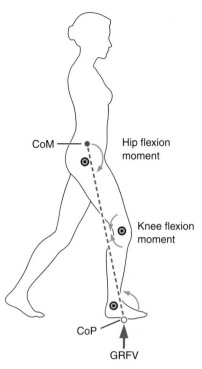

FIGURE 2.3. The ground reaction force vector (GRFV) extends from the center of pressure (CoP) on the plantar surface of the foot to the center of mass (CoM). In this diagram, the GRFV produces external moments represented by curved arrows including a hip flexion moment, knee flexion moment, and ankle dorsiflexion moment.

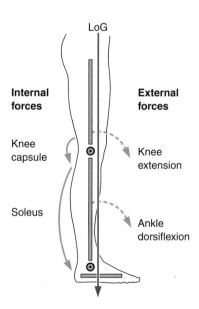

FIGURE 2.4. In normal standing posture, the force of body weight acts through the line of gravity creating external forces that produce knee extension and ankle dorsiflexion moments. To counter these external forces, internal forces are produced by connective tissues and muscle contraction.

restrained by the internal plantarflexion moment produced by soleus muscle contraction. The *magnitude of a moment* is computed as the product of the amount of the force applied and the length of the shortest (perpendicular) distance between the axis of rotation and the line of pull of the force (**Fig. 2.5**). The magnitude of the moment is reported as torque (foot-pounds or newton-meters). The distance between the axis of rotation and the line of action of the force is called the **moment arm**. Prosthetic and orthotic devices can be designed to manipulate the moments acting at a joint to accomplish an orthotic goal and improve function. For example, Mr. Green (Case Study client at the beginning of this chapter) demonstrates knee instability with knee buckling during stance. An ankle foot orthosis (AFO) designed to prevent dorsiflexion beyond a position of neutral or slight plantarflexion will produce an extension moment at the knee by keeping the GRFV anterior to the knee through midstance (Fig. 2.6). When the ankle dorsiflexes (without an orthosis to block it) during stance phase, the GRFV is allowed to move posterior to the knee producing a flexion moment and in the absence of sufficient muscle force to maintain knee extension, knee buckling.

Types of Forces

The five major types of forces are tension (traction or distraction), compression, shear, torsion, and bending. All of these forces, except perhaps torsion, are used in orthotic or prosthetic devices to accomplish their goals. Knowledgeable and effective practitioners who work with clients using orthoses or prostheses must know how and when to apply these forces

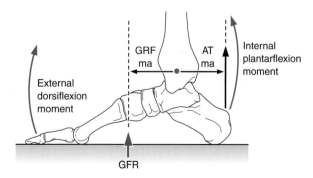

FIGURE 2.5. The external dorsiflexion moment produced by the ground reaction force (GRF × moment arm) is balanced by an internal plantarflexion moment generated by the gastrocnemius/soleus muscle force times the Achilles tendon moment arm (ATma).

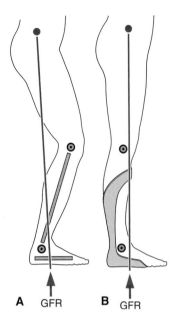

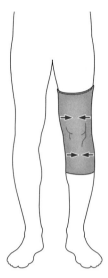

FIGURE 2.7. A neoprene elastic soft knee orthosis provides compression.

FIGURE 2.6. A, The ground reaction force vector (GRFV) produces an external knee flexion moment that contributes to knee buckling. To prevent knee buckling, greater internal hip and knee extensor moments or ankle plantarflexor moments are required. B, An AFO designed to prevent ankle dorsiflexion maintains the GRFV anterior to the knee, which produces an external extension moment and prevents knee buckling.

through devices and how to monitor their effects. Throughout this section, readers are referred to figures in subsequent chapters in this book to view examples of the various types of forces as they are applied in prosthetic and orthotic devices.

Tension (traction) forces are applied perpendicular to a surface or plane within an object which distract or move the surfaces apart or away from one another. An example of an orthotic application of tensile force is a dynamic or static progressive splint that applies end-range tensile loads to shortened connective tissue to trigger mechanical and biological tissue elongation and increase joint range of motion (see Figs. 18.9 and 18.10). *Compression* forces are also applied perpendicularly to a surface or plane, but the direction of the forces is toward one another. A neoprene elastic knee orthosis provides compression forces and may minimize swelling at the joint (see **Figs.** 2.7 and 15.12). A neoprene sleeve can assist with prosthetic suspension (see Table 6.2, neoprene sleeve and Fig. 7.11).

A *shear* force is applied parallel to a surface or plane within an object. Shear forces move or attempt to move one object along the surface of another. *Friction*, a special type of shear force, is also parallel to the

contacting surfaces but is in the opposite direction of the shear and (potential) movement. The magnitude of the friction force on an object is a function of the magnitude of the contact force between the objects and the slipperiness or roughness (coefficient of friction) of the contacting surfaces. The area of contact does not affect the magnitude of friction. Thus, the material and texture of the sole of a shoe influence the amount of friction between the shoe and the floor. Shear and friction forces are important for the prosthetic/orthotic practitioner to consider, because excessive shear and friction between an appliance and a user's skin can contribute to skin breakdown at the appliance–user interface. For example, skin breakdown on a residual limb may be caused by slippage or "pistoning" of a poorly suspended prosthesis on a residual limb (see Fig. 7.22). The various types of prosthetic sockets that employ suction as their primary means of suspension minimize shear between the residual limb and the socket and thus improve comfort (Table 6.2, suction and Fig. 7.31).

A *torsion* force or moment creates rotation of a segment around its long axis and most often describes a rotational force applied to a single object, rather than between two objects. Thus, a torsion force produces a twist within an object. A common anatomical example that describes the effect of a torsion force is the spiral fracture of the humerus caused by application of a twisting force during a forceful tug on the arm, throwing, or a fall on an outstretched arm. Excessive torsional forces applied through a molded plastic orthotic device may contribute to failure of the plastic and ultimate breakage of the appliance.

Bending forces or moments are parallel forces applied to an unsegmented object in a way that results in equilibrium (neither translation nor rotation). When bending forces are applied to a rigid, constrained body, compressive forces develop on the concave surface and tension develops on the convex surface. For example, bending forces with concomitant compression and tensile forces develop in the weight-bearing femur because of its normal bowed shape (**Fig. 2.8**). Patients who require prostheses or orthoses may have bony deformities that also produce these compression and tensile forces. For example, a tibia with a varus deformity is exposed to tensile forces laterally (convex side) and compression medially (concave side). Prosthetic or orthotic components applied to these bowed limb segments must be selected or designed to resist these compression and tensile loads.

When parallel forces are applied to an unconstrained object, some combination of translation and rotation occurs (**Fig. 2.9**). To prevent this translation or rotation, a third "counterforce" is needed. This **three-point bending (counterforce) system** is commonly used in orthoses to control unwanted motion. A three-point counterforce system includes a *middle force* located close to the axis and *two end forces*, which are opposite in direction to the middle force and applied at a distance from the axis. For example, Mr. Green (this chapter's case study client) demonstrates a foot drop that interferes with step initiation and swing. An AFO with a three-point counterforce system (in the sagittal plane) can be used to control the unwanted plantarflexion (**Fig. 2.10A**). However, Mr. Green also exhibits an abnormal varus position at the ankle. Thus, the AFO needs a second three-point counterforce system in the frontal plane (**Fig. 2.10B**) to control the unwanted inversion. In this system, the middle force (lateral to medial direction) is applied directly to the lateral malleolus with proximal and distal end forces applied in the opposite direction (medial to lateral). An orthotic force, however, applied directly at the lateral malleolus (bony prominence) is likely to cause pain and possibly skin breakdown. Thus, an alternative *four-point force system* can be substituted (**Fig. 2.10C**), which is biomechanically sound and more likely to be safe and more comfortable. Two force couples can also compose a four-point bending system. A **force couple** is composed of two parallel forces equal in magnitude and opposite in direction, applied to the same object or rigid segment at different points, resulting in rotation of the segment without translation (Fig. 2.9B). Some functional knee orthoses designed to restrict knee hyperextension and

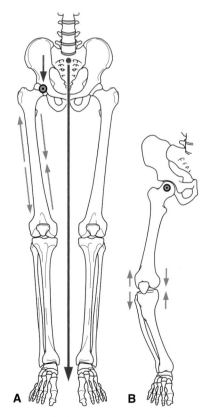

FIGURE 2.8. A, Weight-bearing (WB) applies a bending moment to the femur, which produces both tensile and compressive loads. B, A tibial varus deformity produces medial compression and lateral tensile forces.

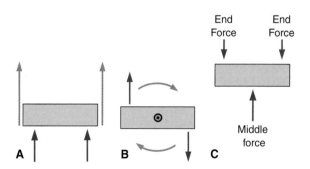

FIGURE 2.9. Application of parallel forces to unconstrained rigid bodies produces translation or rotation. A, Equal parallel forces produce translation. B, Parallel forces in opposite directions form a force couple and produce rotation. C, A three-point counterforce system is used to restrain unwanted rotation or translation.

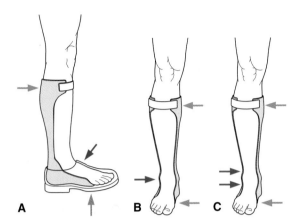

FIGURE 2.10. A, A three-point counterforce system is applied by an ankle foot orthosis to prevent unwanted foot drop (plantarflexion). B, A three-point counterforce system prevents unwanted inversion. C, An alternate four-point force system provides middle and end forces to control inversion and avoids applying force directly over the bony lateral malleolus.

anterior tibial translation employ this type of four-point force system (**Fig. 2.11**, see Fig. 15.13A).

Because prostheses and orthoses function by applying forces to some part of the user's anatomy, practitioners must pay careful attention to the interface between the user and the appliance. **Pressure** (P) is defined as the amount of force (F) per surface area (a) of application (P = F/a). High pressure between an appliance and its user can cause pain and skin breakdown. For example, the orthosis in Figure 2.10B shows the middle force of the three-point counterforce system applied to a small area over the lateral

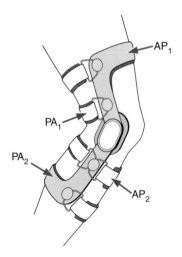

FIGURE 2.11. A four-point force system is used in a knee brace to prevent knee hyperextension and anterior tibial translation. (AP, anterior to posterior force; PA, posterior to anterior force.)

malleolus. This may be painful or cause skin breakdown. If the same force is distributed over a large surface area, it may be more comfortable and safer. The goal of a prosthetic or orthotic device is to apply sufficient force to achieve effectiveness while minimizing pressure to insure comfort and safety of the skin. Various methods to achieve this are discussed later in the chapter and in subsequent chapters.

BIOMECHANICAL PRINCIPLES: APPLICATIONS IN PROSTHETIC AND ORTHOTIC DESIGN AND FUNCTION

Prosthetic and orthotic devices apply forces to body segments to produce, limit, or control or prevent movement in order to achieve improved function for their users. This section describes the methods by which appliances generate and manipulate the forces and moments that are then used to affect movement. Biomechanical and biological factors that must be considered to successfully interface a prosthetic or orthotic device with the user's anatomy are also discussed. Practitioners must understand and apply these principles during prosthetic and orthotic prescription, examination, and evaluation and training in order to achieve the desired functional outcomes, as well as successful appliance fit, function, comfort, and cosmesis.

Methods of Force Application to Produce Movement

Devices or components designed to generate forces that produce movement are called dynamic. There are a variety of ways in which forces can be produced by these *dynamic devices*. These include

- selecting materials and components that store and release energy,
- designing the device and its trimlines to facilitate movement,
- using appliance alignment and componentry to manipulate the GRFV or LoG during weight-bearing function, or
- using functional electrical stimulation (FES) of nonfunctional muscles or amplified myoelectric signals to operate small electric motors to produce motion.

Materials and Componentry to Store and Release Energy

A wide variety of different materials are used in manufacturing prosthetic and orthotic devices. These materials and their properties are described in subsequent chapters. One way to manufacture an appliance that will impart forces to a body part is to construct it of materials that store energy when deformed and release it when unrestrained. Examples of these materials include rubber, some thermoplastics, composite plastics or laminates, such as carbon fiber, and lightweight but strong metals such as titanium. Carbon fiber and other composite materials are often used to accomplish this goal because they are strong, lightweight, and fatigue resistant. A common application of energy-storing materials is in the construction of devices for clients with loss of active plantarflexion. The activity of the plantarflexor muscles is an important component of lower limb support and push-off during the stance phase of gait. This function is lost as a result of lower extremity amputation or muscle paralysis or weakness that may occur with brain injury or peripheral neuropathy. A rigid prosthetic foot or a rigid AFO can provide some midstance support but cannot contribute to a dynamic push-off. However, a prosthetic foot or AFO made of flexible, energy-storing materials deforms during the passive dorsiflexion of midstance when the body glides forward over the stance foot (storing energy) and then releases the energy as a plantarflexion force in late stance during limb unloading. This action of the prosthesis or orthosis facilitates some dynamic push-off (**Fig. 2.12**). In this example, the flexible energy-storing prosthetic/orthotic materials deform similarly to the way in which a diving board is deflected

when a diver lands after the hurtle. During this deflection, the diving board stores energy, which it returns as it pushes the diver into the air (**Fig. 2.13**).

Various prosthetic and orthotic components, such as elastic bands and springs, also act dynamically to produce forces that substitute for missing functions. For example, a client with insufficient or compromised extensor digitorum muscle function in the hand can use a dynamic splint with elastic bands to substitute for lost active extension of the metacarpalphalangeal joints (see Fig. 18.13). A dorsiflexion assist force can be provided for a client with foot drop by choosing an orthotic ankle joint with springs located so that they are compressed during plantarflexion and recoil (producing dorsiflexion) when the limb is unloaded during swing (see Fig. 14.6)

Appliance Design and Trimlines

Appliances are manufactured from a variety of thermoplastic materials that are molded to the client's body. In addition to the mechanical properties of the materials used, the design or shape of the device influences its rigidity or flexibility and thus its ability to limit or facilitate movement. The commonly used molded plastic AFO provides an example of the effect of trimline location on orthotic flexibility. A molded AFO includes a foot plate (shoe insert) and a posterior calf shell (see Fig. 14.10). The location of the trimlines (edges of the device) determines the width of the

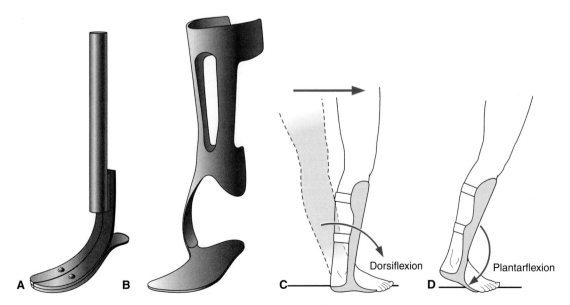

FIGURE 2.12. A dynamic response prosthetic foot (A) and orthosis (B). While the body glides over the stance foot producing dorsiflexion, energy is stored in the appliance (C), which is then released as plantarflexion during limb unloading (D).

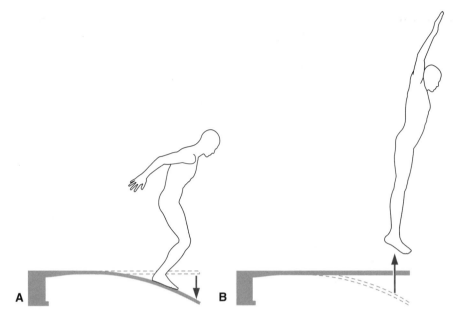

FIGURE 2.13. When the diver lands on the spring diving board, it deflects and stores energy, A. It releases the energy when it recoils, pushing the diver into the air, B.

orthosis at the ankle and the calf shell (**Fig. 2.14**). As the width increases, the orthosis becomes more rigid and more restrictive of motion.[1] When the trimlines are cut to form a narrower, strap-like posterior calf shell, the orthosis is more flexible, allowing it to deform during stance and "spring" into dorsiflexion during swing. Its design allows this one-piece appliance, without moving parts, to behave similarly to the spring-loaded device described earlier.

Designs That Manipulate the Ground Reaction Force Vector or Line of Gravity

A person's body weight acting through the line of gravity and the GRFV produce lower limb joint moments when the line of force application does not pass directly through the joint's axis of rotation (see Figs. 2.2 and 2.3). Prosthetic or orthotic devices can be designed to position the joints in the lower extremity so that the line of gravity or GRFV produces a moment that substitutes for absent or insufficient muscle function. For example, Mr. Green (this chapter's case study client) has significant lower extremity weakness and as a result is experiencing unsafe gait due to right knee buckling (unwanted knee flexion during stance). Although a brace that crosses the knee and locks it into extension would effectively prevent the buckling, it would also cause an inefficient and energy-expensive gait pattern. If the knee can be

positioned so that the GRFV passes anterior to the knee axis during early and midstance, the resulting extension moment may be sufficient to stabilize the knee, substitute for his muscle weakness, and prevent the unwanted knee buckling. An AFO that limits

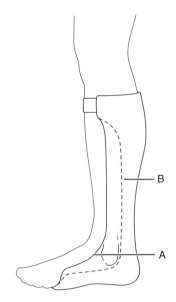

FIGURE 2.14. The rigidity of an appliance is affected by the location of its trimlines. The ankle foot orthosis (AFO) with a wider calf shell (A) is more rigid and more effective in restricting movement. The device with the narrower calf shell (B) is more flexible and can facilitate movement.

ankle dorsiflexion and positions the ankle in a small degree of plantarflexion will manipulate the GRFV and keep it anterior to the knee during most of stance phase. This orthotic manipulation of the GRFV produces an extension moment and eliminates the need for bracing across the knee (see Fig. 2.6).

The alignment of the transfemoral prosthetic knee provides another example of use of the GRFV to substitute for absent muscle control at the knee. Due to amputation, a transfemoral prosthesis wearer does not have normal muscle control at the knee. Energy-efficient knee stability, however, can be achieved during stance by orienting the prosthetic socket so that the prosthetic knee joint axis is located posterior to the GRFV during early stance. As a result, the GRFV produces an extension moment at the knee, contributes to knee stability, and substitutes for the loss of the knee muscles acting at the knee (**Fig. 2.15**).

Functional Electrical Stimulation (FES)

When muscle contraction is too weak to produce enough force for functional activities, an alternative to a conventional orthosis that may be more cosmetic,

less bulky, and less restrictive is FES. FES to either nerve or muscles has been used by itself or in conjunction with an orthosis to improve function in individuals with neuromuscular disorders such as stroke or incomplete spinal cord injury.[2,3] For example, FES to the common peroneal nerve has been used to improve dorsiflexion to enhance limb clearance during swing, gait, speed, and endurance. Additional applications will be discussed in subsequent chapters (see Fig. 14.20).

External Power Sources

Some prosthetic and orthotic devices employ external power sources to produce the forces needed for movement. Two examples of external power sources used in prosthetic or orthotic devices include small electric motors controlled by the user's myoelectric signals and pneumatic muscles attached to orthoses. Although myoelectrically controlled upper extremity prostheses have been in commercial use for many years, pneumatic muscles attached to orthoses are used experimentally at present, but commercial applications in rehabilitation are in development stages. One promising application is a myoelectrically controlled pneumatic muscle attached to an AFO to assist plantarflexion.[4]

Methods of Force Application to Limit, Control, or Prevent Movement

In addition to producing forces to generate or assist needed movements for function, there are other instances when the purpose of an appliance is to limit, control, or prevent unwanted movements. Appliances that control unwanted motions apply the necessary restraining forces through a combination of the mechanical properties of the materials from which they are constructed, their design, and their components. The biomechanical methods used to control or stop unwanted movements include

- using three- or four-point counterforce systems,
- choosing materials or appliance designs that produce high levels of rigidity at unstable joints,
- manipulating the GRFV to produce moments that restrain unwanted movements,
- selecting appliance components that stop or lock movable joints, and
- selecting components that provide mechanical friction or pneumatic and hydraulic resistance when controlled movement is required.

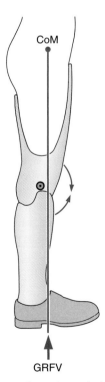

FIGURE 2.15. The transfemoral prosthetic socket is aligned so that the prosthetic knee axis of rotation is posterior to the GRFV, producing an extension moment, which substitutes for knee extensor muscles.

Counterforce Systems and Force Couples

Counterforce systems and force couples were previously described in this chapter in the discussion of types of forces. Three- and four-point counterforce systems and force couples are composed of parallel forces applied in opposite directions (see Figs. 2.9 and 2.11). When employed in the design of rigid prosthetic or orthotic devices, they serve to control or stop unwanted forces that are detrimental to function. Counterforce systems are very simple and are employed in many types of appliances. Figure 2.10 illustrates the use of three-point counterforce systems in the sagittal and frontal planes to stop unwanted ankle plantarflexion (drop foot) and inversion, respectively. Many types of spinal orthoses also employ three-point counterforce control. Examples are shown in Figures 17.5 and 17.9. The spinal orthosis in Figure 17.9 is designed to control unwanted thoracic flexion. Its middle force is applied near the apex of the curve and is directed from posterior to anterior (PA force), while the two end forces are applied anteriorly and are directed posteriorly (AP forces). This design limits and restrains the unwanted spinal flexion bending moment. Force couples are applied to adjacent body or limb segments to prevent rotation at the joints between them. The parapodium, a device used to assist paraplegic children to maintain standing, is an example of the application of two force couples (four alternately applied opposite forces) to control unwanted flexion movement between body and limb segments (see Fig. 16.17).

Appliance Rigidity

To be effective, these parallel three- or four-point counterforce systems must be applied in appliances that are relatively rigid. Appliance rigidity is determined by a combination of the mechanical properties of the material used as well as the appliance design. Most of the metals used in prosthetic and orthotic devices are rigid and thus can be used to apply three- and four-point counterforces and force couples. However, because of the weight of some metals, the cost of others, and cosmesis, metals are used less frequently today in appliance construction than in the past. Thermoplastics, thermosetting plastics, and composite materials are commonly used in the construction of contemporary molded appliances. These molded appliances can provide effective counterforces to limit unwanted movement, provided the appliance has sufficient rigidity. The rigidity of a molded appliance is determined by the mechanical properties of the material from which it is made as well as the cross-sectional area of the material. The material properties of some of the thermoplastic materials commonly used in the construction of prosthetic and orthotic devices are discussed in Chapter 12 (see Table 12.1).

Another method to increase appliance rigidity is to maximize the cross-sectional area of the material in the appliance design. The cross-sectional area is increased by using thicker plastic and by selecting a design that covers more surface area on the limb in the area where control is needed. The appliance labeled in Figure 2.14 as B has less cross-sectional area than the one labeled A. The orthosis with greater cross-sectional area (A) is more rigid and better able to provide effective counterforce to control unwanted ankle motion.[1] Other orthotic and prosthetic designs that increase cross-sectional area and rigidity are discussed in subsequent chapters that focus on specific devices.

Designs That Manipulate the GRFV or LoG

A person's body weight and the GRFV produce lower limb joint moments when the line of force application does not pass directly through the joint's axis of rotation (see Figs. 2.2 and 2.3). Manipulation of the GRFV to replace or substitute for a missing function is discussed earlier in this chapter. Prosthetic or orthotic devices are also designed to position the joints in the lower extremity so that the line of gravity or GRFV produces an external moment that restrains an unwanted movement. An example of an unwanted, deleterious movement in the lower extremity is knee hyperextension. Repetitive or sustained knee hyperextension over time can cause ligament injury and lead to an unstable, painful joint. One approach to restraining or limiting this unwanted hyperextension is to position the lower extremity so that the GRFV passes posterior to the knee joint axis, producing a knee flexion moment. This can be accomplished by using an orthosis that positions the ankle in a small amount of dorsiflexion and prevents movement into plantarflexion (see Fig. 14.12). Another method of shifting the GRFV posterior to the knee to generate a flexion moment is to add a small heel lift in the shoe on the hyperextending side (see Fig. 13.9C). To accommodate the heel lift, the proximal tibia tilts slightly forward, which allows the GRFV to move posterior to the knee and generate a flexion moment. Alignment alterations are used extensively in prosthetic design to prevent unwanted or unsafe joint motions. These are discussed in detail in Chapters 6 and 7 in the sections on prosthetic alignment.

Components

Some prostheses and orthoses have articulations or mechanical joints where they cross anatomical joints. These mechanical joints may be single or polyaxial but generally allow motion unless there is some componentry present to stop or control it. Appliances with articulations are often chosen when free motion is desired during some aspects of function, but controlled or no motion is required at other times. Components that can be added to mechanical joints to restrict joint motion are called stops or locks. A component called a *stop* prevents motion in a particular direction but allows movement in the other directions at the joint. For example, an orthosis with a plantarflexion stop is one that has components or has been designed to stop plantarflexion at a desired point in the ankle range of motion (ROM), but allows free dorsiflexion (see Figs. 14.5B and 14.18A). *Locks* are components that when present at a mechanical joint can be engaged to lock the joint in a selected position, preventing all movement at the joint while it is engaged. The lock, however, can be disengaged, thus permitting unrestrained motion when desired (see Fig. 15.5). There are many different kinds of stops and locks that are discussed in the chapters in this text that discuss specific prosthetic and orthotic componentry.

Methods to Control Motion Without Stopping It

At certain times during functional activities, it is desirable to restrain, control, or slow joint movements without totally stopping them. A variety of prosthetic and orthotic designs and components are available to provide controlled movement. At times, locking or stopping joints and using mechanical components to hold them in selected positions may be necessary and the only alternative. However, whenever possible, practitioners usually prefer to design appliances that permit normal or near-normal motions, while only blocking or stopping deleterious or unsafe motions or loads.

During many functional activities, muscles act eccentrically to control joint and body segment movement, rather than to produce it. For example, during swing phase of gait, when the knee is extending, the hamstrings contract to dampen or slow knee extension, which is produced by momentum rather than muscle contraction. Resistance to joint movement in prosthetic and orthotic joints can be produced by friction from mechanical, pneumatic, or hydraulic sources (see Table 6.4, fluid controlled). Movement can also be slowed or controlled when a moving component contacts a compressible material and engages the resistance that the material offers to compression. This is accomplished by using various cushioning materials such as rubber, synthetic rubber materials, and foamed thermoplastics to act as a dampening device or bumper. For example, an extension "bumper" may be used in a prosthesis to soften an abrupt terminal impact at the end of knee extension during swing. Another common application of the damping effect of compressible materials is the usage of a cushion heel in a solid-ankle prosthetic foot or on the heel of a shoe used with a rigid orthosis (see Table 6.1, SACH and Fig. 13.10F). This heel cushion controls the lowering of the forefoot to the ground during initial contact and weight acceptance. Other methods to dampen excessive plantarflexion at initial contact include the use of deformable energy-storing composite materials, such as carbon fiber (see Table 6.1, dynamic response) or hydraulics (see Table 6.1, hydraulics).

Biomechanical Factors That Affect the Appliance–User Interface

Appliances are designed to produce or control forces and movements in order to improve function. But, the best designed appliance cannot improve function if its user cannot tolerate those forces. Thus, in addition to understanding how prosthetic and orthotic devices apply and manipulate forces to produce or control joint movements, practitioners must understand the interface between the appliances and their users and how to make the application of the device's forces safe, comfortable, and effective. To optimize function and comfort, devices must be designed to apply the least effective force. That is, appliances must apply sufficient force to effectively accomplish their goals, but no more. Excessive force is likely to cause pain and skin breakdown, requiring discontinuance of appliance usage or abnormal movement patterns that make functional activities energy inefficient and impractical. To accomplish this balance between effective control and comfort, practitioners must understand and apply the following biomechanical principles:

■ minimize the magnitude of the force requirement by maximizing the length of the moment arm through which the force acts,

- minimize the pressure between the appliance and the user's anatomy, and
- minimize friction and abnormal movements between the appliance and the user with appropriate mechanical–anatomical alignment.

Lever Arm Length

Appliances that apply forces using counterforce systems or force couples function like first-class levers (like a "seesaw"). Thus, the moment applied by the appliance to the user's anatomy is equal to the product of the magnitude of the force and the length of the lever arm (distance from the point of force application to the CoR of the moving joint). Designing an appliance with the longest practical lever arm means that the same control moment can be generated with a smaller force. Reducing forces is an important method of minimizing the pressure exerted by an appliance on body tissues, thus increasing user comfort while wearing the device. For example, an orthosis designed to protect knee joint structures is depicted in **Figure 2.16A**. Although it demonstrates a three-point counterforce system, it is not tolerable to the wearer due to contact pain. Another orthosis for the same problem is diagrammed in **Figure 2.16B** with the same design but longer lever arm length. Less force is required in the second appliance because the lever arm length is greater than in the first device.

Individuals with amputations contract the muscles of their residual limb to produce force couples to control their prostheses. The moment exerted by a force couple is determined by the product of the amount of the forces applied and the distance between them, which in the case of a residual limb is determined by the length of the long bone of the skeleton within the residual limb (**Fig. 2.17**). As a result, individuals with longer residual limbs have greater leverage and can produce greater moments with the same force application compared to individuals with shorter residual limbs. Thus, individuals with short residual limbs may require prostheses with components that provide

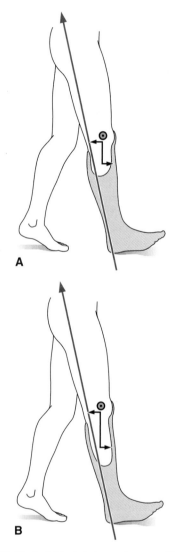

A

B

FIGURE 2.17. The individual, A, has a shorter residual limb (and lever arm) and needs to generate more muscle force to produce the same internal moment as the individual in B with a longer residual limb and lever arm.

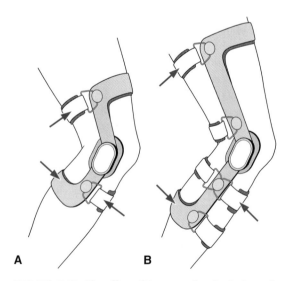

A   **B**

FIGURE 2.16. The effect of lever arm length. Both appliances (A and B) have the same three-point counterforce design. Applying force through a greater distance (lever arm length), as in appliance B, reduces the amount of force required to produce equivalent effects.

more control of the prosthetic joints than those with longer residual limbs.

Pressure

Various biological tissues have different tolerances for the application of external forces. Anatomical sites that are padded with layers of fat and muscle are able to tolerate higher forces than are bony prominences or areas containing superficial blood vessels and nerves. As a result, when appliances are designed and fabricated, careful attention must be paid not only to how forces are applied, but also to where they are applied. Forces over pressure-sensitive areas are reduced by depressions or hollowed-out areas (relief areas) that contour to the pressure-intolerant structures. Additional pressure relief can be designed into the appliance by adding built-up areas or relief additions over nearby pressure-tolerant areas. This combination of relief depressions and additions helps to redistribute loads from pressure-sensitive structures to pressure-tolerant ones. A specific weight-bearing transtibial prosthetic socket demonstrates application of these principles of relieving the pressure-sensitive structures, such as the tibial crest and fibular head (see Figs. 6.9 and 6.10). Many foot orthoses are designed to provide relief to the pressure-sensitive metatarsal heads (see Fig. 13.16).

Another method to reduce tissue pressure at the interface with the device is to increase the total contact area over which the force is applied. Pressure is determined by the magnitude of the applied force divided by the surface area to which the force is applied (P = F/a). Thus, increasing the total contact area between the appliance and the user's body surface distributes the applied force over a larger area and decreases the contact pressure. An appliance that is in total contact with the user's body and is contoured with relief areas to minimize pressure on pressure-sensitive anatomy is more likely to be comfortable and safe (see Figs. 17.11 and 17.12). Practitioners must be aware, however, that users of total contact, contoured appliances who have skin insensitivity or experience periods of fluctuating limb edema may be at risk for skin breakdown, despite the best intimate total contact at the time of fitting.

Alignment Between the Appliance and the User's Anatomy

When prostheses or orthoses have articulated mechanical joints that move along with anatomical joints contained within the appliance, congruency between the mechanical and anatomical joint axes is imperative. If the anatomical and mechanical axes do not coincide, undesirable forces, including compression and shearing, are generated at the soft tissue interface as the joints move together about different axes (**Fig. 2.18**). This can cause discomfort, skin breakdown, and poor function. Because most anatomical joints have multiple axes, triplanar axes, or instantaneous centers of rotation, and most mechanical axes are uniaxial (single axis), establishing congruence is not always easy. Biomechanists along with clinicians have established estimates of the locations of anatomical joint axes by using external anatomical landmarks (see Table 2.1). Using these anatomical guidelines, practitioners can identify reasonable congruency between anatomical and mechanical joints and minimize unwanted, deleterious forces. Mechanical polycentric axes are available for some joints, which also reduce unwanted forces and appliance migration (see Fig. 15.3D and E).

CHARACTERISTICS OF NORMAL GAIT: IMPLICATIONS AND APPLICATIONS FOR PROSTHETIC AND ORTHOTIC USE

The ability to prescribe prosthetic and orthotic devices and fit and train clients in their use requires a thorough understanding of and the ability to critically analyze

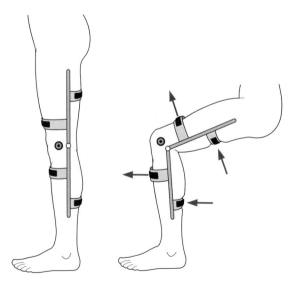

FIGURE 2.18. Effects of misalignment between anatomical and mechanical joint axes during movement. The mechanical axis seeks to align with the anatomical axis, which produces appliance migration, compression and increased pressure (posterior), or gapping (anterior).

impaired function. **Functional analysis** requires the practitioner to methodically observe a client performing a functional activity, break the activity into component parts, compare the movements in each component to "typical" or effective movement, and identify impairments that limit or restrict the overall function. Then, based on his or her knowledge, evidence from the research literature, and experience, the practitioner must select methods to minimize or eliminate the impairments and retrain the client to effectively, efficiently, and safely perform the problem functional activity. This skill of functional analysis and training is an important and foundational part of designing rehabilitation programs and selecting effective interventions. When the impaired function is gait, functional analysis is performed as *gait analysis*. Gait analyses are performed as observational or instrumented gait analyses. In an observational gait analysis, a clinician uses a methodical process to visually evaluate an individual's gait to identify kinematic, spatial, and temporal differences from typical gait. These qualitative differences or abnormalities are called gait deviations. Prosthetic gait deviations and their causes are described in Chapter 7. Instrumented gait analysis employs instrumentation to quantitatively measure various parameters that describe gait, including kinematic, kinetic, distance, time, and electromyographic characteristics. Additional functional activities that are observed and analyzed by clinicians working with prosthetic and orthotic wearers include functional analyses of running and ascending and descending stairs. The knowledge base that clinicians use when performing observational gait analyses is reviewed below. Keywords listed at the end of this chapter can be used to guide a literature search to learn more about the analysis of running and ascending and descending stairs.

Bipedal locomotion, or ambulation, in humans is a cyclical process that, once started, occurs as a repetitive sequence of events and movements of the upper and lower extremities and trunk. This basic repeating sequence is called the **gait cycle**. This repeating gait cycle has been studied and described in a variety of ways. This section provides an overview of the aspects of the gait cycle and gait analysis that practitioners who work with users of prosthetic or orthotic devices apply in clinical decision making regarding devices.

The Fundamental Tasks of Gait

The general *purpose of locomotion* is mobility and forward progression. Winter lists specific fundamental tasks that must be accomplished during effective locomotion.[5] These tasks are

- to support the body and prevent collapse of the weight-bearing lower limb,
- to maintain upright posture and balance,
- to control the foot to insure ground clearance while the leg is moving forward and to insure a safe and "soft" initial contact with the ground,
- to generate the mechanical energy to produce, maintain, or increase the forward propulsion of the body, and
- to provide shock absorption and stability to slow the forward propulsion of the body.

The Gait Cycle

The basic unit of gait, the **gait cycle**, includes all the movements in both extremities that occur from the initial contact with the ground of one foot to the next time the same foot strikes the ground. The period of time when each foot is in contact with the ground is called *stance phase,* and the period of time when the foot is off of the ground and the limb is advancing is called *swing phase.* At a comfortable, self-selected walking speed, stance phase usually occupies 60% of the gait cycle and swing phase the remaining 40%. During walking, each gait cycle includes two periods of *double limb support,* when both feet are on the ground at the same time. These periods of double limb support occur at the beginning and end of each stance phase and each is about 10% of the gait cycle. The period between the double limb support periods is termed *single limb support,* when only one foot contacts the ground and the contralateral limb is advancing. In bipedal locomotion, the faster one walks, the shorter the periods of double limb support become, until running begins when the gait cycle no longer has any periods of double limb support. Conversely, slower gait speeds increase the time spent in double support for both steps in a gait cycle.

The stance and swing phases of gait are further broken down into events and subphases. At normal, free (self-selected or comfortable) walking speed, these events and subphases usually occur at predictable times that are often described in terms of a percentage of a whole gait cycle (100%), where 0% denotes the initial ground contact, 60% marks the end of stance phase, and 100% marks the end of swing phase. **Figures 2.19 and 2.20** summarize the events and phases of the gait cycle, describe observations to identify each, and provide an estimate of when each

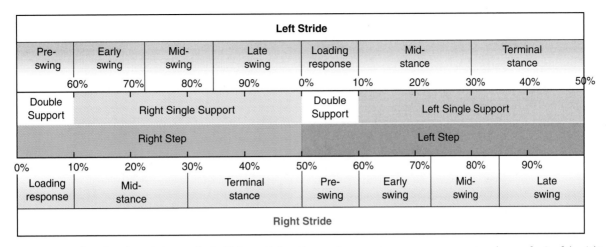

FIGURE 2.19. The gait cycle and phases of gait. Right and left strides are drawn to demonstrate co-occurring phases of gait of the right and left lower extremities.

occurs in the gait cycle. This terminology is used throughout this text to describe normal walking gait.

Kinematics of Gait

Kinematics describes movement in terms of displacement, velocity, and acceleration. This section reviews the kinematics of gait only in terms of displacement, including the distance and temporal (time duration) characteristics of gait followed by a description of the discrete movement patterns of individual joints during gait.

Time and Distance Characteristics of Gait

Stride length is the distance traveled during one gait cycle. A stride is measured as the linear distance from one heel strike (or initial ground contact) to the next heel strike of the same extremity. Each stride is composed of two steps, a right and a left step. *Step length* is the linear distance measured from the heel strike, or initial ground contact, of one foot to the next heel strike of the contralateral foot. *Step width* represents the base of support and is measured as the perpendicular distance between similar points on both feet, measured during two consecutive steps. *Foot angle* is the angle measured between the long axis of the foot and the line of forward progression. Although there is much variation in these parameters among individuals, within an individual there is usually side-to-side symmetry (**Fig. 2.21**). Thus, asymmetric step length, width, or foot angle should key the observer to look for the cause of the asymmetry. Asymmetric step

length is often observed in individuals who use a unilateral prosthetic or orthotic device. Although there are many causes for asymmetrical step lengths, individuals who use a unilateral prosthetic/orthotic device often spend less time in stance phase on the involved side, which shortens swing time and thus step length on the noninvolved side (**Fig. 2.22**).

The primary *temporal characteristics* of the gait cycle are walking speed and cadence. *Walking speed* is the distance covered in a period of time, usually reported in research studies as meters per second (m/sec). Treadmills in the United States, however, usually show speed as miles per hour (10 meters equals 0.006 mile). Most sources report typical stride time for an unimpaired adult as about 1 second and normal walking speed as about 3 to 4 miles per hour (mph) or about 1.3 m/sec. *Cadence* is the number of steps per minute. Walking speed is a function of cadence and step length. Increasing either or both cadence and step length will increase walking speed and, as a result, reduce stance time and swing time. Although both stance and swing time are reduced as walking speed increases, stance time is reduced more. Thus, as walking speed increases, the swing-to-stance-time ratio (normally about 0.6) approaches 1.

Similarly, gait speed decreases when either step length or cadence is reduced. A commonly observed effect of aging on gait is a reduction of gait speed, typically caused by decreased step length, rather than reduced cadence.[6–8] Slower gait speed is also common among individuals with impairments that require the use of prosthetic or orthotic devices.

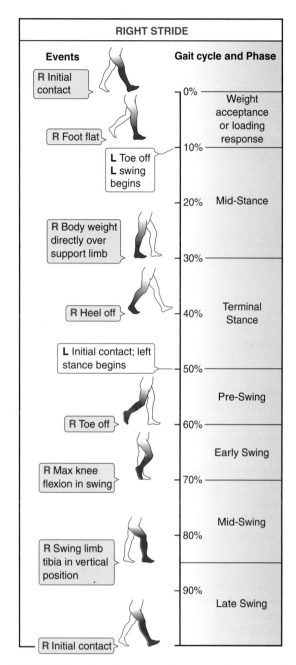

FIGURE 2.20. Observable events that occur during gait. The events that are used to divide the gait cycle (or stride) into phases are described.

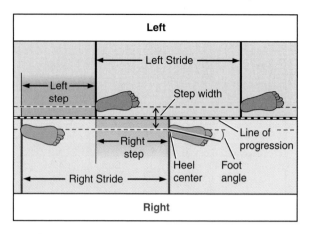

FIGURE 2.21. Commonly described distance measurements of the gait cycle. Note the typical symmetry between right and left sides.

Angular Displacement of Joints During Gait

The joints of the upper and lower extremity and trunk go through repetitive movement patterns of joint excursions during the gait cycle. Because joint movements in the lower limb occur under closed chain conditions during stance, insufficient joint ROM in one joint requires compensation at another joint or joints. These compensations produce abnormal movement patterns called gait abnormalities or deviations. **Table 2.2** lists the values of the typical peak joint excursions that occur in the sagittal plane during normal adult gait at free walking speed. Thus, these joint measurements also represent the joint passive ROM requirements for normal joint movement patterns to occur during gait. Joint excursions in the frontal and transverse planes during gait are much smaller and more variable. Because there is much intra- and interindividual variability in the specific amount of joint movement that occurs during the gait cycle, the *pattern of movement* for each joint is presented and discussed rather than specific ranges of joint motion. Practitioners observing gait in clients with gait impairments are encouraged to observe these *overall patterns of movement* at each joint, rather than focus on the presence of a particular amount of ROM during particular intervals during gait.

Sagittal Plane Movement Pattern

The patterns of sagittal plane movement through the gait cycle are drawn in **Figure 2.23**.[9] The *hip* demonstrates a single cycle of motion starting at initial contact in maximum flexion (~25°). It reaches maximum extension during late stance at about 50% of the gait

Individuals who walk slowly may do so for a variety of reasons, including cardiovascular or pulmonary diseases or deconditioning that make it difficult to meet the energy requirement for walking as well as neuromusculoskeletal impairments such as reduced muscle strength, joint ROM, or balance.

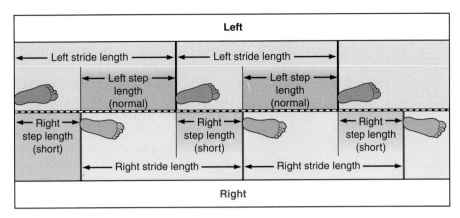

FIGURE 2.22. Step and stride length measurements from an individual using a unilateral prosthetic/orthotic device, with an asymmetrical gait pattern. The right steps are short, and thus, the left side is probably the involved side. Although right and left steps are unequal, right and left strides are equal, as long as the individual is walking in a straight line.

cycle when the contralateral foot contacts the ground and then begins flexing again in pre-swing. It reaches maximum flexion a second time in late swing at about 80% to 85% of the gait cycle. The pelvis rotates anteriorly whenever the hip extends. This combination of hip extension and anterior pelvic rotation gives the appearance that the hip joint is extending more than it actually does.

The *knee* exhibits two cycles of flexion and extension during a gait cycle. The first flexion–extension cycle occurs during stance phase. At initial contact, the knee is only a few degrees from full extension. It rapidly flexes to about 15° to 20° for foot flat (at ~10% of gait cycle) and then begins to extend again, reaching maximum extension at about 40% of the gait cycle when the heel lifts off of the floor and knee flexion begins again. During swing phase, the knee goes through the second flexion–extension cycle. The knee flexes through early and midswing and reaches maximum flexion (~60°) at about 75% of the gait cycle. The knee extends again through terminal swing to reach near full extension just before initial contact.

The *ankle* also goes through two cycles of dorsiflexion and plantarflexion. During stance phase, the

TABLE 2.2	Sagittal Plane Joint Range of Motion Requirements for Typical Adult Walking Gait	
Joint	**Max ROM (°)**	**When It Occurs in the Gait Cycle**
Hip	25° flexion	Terminal swing Initial ground contact
	20° extension	Terminal stance (~50% in gait cycle)
Knee	0°	Initial ground contact
	60°	Heel off (~40% of gait cycle) Initial (early) swing
Ankle	10° dorsiflexion	Late stance before heel off occurs
	20° plantarflexion	Toe off
Subtalar*	4° to 6° pronation	Loading response (weight acceptance)
	4° to 6° supination	Heel off through toe off

* Motion at the subtalar joint is triplanar (supination and pronation) with component motion occurring in all three planes.

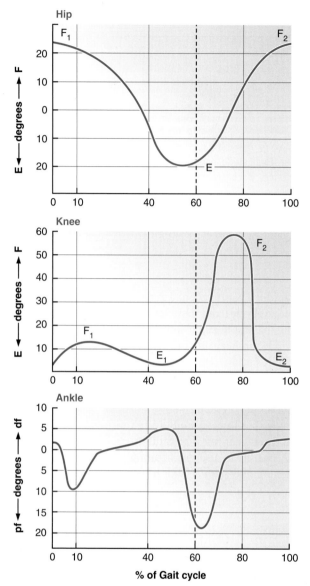

FIGURE 2.23. The patterns of sagittal plane movement at the hip, knee, and ankle through the gait cycle. (F, flexion; E, extension; df, dorsiflexion; pf, plantarflexion.)

from the ground. During swing, the ankle assumes a position around neutral or slight plantar or dorsiflexion that is sufficient to clear the foot as it advances over the ground.

Observation of the sagittal plane patterns of movement of all three joints together (see Fig. 2.23) demonstrates that there is only a brief interval following toe-off (60% of gait cycle) when all three joints move in the same direction at the same time to pull the limb away from the ground. At this moment, the hip and knee are flexing and the ankle is dorsiflexing. At all other times in the gait cycle, the joints must move independently, so that as one or two joint(s) move the foot away from the ground, other(s) move it toward the ground. For example, during swing phase when the limb is reaching for initial contact of a new step, the hip is flexing with ankle doriflexion (moving the foot in the same direction away from the ground), but the knee must extend. Mr. Green, the patient with right hemiplegia described in the case presentation at the beginning of this chapter, has difficulty with this task. His inability to initiate volitional movements independently in his involved right hip, knee, and ankle contributes to his gait difficulties. In particular, he has difficulty

- during midstance when he needs to produce hip and knee extension with dorsiflexion,
- in preswing when he needs to produce plantarflexion with hip and knee flexion, and
- during terminal swing when he needs to extend his knee with hip flexion and ankle dorsiflexion.

Many individuals with neuromuscular disorders experience difficulty dissociating volitional movement at the joints within a limb, which may cause gait deviations that make gait slow, inefficient, or unsafe. The inability to dissociate movements within a limb may require special consideration when developing an orthotic prescription or gait training program for an individual using an orthosis.

Frontal Plane Movement Pattern

Frontal plane motions (abduction and adduction) are much smaller, more variable, and less studied than sagittal plane motions during gait. The movements of the *hip* in the frontal plane are illustrated in **Figure 2.24**. Hip position in the frontal plane is influenced by the movement of the pelvis toward the weight-bearing side to keep the CoM over the base of support (producing adduction of the hip on weight-bearing side) and by the drop of the pelvis on the non-weight-bearing side

ankle plantarflexes (~15°) during the first 10% of the gait cycle to achieve foot flat and loading respsonse (weight acceptance). As body weight is shifted onto the limb and the body advances or glides over the stance foot, the ankle dorsiflexes and achieves maximum dorsiflexion just after the knee reaches full knee extension (~40% of gait cycle). The second cycle begins with ankle plantarflexion in terminal stance and preswing (push off) and reaches maximum plantarflexion (~20°) just after toe-off. The ankle then moves again into dorsiflexion as the limb pulls away

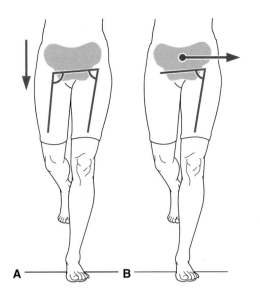

FIGURE 2.24. A, During weight acceptance, the hip of the weight-bearing (WB) limb adducts slightly due to pelvic drop on the non-WB side. B, Lateral shifting to side of the WB limb to keep the body's CoM within the base of support also contributes to adduction.

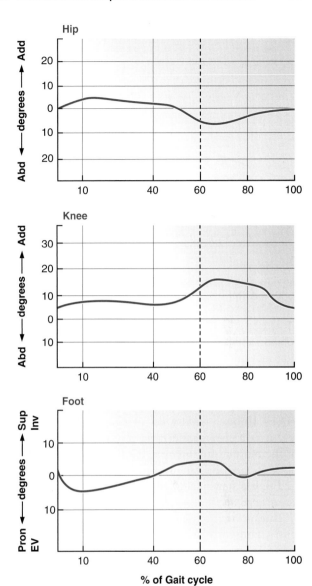

FIGURE 2.25. The patterns of frontal plane movement at the hip, knee, and subtalor joints through the gait cycle. (Add, adduction; Abd, abduction; Sup, supination; Inv, calcaneal inversion; Pron, pronation; Ev, calcaneal eversion.)

(producing slight abduction). The hip is in a position close to neutral at initial contact and then moves into adduction during weight acceptance. Adduction continues until late stance and the beginning of double support. When limb loading begins on the contralateral side (double support), hip abduction begins ipsilaterally in response to lateral pelvic shift to the new weight-bearing limb (see Fig. 2.25). The *knee* has little frontal plane movement as long as there is good ligamentous stability. Frontal plane movement of the *foot* reflects the calcaneal inversion and eversion component of closed-chain supination and pronation (**Fig. 2.25**). The general pattern of movement in the foot during gait includes subtalar pronation (frontal plane eversion) during early stance/weight acceptance and subtalar supination (frontal plane inversion) during mid- and late-stance phase. This pattern of movement helps to keep the plantar aspect of the foot in contact with the ground through stance phase, allows the foot to be flexible during weight acceptance to absorb or dissipate the impact of limb loading, and makes the foot more rigid to facilitate push-off during late stance.

Transverse Plane Movement Pattern

Like movement in the frontal plane, transverse plane movements are also very small and variable. Transverse plane movements at the *hip* joint (internal and external rotation) are a function of transverse plane motion of the pelvis and the femur in the closed chain (**Fig. 2.26**). Forward rotation of the pelvis about the stance limb (Fig. 2.26A) accompanies hip flexion during swing and reaches maximum forward rotation at foot initial contact. This forward pelvic rotation that occurs with hip flexion produces a greater step length than is possible from hip flexion alone. The forward pelvic advancement also contributes to lateral rotation of the advancing leg. At the same time the opposite hip (of the stance limb) is in maximum extension, the pelvis is in relative backward rotation and the femur is rotated medially (Fig. 2.26B). Independent femoral

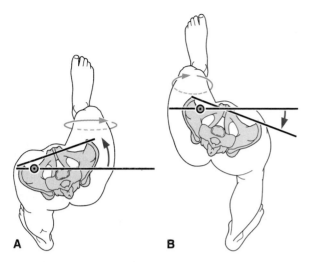

FIGURE 2.26. During gait, step length is increased as a result of pelvic forward (A) and backward (B) rotation about the stance limb (⊙). The stance leg also experiences medial rotation at the hip.

rotation about its long axis also contributes to the rotation movement that occurs at the hip joint. At initial contact, the femur is oriented close to neutral. It rotates internally (medially) during weight acceptance and midstance. It then begins to rotate laterally, which continues through midswing when medial rotation resumes. Despite considerable variability, the direction of the movement pattern at the hip in the transverse plane is medial rotation from initial contact through mid to late stance followed by lateral rotation through late swing.

During the closed-chain conditions of stance phase, transverse plane movement at the *knee* is influenced by motions occurring at the foot and sagittal plane motion at the knee. Pronation of the foot is linked to tibial medial rotation and knee flexion, which together facilitate shock absorption during loading response. Later in stance as the foot supinates, the tibia rotates laterally and the knee extends, allowing the body to roll forward, smoothly transferring weight onto the opposite limb.

Movement Patterns of the Trunk

The head and trunk also participate in the cyclic movement patterns that occur during the gait cycle. In the sagittal plane, the trunk displays slight flexion (forward lean) and extension during the gait cycle. The trunk is more erect during single limb support and is slightly flexed during double-limb support. In the frontal plane, the trunk leans slightly toward the stance limb with each step in order to keep the CoM

over the stance foot and maintain balance. In the transverse plane, trunk forward rotation is concomitant with forward pelvic rotation on the opposite side. Additionally, the shoulder flexes with forward trunk rotation on the same side. The linked but opposite rotation that occurs between the trunk and pelvis is necessary for efficiency of movement during gait. Individuals who are unable to rotate their trunk and pelvis separately due to back pain, muscle rigidity, or restrictions caused by a prosthetic or orthotic appliance expend more energy during walking.

Muscle Activity During Gait

Muscle activity during gait has been studied extensively with electromyography (EMG).[10] The primary muscles contracting during gait and when during the gait cycle they are most active are summarized in **Figure 2.27**. During gait, muscles contract primarily in short bursts of activity, most often at times of transition between phases: swing to stance or stance to swing (**Fig. 2.28**). Typically, muscles first contract eccentrically to decelerate the limb or a limb segment, followed by a concentric contraction, which initiates the affected joint's forward movement or movement in the opposite direction. Most often, the joint affected by a concentrically contracting muscle continues to move after active muscle contraction has ceased due to the kinetics or momentum of the movement. Illustrations of these principles of muscle activity during gait are presented in the following descriptions of the muscular control of the joints of the lower limb during walking.

At the *transition from swing to stance*, several muscles have a burst of activity. These include the gluteus maximus, the hamstrings, the gluteus medius, the quadriceps, and the dorsiflexor muscles (see Figs. 2.27 and 2.28). The *gluteus maximus* and *hamstrings* contract eccentrically to decelerate the flexing hip at the end of swing phase. Their continued contraction helps to initiate hip extension in early stance. Additionally, the effect of the gluteus maximus on the femur during early single limb support helps to fix the femur and accelerate the knee into extension. Individuals who have difficulty maintaining knee extension during midstance due to quadriceps weakness can compensate by maximizing this effect of the gluteus maximus in contributing to knee stability. The *gluteus medius* also has a burst of activity during this same time frame. It begins contracting just before initial contact, peaks during weight acceptance, and

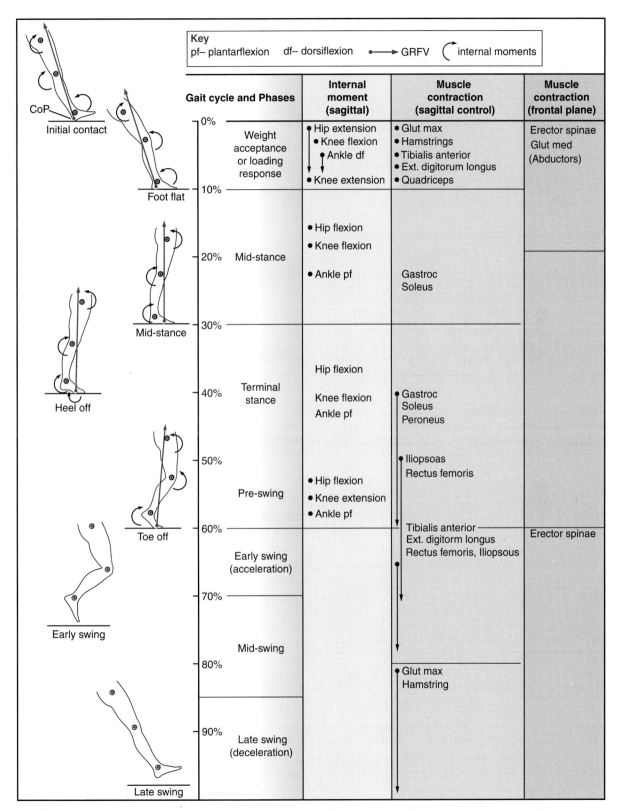

FIGURE 2.27. Muscle activity during the gait cycle. Curved black arrows indicate the internal moments, primarily produced by muscle contraction. The ground reaction force vector (GRFV), which produces external moments, is shown as red arrows extending from the center of pressure (CoP) on the sole of the foot to the center of mass.

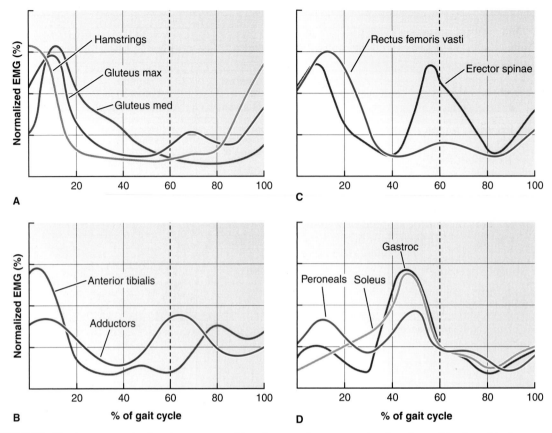

FIGURE 2.28. Muscles contract in short bursts at transitions between the stance and swing phases. Muscle activity is expressed as electromyographic data as a percent of a maximum voluntary isometric contraction.

continues to contract at a lower level until loading begins on the opposite leg. It provides frontal plane stability to the pelvis through stance phase. Individuals who use lower extremity prostheses or orthoses must have good strength and control of their gluteus muscles, as well as the core muscles that stabilize the trunk, for effective dynamic balance during walking. Muscle activity at the knee demonstrates cocontraction of the quadriceps and hamstring muscles during loading response and early midstance. The *quadriceps* is essential in controlling the knee during the early part of stance. During late stance, however, quadriceps activity is low and the increasing activity of the *soleus* contracting under closed-chain conditions contributes to maintaining knee extension stability. The *dorsiflexor muscles* demonstrate a burst of activity at initial contact and loading response to control the descent of the foot to the ground.

At the *transition from stance to swing phase*, the hip flexor and the plantarflexor muscles are of primary importance. The *hip flexors* contract at the end of

stance phase to decelerate the extending hip and to initiate hip flexion to pull the limb away from the floor and begin swing phase. This hip flexion also initiates passive knee flexion for early swing with very little contribution from the hamstrings. The *plantarflexor muscles* gradually increase their activity through stance and produce a burst of activity from heel off to toe off. This plantarflexor muscle activity provides the majority of lower extremity support and balance during late-stance phase. Individuals who lack active plantarflexion either due to weakness or amputation may demonstrate shorter contralateral step length, reduced gait speed, and impaired balance. The activity of the hip flexor and the plantarflexor muscles produces the majority of the force for knee flexion during swing phase. Although the knee moves through an excursion of about 60° of ROM, most of swing phase proceeds with no muscle activity at the knee. Prosthetic designs for clients with transfemoral amputation take advantage of this in that no prosthetic mechanism is required to produce knee flexion for swing phase as long as the individual is able to flex the hip and walk fast enough to produce some momentum. During swing phase, the *dorsiflexor muscles* contract at a continuous low level to hold the foot away from the ground and to maintain the ankle joint at a position around neutral.

Kinetics of Gait

Kinetics refers to the forces, moments, and power produced during gait. During the limb movements that occur during locomotion, the lower extremities sustain large and repetitive loads that increase as the weight of the individual and the speed of walking or running increases. During locomotion, **internal moments** are produced by the contraction of muscles and the viscoelastic properties of joint capsules and ligaments in order to offset the effect of **external moments** that are generated by GRFs. Internal moments that are typical in the sagittal plane at the hip, knee, and ankle during normal walking are summarized in Figure 2.27. These internal moments are consistent with the muscle activity discussed in the previous section: the contraction of the hamstrings, quadriceps, and plantarflexor muscles produce extensor internal moments and the hip flexor and dorsiflexor muscles produce flexion moments or moments that pull the limb away from the ground. Winter studied these internal moments and developed the concept of the **support moment** (Fig. 2.29).[11] The support moment is the sum of all the sagittal plane internal moments acting at the hip, knee, and ankle that tend to push the body away from the ground and support the body.[11] He notes that during most of stance phase, this summed moment is an extensor moment, or a moment that supports the body weight and prevents limb collapse during weight bearing. He also describes that the relative or proportional contributions to the support moment from the hip, knee, and ankle are inconsequential, *as long as the sum from the three joints is an extensor moment.* Thus, an individual, such as our case study client, Mr. Green, who has significant distal (plantarflexion) weakness can maximize the contributions from the hip and knee to the overall support moment in order to compensate and achieve safe gait. Further review of the support moment and its components (Fig. 2.29) shows that the hip and knee are primarily responsible for limb support in early stance (0% to 20% of the gait cycle), but *plantarflexion is the major factor in limb support from mid through the end of stance phase.* Thus,

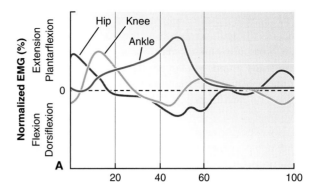

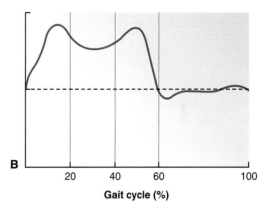

FIGURE 2.29. A, The sagittal plane internal moments at the hip, knee, and ankle with the extensor moments oriented in the positive direction (above zero). B, When the three joint moments are summed, an extensor curve called the support moment is formed.

individuals with impaired plantarflexion strength due to paralysis or amputation may experience mid- to late-stance phase support and balance problems or difficulty maintaining forward motion on the involved side. These individuals may benefit from exercises to improve plantarflexion strength. If this is not possible, they may benefit from learning to compensate by increasing hip and knee extension force. Another alternative when neither of these options is possible is the selection of prosthetic/orthotic componentry that substitutes, at least partially, for this very important support function.

External moments are largely a result of the GRFV, which extends from the CoP on the plantar surface of the foot to the CoM of the body (see Fig. 2.3). These force vectors usually pass eccentrically to the joint axes and thus produce an external moment at the joint that must be countered by internal moments (muscle, ligaments). Figure 2.27 diagrams the typical GRFV in selected stages of the gait cycle. When the sources of internal forces, such as muscle contraction, are insufficient to restrain the external moment, abnormal movements may occur. For example, our case study client, Mr. Green, has significant weakness of his right lower extremity that results in knee instability and near buckling. Because he has hip and knee extensor and plantarflexor weakness, the GRFV remains posterior to the knee axis of rotation during midstance, generating a flexion external moment. Solutions for Mr. Green's knee buckling problem may include strengthening exercises for the hip and knee extensor and plantarflexor muscles, using an orthosis that will manipulate the GRFV so that it is anterior to the knee axis (see Fig. 2.6), or a combination of the two approaches.

Factors That Influence Gait

The descriptions of normal gait presented in this chapter are based on the study of normal adults walking at their comfortable, free walking speeds. Many factors, however, influence the kinetic and kinematic characteristics of a specific individual's gait, including the neuromusculoskeletal impairments of the individual and their use of appliances or assisted devices. Extensive descriptions of studies that examine these factors are available but are beyond the scope of this text.[12] Two of these factors, however, have been shown to have a significant affect on gait and must be considered when evaluating the gait of individuals walking with or without prosthetic or orthotic appliances. These factors are walking speed and the age of the walker. Practitioners who observe clients and make judgments about gait abnormalities must consider these factors and their effects on "normal gait" when identifying gait problems and prescribing solutions to improve gait.

Walking Speed

Cadence, step length, and stride length all increase as gait speed increases, and conversely, they decrease at slower speeds.[9,13] Likewise, the amount of joint excursion increases with increasing gait speed and decreases with reduced speeds. The energy requirement (oxygen consumption) for ambulation and speed of gait also influence one another. For example, individuals, whether impaired or unimpaired, usually self-select the walking speed that is most energy efficient for them. Thus, individuals with gait impairments typically walk at slower than typical speeds and use more energy when compared to unimpaired individuals. Interestingly, individuals without impairments consume more oxygen when walking either faster or slower than their self-selected comfortable walking speed. Many people who use prosthetic or orthotic devices for ambulation walk at slower rates and expend more energy during walking when compared to unimpaired individuals. Thus, practitioners must expect that this slower walking speed will contribute to reduced step and stride length, cadence, and joint excursion and take this into consideration when identifying gait abnormalities. For example, individuals who walk very slowly may have difficulty with foot clearance during swing because the resultant reduced step length and hip flexion do not produce sufficient knee flexion during swing phase.

Faster walking speeds also produce greater GRFs, which leads to alterations in muscle activity and patterns of muscle contraction during gait. Although the relationship between walking speed and muscle activity may differ among specific muscles, generally faster walking speeds result in higher peak muscle activity. Walking speed also affects the duration of muscle activity, which increases with both very fast as well as very slow walking. Clinicians performing gait training with clients at various ambulation speeds must recognize and accommodate these effects of gait speed on muscle activity.

Maturation and Aging

A discussion of the development of mature gait in children is beyond the scope of this textbook; however, in general, most authors report that the distance and temporal characteristics of gait reach adult values by about age 7 years in typically developing children. Sutherland suggests that certain gait characteristics can be used to identify mature gait in children. These include increased duration of single-limb stance, walking speed, and step length as well as decreased step width and cadence.[14]

Reports on the effect of healthy aging on gait are variable; however, a few findings are consistent. It appears that in older adults, the self-selected comfortable walking speed is slower, stride length is shorter, and stance time is longer.[6,7] Some have also reported that older persons have reduced plantarflexion power generation and may also exhibit reduced dorsiflexion and hip extension ROM during gait.[8] It is very difficult, however, to determine if these alterations of gait are the true consequence of aging alone or result from neuromusculoskeletal impairments that are common among elders. Others suggest that the reduced joint excursions, step length, and GRFs observed in elders may simply be a result of their slower walking speeds.[6,7] In order to insure the best functional outcome, practitioners making decisions about prosthetic or orthotic appliances for maturing children or elders must consider and test all these factors before making definitive appliance prescriptions.

Biomechanical Aspects of Balance

Balance, or the ability to control and maintain upright postures, requires an individual to maintain his or her CoM within his or her base of support (BoS). In standing postures in typical adults, the CoM is located slightly anterior to the second sacral vertebra, while in young children in standing posture the CoM is located at about the level of the 12th thoracic vertebra. The location of the CoM, however, is not fixed and is affected by changes in position, limb and trunk movements, as well as adding things to the body, such as carrying an object.[15] For example, if an individual is wearing a leg cast or heavy orthosis or prosthesis, the CoM moves lower and toward the additional weight.[16] Similarly, if an individual loses a limb or part of a limb to amputation, there is a concomitant shift in the location of the CoM away from the amputated limb segment. The amount of the shift of the CoM is determined by the amount and mass of the limb loss or the addition of weight. This shift in CoM may disrupt balance and the ability of the individual to respond accurately to postural disturbances. Thus, practitioners who train individuals to use prosthetic or orthotic devices must expect balance deficits and include balance training as part of functional training both with and without the appliances.

Although only a small amount of muscle activity is required to maintain erect standing posture, control of posture is complex and requires somatosensory (including tactile sensation and proprioception), visual, and vestibular inputs that are processed in the central nervous system. Loss or alteration of any of these inputs by amputation or injury affects the body's ability to control posture effectively and efficiently. To maintain balance and erect posture, the body responds to perturbations or postural challenges with centralized patterns of muscle activity called fixed-support synergies (ankle or hip strategies) or change in support strategies (stepping or grasping synergies).[17] The ankle and hip strategies are discrete bursts of muscle activity that occur in a distal to proximal pattern in response to forward or backward perturbations. An individual with amputation or impaired muscle control or sensation may not be able to use these balance recovery strategies and thus may be more susceptible to balance loss and falls. Practitioners who prescribe prosthetic or orthotic devices must anticipate these balance impairments and select components that maximize mobility while insuring safe postural stability. Because a strong relationship has been identified between balance and walking ability in individuals with lower limb amputation, therapists who train clients in the use of prosthetic and orthotic devices must include therapeutic activities to improve balance in all aspects of functional activity.[18]

SUMMARY

The biomechanical assessment of functional activities and gait analysis are important basic skills for practitioners who work with individuals who use prosthetic or orthotic devices. Practitioners must use their biomechanical knowledge to understand the effects of an individual's impairments on his or her function as well as to determine ways in which devices can be designed to apply forces to improve function. A thorough understanding of biomechanics is also necessary to work effectively with prosthetists and orthotists to develop appliance prescriptions that are effective and efficient and maximize the client's function.

KEYWORDS FOR LITERATURE SEARCH

For each search topic choose relevant search terms from each category and use the Boolean term "AND" to narrow your search to your area of interest.

Biomechanical Assessment of Gait

Gait (limit all searches to humans)
Gait analysis/gait AND biomechanics
Walking/physiology
Locomotion/physiology

Type of Gait Assessment
Gait disorders
Biomechanics
Mechanical energy
Muscle, skeletal/physiology
Kinetics
Kinematics

Conditions of Interest (just a few are listed for examples)
Cerebral palsy
Arthritis
Spinal cord injury
Stroke/rehabilitation, surgery, therapy

Intervention
Artificial limbs
Orthotic devices

Functional Analysis of Running and Stair Climbing

Activities
Running
Stair ascent, ascending stairs
Stair descent, descending stairs
Stair climbing, stair locomotion, stair ambulation

Characteristics
Kinematics
Kinetics
Mechanical power, power
Electromyography, EMG
Biomechanics

Populations
Lower limb amputees, above-knee amputees, transtibial amputees, transfemoral amputees
Orthotic devices
Artificial limbs
Any particular client population of interest; cerebral palsy, hemiplegia, etc

7. Himann JE, Cunningham DA, Rechnitzer PA, et al: Age-related changes in speed of walking. Med Sci Sports Exerc 20:161–166, 1988.
8. Winter DA, Patla AE, Frank JS, et al: Biomechanical walking patterns in the fit and healthy elderly. Phys Ther 70:340–347, 1990.
9. Murray MP: Gait as a total pattern of movement. Am J Phys Med 46:290–333, 1967.
10. Winter DA, Yack HJ: EMG profiles during normal human walking: stride-to-stride and inter-subject variability. Electroencephalogr Clin Neurophysiol 67:402–411, 1987.
11. Winter DA: Overall principles of lower limb support during stance phase of gait. J Biomech 13:923–927, 1980.
12. Olney SJ: Gait. In PK Levangie, CC Norkin, eds. Joint Structure and Function: A Comprehensive Analysis, 4th ed. FA Davis, Philadelphia, 2005, pp 559–564.
13. Andriacchi TP, Ogle JA, Galante JO: Walking speed as a basis for normal and abnormal gait measurements. J Biomech 10:261–268, 1977.
14. Sutherland DL, Olshen R, Cooper L, Woo SL: The development of mature gait. JBJS (AM) 62:336–352, 1980.
15. Panjabi MM, White AA: Biomechanics in the Musculoskeletal System. Philadelphia, Churchill Livingstone, 2001.
16. Nordine M, Frankel VH: Basic Biomechanics of the Musculoskeletal System, 3rd ed. Philadelphia, Lippincott Williams & Wilkins, 2001.
17. Horak FB, Henry SM, Shumway-Cook A: Postural perturbations: new insights for treatment of balance disorders. Phys Ther 77:517–533, 1997.
18. van Velzen JM, van Bennekom CAM, van der Woude LHV, et al: Physical capacity and walking ability asfter lower limb amputation: a systematic review. Clin Rehabil 20:999–1016, 2006.

REFERENCES

1. Sumiya T, Suzuki Y, Kasahara T: Stiffness control in posterior-type plastic ankle-foot orthoses: effect of ankle trimline. Part 2: Orthosis characteristics and orthosis/patient matching. Prosthet Orthot Int 20:132–137, 1996.
2. Kottink A, Oostendorp L, Buurke J, et al: The orthotic effect of functional electrical stimulation on the improvement of walking in stroke patients with a dropped foot: a systematic review. Artif Organs 28:577–586, 2004.
3. Kim C, Eng J, Whittaker M: Effects of a simple functional electric and/or hinged ankle-foot orthosis on walking in persons with incomplete spinal cord injury. Arch Phys Med Rehabil 85:1718–1723, 2004.
4. Ferris D, Gordon K, Sawicki G, et al: An improved powered ankle-foot orthosis using proportional myoelectric control. Gait Posture 23:425–428, 2006.
5. Winter DA: Biomechanics of normal and pathological gait: implications for understanding human locomotor control. J Motor Behav 21:337–355, 1989.
6. Finley FR, Cody KA, Finzie RV: Locomotion patterns in elderly women. Arch Phys Med Rehabil 50:140–146, 1969.

Psychosocial Issues

3

OBJECTIVES

At the end of this chapter, all students are expected to:

1. Recognize, discuss, and respond appropriately to the anxieties, frustrations, and coping mechanisms used by individuals who need an external device for function.
2. Compare and contrast the psychosocial and cultural responses to changes in body image among clients of all ages.
3. Differentiate between phantom sensation and phantom pain, and discuss the effects of the phantom on prosthetic adjustment and function in clients of different ages.
4. Discuss the major approaches to the treatment of disabling phantom pain.

CASE STUDIES

Janice Simmons, a 65-year-old woman, had a left transtibial amputation yesterday secondary to diabetic gangrene and a nonhealing ulcer on the plantar surface of the right foot.

Linda Bean is a 12-year-old female who underwent a transfemoral amputation yesterday secondary to grade IIB osteogenic sarcoma of the proximal right tibia; the tumor was not appropriate for tumor resection and reconstruction.

Tyrone O'Neal, a 17-year-old high school football player, sustained a T_8 fracture in an auto accident when he was thrown from the car. The accident occurred 3 months ago, and he received immediate decompression and spine stabilization surgery at a trauma center. Despite prompt treatment, he has a complete spinal cord injury (ASIA level A) with neural motor and sensory levels of T_{12} bilaterally.

Janice Dione, a 12-year-old child, was just diagnosed with Adolescent Idiopathic Scoliosis. She has a double thoracolumbar curve. The thoracic curve, which is the primary curve, is a right 30° curve with the apex at T_9; the secondary lumbar curve is a left 26° curve at L_3. She is premenarche, and her iliac apophyses are rated as Risser 1. Janice is very athletic and participates in many very active sports, including soccer and gymnastics.

Case Study Activities

1. Compare and contrast the possible emotional responses of the patients presented above. What similarities and differences would you expect and why?
2. What would you expect the major psychosocial and economic concerns to be for each of the clients?
3. Which of the above patients are likely to experience phantom sensation or pain? Why? How may that affect their rehabilitation?
4. In laboratory or group sessions, role-play the initial and ongoing contact between the therapist/assistant and the client.

GENERAL CONCEPTS

Our perception of our body is an integral part of how we see ourselves, our **self-concept**, our ego, how we perceive our place in the world, and how we think others see us. A change in **body image** may affect our self-concept, our psychological reactions, and our ability to adjust to the change; it will be influenced by our cultural and social heritage and current environment. Body image and our reactions to disability are complex structures that have been well explored in numerous texts and papers in the psychosocial literature. The role of the therapist and assistant is to recognize the effects of changes in body image and help facilitate the client's adjustment to the change.

The physical and psychological effects of a change in body image are the result of many complex and interrelated aspects of the client's life. The effect is related, among other things, to how well the person can continue to pursue previous vocational, social, and leisure activities. It is also related to whether the change occurred gradually or suddenly. The individual with vascular disease who is amputated at the transtibial level after many months of ulcer care may view the loss differently from the individual who is amputated at the same level following an automobile accident. The former may actually welcome the amputation as an end to many months of treatments and disability. The latter may view it as a loss of self-concept and ability. As Dench and associates indicated, the sudden loss of body image has a shock value; the person is unprepared for the disruption and may go into depression, taking longer to adjust than the individual with vascular disease.[1]

There is a strong link between psychosocial adjustment and physical rehabilitation. Individuals who are dissatisfied with their body image may not be as motivated to reach their highest level of rehabilitation. In a study of individuals with and without physical disability, Tam reported higher self-concept ratings among individuals without disability.[2] How an individual will respond to changes in body image and to disability depend on many factors. **Table 3.1** outlines the major categories as discussed by Dench.[1]

TABLE 3.1	Categories of Responses to Body Image Loss*
Category	**Factors**
Prior loss	Previous disabilities (ulcers, other amputations, injuries)
Current loss	Permanent or improvable Other lifestyle issues (eg, cancer) Visible or hidden
Prognosis	Potential for return to functional lifestyle Degree of lifestyle disruption Availability of treatment Pain
Pattern of development	Dealing with previous disabilities Sudden or gradual onset Age and peer influences
Values	Family values Cultural aspects Patient beliefs, self-esteem Patient attitudes toward self-image and disability Societal values
Control	Ability to exert personal control Importance of personal control
Stigma	Perception of blame for problem Religious beliefs related to disability
Social support	How the disability affects previous social support Family reaction and available support

Adapted from Dench ME, Noonan AC, Sharby N, Ventura SH: Psychosocial aspects of health care, 2nd ed. New Jersey, Pearson Prentice Hall, 2007.

Badura-Brzoza and associates compared psychosocial adjustment of a group of individuals amputated for dysvascular problems with a control group using standardized psychological tests. They reported higher levels of anxiety and depression among the amputated group, particularly among individuals identified as having neurotic personality problems.[3] Other studies have supported those findings and provided evidence of the need for psychological support for individuals with amputations and similar permanent disabilities. Darnall and associates[4] used telephone interviews and a standardized scale to evaluate the extent of depression in a large sample of amputees. They reported that 28.7% of their sample exhibited severe depressive symptoms. Contributing factors included recent divorces, low income, altered lifestyles, and comorbidities. Individuals with higher levels of education were less likely to exhibit severe depression. Of the individuals with severe depression, only 44% had received mental health service within the past year.

However, not all individuals who undergo amputation or sustain disabilities requiring orthotic use are maladjusted or maintain evidence of severe depression. Certainly a sense of loss, some depression, and sometimes anger and denial accompany such incidents. Desmond and MacLachlan[5] in a study of veterans in the United Kingdom identified beneficial coping strategies. In general, they found that seeking social support, time since incidence, and using problem-solving strategies were positive coping mechanisms, but avoidance and denial were negative coping mechanisms.

STAGES OF ADJUSTMENT

Individuals who experience a disability may go through several stages in the process of acceptance and adjustment depending on the severity and the permanence of the disability. Bradway, Malone, and associates suggested four stages of emotional adjustment to amputation.[6] The first occurs before surgery when the individual begins to be aware that an amputation may happen. It is not unusual to have a client being treated for a vascular ulcer say to a therapist or assistant, "I'm afraid I may lose my foot." Our first instinct is to say: "Oh no, no, don't even think that!" While temporarily reassuring, such a response is not particularly helpful. A reflecting response, such as "I can understand your concerns about your foot," may encourage the client to explore feelings about a possible amputation and raise questions or concern about prosthetic replacement, pain, financial limitations, and dependency. Grief may be the first reaction to the official initial announcement that an amputation is necessary.

The second stage, immediately after surgery, is usually of short duration. Individuals who have undergone emergency or traumatic amputation may appear euphoric and overly cheerful. Individuals who anticipated the amputation may express relief at having an outcome and being able to start on the rehabilitative process. There may be some expression of grief as well. A part of the body has been irrevocably lost, and the person may feel incomplete and mourn the lost extremity. The person may experience insomnia and restlessness and have difficulty concentrating. There is little evidence, however, that attitude toward the amputation at this stage has any relationship to an eventual level of emotional or functional adjustment.[6]

The third stage occurs as the person becomes involved in the postoperative program and really faces the permanence of the loss. Younger individuals may deny the amputation by trying to exhibit physical capabilities in the use of wheelchair or crutches. Many individuals mourn, not specifically the loss of the limb, but the anticipated loss of a previous lifestyle. Individuals may mourn or fear the possible loss of a job or the ability to participate in a favorite sport or other activity. Men who lose a limb often fear the loss of sexual capability and potency; some may equate the loss of the limb to castration. In the early stages, the client's grief may alternate with feelings of hopelessness, despondency, bitterness, and anger. Throughout this stage, the client may have questions, and it is important that he or she knows what to expect during the entire process. The steps of rehabilitation and the expectations should be carefully explained, but only as the person asks questions or appears ready for the information. Overloading the individual with a plethora of information too early will insure only that the information will not be heard. It is a common mistake among less-experienced therapists and assistants to try to educate the patient in all aspects of rehabilitation. It is important for the individual to know and understand as much as possible about the future, but overwhelming a person with too much information at one time may only increase the feeling of helplessness.

Individuals with disability who have made satisfactory adjustments and successfully completed rehabilitation can support and encourage the new client in private or group sessions. Treating the individual in an area with clients in later stages of rehabilitation is often helpful. Showing the client a prosthesis or orthosis and using films or slides may also help. Understanding the device's function and use may help the client feel more comfortable and accepting of the need for the device.

The final stage is related to reintegration into a functional lifestyle. Clients have various attitudes toward the prosthesis or orthosis. Some are particularly concerned about its appearance, hoping that it will conceal their disability and give the illusion of an intact body. Others are concerned primarily with the restoration of function. If individuals with amputations have been told that the prosthesis will replace their own limb, then they may have unrealistic expectations that appearance and function will be as good as in the nonamputated extremity.

A client may not follow any of the stages or sequences described above. It is important to remember that the individual's basic personality and ability to adjust to the demands of everyday life are the greatest determinant of that person's ability to adjust to disability.

SEXUAL ISSUES

A major trauma, amputation, or disability affects one's self-concept and how one views one's attraction to existing or potential partners. Although sexual issues have been extensively studied among patients with neurological problems such as stroke and spinal cord injuries, there is little in the literature of the sexual problems of individuals following amputation or injuries requiring the use of orthoses.

Adolescent and young adults with chronic or "visible" disabilities may have difficulty developing a positive sexual image. They may not have the opportunities to participate in activities that help develop social skills. Older adults may find decreased sexual abilities from illness and chronic disability. Men tend to focus on physical sexual function and may find a reduction in their abilities either directly or indirectly as a result of their disability. Both men and women may find that their disability may interfere with their ability to attain their usual sexual positions, and they may not experience pleasure or fulfillment.[1] Clients rarely feel comfortable discussing these concerns with their therapist or even their physician. Concerned with the ability to regain physical function, busy rehabilitation staff rarely consider or provide assistance

for sexual concerns. In a small, self-reported study of amputees in Japan, Ide and associates[7] reported that the presence of an understanding partner and being able to discuss sexual concerns were related to satisfaction in their sexual activities.

PAIN

Pain is frequently associated with injury and disability. Pain associated with various prosthetic or orthotic situations is discussed in appropriate chapters. Chronic pain, however, can have substantial psychosocial adjustment to disability and rehabilitation outcome. **Chronic pain** is generally defined as consistent or episodic pain that persists for at least 6 months or more. Chronic pain has been further subdivided into three major categories[8]: pain related to an ongoing disease process (eg, cancer); pain related to specific injury to the peripheral or central nervous system (eg, phantom pain); and pain that cannot be completely explained by a known diagnostic entity or that cannot be related to a known diagnostic entity (eg, fibromyalgia or generalized residual limb pain). An exploration of the multidimensional constructs of chronic pain is beyond the scope of this text; however, it is important to know that chronic pain can have a major influence on rehabilitation outcomes and needs to be identified early and treated by a team knowledgeable in this area.

THE PHANTOM

Phantom sensation and phantom pain are not unique to individuals with amputations. The phantom, the sensation that the absent limb is still there in some form, is a common and well-known sequelae of amputation. Individuals with complete paralysis of one or more limbs may also experience phantom sensation or pain. Phantom sensation has been around as long as individuals survived the loss of a limb, but the first detailed description of the phenomenon is attributed to Ambroise Pare (around 1551).[9] This coincides with improvements in amputation surgery developed by Dr. Pare that resulted in greater survival rate. The term "phantom limb" is attributed to Silas Weir Mitchell (in 1866), a civil war surgeon who established a major treatment center for amputees and published an account of their experiences through the eyes of a fictional soldier. Even though the term and the phenomenon have been long recognized, there has been little agreement on the cause. Early theories postulated responses to nerve stimulation either peripherally or centrally as the causative factor, although attempts to treat severe phantom pain through nerve blocks, reamputation, or similar methods were generally unsuccessful.[10] More recently, Melzack[11] believed that clients view the phantom as an integral part of themselves regardless of where it is felt in relation to the body, and that phantom sensation and pain originated in the cerebrum as the brain continuously generated patterns of impulses indicating a whole body. Melzack did not believe that children with congenital or acquired amputation at very early ages had phantom sensation.[11] However, studies have shown the phantom to be present in as many as 80% of amputees, including some congenitally amputated adults and some young children.[12] Currently, researchers are looking into areas of sensory reintegration and reorganization and are looking at reorganization in the somatosensory cortex.[13] More detailed information regarding current theories and research can be found at http://en.wikipedia.org/wiki/Phantom_limb.

Physical therapists (PTs) and physical therapist assistants (PTAs) need to recognize the prevalence of the phantom and be ready to answer questions and help the patient adjust to this strange sensation. The phantom that usually occurs immediately after surgery is often described as a tingling, pressure sensation, sometimes a numbness. The distal part of the extremity is most frequently felt, although, on occasion, the person will feel the whole extremity. The sensation is responsive to external stimuli such as bandaging or rigid dressing; it may dissipate over time or the person may have the sensation throughout life. Phantom sensation may be painless and usually does not interfere with prosthetic rehabilitation. It is important for the client to understand that the feeling is quite normal. Phantom sensation is prevalent in the majority of individuals following amputation and may last for many years.[12]

Phantom pain is characterized as a cramping or squeezing sensation, a shooting pain, or a burning pain. Some clients report all three. Pain may be localized or diffuse; it may be continuous or intermittent and triggered by some external stimuli. It may diminish over time or become a permanent and often disabling condition. In the first 6 months following surgery, phantom pain is thought to be related to preoperative limb pain in location and intensity. That relationship does not last, however, and preoperative pain is not believed to be related to long-term

phantom pain.[13] In a recent study, about 72% of the respondents indicated they felt phantom limb pain at some time. Only 30% reported severe pain, and 32% indicated the pain was severely bothersome.[13]

There has been some interesting work in the management of phantom pain in the upper extremity using a mirror box system. The mirror box is a box that is halved by a mirror. The person puts the unamputated arm on the mirrored side and the amputated arm on the other, or covered, side. The person can see only the mirrored side that produces a "stereoisomeric image" of the other limb. For example, if the individual had an amputated lower right arm, he or she would put both arms on opposite sides of the mirror and then the right half would be covered. The mirror mimics the left arm's actions, and the participant perceives this manipulated reflection as his or her right arm. Because the subject is seeing the reflected image of the unamputated hand moving, it appears as if the phantom limb is also moving. Through the use of this artificial visual feedback, it becomes possible for the individual to "move" the phantom limb and to unclench it from potentially painful positions.[13] Ramachandran and Blakeslee reported some success in using the mirror box over a long period in treating phantom pain. The mirror box technique has come into general use to treat a wide variety of "phantom" pain related to other injuries such as brachial plexus damage or stroke. Mirror boxes can now be purchased commercially or contructed.[14] Zuckweiler reported on three cases of phantom pain or sensation treated with a series of mental imagery sessions over a period of several weeks.[15] The sessions were designed to teach each person how to use mental imagery to control the phantom and eliminate the pain; all three individuals reported being able to successfully resolve their phantom by using the mental imagery. More recently, Murray and associates reported the use of virtual reality with three individuals complaining of chronic severe phantom pain.[16] Two patients had lost an upper extremity, and one had lost a leg below the knee. The virtual reality environment created a virtual missing limb that the individual had to use to complete a series of tasks, such as moving colored tiles or kicking a ball. All three patients reported a decrease in their pain during the sessions, but the benefits lasted only a few days. The most improvement was reported by the person with the most recent amputation. The benefits also appeared greater for those with upper extremity amputations. The authors suggested that the results indicated the need for further study.

Disabling or intractable phantom pain is relatively infrequent, but no consistent treatment has been found to be effective. Sherman[17] studied phantom pain and reviewed more than 60 medical, surgical, and psychological treatments as well as the use of alternative approaches. Little or no significant effects were found in these treatments, and nonconsistently helpful treatments have been reported in the literature. Limited success has been reported in the use of perioperative epidural analgesia. Some studies have shown some success, while others have not indicated long-term effects.[8] For the therapist and assistant working with an individual with phantom pain, the most effective approach would be to help the patient understand and accept the phenomena while focusing attention on the rehabilitation program.

AGE CONSIDERATIONS

Children

Shock is the usual parental reaction to the birth of a child with a congenital anomaly, to an amputation, or to the need to use an external device on a long-term basis. Parents may go through periods of denial and anger and experience feelings of guilt and shame before accepting their child's disability. Some parents may be overwhelmed and inconsolable; others may not fully appreciate the implications of disability. Rehabilitation team members should be concerned with parental adjustment, because parental acceptance will likely correlate with the child's adjustment.

Children generally adapt fairly easily to an orthosis or prosthesis. Children with congenital amputations are fitted as soon as they are developmentally ready for the prosthesis. A child with an upper extremity loss can be fitted as soon as he or she starts bilateral hand activities, and the child with a lower limb loss can be fitted as he or she starts to pull to stand. For a child, the major issue is comfort, and as long as the appliance is comfortable, it will generally be incorporated into the child's lifestyle. The more normally the parents can treat the child, the easier will be the adjustment and development.

Regardless of age, the child's emotional reactions must be considered by the rehabilitation team. Too often, detailed discussions about the issues, devices, and care are conducted with the parents, and the child is overlooked. The child should be aware of what to expect. Misinformation or distortions should be detected and corrected. Mourning is a normal process for the child as well as the adult. Children, when depressed, are likely to regress to a more infantile level of behavior and must be given the opportunity to express their feelings through play or talk. The early adolescent may grieve over the loss of self image, while the adolescent may be afraid of rejection and social ostracism. Adolescence is a dynamic phase during which profound changes lead people to feel sexually attractive and capable of reproduction. Self-esteem is very vulnerable at this time. The adolescent may feel inadequate after disability and needs reassurance from significant others. Compliance with orthotic wear may become an issue. Contact with other young clients may be quite constructive. Involvement in sports programs is especially helpful. Reaction to physical disability is affected by the child's previous experiences and the reactions of family members. Parental reaction profoundly influences the way the child copes.

The Elderly

The elderly individual with a disability is motivated to seek effective rehabilitation services and a meaningful lifestyle. Maintaining independence is a critical issue with the older adult. Any disability requiring the use of an external device, especially amputation, may be seen as the end of an independent lifestyle. To some extent, the reaction will be affected by the previous level of pain and disability and the sudden or gradual onset of the disability. Individuals who have suffered considerable pain may be grateful that the pain has ended. Clients who underwent extensive medical and surgical procedures may experience a sense of failure that the efforts were not successful. If preoperative attitudes are unrealistically hopeful, then postoperative disturbances may be more severe. The elderly person should not be led to expect a total cure. Learning to use an artificial limb or an orthosis may be a slow and discouraging ordeal, and the client may not express distress or depression in front of the optimism of others. However, the PT and PTA must keep in mind that the majority of older individuals, particularly those amputated at transtibial levels, make excellent adjustments to prosthetic function.[18]

Elderly individuals are subject to considerable stress from concerns about financial limitations, loss of control over their lives, and fear of becoming dependent. An elderly individual who requires an amputation or who sustains a severe disability must often cope with multiple physical problems. Loss is a part of normal aging—loss of physiological capabilities, loss of a spouse or friends, loss of the self-esteem related to one's career or job, and now, loss of function. It is helpful to give the client as much control over decision making as possible, to provide opportunities to be involved in goals setting and sequencing of activities. As with any client, PTs and PTAs need to be aware of the stressors affecting the clients and assist with coping by being reflective listeners and enablers.

Cognition and Motivation

It is a myth that elderly individuals cannot learn a new skill, have difficulty remembering, and cannot achieve at the same level as younger individuals. Some elderly individuals may have difficulty learning a new skill, but many are able to adapt successfully to a disability such as an amputation and lead a full and normal life. Although some suffer from dementia, others who are labeled as having dementia because of confusion in the acute care setting may actually only be responding to medications, metabolic imbalances, infection toxicity, insecurity in a strange environment, or the sequelae of anesthesia. It is important to remember that cognitive dysfunction does not preclude satisfactory rehabilitation. Understanding the client's cognitive capabilities helps the PT and PTA structure learning experiences appropriately. Goal-oriented statements may be clearer than step-by-step instructions. We do many activities almost automatically—getting up from a chair, turning in bed, and walking. Most of us have developed particular patterns of movements over the years. The therapist/assistant can draw on such patterns by suggesting the movement goals (see Chapter 7).

MOTIVATION AND COMPLIANCE

Motivation and **compliance** are closely interrelated, but compliance is not obedience. Everyone is motivated toward some goal. To the extent that the client's and the health professional's goals are congruent, and the client performs as the health professional expects, the client is said to be motivated and compliant. However, if the client has different goals and does not follow the program the health professional has outlined, the client is considered to be noncompliant. This is one reason why it is important to clarify the client's goals and organize the rehabilitation program to help the client meet those goals. Kemp developed a formula of motivation that takes into account the

client's wants, beliefs, rewards, and the cost of the performance.[19]

$$\text{Motivation} = \text{Wants} \times \text{Beliefs} \times \text{Rewards}$$

COSTS

The client's wants are essentially the client's goals, what the client wants to accomplish. Beliefs relate to what the client thinks of the activity, the future, and the disability. Rewards are the outcomes, the pleasure, accomplishments, and positive feelings the client obtains from the activity or program. Finally, the cost stands for the consequences of participation in an activity. Is the activity painful? Is it very energy demanding? Does it interfere with other more pleasurable activities?[18] The PT or PTA must consider all the elements of the equation in establishing a rehabilitation program and in planning simple activities such as home exercises.

CAREGIVERS

In most instances, the PT and PTA will be working with a caregiver as well as with the client. The caregiver is an integral part of the team and must be involved in the rehabilitation program. Caregivers can be members of the family, close friends, neighbors, or paid helpers. Caregivers have their own emotional reactions to the amputation and the client's illness. Caregiving is a demanding and often tiring activity that can upset family balance and create considerable stress. The PT and PTA need to be open to the needs of the caregiver and work closely with him or her. It is important to determine the caregiver's goals, fears, and concerns. Is the caregiver afraid of handling the client or the residual limb? Is the caregiver resentful of the time demands that caregiving imposes? What was the premorbid relationship between the client and the caregiver?

The therapist and assistant can provide useful information to the caregiver regarding the disability and prognosis, as well as helping techniques for coping with daily life. Providing time for the caregiver to ask questions and voice concerns can be an integral part of the therapeutic intervention. Many caregivers are afraid of "doing something wrong" and need to develop confidence in their caregiving skills. Effective teaching strategies need to be used with caregivers as well as clients to insure a smooth transition into the home program.[20]

SUMMARY

PTs and PTAs learn a great deal about helping patients and caregivers cope with the emotional issues related to disability. Chronic disability, the use of assistive devices, and amputations present special problems. Therapists need to understand issues related to body image, the phantom, and the changes that occur in individuals of all ages with disabilities requiring the use of orthotic or prosthetic devices.

KEYWORDS FOR LITERATURE SEARCH

Body image

Chronic pain

Depression

Motivation

Phantom sensation/pain/limb

Sexual response to disability

REFERENCES

1. Dench ME, Noonan AC, Sharby N, Ventura SH: Psychosocial aspects of health care, 2nd ed. New Jersey, Pearson Prentice Hall, 2007.
2. Tam SF: Comparing the self concepts of person with and without physical disabilities. J of Psych 132(1):78–86, 1998.
3. Badura-Brzoza K, Matysiakiewicz J, Piegza M, Rycerski W, Niedziela U, Hese RT. Sociodemographic factors and their influence on anxiety and depression in patients after limb amputation. [Polish] Psychiatria Polska 40(2):335–345, 2006 Mar–Apr.
4. Darnall BD, Ephraim P, Wegener ST, Dillingham T, Pezzin L, Rossbach P, MacKenzie EJ: Depressive symptoms and mental health service utilization among persons with limb loss: results of a national survey. Arch Phys Med Rehabil 86(4):650–658, 2005 Apr.
5. Desmond DM, MacLachlan M: Coping strategies as predictors of psychosocial adaptation in a sample of elderly veterans with acquired lower limb amputations. Soc Sci Med 62(1):208–216, 2006 Jan.
6. Bradway JK, Malone JM, Racy J, Leal JM, Poole J: Psychological adaptation to amputation: an overview. Orthot Prosthet 38(3):46–50, 1984.
7. Ide M, Watanabe T, Toyonaga T: Sexuality in persons with limb amputation. Prosthet Orthot Int 26(3):189–194, 2002 Dec.
8. Ehde DM, Smith DG: Chronic pain management. In Smith DG, Michael JW, Bowkey JH (eds): Atlas of amputations and limb deficiencies: surgical, prosthetic and rehabilitation principles, 3rd ed. Rosemont, IL, AAOS, 2004, pp 711–726.
9. Wade N: The legacy of the phantom limb paper read at a conference: The Phantom Limb: a neurobiological diagnosis with aesthetic, cultural and philosophical implications. London 2005, as published on http://www.artbrain.org/the-legacy-of-phantom-limbs/.
10. Finger S, Hustwit MP: Five early accounts of phantom limb in context: Pare, Descartes, Lemos, Bell, and Mitchell. Neurosurgery 52(3):675–686, 2003 Mar.
11. Melzack R: Phantom limbs. Scientific American 266(4):120, 1992.
12. Racy J: Psychological adaptation to amputation. In Smith DG, Michael JW, Bowkey JH (eds): Atlas of amputations and limb deficiencies: surgical, prosthetic and rehabilitation principles, 3rd ed. Rosemont, IL, AAOS, 2004, pp 727–738
13. Ramachandran VS, Hirstein WL: The perception of phantom limbs: the D. O. Hebb Lecture. Brain 9(121):1603–1630, 1998.
14. Ramachandran VS, Blakeslee S: Phantoms in the brain: probing the mysteries of the human mind. New York, William Morrow, 1998.
15. Zuckweiler RL: Zuckweiler's image imprinting in the treatment of phantom pain: case reports. JPO 17:113–118, 2005.
16. Murray CD, Patchick EL, Caillette F, Howard T, Pettifer S: Can immersive virtual reality reduce phantom limb pain? Stud Health Technol Inform 119:407–412, 2006.
17. Sherman RA: Phantom pain. New York, Plenum Press, 1997.
18. Gauthier-Gagnon C, Grisé MC, Potvin D: Enabling factors related to prosthetic use by people with transtibial and transfemoral amputation. Arch Phys Med Rehabil 80(6):706–713, 1999.
19. Kemp BJ: Motivation, rehabilitation, and aging: a conceptual model. Top Geriatr Rehabil 3(3):41–51, 1988.
20. May BJ: Caregivers. In May BJ (ed): Home health care and rehabilitation. Concepts of care, 2nd ed. Philadelphia, F.A. Davis, 1999, pp 261–280.

Amputations and Prostheses

Amputation Surgery of the Lower Extremity

4

OBJECTIVES

At the end of this chapter, all students are expected to:

1. Discuss the implications of etiology and incidence of amputation surgery.
2. Describe the process of amputation surgery in relation to residual limb characteristics and patient function.
3. Describe the functional results of amputation surgery.

CASE STUDIES

The following clients have been referred to physical therapy for postsurgical care:

Janice Simmons, a 65-year-old woman, had a left transtibial amputation yesterday secondary to diabetic gangrene and a nonhealing ulcer on the plantar surface of the right foot.

John Adams, a 72-year-old man, had a right transfemoral amputation yesterday secondary to chronic arteriosclerosis obliterans.

Richard Canto, a 19-year-old Army soldier who underwent traumatic transtibial amputation secondary to a road bomb encounter in Iraq 2 days ago; he was evacuated to an Army hospital in Germany where efforts to save the limb failed. He also sustained some shrapnel injuries to his chest and right arm, but these are not considered serious.

Linda Bean is a 12-year-old female who underwent a transfemoral amputation yesterday secondary to grade IIB osteogenic sarcoma of the proximal right tibia; the tumor was not appropriate for tumor resection and reconstruction.

Case Study Activities

All Students

1. For each client, describe what the surgeon will do with the bone, blood vessels, nerves, muscle tissue, and skin during each amputation. Review the surgery depicted at www.ampsurg.org.

Physical Therapy Students

1. Identify what you need to know about amputation surgery to select appropriate tests and measures and develop a postsurgical plan of care.

Physical Therapist Assistant Students

1. Identify what you need to know about amputation surgery to implement selected postsurgical interventions.

EPIDEMIOLOGY AND ETIOLOGY OF AMPUTATIONS

It is estimated by the Centers for Disease Control and Prevention that there are approximately 1.8 million people living in the United States with the loss of one or more limbs. One out of every 200 people has had one or more amputations. The majority of amputations, approximately 82%, are due to peripheral vascular disease, with more than 50% of these due to complications of diabetes. Among lower extremity amputations, over 90% are due to vascular diseases.[1] Other causes of amputation include trauma, tumors, and congenital malformation. Among upper extremity amputations, the leading cause is trauma.

Dillingham and associates[1] studied the rates and trends in amputation from 1988 to 1996 and found a 27% increase in new amputations for vascular disease, while amputations for all other causes showed a decrease. In 2004, the last full year for which data are available, there were 114,548 hospital discharges with a primary diagnosis of amputation.[2] Dillingham and associates further indicated that hospital discharges for dysvascular amputations increased about 3% per year for the study period.

The risk of amputation for dysvascular disease increases with age, sex, and race. Dillingham and associates[1] found that amputations among blacks over the age of 85 were 1057.8 per 100,000 individuals, while the rate for middle-aged blacks (45 to 54 years of age) was 90.4 per 100,000 people. The rate of amputation was also higher for women over the age of 85, with 361.8 amputations per 100,000 as compared to 29.2 amputations per 100,000 in the 45 to 54 age groups. The risk of amputation was also higher for nonblack men in the older age groups but at a much lower rate of incidence. Other studies revealed a similar rate of amputation among blacks as compared to other racial and ethnic groups.[3–6] Researchers have made several suggestions for the disparity in amputation rate along racial lines. Rucker-Whitaker and colleagues[7] suggested lower-income African Americans had less access to **revascularization** procedures. Others have supported the suggestion of a low-income bias toward amputation rather than other procedures as well as a greater incidence of diabetes among African Americans.[4–6] There are, of course, other factors contributing to the incidence of amputation among individuals with diabetes or nondiabetic peripheral vascular disease. Imran and associates[8] found a direct relationship between poor glycemic control and recurring foot ulcers and incidence of major amputations among individuals with diabetes. Several studies have also found that poor glycemic control was a strong predictor of major amputation as well as peripheral neuropathy, smoking, and renal or retinal disease.[9–12]

IMPLICATIONS

There are approximately 20.8 million children and adults in the United States with diabetes,[13] and approximately 5% of the adult population is affected with some form of peripheral vascular disease. Many of the patients we treat for a wide variety of nondiabetic or vascular disease–related problems will also have peripheral vascular disease with or without diabetes. Recent studies have shown a relationship between early patient education and proper foot care and a reduction or delay in the incidence of amputations.[14,15] As physical therapists, it is our responsibility to determine all of our patients' problems, both actual and potential, and initiate an appropriate program of education and prevention. There are many guidelines available for patient education in proper footwear, foot care, and disease management.[13]

LEVELS OF AMPUTATION

Figure 4.1 outlines the major levels of amputation. (Upper extremity amputations are discussed in Chapter 11.) Many factors affect the selection of level of amputation. In vascular disease, amputation usually results after limb salvage procedures have failed; level is selected on the basis of anticipated viability of tissue for healing. Postoperative patient function is always a consideration, and surgeons try to amputate at the lowest level possible. Controversies exist between surgeons when determining the most appropriate level in the presence of vascular disease. The

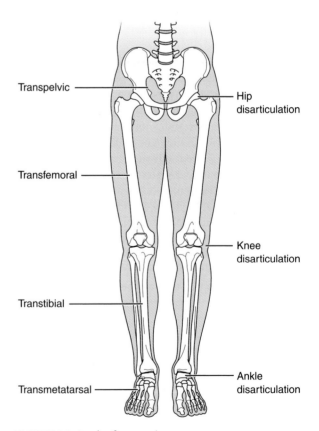

Transpelvic

Transfemoral

Transtibial

Transmetatarsal

Hip disarticulation

Knee disarticulation

Ankle disarticulation

FIGURE 4.1. Levels of amputation.

vascular surgeon is often more concerned with primary healing and may opt to amputate at a **transfemoral** level, although successful prosthetic rehabilitation is more frequent when the amputation is performed at a transtibial level. Initial amputations for vascular disease may be in the foot, a toe, or a single ray, or amputation through the metatarsals. Success rates for partial foot amputation vary greatly and are dependent on test results indicating **patency** of major vessels in the area. Most surgeons will not perform a disarticulation at the ankle or knee, believing that poorer circulation may interfere with healing. However, there have been some studies to indicate that ankle or knee **disarticulation** may be successful among some individuals with dysvascularities.[16,17]

Level selection for traumatic amputations or for major tumors is determined by the nature of the injury and the viability of tissues. Surgeons have generally been reluctant to amputate, even in the presence of multiple and severe traumatic injuries of the lower extremities. New and complex limb salvage procedures, improved emergency care, and surgeons who specialize in traumatology have enabled the reconstruction of even the most mangled lower limbs. However, long-term heroic limb salvage efforts may impose considerable physical, mental, and financial costs to the patient and family and must be considered in the decision making. Algorithms have been developed to help guide the physician in determining when to attempt limb salvage and when to amputate.[18] The incidence of amputation for tumors has decreased markedly with the advent of improved detection, multiagent chemotherapy and adjuvant radiation therapy. Whenever possible, the tumor is excised followed by some form of skeletal reconstruction. Five-year survival rates have been about the same for individuals undergoing amputation and those having segmental excisions. Amputations are generally performed on individuals with large tumors who do not respond well to chemotherapy and radiation.[19]

GENERAL PRINCIPLES

Several principles of amputation surgery apply to all levels of amputation. Generally, surgeons want to save as much length as possible while providing a residual limb that is able to tolerate the stresses of prosthetic ambulation. Sometimes, compromises are necessary between keeping bone length and avoiding scars and other deformities that may interfere with prosthetic fitting (**Fig. 4.2A,B**). Newer prosthetic components

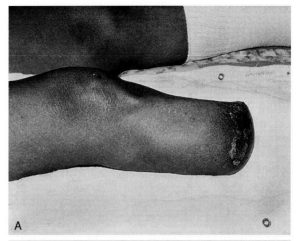

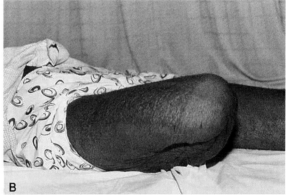

FIGURE 4.2. (A) Residual limb after transtibial amputation. **(B)** Residual limb after transfemoral amputation.

including gel liners and socks that provide a close-fitting and shock-absorbing interface between residual limb and socket have greatly increased the ability to comfortably prosthetically fit an individual with a bony or scarred residual limb (see Chapter 6).

Amputating a limb involves severing both small and large nerves; when severed, all peripheral nerves put out new tendrils that form into small neoplasms of nerve ends (**neuromas**). If small and embedded in soft tissue, the neuroma does not usually cause a problem. If the neuroma is large, superficial, or becomes squeezed against a bone, it can cause pain that may interfere with prosthetic wear. To mitigate against the possibility of neuroma pain, the surgeon pulls down the major nerves firmly, resects them sharply, and allows them to retract into the soft tissue.

Muscle and soft tissue are differentially handled depending on the level of amputation. When a muscle is severed, it loses its distal attachment and, if left loose, will retract, atrophy, and scar against adjacent structures. Without attachment at both ends, a muscle is unable to function. There are two ways muscle can be managed. **Myoplasty** refers to the attachment of anterior and posterior compartment muscles to each other over the end of the bone. Myoplasty is usually performed in through-the-bone amputations and incorporated with myofascial closure to provide muscle stability, making sure the muscles do not slide over the end of the bone.

Myodesis refers to the anchoring of muscles to bone. Myodesis is more rarely performed as it requires a longer surgical procedure and causes more trauma to the bone. In both instances, muscles are stabilized under a little tension to provide a well-shaped residual limb.

Skin **flaps** are usually as broad as the distal end of the limb and are shaped to allow the corners to retract smoothly. Types of postsurgical dressings vary and are discussed in more detail in Chapter 5. A drain is often inserted just under the incision to allow for the evacuation of excess fluid. The drain is usually removed 1 or 2 days after surgery.

TRANSTIBIAL (BELOW KNEE)

The **transtibial** is the most common level of extremity amputation for peripheral vascular disease. Prosthetic rehabilitation is more successful and postoperative mortality lower with transtibial compared to transfemoral amputations whether or not the patient has diabetes. However, mortality rates are consistently higher among individuals with diabetes and higher among individuals with diabetes and renal disease requiring dialysis. Aulivola and colleagues[20] reported an 8.6% worse rate of 30-day survival for individuals undergoing transfemoral amputations as compared to transtibial amputations. Long-term survival also favored individuals amputated at the transtibial level, with 74.5% surviving at 1 year and 37.8% at 5 years as compared to 50.6% and 22.5%, respectively, for those amputated at the transfemoral level. Perioperative morbidity was also higher among those undergoing transfemoral amputations and worse in individuals with renal failure. Other studies have supported these findings. Generally, among patients amputated for vascular diseases, individuals with diabetes have a worse survival and rehabilitation rate than those without diabetes. Individuals requiring transfemoral amputation do significantly worse than those amputated at transtibial levels. Among individuals with diabetes who require amputation, those with significant levels of renal disease requiring dialysis have poorer survival rates than all other groups.[21–25]

Not surprisingly, reamputation rates are higher for individuals with partial foot over transtibial amputation. Reamputation rates for transtibial amputations to transfemoral level have been variously reported but appear to be generally less than 10%. There are many factors that affect reamputation rates, including severity of dysvascularity, glycemic control among individuals with diabetes, infection at the time of amputation, and socioeconomic level.[26] Reamputation of the contralateral limb increased over time and was fairly high for individuals with diabetes. The rate rose by year, reaching 53% by 5 years following initial major amputation.[26]

An earlier study indicated that primary healing rates have remained relatively constant over the years, ranging from 30% to 92% with a reamputation rate of 4% to 30%. The authors also suggested that primary healing at transtibial levels improved to 90% if the popliteal pulse was present.[27] The greater prosthetic rehabilitation potential for the transtibial level of amputation supports a greater ratio of transtibial versus transfemoral amputations.

Level of Transtibial Amputation

The desirable length for a transtibial amputation is a matter of controversy. Some surgeons advocate leaving as much bone length as possible, believing that the longer lever arm will decrease the energy required for effective ambulation. Others state that individuals with very long residual limbs develop distal skin problems because of the lack of subcutaneous padding.[28] Level selection is the purview of the surgeon who may or may not be well informed on prosthetic components and the importance of knee function in continued mobility. The longer the residual limb, the better control the patient will have of prosthetic function and the smoother the gait, thereby reducing the amount of energy required for mobility (see Chapter 7). The tibial tubercles is the shortest level of transtibial amputation compatible with knee function. Generally, the fibula is cut about 1 cm shorter than the tibia to provide a conical shape to the residual limb. Both the tibia and fibula are beveled distally, the tibia anteriorly and the fibula posterolaterally, to prevent any soft tissue impingement during prosthetic wear. The ends of the bone must be carefully filed to prevent any sharp edges.[28] Therapists can palpate these smooth edges after healing (**Fig. 4.3**).

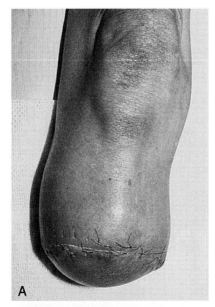

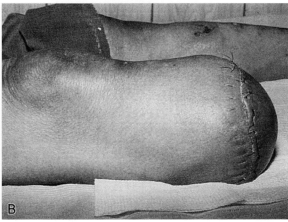

FIGURE 4.3. (A, B) Residual limb from a transtibial amputation, showing the anterior suture from a long posterior flap. *(From May BJ: Assessment and treatment of individuals following lower extremity amputation. In O'Sullivan SB, Schmitz TJ (eds): Physical rehabilitation: assessment and treatment, 3rd ed. Philadelphia, F.A. Davis, 1994, p 377, with permission.)*

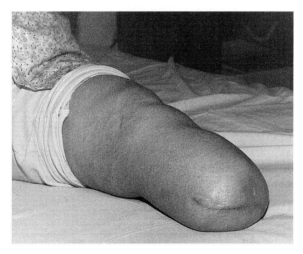

FIGURE 4.4. Residual limb from a transtibial amputation with suture of equal length flaps. *(From May BJ: Assessment and treatment of individuals following lower extremity amputation. In O'Sullivan SB, Schmitz TJ (eds): Physical rehabilitation: assessment and treatment, 3rd ed. Philadelphia, F.A. Davis, 1994, p 377, with permission.)*

SKIN FLAPS/INCISIONS

Amputations may be either closed or open. In an open amputation, the distal end of the residual limb is left open. An open amputation is used in the presence of infection or if there is not enough tissue to provide good closure primarily. In a closed amputation, the surgeon may use one of several different flaps and incisions, the first two are the most common.

Equal length anterior/posterior flaps **(Fig. 4.4)** are generally used when conserving bone length or when primary healing is not an issue. Anterior and posterior skin flaps place the scar in a medial/lateral direction at the end of the residual limb. The flaps are shaped at closure to reduce excessive tissue or "dog ears" at the corners.

A long posterior flap is used when vascularity at the distal end is of concern or when more padding is needed distally **(Fig. 4.5)**. The skin over the posterior leg has a better blood supply than the skin over the anterior leg. The anterior skin flap is cut at approximately the level of anticipated section of the tibia and the posterior flap is 13 to 15 cm longer to ensure adequate coverage without undue tension. It is advocated that skin and subcutaneous tissue not be separated from the muscular fascia to preserve skin perfusion.

Skew sagittal flaps **(Fig. 4.6)** are sometimes used in severe dysvascular situations to utilize the collateral circulation of medial and lateral tissue. Skew flaps result in an anterior–posterior incision.

END-BEARING AMPUTATION

In some instances, the surgeon will try to provide for improved end bearing of the residual limb by leaving the fibula the same length as the tibia and creating a bony bridge between the two distal ends. This technique has been used in traumatic amputation to provide better prosthetic control and sensory feedback. There is little research data yet to support the value of

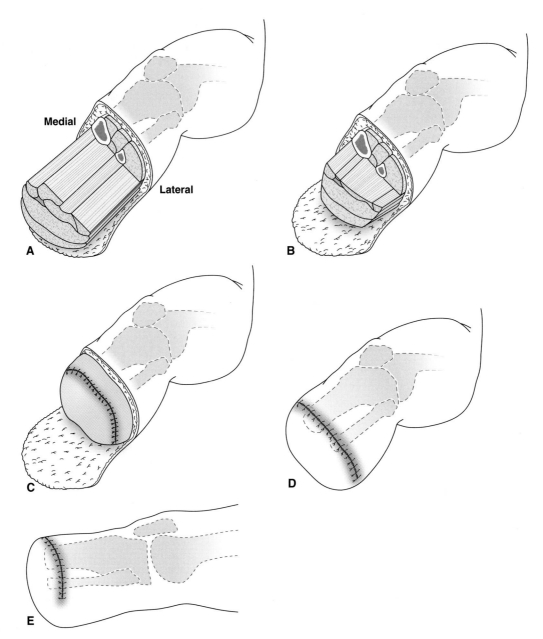

FIGURE 4.5. Transtibial amputation with long posterior skin flap. **(A)** The surgeon leaves a long posterior skin flap. **(B)** The surgeon bevels and contours the flap for a smooth distal end. **(C)** After myoplasty, the soft tissues are approximated. **(D)** The final suture is over the anterior part of the residual limb. **(E)** The relationship of the tibia and fibula.

this procedure.[28] Tisi and Callam[29] reviewed a number of studies and databases comparing the skew sagittal flap to the more traditional long posterior flap for dysvascular amputations and found no difference in healing rates or rehabilitation.

Although the physical therapist and physical therapist assistant have little input into the surgical technique, they need to understand what the surgeon has done to provide for effective postsurgical handling.

TRANSFEMORAL (ABOVE KNEE)

Historically, transfemoral was the most common amputation level for individuals with impaired circulation and gangrene of the foot and toes (**Fig. 4.7**). The improved circulation above the knee increased the chances of primary healing. However, as indicated in Chapter 7, ambulation with a transfemoral prosthesis requires considerable energy, and many individuals with vascular disease never become functional walkers. In the past

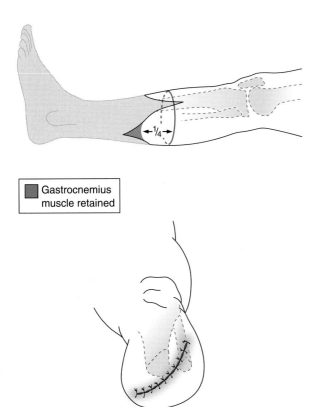

Gastrocnemius muscle retained

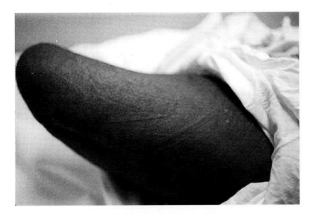

FIGURE 4.6. Skew flaps.

FIGURE 4.7. Transfemoral residual limb.

30 years, the trend has changed as research indicated that amputations at the transtibial level can heal primarily and prosthetic rehabilitation is more successful among individuals with transtibial amputations as compared to those with transfemoral amputations. Today, more transtibial than transfemoral amputations are performed for vascular problems. The ratio has remained fairly stable over the years at three transtibial amputations for every one transfemoral amputation.[30]

The transfemoral level is indicated if gangrene has extended to the knee or the patient's circulatory status precludes healing at the transtibial level. Trauma is the other major cause of transfemoral amputation, with some procedures also done for osteomyelitis or tumors. Survival and functional prosthetic rehabilitation rates are considerably lower among individuals with dysvascular disease following transfemoral amputation. Individuals requiring this level of amputation usually have multiple system problems, have been ill for longer periods, and have less energy reserves than individuals amputated at transtibial levels. Individuals amputated for trauma are younger and are generally healthy; however, they may have sustained multiple injuries as part of the trauma, particularly those who sustained major traumas from war. Today, soldiers survive severe bomb and blast injuries with improved emergency and evacuation procedures to major trauma centers. Although sophisticated limb salvage procedures may reduce the necessity for amputation in many instances, the violence of current weapon systems results in more multiple amputations.[31]

It is critically important to prosthetic stability in gait to maintain the femoral shaft axis as close to normal as possible. However, this is difficult to achieve surgically, because the attachments of the major adductor muscles are mostly lost. The adductor magnus is in the best mechanical position to maintain normal adduction, but its femoral attachment is lost during amputation. Some surgeons advocate using myodesis to attach the adductor magnus to the femur at the level of amputation to help maintain normal alignment so important to a proper prosthetic gait pattern.[32] Some surgeons believe that myoplasty of the quadriceps and hamstring muscles provides adequate stabilization, but others recommend myodesis of the quadriceps muscle with the hamstring tendons attached to either the adductor magnus or quadriceps. This is advocated to provide a well-balanced dynamic residual limb and to maintain as much muscle function in the residual limb as possible.[31] The residual limb should be maintained in extension and adduction during surgery to maintain proper muscle tension and alignment. Flaps of equal length or a long medial flap in the sagittal plane are often used.[31]

OSSEOINTEGRATION

Osseointegration is the direct attachment of a prosthesis to the body, usually through an implant in the amputated bone. The concept has been used in dental practices for many years and has been tested with transfemoral amputees in various centers for several decades. The advent of new commercially available implants and attachments is making the technique more common. Patient selection is critical, as the process of preparing the bone for the eventual loads is slow. The surgery is a two-step process: first, the limb is amputated, and the implant is placed within the end of the bone. Later, the incision is reopened, and the externally protruding connector is placed. The postsurgical program is long and demanding, and it may be as long as 18 months before a fully definitive prosthesis can be used. At this time, most osseointegration is done as clinical trials with well-informed volunteers.[33] Sullivan and associates, reporting on follow-up with 11 cases done in the United Kingdom, stressed the importance of carefully selecting appropriate candidates, although, with the right person, the procedure resulted in more effective and comfortable prosthetic wear.[34] Considerable work has also been done in this area in Europe, particularly Sweden. Hagberg and associates reported on a survey of 18 individuals (8 males, 10 females) who were fitted with limb-anchored prostheses up to 15 years after initial amputation for trauma or tumor. On follow-up, 17 of the 18 reported a preference for the osseoanchored limb, citing better prosthetic control, better function, and longer wearing times.[35] In a further study, Frossard and associates[36] compared the temporal gait characteristics (cadence, support phase, and swing time) of 12 individuals fitted with osseointegrated prostheses to similar characteristics of individuals fitted with socket-type prostheses. While preliminary because of the small sample, the authors reported that those fitted with osseointegrated prostheses exhibited similar or improved gait characteristics with slightly longer prosthetic support phase, more even stride length, and a slightly quicker swing phase. The authors emphasized that further study was necessary.

OTHER LEVELS

See Chapter 8 for details on the surgery and management of patients with other levels of amputation, including partial foot, ankle, knee and hip disarticulations, and **transpelvic.**

SUMMARY

The physical therapist and physical therapist assistant must understand the basic procedures in amputation surgery to work effectively with the postsurgical client and to provide guidance for proper residual limb management. When possible, clinicians are encouraged to read the operative report to note any unusual findings or surgical variations. Observing surgery is also instructive.

KEYWORDS FOR LITERATURE SEARCH

Amputation stump

Amputation surgery

Limb amputation

Osseointegration

Residual limb

Transfemoral

Transpelvic

Transtibial

Vascular surgery

REFERENCES

1. Dillingham TR, Pezzin LE, Mackenzie EJ: Limb amputation and limb deficiency: epidemiology and recent trends in the United States. South Med J 95(8):875–883, 2002.
2. U.S. Department of Health and Human Service, Agency for Healthcare Research and Quality: Outcomes by 157 Amputation of lower extremity, 2004, www.hcup.ahrq.gov.
3. Feinglass J, Rucker-Whitaker C, Lindquist L, McCarthy WJ, Pearce WH: Racial differences in primary and repeat lower extremity amputation: results from a multihospital study. J Vasc Surg 41(5):823–829, 2005 May.
4. Lavery LA, Ashry HR, van Houtum W, et al: Variation in the incidence and proportion of diabetes-related amputations in minorities. Diabetes Care 19:48–52, 1996.
5. Wachtel MS: Family poverty accounts for differences in lower-extremity amputation rates of minorities 50 years old or more with diabetes. J Natl Med Assoc 97(3):334–338, 2005 Mar.
6. Lavery LA, van Houtum WH, Ashry HR, et al: Diabetes-related lower-extremity amputations disproportionately affect blacks and Mexican Americans. South Med J 92:593–599, 1999.
7. Rucker-Whitaker C, Feinglass J, Pearce WH: Explaining racial variation in lower extremity amputation: a 5-year retrospective claims data and medical record review at an urban teaching hospital. Arch Surg 138(12):1347–1351, 2003 Dec.
8. Imran S, Ali R, Mahboob G: Frequency of lower extremity amputation in diabetics with reference to glycemic control and Wagner's grades. JCPSP, J Coll Physicians Surg [Pakistan] 16(2):124–127, 2006 Feb.
9. Miyajima S, Shirai A, Yamamoto S, Okada N, Matsushita T: Risk factors for major limb amputations in diabetic foot gangrene patients. Diabetes Res Clin Pract 71(3):272–279, 2006 Mar.
10. Resnick HE, Carter EA, Sosenko JM, et al: Strong Heart Study. Incidence of lower-extremity amputation in American Indians: the Strong Heart Study. Diabetes Care 27(8):1885–1891, 2004 Aug.

11. Centers for Disease Control and Prevention (CDC). History of foot ulcer among persons with diabetes—United States, 2000–2002. MMWR, Morbidity & Mortality Weekly Report 52(45):1098–1102, 2003 Nov 14.

12. Young BA, Maynard C, Reiber G, Boyko EJ: Effects of ethnicity and nephropathy on lower-extremity amputation risk among diabetic veterans. Diabetes Care 26(2):495–501, 2003 Feb.

13. ADA: Resources for Health Professionals. American Diabetes Association. www.diabetes.org.

14. Driver VR, Madsen J, Goodman RA: Reducing amputation rates in patients with diabetes at a military medical center: the limb preservation service model. Diabetes Care 28(2): 248–253, 2005 Feb.

15. Valk GD, Kriegsman DM, Assendelft WJ: Patient education for preventing diabetic foot ulceration. [Update of Cochrane Database Syst Rev. 2001;(4):CD001488; PMID: 11687114].

16. Pinzur MS, Bowker JH: Knee disarticulation. Clin Orthop Related Res (361):23–28, 1999 Apr.

17. Siev-Ner I, Heim M, Warshavski M, Daich A, Tamir E, Dudkiewicz IA: Review of the aetiological factors and results of trans-ankle (Syme) disarticulations. Disabil Rehabil 28(4):239–242, 2006 Feb.

18. Archdeacon MT, Sanders R: Trauma: limb salvage versus amputation. In Smith DG, Michael JW, Bowker JH (eds): Atlas of amputations and limb deficiencies: surgical, prosthetic, and rehabilitation principles, 3rd ed. Rosemont, IL, American Academy of Orthopaedic Surgeons, 2004, pp 69–76.

19. Mnaymneh W, Temple HT: Tumor: limb salvage versus amputation. In Smith DG, Michael JW, Bowker JH (eds): Atlas of amputations and limb deficiencies: surgical, prosthetic, and rehabilitation principles, 3rd ed. Rosemont, IL, American Academy of Orthopaedic Surgeons, 2004, pp 55–68.

20. Aulivola B, Chantel NH, Allen DH, et al: Major lower extremity amputation: outcome of a modern series. Arch Surg 139:395–399, 2004.

21. Schofield CJ, Libby G, Brennan GB, MacAlpine RR, Morris DD, Leese GP: Mortality and hospitalization in patients after amputation: a comparison between patients with and without diabetes. Diabetes Care 29:2252–2256, 2006.

22. Subramaniam B, Pomposelli F, Talmor D, Park K: Perioperative and long-term morbidity and mortality after above-knee and below-knee amputations in diabetics and nondiabetics. Anesth Analgesia 100(5):1241–1247, 2005 May.

23. Kazmers A, Perkins AJ, Jacobs LA: Major lower extremity amputation in Veteran Affairs medical centers. Ann Vasc Surg 14:216–222, 2000.

24. Peng CW, Tan SG: Perioperative and rehabilitative outcomes after amputation for ischaemic leg gangrene. Ann Acad Med Singapore 29:168–172, 2000.

25. Ploeg AJ, Lardenoye J-W, Vrancken Peeters M-PFM, Breslau PJ: Contemporary series of morbidity and mortality after lower limb amputation. Eur J Vasc Endovasc Surg 2:633–637, 2005.

26. Izumi Y, Satterfield K, Lee S, Harkless LB: Risk of reamputation in diabetic patients stratified by limb and level of amputation: a 10-year observation. Diabetes Care 29(3):566–570, 2006 Mar.

27. Dormandy J, Heeck L, Vig S: Major amputations: clinical patterns and predictors. [Review] Semin Vascular Surg 12(2):154–161, 1999 Jun.

28. Bowker JH: Transtibial amputation: surgical management. In Smith DG, Michael JW, Bowker JH (eds): Atlas of amputations and limb deficiencies: surgical, prosthetic, and rehabilitation principles, 3rd ed. Rosemont, IL, American Academy of Orthopaedic Surgeons, 2004, pp 481–502.

29. Tisi PV, Callam MJ: Type of incision for below knee amputation. [Review] Cochrane Database of Systematic Reviews. (1):CD003749, 2004.

30. McCollum PT, Raza Z: Vascular disease: limb salvage vs amputation. In Smith DG, Michael JW, Bowker JH (eds): Atlas of amputations and limb deficiencies: surgical, prosthetic, and rehabilitation principles, 3rd ed. Rosemont, IL, American Academy of Orthopaedic Surgeons, 2004, pp 31–46.

31. Gajewski D, Granville R: The United States Armed Forces amputee patient care program. J Am Acad Orthop Surg 14:S183–S187, 2006.

32. Gottschalk F: Transfemoral amputation: surgical management. In Smith DG, Michael JW, Bowker JH (eds): Atlas of amputations and limb deficiencies: surgical, prosthetic, and rehabilitation principles, 3rd ed. Rosemont, IL, American Academy of Orthopaedic Surgeons, 2004, pp 533–540.

33. Robinson KP, Branemark R, Ward DA: Future developments: osseointegration in transfemoral amputees. In Smith DG, Michael JW, Bowker JH (eds): Atlas of amputations and limb deficiencies: surgical, prosthetic, and rehabilitation principles, 3rd ed. Rosemont, IL, American Academy of Orthopaedic Surgeons, 2004, pp 673–682.

34. Sullivan J, Uden M, Robinson KP, Sooriakumaran S: Rehabilitation of the transfemoral amputee with an osseointegrated prosthesis: the United Kingdom experience. P&O Int 27:114–120, 2003.

35. Hagberg K, Branemark R, Gurenberg B, Ridevik B: Osseointegrated transfemoral amputation prostheses: prospective results of general and condition-specific quality of life in 18 patients at 2-year follow-up. P&O Int 32:29–41, 2008.

36. Frossard L, Hagberg K, Haggstrom E, et al: Functional outcome of transfemoral amputees fitted with osseointegrated fixation: temporal gait characteristics. JPO 22:11–20, 2010.

Postsurgical Management

5

OBJECTIVES

At the end of this chapter, all students are expected to:

1. Prioritize all management activities according to the patient's condition and the environmental situation.
   a. Differentiate between early and late postsurgical status.
   b. Handle the **residual limb** to enhance healing and decrease postsurgical pain.
   c. Gather appropriate data accurately throughout the program.
2. Implement a program of intervention appropriate to the goals and the patient's status.
   a. Teach proper positioning.
   b. Describe and demonstrate proper residual limb bandaging and care.
   c. Implement an appropriate program of exercises and mobility training.
   d. Develop an appropriate client education program.
3. Exhibit an understanding of the psychosocial and economical effects of amputation on clients of different ages.
   a. Respond appropriately to patient and family.
   b. Provide guidance and support throughout the program.

Physical Therapy students are expected to:

1. Establish an appropriate physical therapy diagnosis for each person.
   a. Develop and implement a plan of care for the postsurgical period of any lower extremity amputee.
   b. Select appropriate information from the history and system review.
   c. Select, prioritize, and implement appropriate tests and measures in the early and late postsurgical periods
   d. Evaluate data on an ongoing basis to adapt the plan of care as needed.

2. Develop an examination plan throughout the postsurgical period.
3. Evaluate the examination data to
   a. Establish a physical therapy diagnosis
   b. Establish a plan of care
   c. Establish functional outcomes
   d. Implement the plan with any simulated client
4. Take responsibility for making appropriate referrals for effective continuation of care throughout the postsurgical (preprosthetic) program.
   a. In the early postsurgical period, plan for discharge and continuation of care from the onset of treatment.
   b. In the later postsurgical period, ensure proper referral for prosthetic fitting and training using appropriate community resources.

CASE STUDIES

Janice Simmons, 63 years old, underwent a left transtibial amputation yesterday secondary to diabetic gangrene. She had an ulcer on the plantar surface of the first metatarsal that did not heal despite wound care and special shoes.

John Adams, 72 years old, underwent a right transfemoral amputation yesterday secondary to arteriosclerosis. He had a long history of arteriosclerosis with intermittent claudication and rest pain. He had a femoral-popliteal bypass 2 years ago.

Richard Canto, a 20-year-old member of the U.S. Army. While in a firefight in Iraq, he was hit in the left side with fragments from a roadside bomb. Evacuated quickly, he was sent to Germany and then to Walter Reed Medical Center, where attempts to save the leg failed. It was amputated at a transtibial level 1 week ago. The wound was left open because of potential infection. Yesterday, the incision was closed, and he was fitted with an immediate postoperative prosthesis without the **pylon** and foot.

Linda Bean, a 10-year-old, underwent a right transfemoral amputation yesterday secondary to IIB osteogenic sarcoma of the proximal tibia. The tumor by type and location was not suitable for excision, and reconstruction and amputation was considered the best treatment alternative.

Case Study Activities

All Students

1. Compare and contrast the different methods of residual limb postoperative care, identifying the major advantages and disadvantages of each.

Physical Therapy Students

1. What data do you need to make a physical therapy diagnosis of each patient at this time?

INTRODUCTION

The shorter the period of time between amputation and prosthetic fitting, the better are the functional outcomes; the longer the delay, the more likely the development of complications such as joint contractures, general debility, and a depressed psychological state. Individuals may undergo amputation in large medical centers, small community hospitals, military facilities, trauma centers, or general hospitals. Often the type and level of care from amputation to definitive prosthetic fitting are determined by the type of facility, the rehabilitation outlook of the surgeon, and the immediate availability of knowledgeable healthcare providers. Military personnel wounded in battle receive quick evacuation to appropriate facilities and ongoing intensive and high-quality rehabilitation,[1] but many older individuals amputated in general or community hospitals may receive only cursory inpatient physical therapy and no referral for ongoing prosthetic management. In many cases, the physical therapist in the general hospital has not had much experience in the care of individuals following amputation, and may actually only treat a few such patients each year. The therapist may not be aware of the importance of continued care after hospital discharge or the availability of appropriate facilities. Therefore,

it is important for all physical therapists and physical therapists assistants to be competent in the care of these patients and be aware of the critical importance of continued care throughout the postsurgical/preprosthetic period.

The postoperative program can be divided into two phases: the acute or early phase, which is the time between surgery and discharge from the acute-care facility and the postsurgical or preprosthetic phase, which is the time between discharge from acute care and fitting with a definitive prosthesis or until a decision is made not to fit the client. These are not clearly delineated time periods because a person can be fitted with an immediate postoperative prosthesis (IPOP) in the operating room or an early postoperative prosthesis (EPOP) and begin ambulation within a day or two after surgery. However, for those patients not fitted with an IPOP or an EPOP, the time difference is important to delineate between tests and measures and interventions that can be initiated immediately after surgery and those that must be delayed until some degree of residual limb healing has occurred. In all phases, the major goal is to help the client regain the highest level of premorbid function possible, be that to return to gainful employment with an active recreational life, to be independent in the home and community, or even to be independent in the sheltered environment of a retirement center. If the amputation resulted from chronic disease, the goal may be to help the person function at a higher level than immediately before surgery. Ideally, the physical therapist needs to gather a broad area of data to develop the physical therapy diagnosis, establish functional goals, and then develop and implement a plan of care. **Table 5.1** outlines a general postsurgical examination guide. However, implementation of such a guide will vary with each situation and is often not practical in the early postoperative phase as is discussed later in this chapter.

POSTOPERATIVE DRESSINGS

The choice of the postsurgical dressing is, of course, the purview of the surgeon and is dictated to some extent by the cause and level of amputation and the potential for infection. The postoperative dressing protects the incision and residual limb, fosters incisional healing, controls postoperative edema, and controls postoperative pain. Edema control is critical as excessive edema in the residual limb compromises healing and causes pain. The postoperative dressing may take many forms as outlined in **Table 5.2.**

TABLE 5.1	General Postsurgical Data Gathering Guide
History	1. General demographic data 2. Family and social data 3. Preamputation status (work, activity level, degree of independence, lifestyle) 4. Prosthetic goals (desire for prosthesis, anticipated activity level, and lifestyle) 5. Financial (available payment for prosthesis) 6. Prior prosthesis (if bilateral) 7. Other as appropriate to specific client
General Systems Review	1. Cause of amputation (disease, tumor, trauma, congenital) 2. Associated diseases/symptoms (neuropathy, visual disturbances, cardiopulmonary disease, renal failure, congenital anomalies) 3. Current physiological status (cardiovascular, neurological, urinary) 4. Medications
Integumentary	1. Scars (healed, adherent, invaginated, flat) 2. Other lesions (size, shape, open, scar tissue) 3. Moisture (moist, dry, scaly) 4. Sensation and location (absent, diminished, protective, hyperesthesia) 5. Grafts (location, type, healing) 6. Dermatologic lesions (psoriasis, eczema, cysts)
Residual Limb Length	1. Bone length (transtibial limbs measured from medial tibial plateau; transfemoral limbs measured from ischial tuberosity or greater trochanter) 2. Soft tissue length (note redundant tissue)
Residual Limb Shape	1. Cylindrical, conical, bulbous end, etc 2. Abnormalities ("dog ears," adductor roll) 3. Specific circumferential measurements
Vascularity (both limbs if amputation cause is vascular)	1. Pulses (femoral, popliteal, dorsalis pedis, posterior tibial) 2. Color (red, cyanotic) 3. Temperature 4. Edema (circumference measurement, water displacement measurement, caliper measures) 5. Pain (type, location, duration) 6. Trophic changes 7. ABI (ankle-brachial index) reading
Range of Motion (ROM)	1. Residual limb (specific for remaining joints) 2. Other lower extremity (gross for major joints; specific for hip; ankle and any area of obvious impairment)
Muscle Strength	1. Residual limb (specific for major muscle groups) 2. Other lower extremities (gross for most joints unless obvious impairment dictates otherwise)
Neurological	1. Pain (phantom [differentiate sensation or pain], neuroma, incisional, from other causes) 2. Neuropathy 3. Sensory testing 4. Cognitive status (alert, oriented, confused) 5. Emotional status (acceptance, body image)

Continued

TABLE 5.1	General Postsurgical Data Gathering Guide—cont'd
Functional Status	1. Transfers (bed to chair, to toilet, to car) 2. Balance (sitting, standing, reaching, moving) 3. Mobility (ancillary support, supervision, closed and open environments, steps, curbs) 4. Home/family situation (caregiver, architectural barriers, hazards) 5. Activities of daily living (bathing, dressing) 6. Instrumental activities of daily living (cooking, cleaning)

TABLE 5.2 Postsurgical Dressings		
Type of Dressing	**Advantages**	**Disadvantages**
Compressible soft dressing	Easy to apply Inexpensive Easy access to incision	Little edema control Minimal RL (residual limb) protection Requires frequent rewrapping
Shrinker	Easy to apply Inexpensive	Not used until sutures are removed Requires changing as RL shrinks
Semirigid dressing	Better edema control than soft dressing RL protection	Needs frequent changing Cannot be applied by patient No access to incision
IPOP	Excellent edema control Excellent RL protection Control of RL pain	No access to incision More expensive than other dressings Requires proper training for use

Immediate Postsurgical Prosthesis (IPOP)

In the early 1960s, orthopedic surgeons in the United States started experimenting with immediate postoperative prosthetic fitting, a technique developed in Europe that consisted of fitting the client with a plaster prosthetic socket. An attachment, at the distal end of the dressing, allowed the addition of a foot and pylon for limited weight-bearing ambulation[2–4] (Fig. 5.1). The rigid dressing may still be made of plaster, but more sophisticated appliances have become available. Many surgeons prefer a lightweight copolymer shell with a soft lining that covers from the end of the residual limb to mid-thigh, holding the knee in extension. These prefabricated shells are removable for wound inspection, and some allow the eventual attachment of a pylon and foot. As the residual limb shrinks, additional lining or socks can be added to maintain an appropriate fit.[5,6] The Air Limb (Fig. 5.2) is another example of a commercially available IPOP. Commercial devices are generally adjustable for different size residual limbs and often are used as EPOP as well as IPOP. Use of immediate postoperative rigid dressings varies greatly. Generally, orthopedic surgeons use the technique more than vascular surgeons, despite documented benefits to healing and rehabilitation.[6] Although specific protocols vary between surgeons and centers, generally, the IPOP is changed weekly for 3 weeks to ensure proper fit and to inspect the incision. After the sutures are removed, usually at about 3 weeks, an EPOP or a temporary prosthesis may be applied or the patient may be fitted with an elastic shrinker.[6] EPOPs are similar to IPOPs in design except that pylon and foot are attached, and they are applied several days following surgery. They are usually removable. The effects of IPOP and EPOP on the management of patients in the early postoperative phase will be discussed later in this chapter.

Semirigid Dressing

Semirigid dressings (SRDs) are made of a paste compound of zinc oxide, gelatin, glycerin, and calamine and are applied in the operating or recovery room.[7]

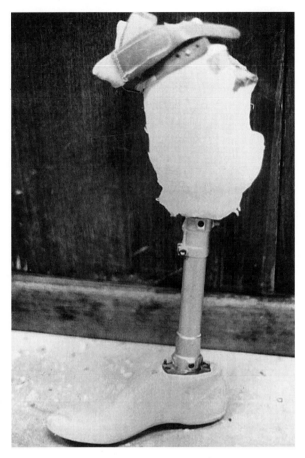

FIGURE 5.1. Rigid postoperative dressing with pylon and prosthetic foot attached.

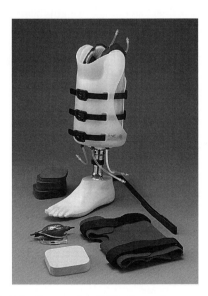

FIGURE 5.2. Commercial IPOP (immediate postoperative prosthesis) kit. *(Photograph from Air Cast, with permission.)*

The dressing adheres to the skin, eliminating the need for a suspension belt, and allows slight joint movement. The SRD has been shown to be more effective than the soft dressing in helping reduce postoperative edema.[7] It does not appear, however, to be in broad use today.

Air Splint

Little first reported the use of an air splint to control postoperative edema as well as aid in early ambulation.[8,9] The air splint is a plastic double-wall bag that is pumped to the desired level of rigidity. The residual limb is covered with an appropriate postoperative dressing and inserted in the bag. The air splint allows for wound inspection, but the constant pressure does not intimately conform to the shape of the residual limb, and the plastic is hot and humid, requiring frequent cleaning. There is little evidence in the literature that either the semirigid dressing or the air splint are in common use today.

Soft Dressings

The soft dressing is the oldest method of postsurgical management of the residual limb. Immediately after surgery, the soft dressing consists of sterile gauze wrapped directly over the incision which is then covered with either a compressive elastic bandage wrapped in a figure-eight pattern, or plain gauze (**Fig. 5.3**). Later, the soft dressing can be either an elastic wrap or a shrinker. The soft dressing is probably

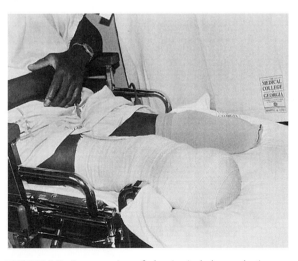

FIGURE 5.3. Postoperative soft dressing includes an elastic wrap over gauze pads.

the most frequently used and is generally indicated in cases of local infection. Elastic wrap needs frequent rewrapping; movement of the residual limb against the bedclothes, bending and extending the proximal joints, and general body movements cause slippage and wrinkling. Wrinkles in the elastic bandage create uneven pressure on the residual limb, which can lead to skin abrasions and breakdown. If not applied properly, the elastic wrap can create a tourniquet and interfere with healing. Covering the finished wrap with stockinet helps reduce some of the wrinkling. However, careful and frequent rewrapping is the only effective way to prevent complications. Nursing as well as the therapy staff need to assume responsibility for frequent inspection and rewrapping of the residual limb while the client is in the hospital.

Shrinkers are sock-like garments knitted of rubber-reinforced cotton; they are conical or cylindrical in shape and come in various sizes (**Fig. 5.4**). Shrinkers should not be used until after the sutures have been removed and drainage has stopped, as the act of donning the shrinker can put excessive distracting pressures at the distal end of the residual limb, and wound drainage will soil the shrinker. The shrinker is easy to don and is probably as effective as the elastic wrap but is less effective than the rigid or semirigid dressing in controlling edema. As the residual limb becomes smaller, a new shrinker must be purchased or the existing shrinker made smaller by sewing an additional seam.

Many vascular surgeons prefer delaying elastic wrapping until the incision has healed and the sutures have been removed. Leaving the residual limb without any pressure wrap allows for development of postoperative edema that causes pain and may interfere with circulation in the many small vessels in the

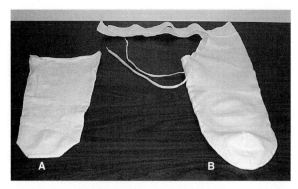

FIGURE 5.4. (A) Transtibial and **(B)** transfemoral residual limb shrinkers.

skin and soft tissue. The therapist needs to discuss the benefits of edema control with the surgeon as early as possible and encourage the use of some form of compression dressing.

EARLY FITTING

The residual limb must attain a stable size if the first definitive prosthetic socket is to fit for a reasonable amount of time. Today's financial limitations imposed by insurance companies and other third-party payers suggest delaying definitive fitting until the residual limb has reached maximum shrinkage. However, regardless of how much shrinkage is obtained prior to fitting, there will always be additional shrinkage after fitting. And, the longer the patient remains without bipedal ambulation, the greater is the potential for debility, contractures, and a lower eventual rehabilitation outcome. The use of a temporary prosthesis or EPOP is helpful in assisting the patient in maintaining a higher activity level during the postsurgical period. The benefits of immediate or early fitting on patient comfort, edema control, residual limb protection, and improved activity levels are well documented and accrue whether or not the patient is allowed early weight-bearing ambulation. In the early postoperative phase, prior to residual limb healing, weight bearing must be limited. The patient must have the necessary balance and control to ambulate with crutches, preferably, and limit the amount of weight placed on the temporary prosthesis. Once incisional healing has been obtained, weight bearing can be increased as tolerated. At all times, the therapist and, eventually, the patient must carefully monitor the residual limb to prevent any injuries or delayed healing.

Patients fitted with IPOPs or EPOPs often wear them both day and night to prevent rebound edema. At night, the pylon and foot are removed for comfort and to avoid torsion stress on the residual limb if the foot becomes entangled in the bedclothes. Patients fitted with temporary prostheses remove them at night and substitute elastic bandages or a shrinker to control edema.

EARLY POSTOPERATIVE CARE

Arbitrarily, the period between surgery and discharge from the acute-care hospital can be designated as the early postoperative period. The pressure to discharge the patient from the acute-care hospital as quickly as possible demands that the therapist focus on the critical aspects of care while gathering data, developing the plan of care, and instituting the program of intervention. The scope and intensity of the program will be dictated by the patient's physiological status, cause of amputation, comorbidities, and response to surgery.

Case Study Activities

Physical Therapy Students

1. Develop an evaluation plan for each patient.
   a. What tests and measures could you perform the day after surgery and which would have to be delayed? Why?
   b. What data are the most critical to gather early after surgery? Why?

Physical Therapist Assistant Students

1. What do you need to know about each patient if some of the postoperative treatment is delegated to you? Why?
2. Can you perform manual muscle testing and take goniometric measurements of the residual limb right after surgery? Why or why not?

Data Gathering

Traditionally, the data-gathering phase includes obtaining the pertinent history and system review, applying appropriate tests and measures, and interviewing the patient and family. It is important for the therapist to prioritize data gathering. What are the most critical data to obtain to develop and begin implementing the plan of care? **Box 5.1** outlines a general data-gathering plan that must be adapted to the specific situation. For all patients, information on the current cardiovascular status, physiological response to surgery, presence of infection, pain level, and medication status indicate to what extent the patient will be able to participate in the therapy program at this time. The person amputated following severe trauma involving other parts of the body will need a different approach from the person amputated for vascular problems without many comorbidities. The type of postsurgical dressing will also influence both data gathering and intervention. The person with a rigid dressing will be able to move more easily in bed than someone with just a soft dressing.

BOX 5.1 | Early Postsurgical Evaluation

- General systems review
- Postsurgical status
  - Cardiovascular
  - Respiratory
  - Diabetes control (if appropriate)
  - Whether OOB
  - Infection
- Pain
  - Incisional
  - Phantom
  - Other
- Vascularity (if appropriate)
- Functional status
  - Bed mobility, transfers, sitting, standing, balance
- Gross range of motion
  - Unamputated extremity
  - Hip, knee flexion and extension
  - Ankle dorsiflexion/plantar flexion
  - Upper extremity to note any limitations that would interfere with functional activities
  - Amputated extremity
  - Avoid joint immediately proximal to amputation
  - May or may not be able to measure hip in transtibial amputation
- Gross strength
  - Unamputated extremities and trunk, all motions
  - Avoid amputated extremity
- Cognition/emotion

Detailed data about the residual limb are not critical at this stage. More important is determining the person's ability to move in bed, sit at the side of the bed, transfer safely, and protect the residual limb while performing these activities. Gross information on the strength and range of motion (ROM) of the upper extremities and the uninvolved lower extremity can be obtained quickly without causing undue stress or fatigue. A detailed manual muscle test and goniometric measurements may not be necessary and depend on the individual situation. At this time, the patient will have limited endurance and responsiveness, regardless of cause of amputation. The presence or absence of any hip flexion contracture bilaterally is very important but cannot always be obtained at this time. With a transtibial amputation, hip ROM may be obtained in the side-lying position if it is difficult for the patient to get prone. ROM of the unamputated hip may not be accurately determined at this time if the person cannot get prone, as the patient should not lie on the amputated side. The patient should be encouraged to move the amputated limb actively and gently, but care must be taken not to stress the incision site. Throughout this phase, the patient must be warned against pushing on the residual limb while moving, even if fitted with a rigid dressing. If wearing a soft dressing, the patient must be taught to protect the residual limb during movements. Simultaneously, the therapist can gather data on the patient's ability to understand and participate in the therapeutic program and the patient's response to the amputation. The therapist can also begin to explore the patient's own goals and expectations. Individuals who underwent an elective amputation will have had time to prepare and think about their future life; those amputated following trauma will need time to adjust their self-image as discussed in Chapter 3.

Diagnosis

The physical therapy diagnosis at this point reflects an individual with limited mobility and functional capabilities. Depending on the specific findings, the individual may also have impaired aerobic capacity, limited endurance, and pain that interfere with function. If the amputation was due to vascular disease, an additional physical therapy diagnosis will focus on the impaired circulation.

Plan of Care

The plan of care is aimed at both the goals to be achieved in this period and the critical findings for each specific patient. In general, the goals for the early postoperative period are for the patient to reach physiological stability and enough functional capacity to be discharged from acute care. General goals are summarized in **Box 5.2**.

Interventions

With only a limited time to reach the goals and the patient's limited endurance, interventions must focus on preparing for discharge from acute care. In general, the early postoperative program will include

■ Positioning to avoid contractures
■ Balance and transfer activities
■ Mobility with crutches or walker
■ Residual limb care and bandaging, if appropriate
■ Care of the remaining lower limb if dysvascular
■ Education on amputation and prosthetics

BOX 5.2 | Early Postsurgical General Goals

■ Healing residual limb
■ Protect remaining limb (if dysvascular)
■ Independent in transfers and mobility
■ Demonstrate proper positioning
■ Begin psychological adjustment
■ Understand the process of prosthetic rehabilitation

Positioning

It is critically important to future mobility to avoid hip flexion contractures bilaterally as well as knee flexion contractures in transtibial amputation. It is never appropriate to place a pillow under the residual limb while in bed. Although the elevated position minimally helps reduce residual limb edema, the flexion position facilitates the development of hip flexion contractures. A person who is not able to stand straight and balance properly over the hips will not become a good prosthetic ambulator. Some patients may already have developed hip flexion contractures, and efforts must be made to decrease these contractures if at all possible. **Figure 5.5** depicts optimum positions for transtibial and transfemoral amputees:

■ Supine—both legs extended and comfortably adducted; no pillow under the residual limb; upper body extended with small pillow under the head and neck
■ Side-lying on unamputated side—nonamputated limb (bottom leg) slightly flexed at hip or knee for balance, pillow between the legs, amputated leg straight (hip and knee at 0 degrees of flexion), pillow behind back for comfort and stability; pillow under upper arm and shoulder if desired
■ Prone (if the patient will tolerate the prone position)—hips and knees straight with a small pillow under the unamputated ankle or the toes over the edge of the mattress; no pillow under the head which is turned in a comfortable position facing the unamputated side; arms positioned comfortably
■ Sitting—knee of the amputated leg straight on board and not hanging in flexion; sitting needs to be on a firm cushion with support for the back; sitting needs to be limited

Balance and Transfer Activities

Sitting balance is tested and worked on as early as the first postoperative day. Most individuals with a unilateral amputation will not have problems with sitting balance, although individuals with bilateral amputations will and will need balance exercises (see Chapter 8). Transfers from bed to wheelchair or from chair to toilet or other chair are best accomplished by leading with the unamputated side with the chair angled to the bed or another chair. Leading with the unamputated side helps protect the residual limb from accidental trauma associated with the transfer. It is also a little safer as the person initiates the movement by standing on the secure leg.

Mobility

Mobility training is an important part of the early program. The more mobile the person, the more active they are likely to be and the better the recovery. In the United States, physical therapists tend to give patients, particularly older patients, a walker for mobility. Although there is more stability in a walker, crutches afford greater flexibility in activities of daily living. Many older individuals can learn to use crutches safely with a little training. In many European countries, walkers are almost unknown, and most patients use crutches.

If the patients had been fitted with an IPOP or an EPOP, then crutches are the ancillary support of choice. With a prosthesis, even with limited weight bearing, a walker forces the patient into an uneven gait pattern. Once learned, this pattern is difficult to change once a definitive prosthesis has been fitted and full weight bearing is allowed. Time taken in the early program to help the person develop the necessary balance and confidence to use crutches will be beneficial in the long run. If the individual has steps leading into the home, crutches will enhance the individual's ability to get into the home. The therapist needs to ascertain the layout of the home and help prepare the patient and family for the highest level of independence possible. Mobility training with an IPOP or EPOP includes teaching the patient how to limit weight bearing on the appliance. A scale is often an effective tool to help the person learn how much pressure is allowed. The patient should be wearing regular well-fitting shoes on both the remaining foot and the prosthetic foot. The shoe must be in good condition and fit properly to avoid undue stress on the remaining foot. The person with vascular insufficiency may need special shoes or inserts to protect the remaining foot (see Chapter 13).

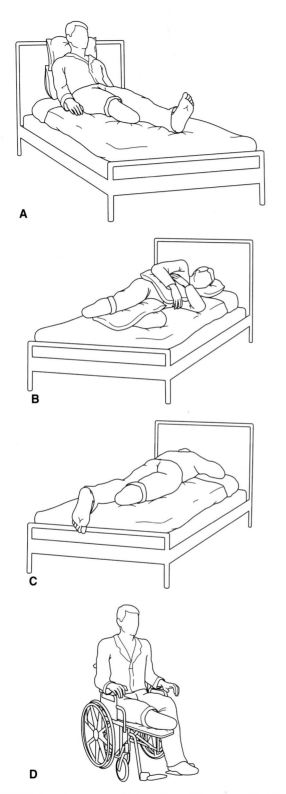

FIGURE 5.5. Proper transtibial positions: **(A)** supine, **(B)** sidelying, **(C)** prone, and **(D)** sitting.

If the patient has not been fitted with any appliance, he or she must be taught a swing-through gait. Try to teach the patient a gentle swing-through gait with control of the forces placed on the remaining extremity. If the amputation was due to vascular disease, care must be taken to make sure the remaining extremity is clean and able to tolerate the stress of single-leg ambulation. Ambulation with slippers or scuffs or even barefoot is contraindicated. The person needs to wear a supportive, well-fitting shoe to protect the foot and remaining limb regardless of whether the amputation was due to vascular disease or other causes.

Residual Limb Care and Bandaging

Although the residual limb will be either encased in a rigid dressing or wrapped in a soft dressing, the patient and family need to understand the ongoing care of the limb. If wrapped in a soft dressing with a compression wrap, careful supervision is necessary to make sure the compression wrap is properly applied, is not forming wrinkles as the patient moves, and is not tighter proximally than distally. The patient and family must understand the importance of avoiding stress on the incision, of moving the limb gently if possible, and of controlling edema. Resistive exercises are contraindicated at this point in time, although gentle active motion is encouraged. The first concern is healing, and stress on the residual limb can interfere with the healing process.

If the residual limb has been placed in an IPOP or EPOP, the need for residual limb bandaging will not be an issue initially, and teaching the patient and family can be delayed for the next level of care. If the residual limb has been placed in a soft dressing, compression residual limb wrapping over the dressing is indicated. It will need to be rewrapped frequently to avoid wrinkles and improper pressure on the residual limb. Methods of residual limb bandaging are outlined later in this chapter.

Care of the Remaining Lower Limb

If the patient has been amputated for vascular reasons, the patient and his or her family must be taught proper foot care and the importance of regularly checking the foot to avoid ulcers or injuries. On evaluation, the sensory level will have been determined, and the patient and family must understand the implications of any sensory loss in the remaining extremity. Proper shoe fitting must be taught as well. Any loss of range of motion or strength must be addressed with a home program. It is important for the patient to have full range of motion in dorsiflexion for good balance in ambulation. Regular and ongoing ambulation will help maintain strength in the remaining lower limb, but a home strengthening program with theraband may be indicated, particularly if the patient is relatively sedentary.

Patient Education

The better the patient and his or her family understand the implications of the amputation and the prosthetic rehabilitation program, the better they will be able to take responsibility for their care and the eventual outcome. Too often, patients are discharged from the acute-care center with no plan for continued therapy. These patients may return to the surgeon's office for suture removal, but the patient is denied the necessary ongoing program that will prepare him or her well for prosthetic ambulation. Many patients "drop through the crack" only to be sent to the prosthetist 6 or more months later with contractures, weak muscles, and limited mobility. These individuals do not do well with prosthetic rehabilitation. The therapist needs to help plan for continued care in a rehabilitation setting, through home health services, or as an outpatient, whatever best fits the situation. The patient needs to understand the importance of continued and ongoing care through this period.

Patient education is an ongoing part of the treatment program. It starts with the initial contact and is integrated throughout the evaluation and all interventions. Education involves the patient and the family. It is desirable to work with a consistent family member, preferably one who will be participating in the ongoing care. This is not always possible, but the therapist must provide written as well as oral information for continuity of care. However, balance must be achieved. Therapists sometimes overwhelm the patient and caregiver with so many forms, home exercise programs, and written materials that neither the patient nor the caregiver can sort them out. Education must be specific and focus on the critical aspects of care. Exercises and positioning need to be reviewed regularly to ensure the concepts are understood. Work with the patient and family to establish a program that is reasonable and achievable.[10]

The patient needs to be taught the importance of continued activity, proper positioning, contracture prevention, ongoing exercises, and how to achieve independence in functional activities with or without a temporary appliance. If amputated for a vascular reason, he or she needs to learn proper foot and residual limb care.

Discharge Planning

As stated earlier, discharge planning needs to start with the onset of treatment. Too often patients are discharged from the acute-care setting without a plan for ongoing therapy. The therapist must take the initiative and discuss options with the patient and family, and then work with the physician to ensure continued care. Ideally, the patient should be referred to an inpatient rehabilitation center to gain independence in functional activities and residual limb care. Stineman and associates, in a study of 2673 older veterans over a 1-year period, reported that patients who received intensive inpatient rehabilitation following amputation surgery had a significantly better 1-year survival rate and home discharge as compared to those who did not receive such therapy.[11]

POSTSURGICAL/PREPROSTHETIC CARE

The period between discharge from acute care and fitting with a permanent prosthesis or until the decision is made that the patient is not a candidate for prosthetic fitting, is usually called the preprosthetic period. The intensity and scope of therapy vary with individual patients and with the place of care.

Data Gathering

Approximately 7 to 12 days after surgery, depending on the condition of the residual limb, the amount of healing, and the postsurgical dressing, specific data regarding the residual limb and adjacent joint can be gathered. Healing is, of course, of primary importance, and residual limb data gathering must be deferred until the residual limb has healed enough to tolerate the stress of handling and resistance. The desired information is outlined in **Box 5.3**. The therapist who assumes responsibility for care at this point will update the initial information by determining the patient's current status as outlined in Box 5.1.

BOX 5.3 | Residual Limb Deferred Data

Transtibial Residual Limb
- Length
  - Medial tibial plateau (MTP) to end of bone
  - MTP to end of soft tissue
- Circumference
  - (TT) Taken every 5 to 8 cm from MTP to end of soft tissue

Transfemoral Residual Limb
- Length
  - Greater trochanter to end of bone
  - Greater trochanter to end of soft tissue
- Circumference
  - Taken every 8 to 10 cm from greater trochanter to end of soft tissue

Both Residual Limbs
- Healing status
  - eg, incision healed, draining, dehiscence, sutures in/out
- Condition
  - eg, edematous, flabby, conical, firm, clear skin

Proximal Joints Range of Motion (ROM)
- Transtibial: goniometric measures of hip and knee amputated side
- Transfemoral: goniometric measurements of hip in flexion/extension; abduction/adduction

Proximal Joints Strength
- Transtibial: gross MMT knee flexors/extensors, hip flexors/extensors, abductors/adductors
- Transfemoral: gross MMT hip flexors/extensors, abductors/adductors

---

Case Study Activities

Boxes 5.4 through 5.7 reflect the preprosthetic data gathered for each of our patients.

All Students

1. Would you expect each of the clients to achieve independent mobility with crutches or a walker prior to definitive prosthetic fitting? Why or why not?

Physical Therapy Students

1. Develop a physical therapy diagnosis for each client.
2. Develop a plan of care for each client for the preprosthetic period.

Physical Therapist Assistant Students

1. What part of the postsurgical intervention program are you comfortable implementing? Why?
2. What information do you want from the physical therapist to treat each person?

Diagnosis

The diagnosis reflects the person's current status following analysis of all the data that have been gathered. The diagnosis informs the goals, plan of care, and interventions. At this point, 1 to 2 weeks after surgery, the patient's status is affected by the

---

BOX 5.4 | Preprosthetic Examination*—Janice Simmons

Ms. Simmons was referred for home health care following discharge from the hospital 7 days after transtibial amputation.

History 63 y.o. female had (L) transtibial amputation 2 weeks ago, secondary to gangrene from diabetic ulcers. Patient has long history of poorly controlled diabetes mellitus and a nonhealing ulcer. Pt has a L transtibial amputation, posterior flap, and soft dressing applied after surgery.

Ms. Simmons lives with her husband in a small house in a Midwestern city. She was a waitress at a local diner until 4 months ago when she had to stop secondary to the ulcer. Her husband is a mechanic in a local plant. She has two children, both grown and out of the house. Ms. Simmons is 5'8" and weighs 172 lb.

Had some physical therapy in hospital. Discharged from hospital 1 week ago and referred to home health care for continued therapy. Nursing completed intake interview and visit. PT only patient.

Medications
Insulin, Ampicillin, Xanax, Darvocet prn

Interview Patient reports that her residual limb hurts occasionally and that she can feel her amputated toes and they are cramped. Husband helps her at home, but she's trying to be active. Was given home exercise program but it isn't clear. Residual limb is poorly wrapped in an elastic bandage.

Examination

Vitals

BP 145/85; pulse 80

Residual Limb Wrapped in an elastic wrap somewhat wrinkled

Sutures in place
Incision healing well, no drainage
Length: 15 cm to end of bone; 15.5 cm to end of limb
Circumference: @ 5 cm from MTP = 32 cm
            @ 10 cm   = 34 cm
            @ 15 cm   = 34 cm

Range of Motion (ROM)
Left limb:
  active and passive knee flexion = 108 degrees; extension = –5 degrees
  active and passive hip flexion = 120 degrees; active extension = –10 degrees; passive = 0 degrees
  active and passive hip abduction/adduction; internal/external rotation = within normal limits
Right limb:
  Right ankle:
    active dorsiflexion = 5 degrees; passive = 8 degrees
    active plantar flexion = 22 degrees; passive = 25 degrees
    active inversion = 15 degrees; passive 20 degrees
    active eversion = 15 degrees; passive 20 degrees
    active and passive knee flexion = 120 degrees; extension 0 degrees
    active and passive hip flexion = 130 degrees; active extension 0 degrees; passive 10 degrees

Muscle Strength Both upper extremities grossly within normal limits.

Left limb:
  knee flexion and extension: G (4/5)
  right hip and knee grossly 4+/5 (Good+/Normal)
Right ankle:
  dorsiflexion 4/5 (Fair+/Normal)
  plantar flexion (NWB) = 4–/5 (Good–/Normal)

Vascular RLE shows evidence of dysvascularity; dry, hairless limb, minimal toenail clubbing, no sores or open areas. Sensation, tested with 10 mg Semmes-Weinstein filament, shows decreased sensation on the plantar surface of the foot and toes and the dorsum of the toes. Wearing scuffed loafer and white sock on right foot. The back of the shoe is broken down and patient wears it like a backless slipper.

Functional Activities
■ Independent in bed to chair transfers
■ Uses walker around house for limited distances with some hesitation. Has a wheelchair

BOX 5.4 | Preprosthetic Examination*—Janice Simmons—cont'd

- Independent in personal care other than bathing
- Unable to get in and out of bathtub, dress or bandage residual limb
- Unable to perform household tasks

Emotional and Mental Ms. Simmons is open and outgoing, stating she wants to get back to work and running the house. She seems to have accepted the amputation, asking questions about prosthetics.

*Although a complete OASIS evaluation would normally be performed on this home health patient, only pertinent data for student activities are included here.

BOX 5.5 | Preprosthetic Examination*—John Adams

Mr. Adams has just been transferred to the inpatient rehabilitation center 5 days following right transfemoral amputation. Mr. Adams is 6'1" tall and weighs 168 lb.

History 72-year-old male had right transfemoral amputation 5 days ago following a right transtibial amputation 3 days before that secondary to a failed femoral bypass. Equal flap procedure amputation closed with sutures, soft dressing. Pt complains of pain in the residual limb and is reluctant to move.

Mr. Adams has a long history of atherosclerosis and cardiovascular disease; he does not have diabetes. He has had bilateral vascular reconstructive surgery within the past 5 years and had cardiac bypass surgery 2 years ago. He lives with his daughter, son-in-law, and their two children. He is a retired high school teacher and has been a widower for 8 years. He has been relatively sedentary for the past year with increasing circulatory problems although he used to like to walk the dog around the neighborhood and play bridge at the local Senior Center.

Medications
Procardia, Coumadin, Capoten, Darvocet, and Lasix

Examination
Vitals
BP 152/82; pulse 79

Range of Motion (ROM) Right hip active (PROM not tested): flexion (supine) 15–110 deg; extension (Thomas position) lacks 15 deg of neutral; abduction 0–20 deg; adduction; 0–5

LLE: Hip and knee motions grossly within normal limits excepts lacks 10 degrees of neutral hip extension (tested supine). Ankle dorsiflexion to 8 degrees, plantar flexion to 20 degrees.

Muscle Strength (patient reluctant to hold against resistance). Both upper extremities grossly in 3+ to 4/5 (F+ –G) range. Left lower extremity grossly in 3+ to 4/5 (F+ –G) range.

Right hip not tested at this point.

Vascular Status Evidence of dysvascularity in LLE. Limb is thin, little muscle bulk, no hair. He has been cleared for a full rehabilitation program from a cardiorespiratory point of view. He is wearing a laced running-type shoe and white sock on the left foot.

Functional Activities Transfer chair to mat and back with moderate assistance of 1 person. Independent in bed mobility. Pushes own wheelchair slowly. Reported to have ambulated one length of the parallel bars while in the hospital and has performed some active motion of the residual limb.

Emotional/Mental Mr. Adams states that he is tired and does not know if he will be able to use a prosthesis.

*Examination results have been limited to key data only to conserve space.

BOX 5.6 | Preprosthetic Examination—Richard Canto

Specialist Canto was initially treated in a military hospital in Germany and transferred to Walter Reed Medical Center 3 days after injury. The amputation was eventually closed, and his shrapnel injuries were treated. He was fitted with an IPOP when the amputation was closed and has been referred to the Rehabilitation Center now that his other injuries have healed enough to allow full participation in rehabilitation. He is now wearing a removable EPOP with pylon and foot attached. It is now 19 days postamputation closure and the sutures have just been removed.

Medications
Tylenol and Keflex

Examination
Vitals
BP 120/65; pulse 60.

Range of Motion (ROM) and Muscle Strength Gross active ROM and muscle strength evaluation of both upper extremities, the left lower extremity, and the right hip are grossly within normal limits.

Residual Limb
Residual limb is healing well, incision is clean.
Length: MTP to end of bone = 18 cm; to end of RL = 18 ½ cm
Circumference: @8 cm = 36 cm
                @10 cm = 37 cm
                @18 cm = 34 cm
ROM Right knee is within normal limits.
Right knee extension = G (4/5)
Right knee flexion = G(4/5)

Functional Activities Richard Canto comes to the rehabilitation gym in a wheelchair although he has crutches with him. He states he has been walking with the IPOP with partial weight bearing but has been limited by his other injuries. He is independent in self-care.

Emotional/Mental Richard is being seen by a mental health professional as part of the total rehabilitation program. He states a desire to regain the strength and endurance he has lost because of the injuries and states he would like to remain in the Army if possible. He was a truck driver before but states he would like to study computers.

BOX 5.7 | Preprosthetic Examination—Linda Bean

Linda Bean has been discharged from the hospital and referred to the outpatient department of the local children's hospital for continued therapy. She is scheduled to start chemotherapy and radiation therapy within 2 weeks. She is 4 days postamputation surgery. The residual limb has been placed in an IPOP with soft spica. Linda is 10 years old, is about 4'5" tall, and weighs about 85 lb.

Linda is the oldest of three siblings living with their parents in their own home. Both parents are attorneys with their own practice. Linda is stated to be a quiet child, not particularly involved in sports but interested in music; she was taking piano lessons prior to discovery of the tumor.

Medications
Tylenol and vistaril

Examination
Vitals
BP 118/70; pulse 68

Range of Motion (ROM) and Strength Gross active ROM and muscle strength of both upper extremities and the left lower extremity appear within normal limits, although the patient was reluctant to participate in therapeutic activities; ROM and strength evaluation of right residual limb deferred. Residual limb reported to be through distal third of the femur.

Functional Activities Linda is brought to the outpatient department by her mother. She is in a wheelchair although she has crutches with her. Her mother indicates that she walks around the house and yard but uses the wheelchair for longer distances. Mother states that she tires easily. She has not returned to school and may have a home teacher while undergoing chemotherapy and radiation therapy.

Emotional/Mental Linda is fairly quiet during the examination period although she complies with requested movements. Her mother indicates that she does not talk much about the amputation, the tumor, or the implications. Tests indicate that all tumor cells were removed and the prognosis is good. Further testing will be done after chemotherapy and radiation therapy. Her mother indicates that the parents have been discussing the possibility of having Linda see a psychotherapist.

cause of amputation and whether or not the person was fitted with an IPOP or EPOP with walking components. The diagnosis reflects functional status, physiological state, and condition of the residual limb.

Plan of Care

The general goals for all patients in the preprosthetic period are outlined in **Box 5.8**, whether or not the patient has been fitted with an IPOP or EPOP. If the person is wearing a nonremovable IPOP, residual limb goals are deferred until a removable IPOP is applied. Generally, patients fitted with nonremovable IPOPs in surgery are refitted with a removable IPOP within 2 to 3 weeks of surgery.

Interventions

The preprosthetic program continues those activities initiated in the postsurgical program, albeit at a higher functional level.

Mobility Activities

Independence in all mobility and functional activities should be achieved as soon as possible. If the patient has been fitted with an EPOP with weight-bearing components, crutch walking with recommended weight bearing is taught. If the patient has not been fitted with an IPOP or EPOP, a temporary prosthesis should be considered as soon as the residual limb is healed enough to tolerate weight-bearing stresses. The person should be encouraged to return to as active a life as possible, including general conditioning activities, while still protecting the residual limb during this healing period. Full weight-bearing prosthetic training is discussed in Chapter 7.

As necessary, balance and coordination are an integral part of mobility training. Patients with a single leg amputation do not usually have a problem with sitting balance, but older individuals may have difficulty with one-legged standing. Care must be taken to protect the remaining extremity from too much stress, but one-legged standing balance is necessary for many self-care activities. One-legged balance activities on a compliant surface are a valuable part of the preprosthetic mobility program (**Fig. 5.6**). Weight bearing through the residual limb is beneficial for balance. If the patient has not been fitted with any appliance, standing balance through the residual limb may be obtained by having the patient kneel on a pillow in a chair or stool of the appropriate height (**Fig. 5.7**).

Emphasis on balance and safety during all mobility activities is a critical component of the rehabilitation program, particularly for individuals with diabetes or other comorbidities. Pauley and associates studied the records of 1267 individuals who had undergone

---

BOX 5.8 | Preprosthetic General Goals

- Independent in residual limb care
  - Bandaging or shrinker application
  - Skin care
  - Positioning
- Independent in mobility, transfers, and functional activities
  - Partial weight-bearing crutch walking if fitted with IPOP or EPOP
  - Full weight bearing when tolerated
  - Single leg ambulation with crutches/walker if fitted with soft dressing
- Demonstrate home exercise program accurately
  - ROM graduating to resistive exercises for all parts of residual lower extremity
  - ROM and strengthening exercises for unamputated lower extremity as needed
- Care of the remaining lower extremity if amputated for vascular reasons

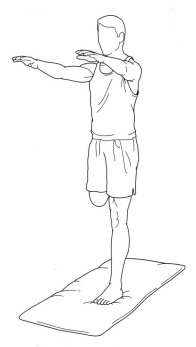

FIGURE 5.6. Standing balance exercise on a compliant surface.

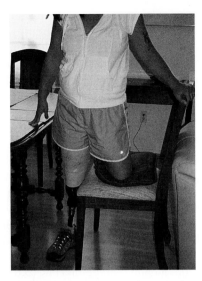

FIGURE 5.7. Kneeling on a pillow on a chair provides an opportunity for some weight bearing.

one or more lower extremity amputation and reported that at least 20% had sustained at least one fall resulting in injury while inpatients in a rehabilitation center. Falls were generally incurred during transfers and were more prevalent among bilateral than unilateral amputees. Poor wheelchair management appeared to be one of the contributing factors.[12] Dyer and associates reported on a multidisciplinary intervention program developed in an inpatient rehabilitation center aimed at decreasing falls among patients with amputations. The program considered environmental factors within the facility, teaching wheelchair management and safety and attention to mobility training. Medication management and specific emphasis on safety were also part of the program, which was reported to be effective in reducing falls among the inpatients.[13]

Residual Limb Care

Regardless if the patient has been fitted with an IPOP, EPOP, or soft dressing, the patient should learn residual limb bandaging or be fitted with a shrinker if the sutures have been removed. The shrinker is easier to apply than the elastic bandage but may not maintain appropriate tension over time. The transtibial shrinker is rolled over the residual limb to mid-thigh and is designed to be self-suspending. Individuals with heavy thighs may need additional suspension with garters or a waist belt. Currently available transfemoral shrinkers incorporate a hip spica that provides good suspension

except with obese individuals. Care must be taken that the client understands the importance of proper suspension, as any rolling of the edges or slipping of the shrinker can create a tourniquet around the proximal part of the residual limb. Shrinkers are easier to apply than elastic bandages and may be a better alternative, particularly for the transfemoral residual limb. However, they cannot be used until the sutures have been removed and complete healing has occurred. Donning the shrinker creates a stretching across the incision line, and sutures can become enmeshed in the shrinker material. Shrinkers are initially more expensive than elastic wraps, but over time, they may provide a better alternative. Patients should have two shrinkers because they need to be worn 24 hours a day except when bathing. Both the shrinker and the elastic bandage are difficult to fit as proximally and medially as desired in the transfemoral limb.

Most methods of residual limb wrapping incorporate figure-eight or angular turns, anchoring turns around the proximal joint, distributing greater pressure distally with a smooth, wrinkle-free application of the bandage. Clients tend to wrap their own residual limb in a circular manner, often creating a tourniquet that may compromise healing and will foster the development of a **bulbous** end. The client can wrap the transtibial residual limb in a sitting position, but it is virtually impossible to properly wrap and anchor the transfemoral limb while sitting. Many clients cannot balance themselves in the standing position while wrapping. The ends of the bandages are better fastened with tape rather than clips or safety pins that can cut the skin and do not anchor well. Care should be taken to avoid anchoring the tape to the skin to avoid potential skin abrasions. Elastic bandages that incorporate hook and loop attachments at each end are difficult to roll properly and can cause excessive pressure secondary to the greater bulk of the ends.

A system of wrapping that uses mostly angular or figure-eight turns was developed specifically to meet the needs of the elderly and has been in use for many years.[14] **Figure 5.8** illustrates the technique.

The Transtibial Residual Limb

Two 4-inch elastic bandages will usually be enough to wrap most transtibial residual limbs. Very large residual limbs may require three bandages. The bandages should not be sewn together so that the weave of each bandage can be brought in contraposition to each other to provide more support. To deter the

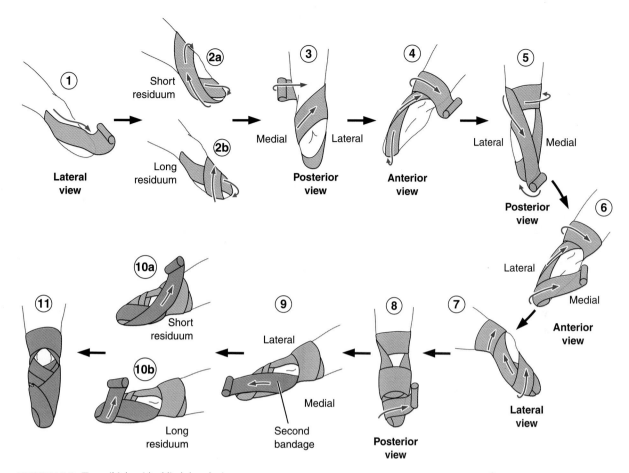

FIGURE 5.8. Transtibial residual limb bandaging.

development of postsurgical edema as much as possible, a firm, even pressure against all soft tissues is desirable. If the incision is placed anteriorly, then an attempt should be made to bring the bandages from posterior to anterior over the distal end so as not to put a distracting pressure on the incision.

The first bandage is started at either the medial or lateral tibial condyle and brought diagonally over the anterior surface of the limb to the distal end. One edge of the bandage should just cover the midline of the incision in an anterior-posterior plane. The bandage is continued diagonally over the posterior surface and then back over the beginning turn as an anchor. At this point, there is a choice—the bandage may be brought directly over the beginning point as indicated in step 2a, or it may be brought across the front of the residual limb in an "X" design as in step 2b. The latter is particularly useful with long residual limbs and aids in bandage suspension. An anchoring turn over the distal thigh is made, making sure that the wrap is

clear of the patella and is not tight around the distal thigh.

After a single anchoring turn above the knee, the bandage is brought back around the opposite tibial condyle and down to the distal end of the limb. One edge of the bandage should overlap the midline of the incision and the other wrap by at least 1/2 inch to ensure adequate distal end support. The figure-eight pattern is continued as depicted in steps 3 through 8 until the bandage is completed. Care should be taken to completely cover the residual limb with a firm and even pressure. Semicircular turns are made posteriorly to bring the bandage in line to cross the anterior surface in an angular line. This maneuver provides greater pressure on the posterior soft tissue while distributing pressure anteriorly where the bone is close to the skin. Each turn should partially overlap other turns so the whole residual limb is well covered. The pattern is usually from proximal to distal and back to proximal starting at the tibial condyles and covering both condyles as well as the patellar tendon. Usually, the patella is left free to aid in knee motion, although with extremely short residual limbs, it may be necessary to cover it for better suspension.

The second bandage is wrapped like the first, except that it is started at the opposite tibial condyle from the first bandage (step 9). Bringing the weave of each bandage in contraposition exerts a more even pressure. With both bandages, an effort is made to bring the angular turns across each other rather than in the same direction.

The Transfemoral Residual Limb

For most residual limbs, two 6-inch and one 4-inch bandages will adequately cover the limb. The two 6-inch bandages can be sewn together end-to-end, taking care not to create a heavy seam; the 4-inch bandage is used by itself. The client is side-lying (**Fig. 5.9**) and that allows a family member or therapist easy access to the residual limb.

The 6-inch bandages are used first. The first bandage is started in the groin and brought diagonally over the anterior surface to the distal lateral corner, around the end of the residual limb, and diagonally up the posterior side to the iliac crest and around the hips in a spica (steps 1 and 2). It is helpful if the initial turns covers the lateral half of the distal end of the residual limb leaving the medial portion open to be covered by the second bandage. The bandage is started medially so that the hip wrap will encourage extension. After the turn around the hips, the bandage is wrapped around the proximal portion of the residual limb high in the groin, then back around the hips (step 3). This is a proximal circular turn, but it does not create a tourniquet as long as it is continued around the hips. Going around the medial portion of the residual limb high in the groin ensures coverage of the soft tissue in the adductor area and reduces the possibility of an adductor roll, a complication that can seriously interfere with comfortable prosthetic wear. In most instances, the first bandage ends in the second spica and is anchored with tape.

If the two 6-inch bandages are not sewn together, the second 6-inch bandage is wrapped like the first but is started a bit more laterally (step 4), in such a

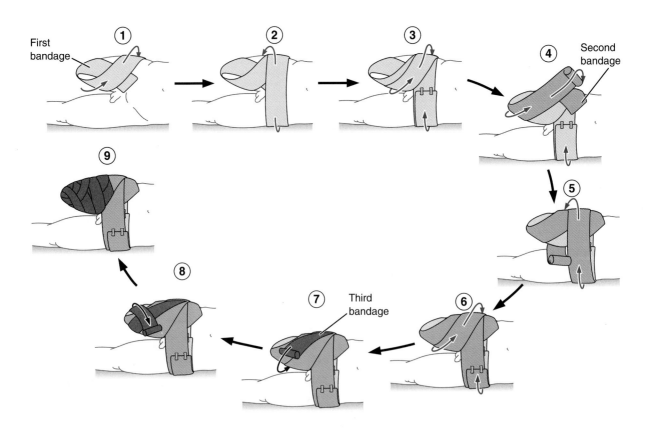

FIGURE 5.9. Transfemoral residual limb bandaging.

manner as to cover all open areas of the residual limb. If they are sewn together, the pattern continues with at least two turns coming high in the groin and going around the hips. Any areas not covered with the first bandage must be covered at this time. The second bandage is also anchored in a hip spica after the first figure-eight and after the second turn high in the groin. More of the first two bandages are used to cover the proximal residual limb, but care must be taken so that no tourniquet is created. Bringing the bandage directly from the proximal medial area into a hip spica helps keep the adductor tissue covered and prevents rolling of the bandage to some degree. At this point the entire residual limb is covered with at least one layer of elastic bandage and the proximal medial area has two layers (step 6).

The 4-inch bandage is used to exert the greatest amount of pressure over mid and distal areas of the residual limb. It is usually not necessary to anchor this bandage around the hips, as friction with the already applied bandages and good figure-eight turns provide adequate suspension. The 4-inch bandage is generally started laterally to bring the weave across the weave of previous bandages (step 7). Regular figure-eight turns in varied patterns to cover the entire residual limb are the most effective.

Bandages are applied with firm pressure from the outset. Elastic bandages can be wrapped directly over a soft postsurgical dressing so that bandaging can begin immediately after surgery. The elastic wrap controls edema more effectively if minimal gauze coverage is used over the residual limb. Several gauze pads placed just over the incision are usually adequate protection without compromising the effect of the wrap. Care must be taken to avoid any wrinkles or folds that can cause excessive skin pressure, particularly over a soft dressing.

Residual limb care also includes maintaining the skin in a soft, pliable condition. Once the sutures are removed, the residual limb is treated like any other body part. Patients should be warned to avoid drying substances on their skin, as a soft, pliable skin is best able to tolerate the stresses of prosthetic fit.

Exercises

The exercise program is designed to help the patient maintain or increase strength as needed. If the patient is ambulatory, proper positioning and resistive exercises for the residual limb are desirable, particularly if not fitted with a temporary prosthesis. Individuals with a transtibial amputation need to emphasize hip and knee extension, hip abduction

and adduction, and knee flexion if no contracture is present. **Figure 5.10** shows a variety of exercises for the transtibial amputee; resistance can be provided by using elastic bands or a cuff weight. Bridging over

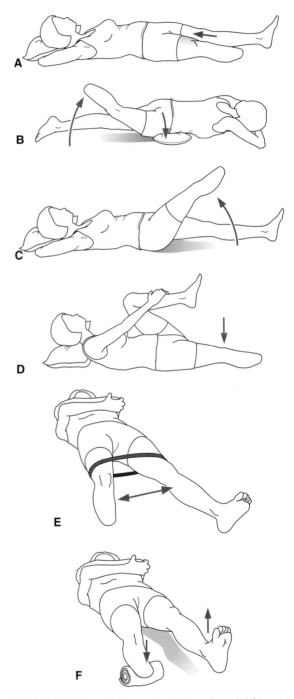

FIGURE 5.10. Transtibial exercises: **(A)** quad set, **(B)** hip extension with knee straight, **(C)** straight leg raise, **(D)** extension of the residual limb with the knee of the other leg against the chest, **(E)** hip abduction against resistance, and **(F)** bridging.

a roll is an excellent exercise to facilitate knee and hip extension. The roll should be placed at the distal end of the residual limb to encourage hip and knee extension. The arms are folded over the chest so the patient does not push with the elbows. The person pushes down with the residual limb on the bolster to lift the buttocks off the mat. Simultaneously, the unamputated leg is lifted slightly off the mat to keep the pelvis level. These particular exercises can only be initiated after residual limb healing has taken place.

Individuals with a transfemoral amputation need to emphasize hip extension and abduction as well as pelvic movements. **Figure 5.11** depicts some exercises that can be done. Again, resistance can be added with an elastic band or cuff weight. The same considerations apply to the bridging exercise as with the transtibial amputee. The roll is placed at the distal end of the residual limb and is usually not as high as with the transtibial amputee. Again, care should be taken that the patient does not arch the back. These exercises should be part of the home program.

Positioning

Patients must be warned to avoid the development of hip flexion contractures. Prolonged sitting is contraindicated, and patients must spend time lying prone and actively working on hip extension bilaterally. If a hip flexion contracture exists, every effort needs to be made to reduce or eliminate it. It is extremely difficult to reduce long-standing hip flexion contractures. Knee flexion contractures are somewhat easier to avoid, except, on occasion, in cases of trauma through the knee. Active knee extension exercises done throughout the day are helpful as is the use of an extension board when sitting.

Patient Education

As before, patient education is an integral part of the preprosthetic program. Discussions regarding prosthetic needs, components, and lifestyle are initiated during this period. A home exercise program is developed, supervised, and evaluated. If amputated for vascular reasons, education regarding proper footwear and the care of the remaining extremity are included.

Discharge Planning

An intense preprosthetic program, while necessary initially, does not necessarily continue throughout the

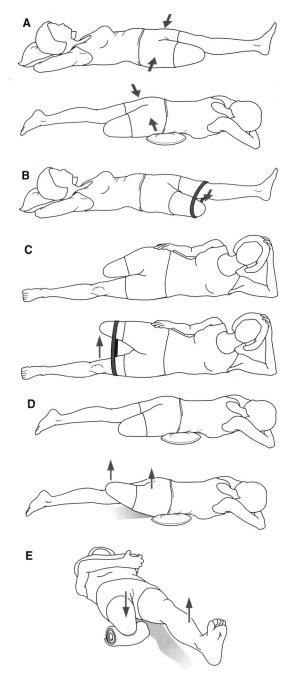

FIGURE 5.11. Transfemoral exercises: **(A)** gluteal sets, **(B)** hip abduction supine, **(C)** hip abduction against resistance, **(D)** hip extension prone, and **(E)** bridging.

preprosthetic program. Once the patient is independent in mobility and self-care activities and is competent in residual limb care, bandaging, or the use of the temporary prosthesis, the patient can be discharged until ready for definitive fitting. If the patient has been fitted with a temporary prosthesis, it is beneficial financially to extend the use of this appliance as long as possible. Adequate fit can be maintained through the use of **stump socks** and socket adjustments. If the patient has not been fitted with a temporary prosthesis, plans should be made for evaluation for prosthetic fitting within 10 to 12 weeks of surgery. Referral to a local amputee clinic is the ideal way to ensure continued and appropriate care; however, many places do not have such clinics, so referral to a prosthetist is desirable. The surgeon may refer the patient to his or her general physician for continued care.

BILATERAL AMPUTATION

The preprosthetic program for the person with bilateral lower extremity amputations is similar to the program developed for someone with a unilateral amputation except for a greater need for balance activities and, of course, ambulation. The special needs of the individual with bilateral amputations are discussed in Chapter 8.

NONPROSTHETIC MANAGEMENT

One of the goals of the preprosthetic period is to determine the individual's suitability for prosthetic replacement. Not everyone with an amputation is a candidate for a prosthesis, regardless of personal desire. The cost of the prosthesis and the energy demands of prosthetic training and ambulation require the use of some judgment in selecting individuals for fitting. Criteria for prosthetic fitting will be explored in more detail in Chapter 7.

Individuals who are not fitted with a prosthesis can become independent in a wheelchair. The therapy program includes all transfer and activities of daily living and education in the proper care of the residual limb. Wrapping the residual limb is no longer necessary unless the person is more comfortable with the limb covered. The program emphasizes sitting balance, moving safely in and out of the wheelchair, and other activities to support as independent a lifestyle as the person's physical and psychological conditions allow.

SUMMARY

The postsurgical program is very important in the rehabilitation of individuals following amputation. The program emphasizes recovery from surgery, rehabilitation to a functional lifestyle, preparation for prosthetic fitting, or evaluation to determine if prosthetic fitting is feasible. The postsurgical program

needs to be coordinated among the hospital and posthospital team members to ensure continuity of care in a most efficient manner.

KEYWORDS FOR LITERATURE SEARCH

Bilateral amputations

Immediate postsurgical fitting

Preprosthetic management

Residual limb

Shrinkers

Stump care

REFERENCES

1. Gajewski D, Granville R: The United States Armed Forces amputee care program. J Am Acad Orthop Surg 14(10): S183–S187, 2006 Sept.
2. Burgess EM: Amputations of the lower extremities. In Nickel VL (ed): Orthopedic rehabilitation. New York, Churchill Livingstone, 1982, p 377.
3. Sarmiento A, May BJ, Sinclair WF, et al: Lower-extremity amputation: the impact of immediate post surgical prosthetic fitting. Clin Orth 68:22, 1967.
4. Harrington IJ, Lexier R, Woods J, McPolin MF, James GF: A plaster-pylon technique for below-knee amputation. J Bone Joint Surg (Br) 73:76, 1991.
5. Walsh TL: Custom removable immediate postoperative prosthesis. JPO (Journal of Prosthetics & Orthotics) 15(4):158–161, 2003 Oct.
6. Bowker JH: Transtibial amputation: surgical management. In Smith DG, Michael JW, Bowker JH: Atlas of amputations and limb deficiencies: surgical, prosthetic, and rehabilitation principles, 3rd ed. Rosemont, IL, AAOS, 2004.
7. MacLean N, Fick GH: The effect of semirigid dressings on below-knee amputations. Phys Ther 74:668–673, 1994.
8. Little JM: A pneumatic weight bearing prosthesis for below-knee amputees. Lancet 1(7693):271, 1971.
9. Little JM: The use of air splints as immediate prosthesis after below-knee amputation for vascular insufficiency. Med J Aust 2:870, 1970.
10. May BJ: Patient education: past and present. J Phys Ther Educ 13(3):3–7, 1999 Winter.
11. Stineman MG & associates: The effectiveness of inpatient rehabilitation in the acute postoperative phase of care after transtibial or transfemoral amputation: study of an integrated health care delivery system. Arch P M & R 89(10):1863–1872, 2008.
12. Pauley T, Devlin M, Heslin K: Falls sustained during inpatient rehabilitation after lower limb amputation: prevalence and predictors. Am J Phys Med & Rehabil 85(6):521–532, 2006.
13. Dyer D, Bouman B, Davey M, Ismond KP: An intervention program to reduce falls for adult in-patients following major lower limb amputation. Healthcare Q 11(3 Spec No.):117–121, 2008.
14. May BJ: Stump bandaging of the lower extremity amputee. Phys Ther 44:808, 1964.

Prosthetic Components

OBJECTIVES

At the end of this chapter, all students are expected to:

1. Compare and contrast the major types of feet, knee joints, socket designs, and methods of suspension for transfemoral and transtibial prosthetic replacements.
2. Describe the function of different classes of components in relation to normal function.

Physical Therapy students are expected to:

1. Make recommendations for prosthetic components for a simulated client.

CASE STUDIES

Our four clients are listed below.

Janice Simmons, a 63-year-old female with a transtibial amputation secondary to diabetic gangrene.

Richard Canto, a 20-year-old male with a transtibial amputation secondary to an explosion while on military duty.

John Adams, a 72-year-old male with a transfemoral amputation secondary to arteriosclerotic gangrene.

Linda Bean, a 10-year-old female with a transfemoral amputation secondary to bone cancer.

Case Study Activities

1. Describe the biomechanics and alignment characteristics of the transtibial and the ischial containment transfemoral sockets.
   a. Differentiate between the quadrilateral and the ischial containment socket.
   b. Describe the major characteristics of variations on the ischial containment socket.
2. Differentiate between different types of prosthetic feet by function.

3. Differentiate functionally between different types of knee components.
4. Reflect on the extent that a person's lifestyle affects prosthetic replacement and selection of components.
5. What components would you select for each of the clients?

GENERAL CONCEPTS

Physical therapists may or may not be involved in recommending specific types of **components** depending on the setting; however, physical therapists must understand the function of different components to train the patient in their use. Technology has led to the development of ever more sophisticated and ever more functional components. The prosthetist is the most knowledgeable person in this area, and physical therapists should develop a good working relationship with all prosthetists in their community.

PROSTHETIC PRESCRIPTION

Any prosthesis needs to be comfortable, functional, and cosmetic, in that order. If the prosthesis is not comfortable, the client will not wear it; pain or discomfort can be the greatest impediment to successful prosthetic rehabilitation. The prosthesis must also be functional. It must allow the individual to perform desired activities that he or she would not be able to do without a prosthesis and do them with the lowest possible expenditure of energy. For most individuals, a well-fitting prosthesis will allow them to perform a greater range of mobility activities than they could on crutches or with a wheelchair. This may not be true for elderly individuals with transfemoral amputations or those with bilateral amputations. When the energy demands for prosthetic mobility are greater than for mobility without a prosthesis, the prosthesis is rarely worn. (See Chapter 7 for more details on energy demands.) Finally, the prosthesis must be as cosmetic as possible. The importance of cosmesis varies with each person and each situation. It is not uncommon for individuals to wear a prosthesis without cosmetic cover, preferring the better foot response to the improved cosmesis. Many individuals have no difficulty wearing shorts with a prosthesis, but for others, appearance is of greater importance. The client's needs and desires must be explored in some detail prior to selecting individual components. It is also very important to educate the client about the many options. The prosthetist will explore all the options with the client and is an integral part of the prosthetic rehabilitation team.

Modern technology and materials have produced a plethora of prosthetic components, some very sophisticated and very expensive. An active individual can have a different prosthesis for sports and for everyday use. Some prosthetic feet adjust to changes in heel height, allowing an individual to switch from sports to dress shoes. Microprocessor knee mechanisms provide multiple controls that make descending stairs, ramps, and curbs automatic, and powered prostheses are just around the corner. Prostheses can be made very lightweight, improving function and reducing energy expenditure. A discussion of each available component and material is well beyond the scope of this book and would probably be outdated by the time the book is published. Therefore, components will be described by type and function rather than individual names, and will focus on components in common use today. Each physical therapist (PT) needs to work closely with local prosthetists to ensure an understanding of the function of the client's particular components. Additionally, the orthotic and prosthetic community has a website (www.oandp.com) that is an excellent starting place for sources of information about different components. Many component manufacturers also include educational materials on their websites to help health professionals understand the function and use of specific components.

THE PROSTHESIS

Any lower extremity prosthesis includes a socket with or without a liner or interface, a method of suspension, and a foot. Transfemoral prostheses also incorporate

a knee mechanism. Most prostheses today use a modular concept in that components of standard design and dimensions are readily interchangeable and adjustable (**endoskeletal**). Through this system, various combinations of components can be tried to find the optimum combination for a given patient. The modular system offers simple and fast maintenance. It also permits more frequent and easier adjustments of alignment. It permits socket interchange without destroying the prosthesis. A flexible foam cover provides an improved appearance and can be removed for adjustments when necessary. Adjustable devices are particularly beneficial to children because the growth process necessitates frequent changes. In some instances, once fabricated, the prosthetic components are covered with a permanent hard lamination (**exoskeletal**). This is not done frequently today but may be used for individuals whose activities require protection for the components. Lower extremity prosthetic components are usually rated for maximum size and weight. Most components are rated up to 250 to 300 lb with some rated for higher weights.

SOCKETS

The prosthetic **socket** is the point of contact between the patient and the prosthesis. The skill of the prosthetist in making the small adjustments necessary to individualize the socket can be critical to the success of prosthetic rehabilitation. Socket design varies with the level of amputation and the configurations of the individual residual limb. Specific socket design is discussed with the appropriate prosthesis. Some general principles of socket design apply to all prostheses. PTs and physical therapist assistants (PTAs) should understand basic design principles to properly evaluate the fit of a prosthesis.

The prosthetic socket must support body weight and hold the residual limb firmly and comfortably during all activities (**Fig. 6.1A,B**). Each area of the residual limb tolerates pressure differently; therefore, tissues are selectively loaded so that the most weight is borne by pressure-tolerant tissue, such as wide and flat bony areas or tendons, and least by pressure-sensitive tissue, such as nerves that are close to the skin and sharp bony prominences. This is accomplished by relief in the form of socket concavity over pressure-sensitive areas and socket convexity over the pressure-tolerant areas. Additionally, the socket needs to grip the residual limb firmly to reduce or eliminate movement between the socket and the skin. The more

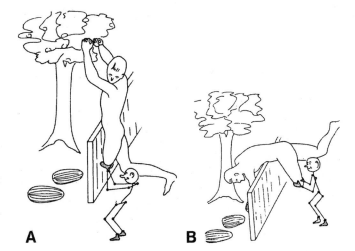

FIGURE 6.1. The prosthesis must **(A)** support the body weight and **(B)** hold the residual limb firmly during all activities. *(From Hall CB: Prosthetic socket shape as related to anatomy in lower extremity amputees. Clin Orthop 37, 1964, with permission.)*

movement occurs between the residual limb and socket, the more insecure the client is during activities and the greater risk of skin abrasions.

There are several ways the prosthetist may fabricate the individual prosthetic socket. Traditionally, the prosthetist casted the residual limb, noting the individual characteristics, then made a positive mold from which the socket was fabricated using special equipment. More commonly today, the prosthetist will scan the residual limb using a digital scanning laser system attached to a computer. Complete cross-sectional and three-dimensional pictures are created along with specific data (**Fig. 6.2**). The prosthetist then sends the images and other data to a central fabrication facility that actually creates the socket using other computers. The computer-created socket designed from the scanned images is more accurate and more cost efficient than the hand-fabricated socket. All prosthetic sockets today are fabricated of some

sort of plastic components. Some are impregnated with carbon filaments for durability and flexibility (**Fig. 6.3**).

The socket is connected to the appropriate foot (transtibial) or knee/foot assembly (transfemoral) with an alignment instrument and a pylon (**Fig. 6.4**). Once the prosthesis is assembled, the prosthetist performs a **static alignment** with the client standing to set the length and to align the foot, or the knee and foot, according to basic alignment principles to maximize comfort and function. The prosthetist will also have the patient walk in the parallel bars to ensure that each part of the prosthesis is aligned for normal function (**dynamic alignment**). At this point, new amputees should be referred to physical therapy for gait training. Unfortunately, this is not always done,

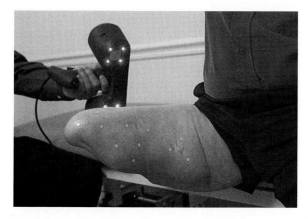

FIGURE 6.2. Digital limb scanner used for socket fabrication.

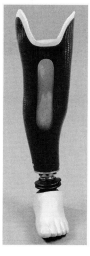

FIGURE 6.3. Total surface-bearing socket reinforced with carbon fiber.

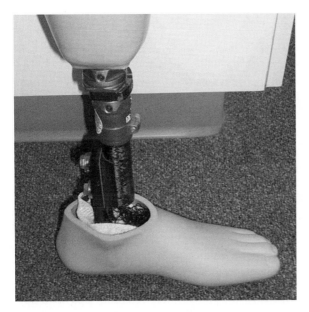

FIGURE 6.4. Transtibial prosthesis on an alignment instrument. A small wrench is used to loosen the four screws under the socket and move the socket as desired.

as some prosthetists try to perform gait training as part of the fitting sessions. The best patient care results from close cooperation between prosthetist and physical therapist, with each providing the care he or she is best educated to perform. (Gait training is presented in Chapter 7.)

Socket Interfaces

A socket interface is something that goes between the residual limb and the socket. Traditionally, in all but suction transfemoral prostheses, cotton or wool stump socks were used as the interface. Constructed of different thicknesses or plies, the socks acted as cushions to protect the residual limb from some of the stresses of prosthetic wear. For many years, polyethylene foam inserts have been used in the transtibial prosthesis along with wool socks. Although they provide a cushioning interface, they do not reduce the shear forces integral to the limb/socket interface. (See Chapter 2 for further discussion of forces.) Today there are a great variety of interfaces, although flexible gel liners may be the most common. Made of silicone or polyurethane materials, gel liners come in different thicknesses and styles (**Fig. 6.5**). Functionally, they all cushion the residual limb, decrease or eliminate shear forces, and help suspend the prosthesis. They are particularly useful for patients with scarred residual limbs, sensitive skin, or

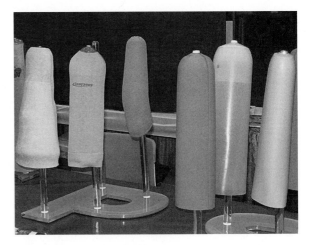

FIGURE 6.5. A variety of gel liners.

areas with grafted skin. Gel liners adhere to the skin and provide intimate contact between the residual limb and the socket. Most gel liners are donned on a clean and dry residual limb, but there are some special liners that require that a powder or liquid be applied to the skin prior to donning. Although most are fabricated of hypoallergenic materials, on rare occasions an individual will encounter irritability with a particular liner. There are some liners particularly fabricated for individuals with sensitive skin. The physical therapist needs to check with the prosthetist or on the manufacturer's website to make sure that proper instructions for donning are given to the patient.

Some gel liners are part of the suspension system as described below. Although many patients have stated a preference for the gel liners, in a study comparing satisfaction with polyethylene inserts, silicone liners, and polyurethane liners, no statistically significant differences were found.[1] Gel liners are not as durable as foam inserts, and patients are usually given two at the time of initial fitting. Newer materials have increased durability in recent years.

Some individuals do not like the feel of the gel liner against the skin and use a thin nylon sheath between the residual limb and the gel liner. These also come in different sizes for different residual limbs. There are silver-impregnated nylon sheaths for people with particularly sensitive skin. There are also small gel-impregnated pads that can be used to provide extra cushioning over a bony prominence or irritated area. Care must be taken when adding these materials, as changes in the thickness of any interface can influence the fit of the socket. (See Chapter 7.)

Suspension

As the patient participates in daily activities, the prosthetic socket moves against the residual limb, particularly in the swing phase of gait. Any movement between the socket and the prosthesis, however minimal, over time can cause discomfort and skin abrasions and interfere with patient function. Movement between the skin and socket is called **pistoning**, and the most effective suspension is the one that eliminates pistoning. Suction suspension is used with both the transtibial and transfemoral prostheses and eliminates all movement between the residual limb and the socket. Essentially, a vacuum is created within the socket to achieve suspension, and a one-way valve is used to prevent air from entering the socket once the vacuum has been achieved, or to eliminate any air that might enter during movement.[2] It was initially used only with the transfemoral prosthesis and only when the residual limb was smooth and pliable and free of scars or abrasions. Initially, the patient donned the prosthesis by pulling the residual limb into the close-fitting socket; as the limb went into the socket, air was expelled, and the valve maintained the vacuum. Newer techniques allow greater use of suction suspension that will be discussed further with the specific prostheses.

The shuttle lock or locking liner system of suspension is also used with both the transtibial and transfemoral prostheses. The flexible roll-on liner has a pin at the distal end that locks into a receptacle at the end of the socket when the patient puts his or her weight into the prosthesis. (See Table 6.2.) This system provides excellent suspension, but on occasion, patients have developed small bursae at the distal end of the residual limb from the constant lifting and dropping of the socket against the end of the residual limb during gait.

There are a variety of belts, straps, and neoprene sleeves that are also used for suspension. They will be discussed with the specific prosthesis.

ANKLE/FOOT MECHANISMS

The prosthetic foot is the foundation of the prosthesis; ideally, it should duplicate the functions of the normal foot. If the prosthetic foot is to replace the normal foot, it should serve the following functions:

- Simulate joint motion and muscle activity: the normal foot allows dorsiflexion/plantar flexion, inversion/eversion, and a smooth rollover from heel contact to toe off.

- Simulate muscle activity: The anatomic foot and ankle have a complex neuromuscular structure that allows for considerable control of mobility activities such as running, jumping, balancing on narrow surfaces, or standing on one foot.
- Shock absorption: the foot needs to absorb the forces generated at heel contact while allowing a smooth progression to foot flat and toe off. Prosthetic feet for transtibial or lower levels need to allow the knee flexion to occur during early stance phase.
- A stable base of support: the foot must stabilize the body during the stance phase of gait as well as during activities such as running, jumping, and so forth.

Traditionally, prosthetic feet have been classified as conventional (SACH), single axis, multiaxis, flexible keel, and dynamic response (also known as energy storage and return [ESAR], energy storing or dynamic elastic).[2,3] Dynamic response feet generally have some sort of spring-like keel that stores energy at heel contact or loading and then releases it in terminal stance. The majority of feet in use today incorporate some sort of dynamic response. They may be articulated or nonarticulated and may be constructed of various materials such as plastics or carbon fiber. Additionally, a foot may incorporate a single-axis ankle, simulating plantar and dorsiflexion limitedly, or multiaxis, additionally simulating inversion and eversion. All these motions are passive, in response to an external stimulus such as heel contact or uneven surface. Most prosthetic feet in use today are actually hybrids, combining characteristics for maximum function. The most common combination is a foot that incorporates a multiaxis ankle with a dynamic response foot. **Table 6.1** outlines the major categories in use today with their advantages and disadvantages as well as looks at future developments.

The SACH foot, the most used foot in the world for more than 50 years, has little place in today's market of technologically sophisticated components. There is a tendency among clinicians to use the traditional SACH foot for elderly individuals who may only walk limitedly. However, there is some evidence that the SACH foot with its rigid keel and lack of response in terminal stance may actually increase double stance time and reduce gait efficiency.[4] The person with limited walking ability and the need for knee stability may actually benefit more from a single-axis foot with dynamic response characteristics. Today, the SACH

TABLE 6.1   Prosthetic Feet

Foot	Description	Advantages	Disadvantages
SACH (solid ankle cushioned heel)	Nonarticulated, rigid wood keel, rubber heel wedge of varying density, rubberized forefoot	Inexpensive, low maintenance, thought to increase plantar flexion at initial contact	No energy return, abrupt dorsiflexion stop after midstance, no adjustment to varied surfaces, thought to maintain a stance phase that was too long
Single axis	Articulated foot with rubber bumpers simulating plantar flexion and dorsiflexion	Fast foot flat enhances knee stability	No energy return, increases knee extension moment at midstance, not for transtibial, requires maintenance
Dynamic response, nonarticulated *From the M+IND Corporation, with permission.*	Nonarticulated, rigid keel with plastic insert that stores and returns a limited amount of energy	Inexpensive, low maintenance, rollover characteristics, good for individuals with limited variation in gait speed and surfaces	Low energy return, little adaption to varied surfaces
Dynamic response, multiaxis	Dorsiflexion/plantar flexion, inversion/eversion with carbon fiber energy return	Varying levels of energy return, adapts to varied surfaces, may allow heel height adjustment, many different models	Heavier than nonarticulated, more expensive, may need more maintenance
Hydraulic	Multiaxis with shock absorption, carbon foot plate with hydraulic controls	Moderate to high energy return, adjusts to varied surfaces, smooth rollover stance phase	Expensive, slightly heavier than some models, not as durable as some feet

TABLE 6.1	Prosthetic Feet—cont'd		
Foot	**Description**	**Advantages**	**Disadvantages**
Powered ankles 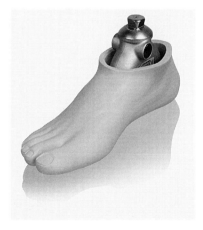 From H. Herr, MIT Education with permission.	Multiaxis provides positive push off in terminal stance and in lifting activities; some battery, some robotic designs	Smooth computer-controlled response to varied surfaces with some active push off at different gait speeds and in ascent and descent activities	Expensive, early design available in limited markets, other designs experimental only, some have problems with weight and battery life

foot is useful mainly for toddlers and infants who have yet to achieve a step-over gait. It is also used in many third-world countries for its low cost, ease of fabrication, and low maintenance.

The only patient who cannot benefit from a dynamic response foot at some level is the individual who does not load the forefoot in normal gait and does not activate the response mechanism. All other individuals should be fitted with a multiaxis ankle and a foot with some dynamic response. The degree of return is determined by the individual's activity level, body weight, and, unfortunately, finances. A more active person may desire a higher level of return, but a lighter weight person may not be able to control the foot adequately. The degree of response is also related to the materials within the foot. Generally, those constructed from carbon fiber have been found to have a higher return than those made from plastics (**Fig. 6.6**).[2] The weight of the foot is also a consideration. Because the foot is at the end of the prosthesis, it is generally thought that the lighter the better. However, too light a foot can reduce the patient's sense of where the foot is in space and may make walking in sand or high grass difficult. Generally, multiaxis feet are somewhat heavier than single-axis feet, but improved function and efficiency mitigate against the problems of weight.[5] There are a great variety of dynamic response feet on the market, including some that incorporate the ability to change heel height on the shoe. Because the prosthesis is aligned with the shoe on the prosthesis, changes in heel height, such as going from a running shoe to a dress shoe, would change the alignment. Many dynamic response feet allow for slight changes in heel height, and some, like the Elation® foot (**Fig. 6.7**), allow for up to 5 centimeters.

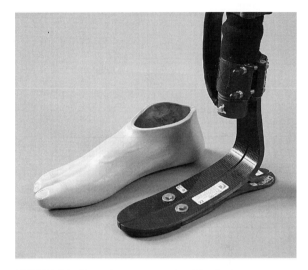

FIGURE 6.6. Dynamic response carbon fiber foot.

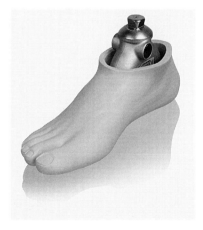

FIGURE 6.7. The Elation® foot allows for changes in heel height. *(Courtesy of Össur America, www.ossur.com.)*

There have been numerous studies comparing the mechanical properties of different prosthetic feet. There have also been many studies on human responses to different feet. The problem is that these studies have little in common, and results are difficult to compare. A mechanical study may show no statistically significant differences between some feet while patients perceive improved function and less fatigue with some feet over others. Hafner and associates found little correlation between patient perception of the function of various feet and statistically significant results of biomechanical studies. They suggested that newer methods of analysis may help the clinician when selecting a foot for a particular patient.[6]

The physical therapist and physical therapist assistant working with the individual patient need to understand the characteristics of the prosthetic foot to evaluate any gait problems that may occur. As with all components, the prosthetist is the most knowledgeable person about the different feet and their characteristics and needs to be involved in any prosthetic prescription.

Today, prosthetic foot motion is responsive and not proactive, while the normal foot provides active motion. There has been considerable research in recent years on the development of a powered ankle that would provide active motion as needed for functional activities. Massachusetts Institute of Technology (MIT) engineers recently revealed a powered ankle that provides active motion for walking, climbing and descending stairs, and hill ascent and descent.[7] Tested on three individuals with transtibial amputations, the powered ankle was found to reduce energy consumption by about 20%, although heavier than passive components. It was also reported by one patient to reduce back discomfort as it did not require as much hip and trunk motion to perform high-level activities (http://www.media.mit.edu/press/ankle/).

Sawicki and Ferris[8,9] developed an experimental robotic pneumatic ankle that simulated the normal motion of the gastroc-soleus muscle. Their study again revealed lower energy use with the powered ankle and indicated that the Achilles tendon played a major part in push off. Össur developed the Proprio® foot (**Fig. 6.8**) incorporating artificial intelligence and specialized sensors to provide some assistance at critical times in gait and when rising from a chair. In limited production out of the United States, it will probably be generally available by the time this book is published.

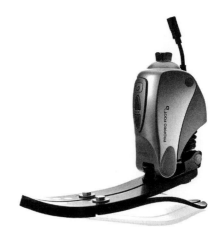

FIGURE 6.8. Össur Proprio® foot. *(Courtesy of Össur America, www.ossur.com.)*

THE TRANSTIBIAL PROSTHESIS

The Socket

The patellar tendon-bearing socket (PTB) is the standard for the transtibial prosthesis (**Fig. 6.9**). The patellar tendon is the major weight-bearing area with stabilizing pressure on the flares of the tibia, the shaft of the fibula, the posterior soft tissue, and, slightly, the distal end of the socket. Areas of relief include the crest and anterior distal end of the tibia and the head of the fibula where the peroneal nerve is close to the skin (**Fig. 6.10**). The medial and lateral walls come above the knee to at least the level of the adductor tubercle of the

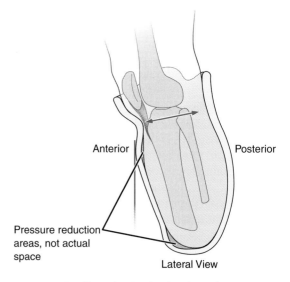

FIGURE 6.9. Patella tendon-bearing (PTB) prosthesis.

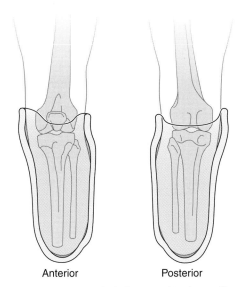

Anterior   Posterior

FIGURE 6.10. Pressure and relief areas within the patella tendon-bearing (PTB) socket.

femur and can be extended to come just above the femoral condyles for better mediolateral knee stability. The anterior wall comes to about mid-patella and is slightly flared above the patellar bar to avoid pressure on the patella. The optimum level for the posterior brim is the popliteal crease, but it must be low enough to allow the client to sit with knee flexed at least 90 degrees, yet high enough to prevent undue bulging of flesh over the brim. The proximal edge is rounded to prevent sharp pressure on the back of the knee; grooves are provided at the medial and lateral corners for the hamstring tendons. The medial groove is deeper because the semitendinosus inserts more distally than the biceps femoris. There is, of course, total contact at the distal end for proprioceptive feedback and proper support of the residual limb. The socket is contoured by the shape of the residual limb and is designed to provide appropriate support throughout.

Many PTB prosthetic sockets use the principle of total surface bearing (TSB), where pressures are distributed throughout the residual limb except for particularly sensitive areas, and there is less weight bearing on the patellar tendon. A variation in the TSB socket is the hydrostatic socket where the cast is made under compression to ensure good distribution of pressures.[10] There is some thought that roll-on liners fit better with the TSB socket design rather than the traditional PTB design. In an early study, patients clearly indicated a preference for a hydrostatic interface.[11] TSB and

hydrostatic designs tend to be used more when the residual limb has matured and is less likely to be subject to large volume fluctuations. There is some thought, however, that minor fluid changes may be more manageable with the TSB type of socket. Gel liners are used with both the TSB and the hydrostatic variations.

Interfaces

Most PTB prostheses are constructed to be used with some sort of an insert or liner—an interface between the residual limb and the hard walls of the prosthesis. The polyurethane foam insert (**Fig. 6.11**) is used specifically with the PTB socket, although gel liners are more common and provide better comfort and protection of the residual limb. The polyurethane foam liner, used with residual limb socks, allows for easy adjustments for fluid changes and is more often indicated for preparatory prostheses or with patients who have major volume changes in the residual limb during the day or from one day to the next. Individuals on renal dialysis tend to have problems with fluid changes. Any of the liners and interfaces mentioned above can be used with the PTB socket.

Suspension

Table 6.2 describes suspensions specific to the PTB prosthesis. Most commonly used today is suction suspension, either with an expulsion valve or a

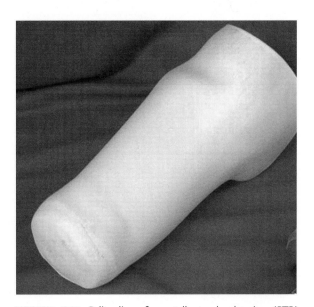

FIGURE 6.11. Pelite liner for patella tendon-bearing (PTB) prosthesis.

TABLE 6.2	Patellar Tendon-Bearing (PTB) Suspension Systems		
Suspension	**Description**	**Advantages**	**Disadvantages**
Suction: valve and sleeve	Expulsion valve in bottom of socket used with lightweight suction sleeve to hold vacuum, sleeve must fit above liner to skin	Secure, comfortable suspension allowing no pistoning; improved proprioception and limb control	Expensive, frequent sleeve replacement, may restrict knee motion to some extent, does not adjust well to volume changes in residual limb, may retain heat and increase perspiration
Suction: valve and liner	Specially designed liner with built-in seals that conform to residual limb plus expulsion valve in bottom of socket	Secure, comfortable suspension allowing no pistoning; allows free knee motion; improved proprioception and limb control	Expensive, liner may need frequent replacement, does not adjust well to volume changes in residual limb, may retain heat and increase perspiration

TABLE 6.2	Patellar Tendon-Bearing (PTB) Suspension Systems—cont'd		
Suspension	**Description**	**Advantages**	**Disadvantages**
Shuttle lock/locking liner	Pin at end of gel liner fits into lock in bottom of socket	Can be donned sitting (although pin locks on weight bearing), secure suspension with no pistoning, use of socks external to liner allows for residual limb volume changes	Some patients find distal pulling on swing uncomfortable, can develop distal bursa, may retain heat and increase perspiration
Neoprene sleeve	Textured, rubberized sleeve that is fitted over prosthesis and rolls over the liner or socks to mid-thigh, some have circular band to increase suspension	Easy to don, inexpensive, suspends well	Sleeve needs frequent replacement, may be hard to don for person with hand problems, circular band may cause residual limb swelling

Continued

TABLE 6.2　Patellar Tendon-Bearing (PTB) Suspension Systems—cont'd

Suspension	Description	Advantages	Disadvantages
PTB-SCSP (patellar tend on-bearing, supracondylar, suprapatellar)	Prosthetic socket covers patella and femoral condyles, medial femoral wedge aids in suspension	May be used for shorter residual limb, good cosmesis	Allows some pistoning, may slip on full knee flexion, not used frequently
Supracondylar cuff	Leather cuff that fits over patella and attaches to medial and lateral wings of socket	Easy to don, simple, inexpensive	Allows some pistoning, circumferential around distal thigh, not used frequently

suction sleeve, the shuttle lock system, or the neoprene sleeve. New suction Iceross Seal-In® suspension liner (www.ossur.com/prosthetics/liners/sealinliner) incorporates five seals that conform to residual limb and socket wall shape to provide secure suspension without an external sleeve. Rarely today, the upper part of the socket is extended to enclose the patella and the medial and lateral condyles of the femur (patellar tendon-bearing, supracondylar, suprapatellar [PTB-SCSP]). Supracondylar cuffs are used in some areas and are not indicated for individuals with dysvascular problem because of the need to attach the cuff around the distal femur.

Pylons

Pylons are the metal pipes that connect the foot to the socket. They are usually made of lightweight carbon graphite materials with a socket connector that allows aligning the socket on the foot (Chapter 7). There are a variety of shock-absorbing and rotational pylon that provide additional shock absorption for active wearers. Some are external to the regular pylon, and others are built into the pylon connection, like the Össur Ceterus® (**Fig. 6.12**). Rotational components absorb some of the sheer forces created by the normal rotational forces of gait. Although these components add some weight to the prosthesis, the benefits make it worthwhile for the active wearer who walks at a fast pace, walks on uneven surfaces, and participates in varied activities. The therapist, patient, and prosthetist must consult to determine if any of these devices is suitable for the individual

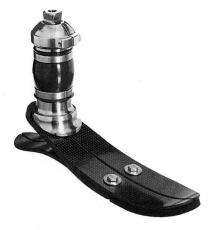

FIGURE 6.12. Össur Ceterus® shock absorbing rotational component. (*Courtesy of Ossur America, www.ossur.com.*)

person. They may or may not be reimbursable by third-party payers.

Alignment

The alignment of the prosthesis refers to the way each component is placed in relation to the other. The prosthesis must be aligned to allow each component to function as close to normal as possible and to make sure forces are distributed appropriately (Chapter 2). The alignment instrument built into the pylon allows the prosthetist to change the anterior-posterior position, the mediolateral position, the rotation of the foot, and the tilt of the socket in any direction, as well as the overall height of the prosthesis. The prosthesis is aligned so that a plumb line dropped from the greater trochanter through the knee to the ankle (TKA) will bisect the knee and come slightly anterior to the simulated ankle so that the weight is distributed evenly between the heel and the forefoot to allow for a smooth transition through stance (**Fig. 6.13A**). The mediolateral alignment must provide a stable surface on the floor as well as create a slight normal genu varum at midstance (**Fig. 6.13B**). The foot is inset enough to allow a reasonably narrow gait base (no more than about 2 inches). The foot is also aligned in about 5 to 7 degrees of external rotation simulating normal toe out. The height of the prosthesis is determined by the length of the other leg so that the iliac crests are level when the patient stands with weight distributed evenly between the legs. The socket is aligned in about 5 to 8 degrees of flexion to assist with the initial knee flexion from heel contact to midstance as well as to put the quadriceps on a slight stretch to help control terminal stance knee recurvatum (**Fig. 6.13C**).[12,13] Specific alignment is, of course, determined by the individual. People with heavy thighs may need the foot more offset; people with very short residual limbs may not tolerate as much inset as needed. If the person has not had any gait training, it is often advisable to institute gait training before alignment is finalized, because the gait pattern will change as the patient develops the balance and prosthetic control for a smooth, energy-efficient gait.

TRANSFEMORAL PROSTHESIS

Sockets

Although the transtibial residual limb generally has areas that allow for contouring and stabilization, the transfemoral residual limb with its single bone well

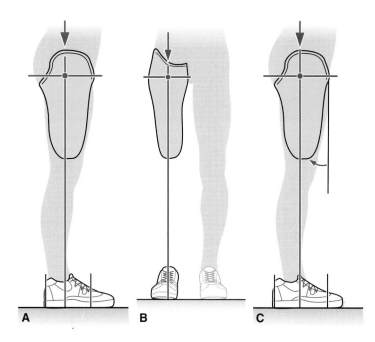

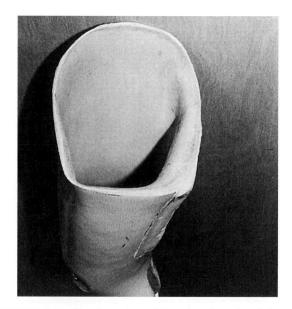

FIGURE 6.13. (A) Anterior-posterior foot alignment. **(B)** Mediolateral foot alignment for narrow base gait. **(C)** The PTB socket is set in about 5 degrees of flexion.

buried in muscle and soft tissue does not. The less stabilization and rotational control, the greater is the energy required for ambulatory activities and the less is the proprioceptive feedback. In particular, the problem of mediolateral stability in stance and the need to control the femur in adduction during stance phase has influenced socket design. Traditionally, the quadrilateral socket has been the socket of choice. Today, the ischial containment socket is the most commonly used, although there is some variation by part of the country and prosthetic facility. Interfaces for the transfemoral prosthesis are the same as for the transtibial limb and need not be discussed further. As indicated below, on occasion, there is no interface between the residual limb and the socket.

The Quadrilateral Socket

The quadrilateral socket (**Fig. 6.14**) was developed in the late 1950s and is named for the shape of the socket. Distally the socket is contoured to provide total contact. Weight bearing is primarily on top of the posterior wall with the anterior wall coming higher in the front to help stabilize the residual limb to maintain its position during walking. The lateral wall is adducted to help control the femur on stance, and the medial wall is perpendicular to provide counterpressure. The quadrilateral socket is

smaller in an anterior/posterior dimension than in the medial–lateral direction. The quadrilateral socket provides minimal medial–lateral and little rotational stability. It is not often prescribed today as the first socket; however, individuals who have worn a quadrilateral socket for many years may be loath to try a different design.

FIGURE 6.14. Transfemoral quadrilateral socket, viewed from above.

The Ischial Containment Socket

The ischial containment socket (**Fig. 6.15**) was developed in the late 1980s and early 1990s to improve pelvic control in stance, increase comfort during weight bearing, and provide for a smoother swing phase of gait. The ischium is contained within the socket, and weight-bearing forces are distributed partially on the ischium and throughout the soft tissue of the residual limb. Compared to the quadrilateral socket, more of the residual limb is contained within the socket, allowing for greater distribution of weight-bearing and stabilizing forces. The narrow medial–lateral dimension and molding over the femoral shaft help keep the ischium and the ramus against the posteromedial wall of the socket as well as contribute to rotational stability. The lateral wall is extended well over the greater trochanter to add to stance phase stability of the pelvis. The socket is contoured for total contact throughout. The ischial containment socket may be constructed of rigid or flexible materials depending on the needs of the patient. Flexible sockets are placed within a rigid frame for support and stabilization with flexible areas that allow muscles to function.[14] The ischial containment is probably the most commonly used socket for transfemoral amputees today. If someone has been wearing a quadrilateral socket for many years, he or she may want to continue to use that design, but most new amputees are fitted with ischial containment sockets.

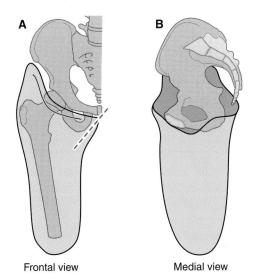

FIGURE 6.15. (A) Frontal view of the femur and pelvis in the ischial containment socket. **(B)** Medial view of the pelvis in the ischial containment socket.

A   B

Frontal view   Medial view

Variations of the Ischial Containment Socket

Over the years, creative prosthetists have made variations in the basic socket design to improve comfort and function. Several of these variations are in use today, and the physical therapist and physical therapist assistant may work with patients with these types of sockets. If a therapist has a patient with a varied socket design, it is always advisable to discuss the design with the prosthetist to ensure that the therapist understands the implications of that design on function.

Although the ischial containment socket helps control medio/lateral stability better than the quadrilateral socket, the need to provide increased stability and residual limb control of the socket has led to the development of the Hanger ComfortFlex™ socket (www.hanger.com) (**Fig. 6.16**). The socket is contoured to lock the pubic ramus and ischium within the socket and provide channels for functioning muscle groups such as the hip adductors and extensors. The socket is made of soft plastic that is meant to fit directly over the residual limb. However, a gel liner or stump sock interface may be used, although such an interface lessens the degree of proprioceptive feedback. The socket is designed to encourage the individual to use remaining musculature actively within the socket during locomotion. The socket can be used for new as well as experienced amputees, although the intimate fit is more effective if the individual has a more mature residual limb. The socket is usually placed within a carbon graphite frame (**Fig. 6.17**) that has the property to tighten during muscle activity and relax during nonactive periods. The intimate fit makes the socket a little more difficult to don; a small turning motion is sometimes required to fit the socket in correctly. Any therapist working with a patient fitted with this socket needs to learn proper donning procedures.

Marlo Ortiz (http://www.oandp.com/articles/2002-11_01.asp), a prosthetist from Mexico, responding to a patient's needs, lowered the posterior wall of the socket to the level of the gluteal fold, thereby leaving the bulk of the gluteus maximus out of the socket. In so doing, he found that the patient was more comfortable sitting, and rather than losing socket stability, the pubic ramus could be more easily and comfortably contained within the socket. The resulting prosthesis also provided for greater range of motion at the hip.[15]

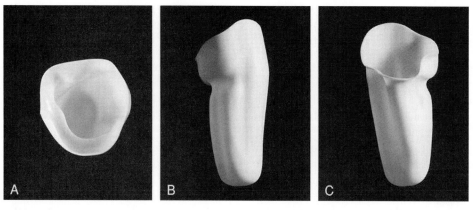

FIGURE 6.16. Three views of the hanger ComfortFlex™ socket: **(A)** top view, **(B)** lateral view, and **(C)** medial view. *(Courtesy Hanger Prosthetics & Orthotics, Inc.)*

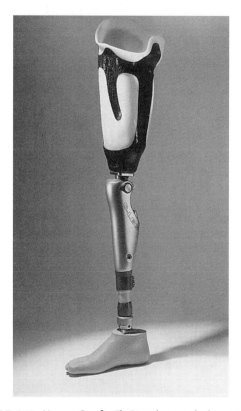

FIGURE 6.17. Hanger ComfortFlex™ socket attached to a Bock "C" leg. *(Courtesy Hanger Prosthetic & Orthotics, Inc.)*

Suspension

Table 6.3 outlines the major suspensions in use today for the transfemoral prosthesis. Suction either with the suspension liner or the hard socket is probably the more common suspension in use today followed by the Silesian band. Donning the hard socket suction prosthesis (**Fig. 6.18**) requires the ability to stand and pull the residual limb into the close-fitting socket. As the residual limb enters the socket, air is pushed out. When the residual limb is fully into the socket, the valve is inserted, creating a negative pressure within the socket. Generally, the patient dons a special pull sock or light cotton sock over the residual limb, pushes the end of the sock out the valve hole, and pulls the sock out of the valve while pushing the residual limb into the socket. The sock is totally removed, making sure all soft tissue is contained within the socket. This requires the ability to stand and balance while pulling the sock out. If the suction liner is used, it can be donned sitting, and then the person stands and puts the residual limb in the liner in the socket, easily pushing the air out the valve hole. When the patient is properly in the socket, the valve is replaced, and air is not allowed to return.

KNEE MECHANISMS

The prosthetic knee has several functions:

■ To support the body weight during stance phase at any gait speed and surface
■ To allow for a smooth and controlled movement of the shank and foot during swing phase at any gait speed and surface
■ To allow for stair climbing and descent, sitting, kneeling, and similar activities

A wide variety of knee mechanisms are on the market today; they perform a great variety of functions and range in complexity from simple to highly complex. None totally duplicate normal knee motion, as, like the foot, they are responsive and not

TABLE 6.3 Transfemoral Suspension Systems

Suspension	Description	Advantages	Disadvantages
Suction (hard socket)	Hard socket worn against residual limb (RL); donning pushes air out, valve maintains vacuum	Allows full freedom of hip motion, total suspension without pistoning, good proprioceptive feedback-through its intimate fit	Suction can be lost through perspiration, potential for skin irritation in a closed medium, requires good balance and coordination for donning, must be donned properly
Soft liner with suction Shuttle lock Lanyard lock	Suction with seal liner as TT (transtibial). Shuttlelock as TT Lanyard from end of liner locks into small attachment in socket	As above, good suspension without pistoning, full hip motion, intimidate fit; easy to don; can be donned sitting	May create heat and perspiration, liner may need replacement regularly
Silesian band	Soft webbing strap that is attached to the lateral socket wall, encircles the pelvis and connects with a strap on the anterior wall	Lightweight suspension, inexpensive, easy to don	Allows some pistoning; difficult to keep clean unless it is detachable; can irritate the waist; difficult to don without good shoulder ROM

Continued

TABLE 6.3	Transfemoral Suspension Systems—cont'd		
Suspension	**Description**	**Advantages**	**Disadvantages**
Total elastic suspension 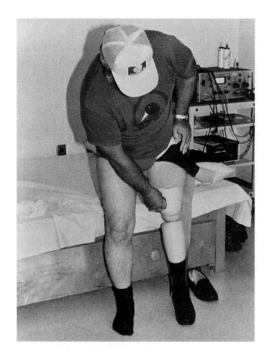	Wide neoprene sleeve attached to proximal socket and goes around waist and pelvis to suspend prosthesis	Inexpensive, adjusts to the size of the individual, provides some rotational control	Allows some pistoning, retains body heat that may lead to skin irritations and discomfort, needs frequent replacement, difficult to keep clean; uncomfortable for individuals with large abdomens

FIGURE 6.18. Donning a transfemoral prosthesis with suction suspension.

proactive. Knee mechanism may be simply mechanical, may function with the use of hydraulic or pneumatic mechanisms, or may be computerized. They range in price from a few hundred dollars to many thousands of dollars. It is beyond the scope of this

text to review all available knee mechanisms. Therapists are encouraged to learn the specific characteristics of the knee mechanism of their patient through discussion with the prosthetist or through the manufacturer website. For ease of discussion, knee mechanisms will be presented in relation to their function and method of control. **Table 6.4** outlines the basic types of knee mechanisms with their advantages and disadvantages.

Knee Control

Basically, knee systems can be divided into those that provide only swing phase control, only stance phase control, or both. Swing phase control refers to the degree of variation of the speed of swing of the prosthetic **shank** in response to varied gait speeds. Think of the shank as a modified pendulum—at toe off, knee flexion is initiated by the forward movement of the body and momentum. Without controls, the knee would flex and then swing back down like a pendulum. A smooth, energy-efficient gait requires that the prosthetic foot be ready for heel contact whether the person is walking slow or fast. It also requires that the prosthetic foot comes off the ground far enough so as not to catch the toe of the foot on the ground as it swings through. (During swing, the prosthetic foot is at 90 degrees because foot mechanisms are reactive and not proactive.)

TABLE 6.4   Knee Systems

Type of Knee	Description	Advantages	Disadvantages
Single axis	Single-speed swing phase control only	Inexpensive, durable, used mainly with children	No variation in swing with gait speed changes, no stance control
Stance phase control	Weight-activated friction brake stabilizes knee even if slightly flexed, limited swing phase control	Good knee stability, durable; indicated mainly for debilitated individuals using slow walking speeds	Weight has to be totally off prosthesis to initiate swing, no adjustments to gait speed changes; requires mostly slow walking
Polycentric	Four bar linkage system provides for moving knee axis	Provides some stance and swing phase control, good for long residual limbs, moving knee axis provides higher toe clearance on swing	Increased weight, needs good voluntary knee control

Continued

TABLE 6.4	Knee Systems—cont'd		
Type of Knee	**Description**	**Advantages**	**Disadvantages**
Manual lock	External system locks knee in extension until released manually	Total knee stability	Stiff knee gait requires considerable energy, used very limitedly
Fluid controlled	Hydraulic system controls knee flexion and extension	Swing and stance phase control, greater variability than polycentric, more normal gait, some are quite light	Expensive, may need more maintenance
Microprocessor	Computer-driven control of swing and stance phase	Quite variable cadence response, allows for easy descent of stairs and hills, closest to normal knee motion	Expensive, responsive only

Stance phase control refers to stability of the knee from heel contact to terminal stance as the person's weight shifts from the heel of the foot to the toes. This is extremely important. Stance phase control is a function of the alignment of the knee axis in relation to the TKA line (alignment control), the type of knee mechanism, and the patient's ability to control the knee by extending the residual limb and moving the pelvis forward at heel contact (voluntary control). (See Chapter 7 for details.) Ideally, the knee axis needs to fall either right on the TKA line or slightly anterior to bring the body weight anterior to the knee at heel contact and create an extension moment. If the patient is not confident that the prosthetic knee will be stable throughout stance phase, the patient will not develop a good energy-efficient gait pattern. Without stance phase control, either alignment, from the knee mechanisms or voluntary, the knee will flex suddenly as weight bearing is initiated. However, too much stance phase control interferes with swing initiation and leads to a halting gait pattern. What is desired is a stable knee during stance phase with an easy flexion of the knee to initiate swing.

Knees can also be divided by the mechanism by which they provide control: single axis, polycentric, fluid control, or microprocessor. The most appropriate knee mechanism for any individual is the one that provides stance phase stability, smooth swing phase initiation, and varied swing phase by gait speed, and requires the least amount of energy for daily activities. There is a balance between stance phase security and swing phase. The effort required to initiate swing phase is increased as more **alignment stability** is built into a prosthesis, thus affecting gait. The amount of alignment stability needed is inversely related to the length and strength of the residual limb. The amount of alignment stability needed is also determined by the type of knee mechanism used.

The single-axis knee is not used very much today except in children if durability is most important. Single-axis stance phase control knees use a weight-activated friction brake system. If the individual puts weight on the prosthesis in less than about 20 degrees of knee flexion, the brake is activated, and the friction will prevent the knee from collapsing. These are indicated for the more debilitated individual who generally walks slowly and does not change gait speed very much. It leads to a slow and somewhat energy-demanding gait. The ultimate stance control is a manual lock knee. This is not indicated for most amputees, because walking with a stiff knee is slow and energy demanding. On occasion, a manual lock knee has been used for bilateral transfemoral amputees, although there are more functional knees available today. (See Chapter 8.)

Polycentric knee joints are usually four-bar linkage systems. They have multiple axes of rotation that change during knee motion. These knees provide some swing phase control by shortening the shank during flexion to allow for better toe clearance and some response to changing gait speeds. They offer some stance phase control by varying stability through the different axes. Most prosthetic companies make one or more versions of the polycentric knee with varying characteristics. In general, the polycentric knee is particularly useful for individuals with long residual limbs or knee disarticulations, or for individuals who do not change walking speed a great deal. They are not the best knee mechanisms for active community ambulators or athletes.

There are a great variety of fluid-controlled knee mechanisms available today. Some provide only swing phase control and others provide both swing and stance phase control. Some units have an additional manual locking system for individuals working around a bench or climbing a ladder. Hydraulic mechanisms provide a normal heel rise and forward swing appropriate to the client's speed of walking. Some, for example, allow separate adjustments for heel rise and terminal swing and provide a high degree of resistance to knee flexion when weight is borne on the prosthesis. The hyperextension moment at the knee that occurs as the individual rolls over the foot disengages the stance control mechanisms, allowing a smooth heel off and knee flexion for swing phase. Many that provide some form of stance control, usually resistance to sudden flexion that allows a slow deceleration, allow the athletic client to walk downstairs step over step. Cost and weight are directly related to the complexity of function. Some are very light, and others add some weight to the prosthesis. Usually the more functions the unit can perform, the heavier it is.

There are several knee units that incorporate a microprocessor. The onboard computer chip provides a more fluid response to changes of cadence. The Otto Bock C-Leg® (www.ottobockus.com) (see **Fig. 6.17**) features an on-board sensor that reads and adapts to the changes in the person's gait cadence. Using a hydraulic-based system driven by the computer, it also incorporates stance phase control by providing resistance to knee flexion at appropriate times. The sensors read and respond to changes up to 50 times a second. Fine-tuning is done by the prosthetist using a computer and specially designed software. The client can move on flat terrain at different gait speeds with confidence as well as maneuver over slopes, stairs, and uneven surfaces. The Ossur Rheo® knee (**Fig. 6.19**) uses a computer-driven magnetorheological system to respond to the individual's walking style. It also responds to the individual's walking speed and the terrain to deliver the appropriate amount of resistance. It can be used with any currently available foot. Computerized knee mechanisms are expensive. They are ideal for community ambulators who have an active lifestyle. They are increasingly used in the general population and are covered by Medicare for active patients.

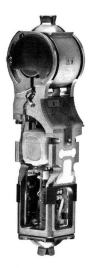

FIGURE 6.19. Rheo microprocessor knee. *(Courtesy of Össur America, www.ossur.com).*

Walking with a transfemoral prosthesis requires more concentration, planning, and concern with the terrain than walking with a transtibial prosthesis. As the person approaches a curb, he or she must make sure he or she can lead with the unamputated leg. Going down steps, step over step, or descending steep hills and ramps requires adaption to the regular gait. The developments of fluid-controlled knee systems, particularly those that included both swing and stance phase control, reduced such demands and allowed the amputee to walk more naturally. The advent of microprocessor knees has reduced such demands even more as the knee responds to a great variety of inputs and controls the knee under many situations. Bunce and associates surveyed 42 C-Leg (Otto Bock Health Care) wearers using several instruments to determine the attitude of the patients toward that particular prosthesis.[16] In general, the subjects indicated that they had a more normal gait with the C-Leg, could walk more automatically, and were less noticeably handicapped than with their previous prosthesis. There have also been a number of studies comparing the C-Leg to several hydraulic knee mechanisms. Hafner and associates studied 17 subjects ranging in age from 21 to 77 years of age as they transitioned from a nonmicroprocessor knee to the C-Leg. They evaluated their functional ability in level walking, stairs, and hills, as well as surveyed the subjects regarding their degree of satisfaction and responses to the C-Leg. They found statistically significant improvement in stair descent and hill descent, and a reduction in stumbles. The amputees reported greater satisfaction with the C-Leg and less cognitive planning when using the microprocessor knee.[17] Similar results were obtained in a study comparing the metabolic usage with the RHEO KNEE®, the C-Leg, and the MAUCH S-N-S®.[18] The two microprocessor knees both led to decreases in metabolic rate with the RHEO KNEE showing a greater decrease. There have been other studies indicating the clinical acceptance and value of microprocessor knee systems.[2] Such knees have only been on the market a few years; research and development continue, and prices decrease as the components come into general use and are accepted by third-party payers. At this writing, Medicare pays for the C-Leg for appropriate consumers.

Alignment

In the transfemoral prosthesis, alignment relates to the position of the socket in relation to the knee/foot assembly. Problems related to the foot/pylon relationship are not as common as in the transtibial prosthesis. (See Chapter 7 for specific gait deviations.) As in the transtibial prosthesis, the prosthetist aligns the socket in relation to basic principles. As stated above, stance phase knee stability is most critical; proper alignment places the knee axis on or just anterior to the TKA line. As in the transtibial prosthesis, the transfemoral socket is set in about 5 degrees of initial flexion primarily to assist with hip extension at initial contact and to prevent excessive extension of the lumbar spine as the person brings his or her weight over the hip joint from heel contact to midstance (**Fig. 6.20**). If the individual has a hip flexion contracture, the socket must be flexed 5 degrees beyond the contracture to allow for some active hip extension. The amount of contracture that can be accommodated depends on the length of the residual limb.

Medial–lateral stability in stance is also very important. In normal gait, the pelvis drops a few degrees toward the unsupported side. This motion is controlled by an eccentric contraction of the hip abductors as they stabilize the pelvis and trunk over the weight-bearing leg. This also helps shift the pelvis over the base of support and contributes to a narrow-based gait. The muscles can function

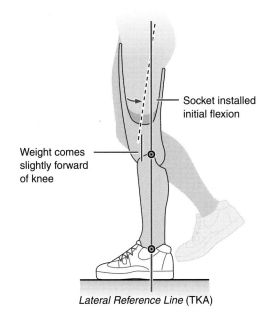

FIGURE 6.20. The transfemoral socket is aligned in a little flexion.

eccentrically, because the femur is stabilized by weight bearing. In the transfemoral amputee, the femur is not anchored to the lower leg fixed on the ground during weight bearing, but rather is loose in the soft tissue of the residual limb contained in the transfemoral socket (**Fig. 6.21**). Therefore, the socket has to provide enough lateral support to stabilize the femur and allow the hip abductors to function eccentrically. In addition to the shape of the socket, the socket is aligned in a little adduction. The

amount of lateral stability that can be built into the socket and into alignment is dependent on the length of the femur. The longer the femur is, the greater the surface over which the forces can be distributed.

OTHER COMPONENTS

In previous years, individuals wearing transfemoral prostheses were limited by the rigid linear relationships of socket to knee to foot. Many activities in daily life are best performed with the knee partially flexed and with some degree of rotation. Golf is one such activity requiring a combination of knee flexion and body rotation. Torsion adapters, rotators, and shock absorbers are available to provide assistance with many activities of daily living (**Fig. 6.22**). Many individuals, particularly in Asian cultures, sit cross-legged on the floor or on cushions. Other people like to rotate their leg and place the foot on the opposite knee. There are rotator mechanisms that can be inserted below the socket that allow full rotation of the knee and shank. A small locking mechanism below the socket allows the individual, while sitting, to unlock the limb and rotate the lower leg at least 90 degrees. This is also useful for getting in and out of a car or narrow seating areas such as a theater.

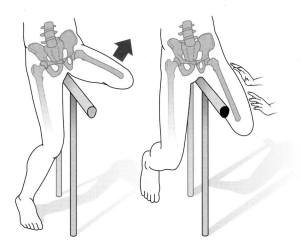

FIGURE 6.21. The socket and alignment must provide mediolateral (ML) stability for the femur.

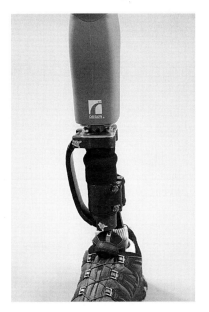

FIGURE 6.22. A shock absorber on the pylon of a transfemoral prosthesis.

SUMMARY

The field of prosthetic components is rapidly changing, and the physical therapist and physical therapist assistant need to work closely with local prosthetists or keep up to date on the Web to understand the characteristics of the particular components. Current research is leading to the development of active components and sensory feedback using computers, myoelectric controls, synthetic muscles and, possibly, neural controls.[19,20] The website, www.oandp.com is a useful entity to find the latest in prosthetic design and developments. Prosthetic checkout and gait training will be much more effective if the therapist understands socket design and the function of the major components.

KEYWORD FOR LITERATURE SEARCH

Artificial limb

C-Leg®

CATCAM

Computerized prosthesis

Prosthetic components

Prosthesis

Prosthetics

Prosthetist

REFERENCES

1. Van de Weg FB, Van der Windt DA: A questionnaire survey of the effect of different interface types on patient satisfaction and perceived problems among trans-tibial amputees. Prosthetics & Orthotics Int 29(3):231–239, 2005 Dec.

2. Michaels JW: Prosthetic suspensions and components. In Smith DG, Michael JW, Bowker JH (eds): Atlas of amputations and limb deficiencies: surgical, prosthetic, and rehabilitation principles, 3rd ed. Rosemont, IL, AAOS, 2004.

3. Hafner BJ: Clinical prescription and use of prosthetic foot and ankle mechanism: a review of the literature. JPO 17:s5–s11, 2005.

4. Gailey R: Functional value of prosthetic foot/ankle systems to the amputee. JPO 17:s39–s46, 2005.

5. Stark G: Perspectives on how and why feet are prescribed. JPO 17:s18–s22, 2005.

6. Hafner BJ, Sanders JE, Czerniecki J, Fergason J: Energy storage and return prostheses: does patient perception correlate with biomechanical analysis? Clinical Biomechanics. 17(5): 325–344, 2002.

7. Au SK, Herr H, Weber J, Martinez-Villalpando EC: Powered ankle-foot prosthesis for the improvement of amputee ambulation. Conf Proc IEEE Eng Med Biol Soc. 2007:3020–3026, 2007.

8. Sawicki GS, Ferris DP: Mechanics and energetics of level walking with powered ankle exoskeletons. J Exp Bio 211: 1402–1413, 2008.

9. Ferris DP, Gordon KE, Sawicki GS, Peethambaran A: An improved powered ankle-foot orthosis using proportional myoelectric control. Gait Posture 23(4):425–428, 2006.

10. Bosker GW, Walden G: Lower-Limb Prosthetics Society: the interfaces between the transtibial residual limb and the socket design. The Academy Today 4(1):2008 February.

11. Kahle JT: Conventional and hydrostatic transtibial interface comparison. JPO 11:85–91, 1999.

12. Kapp SL, Fergason JR: Transtibial amputation: prosthetic management. In Smith DG, Michael JW, Bowker JH (eds): Atlas of amputations and limb deficiencies: surgical, prosthetic, and rehabilitation principles, 3rd ed. Rosemont, IL, AAOS, 2004, pp 503–516.

13. Lannon N: Transtibial alignment: normal bench alignment. ISPO Ortho Letter 11:1–2, 2003 July.

14. Schuch CM, Pritham CH: Transfemoral amputation: prosthetic management. In Smith DG, Michael JW, Bowker JH (eds): Atlas of amputations and limb deficiencies: surgical, prosthetic, and rehabilitation principles, 3rd ed. Rosemont, IL, AAOS, 2004, pp 541–556.

15. Pike A: A new concept in socket design. The Edge, November 2002, http://www.oandp.com/articles/2002-11_01.asp.

16. Bunce DJ, Breakey JW: The impact of the C-Leg® on the physical and psychological adjustment to transfemoral amputation. JPO 19:7–14, 2007.

17. Hafner BJ, Willingham LL, Buell NC, Allyn KJ, Smith DG: Evaluation of function, performance, and preference as transfemoral amputees transition from mechanical to microprocessor control prosthetic knees. Arch Phys Med & Rehab 88:544, 2007.

18. Johansson JL, Sherrill DM, Riley PO, Bonato P, Herr H: A clinical comparison of variable-damping and mechanically passive prosthetic knee devices. Am J Phys Med & Rehabil 84(8):563–575, 2005 Aug.

19. Laferrier JZ, Gailey R: Advances in lower-limb prosthetic technology. Phys Med Rehabil Clinics North Am. 21(1):87–110, 2010 Feb.

20. Versluys R, Lenaerts G, Van Damme M, et al: Successful preliminary walking experiments on a transtibial amputee fitted with a powered prosthesis. Prosthet Orthotics Int 33(4):368–377, 2009 Dec.

Lower Extremity Prosthetic Management

OBJECTIVES

At the end of this chapter, all students are expected to:

1. Describe the factors that mitigate for or against prosthetic fitting.
2. Recognize major gait deviations that may be exhibited by individuals walking with a transtibial or transfemoral prosthesis.
3. Describe the critical components of the prosthetic training program.
4. Compare and contrast the training program for an individual with a transtibial or transfemoral prosthesis.

Physical Therapy students are expected to:

1. Analyze the fit of any prosthesis.
   a. Perform an appropriate prosthetic check out.
2. Establish a physical therapy diagnosis and functional goals for an individual with a transfemoral or transtibial prosthesis.
3. Develop a plan of care for any individual with a transfemoral or transtibial prosthesis.
4. Implement an individualized prosthetic training program for anyone with a transtibial or transfemoral prosthesis.
5. Delegate and supervise physical therapist assistants in the implementation of selected aspects of the prosthetic rehabilitation program.

CASE STUDIES

Janice Simmons, John Adams, Richard Canto, and **Linda Bean** are each ready to b considered for prosthetic fitting.

Case Study Activities

In your small groups, explore your beliefs about the statement: "Everyone has a right to be fitted with a prosthesis."
1. What are the implications of that statement?
2. What conditions have to exist for a patient not to be a prosthetic candidate?
3. What does the research literature reflect on long-term prosthetic use?

Rehabilitation programs for individuals who have undergone an amputation are very variable.

The service person who sustains an injury in a service-related activity is quickly evacuated to the nearest medical center and receives continuous and complete medical services throughout the rehabilitation phase. In Iraq and Afghanistan, wounded soldiers are evacuated to Germany, often within a few hours of injury, and transferred to Walter Reed Medical Center or Brooks Army Medical Center when stabilized for complete medical, surgical, and rehabilitative care. They are fitted with state-of-the-art prostheses and receive rehabilitative care until complete independence for all daily and leisure activities is achieved. Many complete part of their rehabilitation at the Center for the Intrepid, a modern outpatient rehabilitation facility on the campus of Fort San Houston and described later in this chapter. Some are able to return to active military duty.[1] Individuals in the civilian population may also receive continuous care from injury to rehabilitation depending on location, finances, age, cause of amputation, and the proximity of a comprehensive medical center or an in- and outpatient rehabilitation center. In many instances, unfortunately, particularly for older individuals, the surgeon who performs the amputation may not refer the patient for comprehensive care. The patient may eventually be sent to a prosthetist for prosthetic fitting and may never be seen by a physical therapist or may be referred to physical therapy long after the prosthesis has been fitted and the person has developed energy-consuming gait deviations. Ideally, the same continuity of care available to the military member should be available in the civilian population. There are amputee clinics in many major medical centers and patients referred to such programs benefit from the continuity of care. Insurance companies and third-party payers also benefit as the patients return to a fully active life more quickly. In countries with a national health care system, patients are automatically referred for both preprosthetic and prosthetic rehabilitation, but cost factors are also an issue. As was indicated in Chapter 5, the earlier the person can be returned to bipedal ambulation, either through the use of a temporary or definitive prosthesis, the better is the eventual outcome.

CANDIDATE FOR A PROSTHESIS

The first step in the prosthetic management of individuals with lower extremity amputations is to determine who is and is not a candidate for prosthetic fitting. The decision may be made by an amputee clinic team or an individual physician or may be initiated by a physical therapist. The patient and family should be involved in the decision, although many are not aware of the energy demands and balance requirements of prosthetic ambulation. The physical therapist (PT) working in home health or a rehabilitation center is in a particularly good position to make a referral to a local clinic or to discuss prosthetic fitting with the physician.

No general protocol can be applied to determine who will or will not become a successful prosthetic wearer. The decision to fit or not fit an individual involves many factors. The value of a prosthesis in helping the individual achieve desired functional goals must be assessed. Individuals with severe cardiac or respiratory dysfunction, those who were not ambulatory prior to amputation, or those who do not have the capacity to stand and ambulate with some form of assistive device will probably not benefit from prosthetic fitting. On the other hand, individuals who were active community ambulators prior to amputations will certainly benefit from prosthetic fitting and training regardless of level of amputation. In between are individuals where the decision to fit or not fit is not as clear cut. Most unilateral transtibial amputees are candidates for prosthetic fitting. Unilateral transfemoral amputees need better balance, coordination, and endurance to be able to functionally use a prosthesis, but modern components enhance the functional ability of many transfemoral amputees if they receive proper training in prosthetic use. Marzoug and associates in the United Kingdom reported on using refurbished used modular components with individually made sockets as a tool for determining who was and was not a candidate for definite prosthetic fitting among individuals who were doubtful candidates.[2] Each patient received prosthetic training using these lower-cost devices. Thirty-eight percent did well with the temporary appliances and went on to successful fitting and use. Fifty-eight percent decided to abandon prosthetic use for reasons including hip flexion contractures, bilateral amputation, and energy demands. The authors recommend the use of temporary prosthesis as an evaluative tool.[2]

In some instances, family members may demand that their relative be fitted, hoping that prosthetic replacement will make caregiving easier. Unfortunately, family motivation does not translate into patient motivation, and there are individuals who do not want to expend the energy required to learn to use a transfemoral prosthesis. For most unilateral amputees, the decision is not so much whether to fit, but what functional outcome is the patient likely to achieve.

DIAGNOSIS

Patients in need of prosthetic training are referred through an amputee clinic, from a prosthetic facility, or directly from a physician. Regardless of the status of direct access in the state of practice, it is rare for a patient or his or her family to seek services directly from a physical therapist A physician referral is still needed for third-party reimbursement in most states. Therefore, the patient will have an established medical diagnosis but will need one or more physical therapy diagnoses to inform the plan of care. The physical therapy diagnosis focuses on balance, functional abilities, and prosthetic fit and follows the evaluation.

FUNCTIONAL OUTCOMES

Medicare has developed a functional scale called "K level" that guides prosthetists on component reimbursement. There is, of course, a lot of "wiggle room" in the levels, and the physical therapists can provide more detailed information regarding the patient's potential functional outcome (**Box 7.1**). Sometimes, individuals considered to have limited functional potential are fitted with low-cost and low-function components when they might achieve a higher level of function with more functional components. Gailey and associates developed the Amputee Mobility Predictor (AMP),[3] a 20-task inventory designed to measure a patient's physical and psychological potential for prosthetic rehabilitation (**Fig. 7.1**). The AMP is designed for use with patients before or after prosthetic fitting and training. It is relatively simple to administer and score and requires little equipment. The results are linked to the Medicare functional scales and can be used for prosthetic prescription as well as to help establish functional goals. Results are a guide to be used with other data. There are, of course, numerous scales available to determine functional outcomes among the amputee population. Miller and associates evaluated three known scales, the Houghton Scale, the Prosthetic Profile of the Amputee Locomotor Capabilities Index (PPA-LCI), and the Prosthetic Evaluation Questionnaire (PEQ), and found no significant differences between the scales in terms of reliability and validity.[4] Deathe and Miller, reporting that many existing tests were not appropriate for amputees, studied the L Test of Functional Mobility (L Test), an adaption of the Timed Get Up and Go (TUG) test designed specifically for amputees. The test involves a 20-meter walk with two transfers and four turns. Deathe and Miller reported excellent performance in a study involving 93 unilateral amputees.[5] A number of outcome measures specific to the amputee population are detailed in the proceedings of a conference on outcome measures held in 2005.[6]

Establishing functional goals is part of developing a plan of care and the physical therapist, the patient, and relevant family work together to determine the goals. **Box 7.2** lists elements that can influence functional goals.

Premorbid/Preprosthetic Activity Level

Probably the most important aspect is the person's premorbid level of activity. One who worked and led a full active life will likely plan to return to that level of function. Even an individual with diabetes, chronic renal disease, and other limitations who was independent in his or her own home and was able to get around his or her community with some assistance should be able to regain that level. The ability to take care of oneself and ambulate limitedly with an assistive device will be useful to individuals living with relatives or in assisted living centers.

The person's activity level during the preprosthetic period and whether or not the person was involved in a physical therapy program are guides to eventual outcome. Returning to an active lifestyle while the residual limb is healing, participating in an active exercise program to maintain strength and prevent contractures being ambulatory with a temporary prosthesis even with limited weight bearing will all

---

BOX 7.1 | Medicare Functional Classification Levels

- **Functional level 0:** The patient does not have the ability or potential to ambulate or transfer safely with or without assistance, and a prosthesis does not enhance his or her quality of life or mobility.
- **Functional level 1:** The patient has the ability or potential to use a prosthesis for transfers or ambulation on level surfaces at fixed cadence. This is typical of the limited and unlimited household ambulator.
- **Functional level 2:** The patient has the ability or potential for ambulation with the ability to traverse low-level environmental barriers such as curbs, stairs, or uneven surfaces. This is typical of the limited community ambulator.
- **Functional level 3:** The patient has the ability or potential for ambulation with variable cadence. This is typical of the community ambulator who has the ability to traverse most environmental barriers and may have vocational, therapeutic, or exercise activity that demands prosthetic utilization beyond simple locomotion.
- **Functional level 4:** The patient has the ability or potential for prosthetic ambulation that exceeds basic ambulation skills, exhibiting high impact, stress, or energy levels. This is typical of the prosthetic demands of the child, active adult, or athlete.

AMPUTEE MOBILITY PREDICTOR ASSESSSMENT TOOL

Initial instructions: Testee is seated in a hard chair with arms. The following maneuvers are tested with or without the use of the prosthesis. Advise the person of each task or group of tasks prior to performance. Please avoid unnecessary chatter throughout the test. Safety first, no task should be performed if either the tester or testee is uncertain of a safe outcome.
The **Right Limb** is: ☐PF ☐TT ☐KD ☐TF ☐HD ☐intact   The **Left Limb** is: ☐PF ☐TT ☐KD ☐TF ☐HD ☐intact

Task	Description	Score	
1. Sitting balance: Sit forward in chair arms folded across chest for 60s.	Cannot sit upright independently for 60s Can sit upright independently for 60s	= 0 = 1	_____
2. Sitting reach: Reach forward and grasp the ruler. (Tester holds ruler 12in beyond extended arms midline to the sternum)	Does not attempt Cannot grasp or requires arm support Reaches forward and successfully grasps item	= 0 = 1 = 2	_____
3. Chair to chair transfer: 2 chairs at 90°. Pt. may choose direction and use their upper limbs.	Cannot do or requires physical assistance Performs independently, but appears unsteady Performs independently, appears to be steady and safe	= 0 = 1 = 2	_____
4. Arises from a chair: Ask pt. to fold arms across chest and stand. If unable, use arms or assistive device.	Unable without help (physical assistance) Able, uses arms/assist device to help Able, without using arms	= 0 = 1 = 2	_____
5. Attempts to arise from chair. (stopwatch ready): If attempt in no. 4 was without arms then ignore and allow another attempt without penalty	Unable without help (physical assistance) Able requires >1 attempt Able to rise one attempt	= 0 = 1 = 2	_____
6. Immediate standing balance (**first 5s**): Begin timing immediately.	Unsteady (staggers, moves foot, sways) Steady using walking aid or other support Steady without walker or other support	= 0 = 1 = 2	_____
7. Standing balance (30s) (stopwatch ready): For items nos. 7&8, first attempt is without assistive device. If support is required allow first attempt.	Unsteady Steady but uses walking aid or other support Standing without support	= 0 = 1 = 2	_____
8. Single limb standing balance (stopwatch ready): Time the duration of single limb standing on both the sound and prosthetic limb up to 30s. Grade the quality, not the time. Sound side _____ seconds Prosthetic side _____ seconds	Non-prosthetic side Unsteady Steady but uses walking aid or other support for 30s Single-limb standing without support for 30s Prosthetic side Unsteady Steady but uses walking aid or other support for 30s Single-limb standing without support for 30s	 = 0 = 1 = 2 = 0 = 1 = 2	_____ _____
9. Standing reach: Reach forward and grasp the ruler. (Tester holds ruler 12in beyond extended arm(s) midline to the sternum.s)	Does not attempt Cannot grasp or requires arm support on assistive device Reaches forward and successfully grasps item, no support	= 0 = 1 = 2	_____
10. Nudge test (subject at maximum position #7): With feet as close together as possible, examiner pushes lightly on subject's sternum with palm of hands 3 times (toes should rise).	Begins to fall Staggers, grabs, catches self, or uses assistive device Steady	= 0 = 1 = 2	_____

FIGURE 7.1. Amputee Mobility Predictor. *(With permission from Advanced Rehabilitation Therapy, Inc., Miami, Florida.)*

11. Eyes closed (at maximum position #7): If support is required grade as unsteady.	Unsteady or grips assistive device Steady without any use of assistive device	= 0 = 1	_____	
12. Picking up objects off the floor: Pick up a pencil off the floor placed midline 12in in front of foot.	Unable to pick up object and return to standing Performs with some help (table, chair, walking aid, etc) Performs independently (without help from object or person)	= 0 = 1 = 2	_____	
13. Sitting down: Ask pt. to fold arms across chest and sit. If unable, use arm or assistive device.	Unsafe (misjudged distance, falls into chair) Uses arms, assistive device or not a smooth motion Safe, smooth motion	= 0 = 1 = 2	_____	
14. Initiation of gait (immediately after told to "go")	Any hesitancy or multiple attempts to start No hesitancy	= 0 = 1	_____	

			Prosthesis	Sound

15. Step length and height: Walk a measured distance of 12 ft twice (up and back). Four scores are required or two scores (**A & B**) for each leg.
"Marked Deviation" is defined as extreme substitute movements to avoid clearing the floor.
 	
B Foot clearance
	A Swing foot
	  Does not advance a minimum of 12in
	  Advances a minimum of 12in
	
	B Foot does not completely clear floor without deviation
	  Foot completely clears floor without marked deviation
		= 0
		= 1
		
		= 0
		
		= 1
			_____
			
			_____
				_____
				
				_____

16. Step continuity.	Stopping or discontinuity between steps (stop & go gait) Steps appear continuous	= 0 = 1	_____	
17. Turning: 180 degree turn when returning to chair.	Unable to turn, requires intervention to prevent falling Greater than three steps but completes task without intervention No more than three continuous steps with or without assistive aid	= 0 = 1 = 2	_____	
18. Variable cadence: Walk a distance of 12 ft as fast as possible safely 4 times. (Speeds may vary from slow to fast and fast to slow varying cadence.)	Unable to vary cadence in a controlled manner Asymmetrical increase in cadence in a controlled manner Symmetrical increase in speed in a controlled manner	= 0 = 1 = 2	_____	
19. Stepping over an obstacle: Place a movable box of 4in in height in the walking path.	Cannot step over the box Catches foot, interrupts stride Steps over without interrupting stride	= 0 = 1 = 2	_____	

20. Stairs (must have at least 2 steps): Try to go up and down these stairs without holding on to the railing. Don't hesitate to permit pt. to hold on to rail. Safety first: If examiner feels that any risk is involved, omit and score as 0.	Ascending
	  Unsteady, cannot do
	  One step at a time, or must hold on to railing or device
	  Step over step, does not hold onto the railing or device
	Descending
	  Unsteady, cannot do
	  One step at a time, or must hold on to railing or device
	  Step over step, does not hold onto the railing or device
		= 0
		= 1
		= 2
		
		= 0
		= 1
		= 2
			_____
			
			_____	

21. Assistive device selection: Add points for the use of an assistive device if used for two or more items. If testing without prosthesis use of appropriate assistive device is mandatory.	Bed bound Wheelchair Walker Crutches (axillary or forearm) Cane (straight or quad) None	= 0 = 1 = 2 = 3 = 4 = 5	_____	
	Total Score	_____/47		

Abbreviations: PF, partial foot; TT, transtibial; KD, knee disarticulation; TF, transfemoral; HD, hip disarticulation; Pt, patient.

Test ☐ no prosthesis ☐ with prosthesis   Observer _____ Date _____

FIGURE 7.1. CONT'D

BOX 7.2 | **Factors Influencing Functional Goals**

1. Premorbid activity level
2. Preprosthetic activity level
3. Level of amputation
4. Comorbidities affecting balance and endurance
5. Extent of disease or injury leading to amputation
6. Financial situation
7. Relationship of prosthetic components to functional abilities
8. Presence of moderate to severe hip flexion contractures

enhance prosthetic training and eventual functional outcomes. There is little research in this area, and much is needed.

Level of Amputation

Most individuals with transtibial amputations can reach functional independence, frequently as community ambulators. Knee flexion contractures, scars, poorly shaped residual limbs, and adherent skin are not necessarily fitting issues with today's modern components. A knee flexion contracture does not necessarily limit prosthetic ambulation, as many knee flexion contractures can be reduced through walking with a foot aligned to create a knee extension moment at heel strike. Circulatory problems in the nonamputated extremity benefit from bipedal ambulation that reduces stress on that extremity. In some instances, the prosthetic leg becomes the "better" leg, and the person may use a cane to protect the unamputated extremity.

Many people with a unilateral transfemoral amputation can become functional prosthetic users with or without external support. However, the physiological demands of walking with a transfemoral prosthesis are considerably higher than walking with a transtibial prosthesis and not all individuals have the necessary balance, strength, and energy reserves. The transfemoral prosthesis is heavier than the transtibial, and control of the artificial knee may be more difficult with other than a microprocessor knee component. Cost is also a consideration. Long-term studies have regularly supported the fact that individuals with transfemoral amputations, particularly in the dysvascular population, have lower outcomes than the same population of transtibial amputees.[7–9]

Comorbidities/Energy Expenditures

Obviously, the severity of comorbidities can affect functional goals, and these must be assessed on an individual basis. Studies have shown that walking with a prosthesis at any level requires more energy than nonamputee walking.[10] Individuals with transtibial amputations reach a higher level of function and use less energy for ambulation than individuals with transfemoral amputations. Walking speed affects energy utilization; the faster one walks, the more energy is expended. Most individuals select a walking speed that maintains a comfortable level of oxygen consumption. Individuals with transtibial amputations are reported to expend significantly less energy when walking with a prosthesis at a self-selected speed than when walking on crutches without a prosthesis; the difference in energy expenditure for individuals using a transfemoral prosthesis or walking on crutches was not statistically significant.[11] Studies of energy expenditure between individuals using a transtibial or a transfemoral prosthesis vary if walking speed is self-selected or controlled. Most studies of energy expenditure indicate that the higher is the level of amputation, the greater the oxygen uptake value. It is summarized that an individual with a single transfemoral amputation uses at least 49% more oxygen than someone without an amputation, and an individual with bilateral amputations uses up to 280% more oxygen than an individual without an amputation. Additionally, individuals with amputations exhibit a decrease in walking speed and walking efficiency commensurate with the level of amputation.[10]

Comorbidities have, not surprisingly, been found to affect functional outcomes. Fletcher and associates, in a retrospective study, found that patients over the age of 85 with comorbidities had a small likelihood of successful prosthetic ambulation. They further reported that successful prosthetic rehabilitation decreased with increasing age and comorbidities.[9] The more serious the health problems, the less likely for successful rehabilitation. Individuals with unilateral transfemoral amputations are more likely to stop using the prosthesis or use it for only part of the day, than individuals with unilateral transtibial amputations. The higher the level of amputation, the heavier is the prosthesis, and the more artificial joints the person must control to achieve a smooth, energy-efficient gait.

Financial Issues/Components

As stated above, Medicare will reimburse for prosthetic components on the basis of expected functional outcomes. On the other hand, the government will fit war amputees with the latest, most technological advanced prosthetic components, expecting a high outcome level. Individuals not eligible for Medicare are dependent on their own resources or insurance companies for prosthetic payment; unfortunately, many third-party payers often will only authorize the cheapest components that may not provide the function needed for the best outcome. Similarly, many payers, including Medicare, severely limit the amount of training a patient may receive, compounding the problem and limiting the level of achievement the patient may attain. It becomes somewhat of a circular self-fulfilling prophecy. The patient is fitted with a less than optimum prosthesis, receives less than needed training, and achieves a low outcome. The payers cite the number of low-achieving patients as a rationale for fitting, usually older patients, with less than optimum prostheses and not authorizing adequate training, and the circle continues. There is a tendency when working with older individuals with multiple health problems to set the goals too low, and the physical therapist needs to carefully evaluate each patient to set goals at appropriate levels and establish the plan of care. The physical therapist can influence treatment authorization by accurately diagnosing eventual functional outcomes and providing data of the importance of the proper prosthetic components and adequate training for the patient to achieve the desired level.

Hip Flexion Contractures

Hip flexion contractures can be very debilitating and are extremely difficult to reduce. Unlike knee flexion contractures that can be reduced by changes in prosthetic alignment, there is no way to "walk out" a hip flexion contracture. Contractures of less than 25 degrees can usually be accommodated in the prosthetic socket but may affect the patient's ability to properly shift his or her weight and control the prosthesis. Severe hip contractures limit the person's ability to stand upright, balance properly over the lower extremities, and shift the trunk as needed in ambulation. Severe hip flexion contractures require more energy for ambulation and can affect eventual prosthetic outcomes (**Fig. 7.2**).

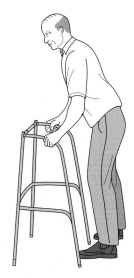

FIGURE 7.2. Hip flexion contractures prevent balanced standing.

CASE STUDIES

Each of the clients is now ready for prosthetic fitting and training.

Janice Simmons is 63 years old and 15 weeks postamputation. She received some home health therapy after discharge from the hospital and has been functioning at home independently using a walker. **Figure 7.3** outlines her current status.

John Adams is 72 years old and is 5 months postamputation. He spent 2 weeks in a rehabilitation center postamputation and then was discharged home. **Figure 7.4** outlines his current status.

Richard Canto is 20 years old and is now 12 weeks postamputation and his other injuries have healed well. He has been ambulatory with a temporary prosthesis and is now ready for definitive fitting. **Figure 7.5** outlines his current status.

Linda Bean is 10 years old and is now 6 months postamputation. She has undergone radiation and chemotherapy. She was fitted with a temporary prosthesis, but training was limited by the radiation and chemotherapy. **Figure 7.6** outlines her current status.

Case Study Activities

1. Do you believe that each of these individuals is or is not a candidate for prosthetic replacement? Why or why not?
2. What components would you recommend?

Ms. Simmons* has indicated she would like a "leg" so she can resume a normal life. She has some financial coverage through her husband's plan at work. She is not sure if she will be able to return to work as a waitress.

Hx: As previously reported.

TEST and MEASURES

Pain: Pt reports occasional burning pain in left (phantom) foot.

ROM: Left lower extremity:
  Active & passive knee flexion = 120 deg; extension = 0 deg
  Active & passive hip flexion = 130 deg; act extension = –5 deg; passive = +5 deg
  Active & passive hip abduction/ adduction and rotation: WNL

  Right lower extremity:
  Active ankle: dorsiflexion = +5 deg; passive = +10 deg; Active and passive plantarflexion = 22 deg
  Active & passive knee: flexion = 120 deg; extension = 0 deg
  Active & passive hip: flexion = 130 deg; active extension = 0 deg; passive = +5 deg

Residual Limb: Residual limb length = 15.5 cm

Circumferential measurement:	5 cm from MTP	$28^3/_4$ cm
	10 cm below	$26^1/_2$ cm
	15 cm below	$25^1/_2$ cm

Appearance: Well healed, nonedematous residual limb; independent mobility skills and is ready for prosthetic fitting.

Vascular Status:
  Right lower extremity: Some clubbing of toenails, hairless throughout lower extremity.
  Decreased protective sensation in the right foot tested with Semmes-Weinstein filament (10g).
  Loss of protective sensation on the plantar surface of first metatarsal.

ADL: Ambulates independently in the parallel bar and with a walker. Reports being independent in self-care and around the house except getting in and out of the bathtub. Has been doing some of the household activities, including some cooking, using her weelchair or walker.

*Examination results have been limited to key data only to conserve space. Some psychosocial and medical information was provided in previous chapters. Students may hypothesize congruent additional information if necessary.

FIGURE 7.3. Current status—Janice Simmons.

PROSTHETIC CHECKOUT

All amputees referred to physical therapy, whether experienced prosthetic wearers bringing a new limb to the amputee clinic or a new patient bringing a new prosthesis for gait training, will need a prosthetic checkout. The evaluation is designed to ensure that the prosthesis fits appropriately and that the wearer is ready to begin to wear the prosthesis. The prosthetic checkout includes a static and a dynamic evaluation; the dynamic evaluation is delayed for new prosthetic wearers until the individual has achieved a stable gait pattern. **Figures** 7.7 and 7.8 depict prosthetic checkout forms for transtibial and transfemoral amputees.

Prior to the prosthetic checkout, a gross assessment of the strength and range of motion (ROM) of the residual and nonamputated limbs provide data helpful to establish functional goals. Observing the patient transfer to and from a wheelchair or ambulate with crutches or walker as he or she enters the department provides information about balance, coordination, and strength. The residual limb needs to be carefully checked to identify any skin problems or painful areas. The prosthetic checkout is performed and the residual limb (RL) again checked carefully to make sure prosthetic pressures are being appropriately distributed. If any problems are identified with the prosthesis, the physical therapist needs to contact the prosthetist and discuss the problem. The prosthetist will have performed his or her own static and dynamic alignment with the patient prior to delivering the limb. Close contact between the prosthetist and the therapist provides an integrated plan of gait training and leads to the most optimum results. Initiating prosthetic training with a prosthesis that does not fit or is not aligned properly is inviting difficulties. As indicated in Chapter 6, today's prostheses carry the alignment mechanism within the pylon so the prosthesis can be adjusted as needed as the patient's gait improves.

Mr. Adams* states that he would like to be able to walk "like before;" the daughter states that he needs a leg to be able to get around more. She states that he spends most of his time in the wheelchair. He complains that his residual limb just aches all over.

Mr. Adams presents as a somewhat thin individual, dependent on family for his care other than self-care. He is on Medicare with a supplement insurance.

TEST and MEASURES

Pain: Pt reports nonspecific residual limb pain of 3 on 10 pt scale. Reports phantom sensation with occasional cramping pain in the right foot.

ROM: Right hip (active):

Flexion = 125 deg; active extension = −13 deg
Abduction = 25 deg: adduction = 10 deg

Right hip (passive):

Flexion = 140 deg; extension = −5 deg
Abduction = 25 deg; adduction = 10 deg

Left lower extremity:

Active & passive hip flexion = 125 deg; active hip extension = −12 deg: passive = −5 deg
Abduction, adduction, and rotation within functional limits.
Active & passive knee flexion = 135 deg; extenson = −5 deg
Active ankle dorsiflexion = 4 deg; passive = 9 deg; active and passive plantarflexion = 28 deg

Muscle strength:

Right hip: flexion: G+ (4+/5); Extension: F (3/5) (measured sidelying; cannot get prone)
abduction = G+ (4+/5); adduction = G (4+/5)

Left lower extremity:

Ankle: dorsiflexion = G (4/5); plantarflexion = G + (4+/5 NWB)
Knee extension = G+ (4+/5); flexion (sidelying) = G+ (4+/5)
Hip flexion = N (5/5); extension (sidelying) = F (3+/5)
Hip abduction = G (4); hip adduction = G (4)

Residual Limb: Residual limb is well healed with no change in measurements for the past 3 weeks. No specific areas of tenderness. Patient had some difficulty with wrapping and was fitted with transfemoral shrinker which he states he wears all the time.

Vascular Status: Left lower extremity is hairless below the knee with evidence of dysvascularity in the foot. It is relatively thin with evident dryness of skin. Patient states it will swell when he sits all day; occasionallly wears an elastic stocking on the leg. He complains of some night cramping. He states he occasionally has some cramping if he stands or walks too much. No evidence of ulcerations. Demonstrates protective sensation in the left foot with Semmes-Weinstein filament testing (10g).

Functional Status: Mr. Adams is independent in all wheelchair transfer activities; generally uses a wheelchair at home except that he uses the walker to go to the bathroom. He is independent in all self-care except for bathing as he cannot get into the bathtub. Mr. Adams is able to ambulate independently in the parallel bars and can use a walker for limited distances in the home.

*Examination results have been limited to key data only to conserve space. Some psychosocial and medical information was provided in previous chapters. Students may hypothesize congruent additional information if neccessary.

FIGURE 7.4. Current status—John Adams.

Mr. Canto* is now 4 months post-amputation; has indicated that he would like to stay in the military if possible. He would like advanced training in computers. He has been on disability leave using the temporary prosthesis and is independent in all activities. He states he wants a permanent leg so he can resume physical training and sports activities. He is interested in the Wounded Warrior program and the Paralympics.

Hx: As previously given.

TEST and MEASURES

Pain: Has occasional pain where shrapnel wounds have healed and has occasional phantom pain in his foot, particularly at night.

Residual Limb: Length: $18\frac{1}{2}$ cm; well healed, nonsensitive, nonedematous
  Circumference: Medial Tibial Plateau (MTP) level = 31 cm;
             5 cm = 33 cm;
            10 cm = 33 cm;
            18 cm = 32 cm.

ROM and muscle strength Right hip and knee within normal limits.

ROM and muscle strength Left lower extremity within normal limits.

Right upper extremity G to G+ strength overall; ROM of joints is grossly WNL.

ADL: Wearing a temporary PTB socket with petite liner and 10 ply of stump socks, pylon, and Flex® foot. Ambulates without external support and is fully independent. Has been active at home, lifting weights and using equipment, although he was advised to delay runnning and highly active sports until fitted with a definitive prosthesis.

*Examination results have been limited to key data only to conserve space. Some psychosocial and medical information was provided in previous chapters. Students may hypothesize congruent additional information if necessary.

FIGURE 7.5. Current status—Richard Canto.

Ms. Bean* has recently completed 3 months of chemotherapy and radiation therapy; she has lost some weight. Adjuvant therapy has been stopped for now and her latest MRI was clear. She has been attending school sporadically during this period and has received home schooling as needed. She was fitted for a shrinker, which she wears. There was some discussion about fitting her with a prosthesis about a month ago but she did not feel strong enough for this while on radiation therapy. She is independent with crutches and lives with her family. All her treatments are through the local Shriner's Hospital who hold a juvenile amputee clinic monthly. She and her family are anxious for her to get a prosthesis and return to a normal life. Prior to her amputation, she was a reasonably active individual although she was not particularly involved in sports activities.

TEST and MEASURES

Pain: Does not report any specific pain other than phantom sensation on occasion.

Residual Limb: Well healed, conical, no edema.
    Length from greater trochanter to end limb = 32 cm
    Circumference: At ischial level = 38 cm;
               5 cm = 36 cm;
               8 cm = 28 cm;
              13 cm = 26 cm;
              28 cm = 26 cm.

Strength: Gross muscle strength of the right hip is within normal limits; gross muscle strength of the left lower extremity appears well within normal limits.

ROM: Active ROM normal in all ranges of both legs.

ADL: Independent on crutches in all ambulation, elevation, and self-care activities.

*Examination results have been limited to key data only to conserve space. Some psychosocial and medical information was provided in previous chapters. Students may hypothesize congruent additional information if necessary.

FIGURE 7.6. Current status—Linda Bean.

General

1. Is the residual limb (RL) free from abrasions, open sores, skin problems?
2. Is the prosthesis as prescribed?
3. Does the liner fit appropriately in the socket?
   Comments:

Standing

4. Does the client have any pain or discomfort when bearing weight in the prosthesis?
5. Is the knee stable? Does the patient have to resist to prevent the knee from being forced into flexion or extension?
6. Is the pelvis level when weight is borne equally on both feet?
7. Is the pylon vertical when weight is borne evenly on both feet?
8. Does the sole of the shoe maintain even contact with the floor?
9. Are tissue rolls around the trimline of the socket excessive?
10. Is there any gapping at the brim of the socket?
11. Is there evidence of total contact?
12. Does the liner fit properly and smoothly?
13. Is suspension maintained as the foot is lifted off the floor?
14. If using a sleeve suspension, does the sleeve extend over the liner or limb socks?
    Comments:

Sitting

15. Is the person comfortable while sitting with the sole of the shoe flat on the floor and knee flexed to at least 90 degrees?
16. Is there adequate flaring of the posterior trimline to accommodate the hamstring tendons?
17. Is the residual limb forced out of the socket excessively?
    Comments:

Walking

18. Is the gait satisfactory? If the gait is not satisfactory, check the deviations.

At Heel Contact:	Ball of the foot more than 1 inch from the floor
	Knee extended
	Unequal stride length
From Heel Contact to Foot Flat:	Knee flexes jerkily
	Knee flexes abruptly
	Maintains knee extension
At Mid-Stance:	Lateral trunk bending exceeds 5 cm
	Shoe not flat on floor
	Lateral displacement of socket exceeds $1/2$ inch
	No lateral or medial socket displacement
Mid Stance to Heel Rise:	Drop off
	Knee flexes jerkily
At Heel Rise:	Knee goes into extension
During Swing Phase:	Vaulting
	Toe drags on floor
	Circumduction

Check With Prosthesis Off

19. After the checkout, is the skin free of any abrasions, blisters, or excessive redness or areas of pressure?
    Comments:

FIGURE 7.7. Transtibial Prosthetic Checkout Form.

General

1. Is the residual limb (RL) free from abrasions, open sores, skin problems?
2. Is the prosthesis as prescribed?
3. Do all joints move freely and smoothly?
   Comments:

Sitting

4. Is the socket securely on the residual limb?
5. Does the length of the shin and thigh correspond to the shin and thigh of the unamputated leg?
6. Can the client sit comfortably without burning or pinching?
7. Is the client able to lean forward and reach his/her shoes?
   Comments:

Standing

8. Does the socket fit properly and comfortably?
9. Is the knee stable when weight is placed on the prosthesis?
10. Is the pelvis level when weight is borne evenly on both legs?
11. Does the socket maintain good contact with the residual limb on all sides as the client shifts his/her weight?
12. If wearing a liner, does it fit smoothly and properly?
13. Is there an adductor roll?
14. Is there pressure on the pubic ramus?
    Comments:

Walking

15. Is suspension maintained during swing phase?
16. Is the socket stable against the lateral shift of the residual limb?
17. Is level walking free of gait deviations? If not, check the deviation observed.

Heel Contact to Foot Flat:	Forceful heel strike
	Knee instability
	Excessive external rotation of prosthesis
Mid Stance:	Lateral trunk bending toward prosthetic side
	Abducted gait
	Lateral gapping of the socket
Mid Stance to Toe Off:	Premature heel rise
	Drop off
	Excessive lumbar lordosis
	Pelvic rise (climbing a hill)
	Delayed swing
Swing Phase:	Circumducted gait
	Lateral heel whip
	Terminal swing impact
	Excessive heel rise
	Medial heel whip
	Lack of knee flexion

Comments:

18. Can prosthesis be removed easily?
19. Is residual limb free of any abrasions or red areas?
    Comments:

FIGURE 7.8. Transfemoral Prosthetic Checkout Form.

Case Study Activity

Individually or in groups, review each item in the transfemoral and transtibial evaluation forms, preferably with a prosthesis. Explain why each item is important and discuss the effect on the client if the item does not meet standards. Be as specific as you can; pain is not an adequate answer, rather state where the pain would be felt and how it would affect function.

TRANSTIBIAL PROSTHETIC CHECKOUT

Table 7.1 depicts key items of transtibial prosthetic checkout and possible issues that may occur with misalignment. Although digitally created sockets generally fit well, the RL may have undergone minor changes since socket measurements were taken and even since the prosthetist fitted the socket. Some individuals experience marked fluid changes from day to day, others may gain weight,

TABLE 7.1	Static Transtibial Prosthetic Checkout	
Checkout Item	**What to Check**	**Issues**
General Residual limb	Look for skin irritations, bony prominences, etc	Areas that may not tolerate socket pressures
Prosthesis	Compare limb to prescription, if available	Discuss changes with prosthetist
Liner	Pelite liner fit to top of socket, gel liner rolls to mid-thigh	Improperly fitting liner may cause pain, abrasions, gait deviations
Sitting Sit with knees flexed to 90 degrees and foot flat	The residual limb tends to move up a little when person sits, sleeve or liner needs to stretch adequately to prevent excessive pressure	Pressure on knee or bony prominences in socket, patient may keep leg extended
Posterior flaring	Check for pressure on the hamstrings when sitting	Client will keep leg outstretched when sitting or complain of pain
Residual limb when sitting	The stump will rise out of the socket a little when sitting	May indicate a socket that is too small or the client is wearing too many socks
Standing Pain on weight bearing	Check limb/socket interface, particularly bony prominences	Excessive pressures can lead to skin problems and gait deviations
Knee stability	Patellar tendon-bearing (PTB) socket aligned in 5 to 8 degrees of flexion	Too much flexion will lead to counter knee extension and anterior distal pressure, too little flexion can lead to end bearing
Equal length (see **Fig. 7.12**)	Palpate the iliac crests with client standing evenly on both feet	A long or short prosthesis will lead to gait deviations

Continued

TABLE 7.1 Static Transtibial Prosthetic Checkout—cont'd

Checkout Item	What to Check	Issues
Vertical pylon	On weight bearing, check the pylon connecting the socket and foot; best viewed from behind the patient	See medial and lateral leaning pylons on gait deviations; if the patient has large thighs or is not bearing weight evenly, pylon may lead medially
Shoe level on floor	Check that the foot is fully on the floor on weight bearing	May indicate a foot that is too dorsiflexed or plantarflexed
Tissue rolls	Check the edges of the residual limb (RL) at the socket line	Excessive rolls may indicate a socket that is too tight proximally
Gapping at the brim	Check the edges of the RL at the socket line	Gapping may indicate a socket that is too large proximally or not properly molded
Is there evidence of total contact?	Put a little ball of play dough at the end of the socket below the liner, - then have the client weight bear, the displacement of the play dough indicates the extent of total contact	Too little contact can cause distal end skin problems and a stretching pain, too much can cause excessive pressure at the end of the stump and pressure pain
Liner	Stump/socket interface: gel liner, socks, nylon sheath, etc	Liners, socks, etc, have a limited life span; wrinkles, holes, or worn areas create skin abrasions
Suspension	Check that there is not excessive movement of the prosthesis away from limb when weight is removed, place a finger lightly at edge of socket and have the patient lift the limb straight up	Too much movement between residual limb and socket creates abrasions and can lead to toe drag on swing, there should be no movement with suction or shuttlelock suspension
Sleeve suspension (nonsuction)	The sleeve should be in direct contact with the skin for at least 2 inches above any socks or liner	Failure to have skin-to-sleeve contact will lead to loss of suspension and pistoning

and still others may lose weight. The physical therapist must ensure that the socket fits properly each day, and the patient must be taught to feel how the socket should fit. The prosthetist will have reviewed **donning** and **doffing** procedures; however, the process must be reinforced throughout the checkout and training period (**Fig. 7.9**).

SOCKET FIT CONSIDERATIONS

Comfort is a critical factor; if the patient is not comfortable, he or she will not learn to bear weight properly and will not be able to develop a smooth step-over-step gait. Comfort should be assessed throughout the process. Care must be taken to

determine if reported discomfort comes from an issue with socket fit, prosthetic misalignment, or a RL problem such as a neuroma. RL problems will be discussed later in this chapter. Generally, if the patient reports excessive pressure or pain at the distal end of the residual limb, the patient is going too far in the socket either because of residual limb shrinkage or weight loss. This problem is easily remedied by adding socks between the liner and the socket. If the patient complains of a stretching sensation distally or does not seem to have **total contact**, it may be because the residual limb is more edematous than when fitted or the patient has gained weight. This is not as easily remedied unless the patient is wearing too many socks. If the

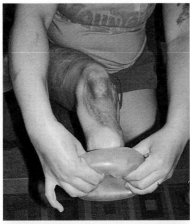

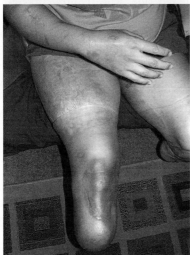

FIGURE 7.9. Patient donning a flexible gel liner.

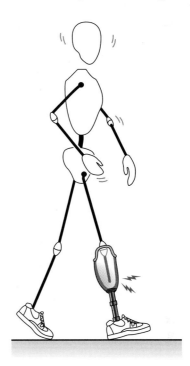

FIGURE 7.10. Heel contact to foot flat: Extension force on knee creating anterior distal pressure.

residual limb is edematous, wrapping or using intermittent compression may reduce the swelling adequately for socket fit. If not, the prosthetist needs to be contacted to see if any adjustments can be made. Weight control is an issue as patients who may have lost weight because of illness or trauma may now gain weight and lose socket fit.

The patellar tendon-bearing (PTB) socket is aligned in 5 to 8 degrees of knee flexion to allow for better weight bearing on the patella tendon and to enhance normal knee motion from heel contact to foot flat. Excessive socket flexion creates knee instability; the client extends the knee to counteract the instability and drives the anterior distal end of the tibia that is close to the skin against the wall of the socket, causing pain and possible abrasion (**Fig. 7.10**). Insufficient socket flexion reduces the

weight-bearing potential of the patellar tendon and can lead to pressure at the end of the residual limb.

Total contact of the residual limb with the liner and socket provides for some kinesthetic feedback and improves the distribution of pressure appropriately throughout the residual limb. Lack of total contact can lead to skin problems. The intimate fit of the gel liner reduces the possibility of lack of total contact unless the patient does not put the liner on properly.

The prosthesis must be held on firmly by the suspension mechanism. Suspension is not usually a major problem with suction or shuttlelock systems but may occur with the sleeve or supracondylar cuff. Pistoning, which is the excessive drop of the socket away from the residual limb during swing, can be checked if the therapist puts a finger lightly at the socket brim and asks the patient to lift the leg straight up off the ground (**Fig. 7.11**). Any drop in the socket can be palpated.

Alignment

The length of the residual limb should match the length of the unamputated extremity. The therapist determines equal leg length by palpating both iliac

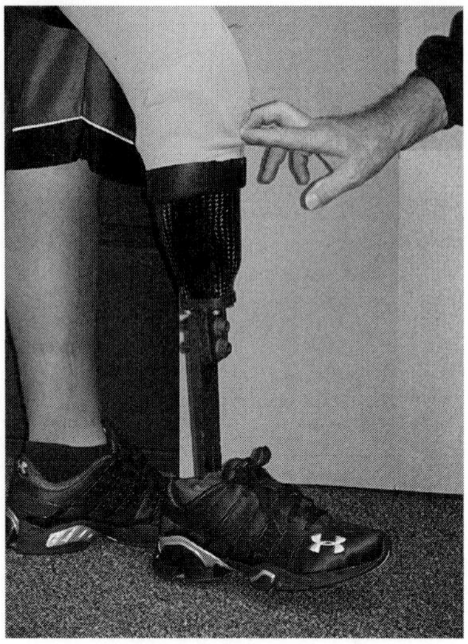

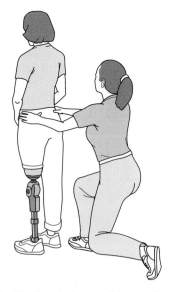

FIGURE 7.11. Checking for pistoning with sleeve suspension.

crests with the patient standing with his or her weight equally on both legs (**Fig. 7.12**). The foot of the prosthesis should be flat on the floor when the patient is standing with the weight equally on both feet. The pylon should be perpendicular to the floor; however, if the patient is not bearing equal weight on both legs, the pylon will not be perpendicular. Likewise, if the person is obese or has large thighs, some genu valgus may be necessary, and the pylon will lean medially.

FIGURE 7.12. Checking the length of the prosthesis by checking for a level pelvis.

TRANSTIBIAL GAIT ANALYSIS

Normal Prosthetic Gait

Prosthetic gait analysis requires an understanding of normal gait characteristics, including the phases of gait, floor reaction forces, and an understanding of normal muscle activity in gait. Prior to studying prosthetic gait, the student is advised to review prior study of normal gait.[12] Prosthetic gait is determined by several factors: the level of amputation, the technical capabilities of the prosthetic components, the strength of the muscles of the involved extremity, and the range of motion of the hip or the hip and knee on the amputated side. Knee contractures greater than 10 degrees as well as hip flexion contractures adversely affect the prosthetic gait pattern and energy expenditure.[13]

Gait analysis is best done when viewing the client walking both from an anterior-posterior (AP) and a lateral (prosthetic side) point of reference. The therapist needs to obtain an overall impression of the gait and then focus on each part of the body individually to ensure a thorough analysis.

Weight Acceptance, Lateral View

The shock-absorbing capability and the speed of plantar flexion vary according to the type of foot (Chapter 6). At weight acceptance, the knee is slightly flexed, and the ball of the prosthetic foot should be no more than 4 cm from the floor. The pelvis and trunk are erect with the body weight transferring from the intact leg to the prosthetic leg smoothly.

Weight Acceptance to Foot Flat, Lateral View

Progressing toward foot flat, the knee flexes about 6 to 10 degrees as compared to about 18 degrees in normal gait. The heel of the prosthetic foot may be seen to compress about 1.5 to 2 cm depending on the person's weight and type of foot. Throughout this part of gait, the quadriceps contract vigorously to control knee flexion. The hip functions relatively normally, and the trunk remains balanced over the point of support.

Midstance, Anterior-Posterior View

At midstance, the client bears full weight on the prosthesis. The pelvis and upper body remain balanced over the prosthesis with no more than 2.5 cm of head or trunk sway toward the prosthetic side. The overall gait base is no more than 5 cm wide. There is minimum lateral socket displacement. On the alignment instrument, the pylon is perpendicular to the floor. The foot is flat on the floor.

Midstance, Lateral View

The limb and body continue to move forward over the foot with the amount of dorsiflexion determined by the type of foot. Dynamic feet allow a longer period of foot flat than the solid ankle cushioned heel (SACH) foot. The extent of muscle activity also varies by the type of feet, with dynamic feet allowing a greater arc of dorsiflexion and a smoother transition.[13]

Midstance to Toe Off, Lateral and Anterior-Posterior Views

The transition from single-leg to double-leg support involves an unloading of the prosthetic leg and a loading of the unamputated leg. The transition is also affected by the type of foot, although no prosthetic foot yet goes into active plantar flexion, resulting in some abruptness in transition. There is increased demand on the unamputated limb in weight transfer.

Swing Phase, Lateral View

The knee flexes easily and allows the toe to clear the floor. The socket remains securely on the residual limb. Step length is the same on each side.

Swing Phase, Anterior-Posterior View

The shank and foot swing in the line of progression, and the pelvis remains level.

Transtibial Gait Deviations

Gait deviations may be due to an improperly fitting socket, a malaligned prosthesis, a painful residual limb, inadequate training, or poor walking habits. Gait deviations increase energy consumption, can cause discomfort in the residual limb, and limit functional outcomes. It is desirable to identify gait deviations as early as possible so they can be remedied before problems become permanent. Depending on the length of the residual limb and the type of suspension, a slight lateral movement of the socket may be seen at midstance. This movement is the result of the adduction of the femur and the slight valgus position of the normal knee. Normal floor reaction forces create a slight varus movement of the knee at midstance. As long as

the movement is slight and does not affect comfort or stability, it is considered normal. Careful observation is required, as most deviations are not clear cut and some may be due to physiological or anatomical elements. The most common gait deviations that may occur with current components are listed here.

Initial Contact to Foot Flat

Excessive Knee Extension

In the normal gait pattern, the knee flexes smoothly 8 to 10 degrees from heel contact to midstance. Flexion reduces the excursion of the body's center of gravity, allows for absorption of the floor reaction forces generated at heel strike through the joints of the lower limb, and reduces the amount of energy required in gait. Keeping the knee extended increased the amount of energy expended in walking; the deviation can best be seen from the side, observing the prosthetic knee from initial contact to midstance.

The client reports a sense of walking up a hill. Maintaining an extended knee with a socket aligned in flexion may lead to anterior distal pain and skin abrasion. Extension in this phase of gait leads to pelvic displacement and may appear as if the prosthesis is too long.

The major prosthetic causes are too long a **toe lever arm**, insufficient flexion of the socket, or too soft a heel support. The deviations can be differentiated by watching the heel from initial contact to midstance. Knee extension may also be the result of inadequate gait training or weakness of the quadriceps.

1. Too long a toe lever arm (posterior displacement of the socket over the foot) (**Fig. 7.13**): Posterior displacement of the socket brings the center of gravity line posterior, thereby increasing the length of the anterior segment or toe lever arm. If the foot is set too far anteriorly under the socket,

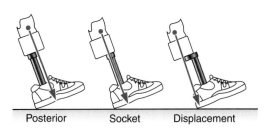

Posterior   Socket   Displacement

FIGURE 7.13. An overlong toe lever arm is created when the socket is placed too far posterior on the foot. The first placement is correct. The other two are different degrees of incorrect placement.

the length of the toe lever arm is increased and that of the heel level arm is decreased. As the client progresses from initial contact to foot flat, the center of gravity moves anterior to the axis of rotation of the knee very quickly, forcing the knee into extension. The client feels as if he or she is walking up a hill as the length of the anterior support component is increased.

2. Insufficient socket flexion: If the socket is not aligned in the desired 5 to 8 degrees of flexion, the patient will not be able to allow the knee to flex normally in this phase of gait.

3. Too soft a heel support: A heel wedge or plantar flexion bumper that is too soft for the client's weight will allow the prosthetic foot to plantar flex too fast. This premature contact of the foot with the floor tends to keep the knee in extension rather than allow normal rolling over the foot. This deviation is more common with single-axis feet such as the Seattle foot and more rarely seen with multiaxis or dynamic response feet.

4. Inadequate training: Individuals who have not been properly trained to use the prosthesis and have not developed confidence in their ability to control the limb may keep the knee in extension. Usually, a brief period of instruction with early follow-up will suffice to establish a satisfactory walking pattern.

Knee Instability

Knee stability is critically important to a smooth, energy-efficient gait. A client who does not feel stable and fears the knee will buckle will be loath to trust the limb will likely shorten stance phase on the prosthetic side. Knee instability can be seen at initial or terminal stance depending on the prosthetic cause (**Fig. 7.14**). The major prosthetic causes of knee instability include too short a toe lever arm, too hard a heel support, or too much socket flexion The short toe lever arm is described under terminal stance.

1. Too hard a heel support; dorsiflexed foot, higher heel shoe: The compressibility of the prosthetic foot, the density of the plantar flexion bumper, or the rigidity of the dynamic response foot is determined by the size, weight, and activity level of the client. If the foot characteristics do not match the patient, the necessary amount of plantar flexion and shock absorption will not take place, and the knee on the prosthetic side will be forced into excessive flexion from initial contact to midstance. The client may try to maintain knee stability by

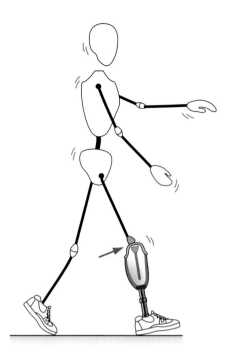

FIGURE 7.14. Heel contact to foot flat: knee instability.

extending the knee against the flexing forces, thereby creating excessive pressure at the anterior distal end of the residual limb and, possibly, the posterior proximal brim of the socket.

Midstance

Excessive Rising or Dropping of the Hip on the Prosthetic Side

1. Too long a prosthesis: If the prosthetic leg is longer than the sound leg, the client will raise the center of gravity over the support joint during stance phase. The deviation can best be seen from the rear by watching the prosthetic hip and shoulder during midstance. The client may also have difficulty bringing the prosthetic leg forward in swing and will either bend the knee excessively or raise the body up on the toe of the sound leg to allow room to clear the prosthetic foot. The latter deviation is called vaulting.

2. Too short a prosthesis: If the prosthetic leg is shorter than the sound leg, the person will seem to be walking in a hole on the prosthetic side (**Fig. 7.15**). The hip and shoulder on the amputated side drop at the beginning of stance phase. The deviation can best be observed from the rear by watching the hip and shoulder at midstance.

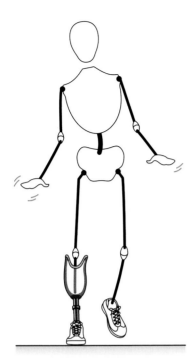

FIGURE 7.15. Midstance: Prosthesis too short.

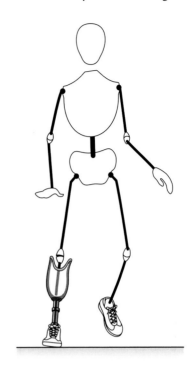

FIGURE 7.16. Midstance: Wide-based gait.

Some individuals prefer the prosthetic leg to be just slightly shorter than the sound leg, especially those who have had discrepancy in leg lengths for their whole lives. While ideally the legs should be the same lengths, comfort and function must be the guide in determining appropriate length alignment. This deviation is sometimes confused with "drop off" that occurs at terminal stance. In drop off, the prosthetic knee may have a tendency to buckle that usually does not occur with a prosthesis that is too short.

Wide-Based Gait

If the base of support is moved laterally, support is lost medially during single foot stance (**Fig. 7.16**). The client attempts to move the pelvis laterally to reach the support point, exhibiting a wide-based gait with the hips and the shoulders dropping laterally during stance phase. Excess pressure will be felt at the proximal lateral brim of the socket and the medial distal end of the residual limb. Two prosthetic causes are an outset foot and a medial leaning pylon. Both deviations can best be seen in the front or rear view, noting particularly the movements of the trunk and shoulders in stance. The outset foot can be differentiated from the medial leaning pylon by looking at the pylon at midstance. The gait deviation may

sometimes be noted if the person does not shift the weight properly over the prosthesis on stance. This training problem can be differentiated from a prosthetic problem by looking at the pylon at midstance and noting the width of the gait base.

1. Outset foot: Dynamically, the foot is usually set 1 cm medial to a line from the center of the posterior wall to the floor. If the foot is set too far lateral to the line, the client will lose support medially during stance. The sole of the shoe usually remains flat on the floor when the foot is outset.
2. Medial leaning pylon: Proper dynamic alignment places the pylon perpendicular at midstance (Fig. 7.17). If the top of the pylon is medial to the bottom, the pylon is said to lean medially. The client exhibits a wide-based gait and seems to lose support medially as in an outset foot, but if the problem is a medial leaning pylon, the foot will have more pressure on the medial side.

Narrow-Based Gait and Excessive Lateral Thrust of the Prosthesis

A narrow-based gait and thrust of the prosthesis laterally away from the knee at midstance often occur together and derive from the tendency of the prosthesis to rotate around the residual limb. If the base of

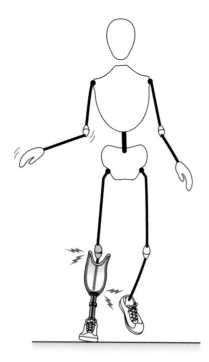

FIGURE 7.17. Midstance: Medial leaning pylon results in excessive pressure on the proximal lateral and distal medial areas of the residual limb.

support (the prosthetic foot) is moved medially, support is lost laterally during single-foot stance. Because there is no support for the pelvis in its normal alignment, it drops. In an attempt to maintain the pelvis level, the client may overcompensate and lean away from the prosthetic side on stance, or may allow the drop to take place and lean laterally over the prosthesis on stance. In both instances, there is excess movement of the pelvis and shoulder either toward or away from the prosthesis. This gait deviation simulates a weak gluteus medius gait. The client will report increased pressure at the medial proximal and lateral distal end of the socket. The socket may be seen to move laterally at midstance, opening a gap between the residual limb and the top of the socket. A slight lateral thrust of the knee on stance is considered normal; an excessive lateral thrust can cause injury to the knee joint. Two major prosthetic causes of this deviation are an excessively inset foot and a lateral leaning pylon. Both deviations can best be seen from the rear. In all deviations involving the alignment of the pylon, it is important to note the position at midstance and not at any other part of the **gait cycle.**

1. Improper mediolateral tilt of the socket (lateral leaning pylon): If the socket is set in abduction and the top of the pylon is more lateral than the

bottom at midstance, the pylon is said to lean laterally (**Fig. 7.18**). This increases pressure at the medial brim. In addition, the prosthetic foot is not flat on the floor and the weight is borne on the lateral border of the foot. These circumstances can be remedied by adducting the socket.

2. Inset foot: An inset foot results when the prosthetic foot is placed too far medial to the dynamic alignment line. At midstance, the sound extremity is swinging through the air so that all of the body weight is supported by the prosthetic foot on the floor. If this supporting foot is too far medial to the line of action of forces transmitted through the socket, a force couple is created that tends to rotate the socket around the stump. In almost all instances, this lateral thrust can be minimized or eliminated by "out-setting" the prosthetic foot slightly.

Terminal Stance

Knee Instability

1. Short toe lever arm (drop off): The toe lever arm provides support from midstance to terminal stance and allows the client to roll over the foot in a smooth manner (**Fig. 7.19**). The **heel lever arm** provides support from initial contact to midstance,

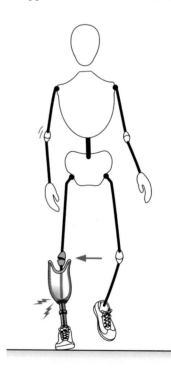

FIGURE 7.18. Midstance: Lateral leaning pylon results in excessive pressure on the proximal medial and distal lateral areas of the residual limb.

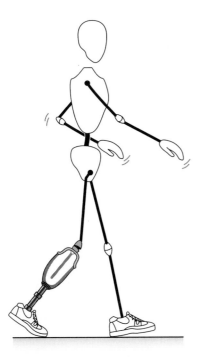

FIGURE 7.19. Terminal stance: Drop off.

allowing smooth descent of the prosthetic foot and controlled knee flexion. Just prior to heel-off during normal gait, the knee is extending. At heel-off or immediately thereafter, knee flexion begins. This change from extension to flexion coincides with the passing of the center of gravity over the metatarsophalangeal joints. If the body weight is carried over the metatarsophalangeal joints too soon, the resulting lack of anterior support allows premature knee flexion or drop off. If the foot is placed too far posterior under the socket, the toe lever arm will be shortened, and the client will not be supported in the terminal stance phase (**Fig. 7.20**). This premature loss of support causes the prosthetic knee to flex and the hip to drop sharply just before the end of stance. This deviation is called "drop off." It can

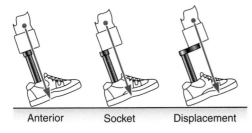

Anterior   Socket   Displacement

FIGURE 7.20. Too short toe lever arm is caused by placement of the socket too far forward on the foot. The first placement is correct. The other two are different degrees of incorrect placement.

best be seen from the lateral viewpoint by watching the hip and knee in terminal stance.

Knee Extension: Vaulting

1. Long toe lever arm: If the body weight is carried forward over a long toe lever arm, the knee joint remains in extension during the latter part of the stance phase and the client complains of a "walking uphill" sensation, because the center of gravity is carried up and over the extended knee (**Fig. 7.21**). This prosthetic problem may best be seen laterally.

Swing Phase

Pistoning (Loss of Suspension)

If the suspension mechanism is loose or inadequate, the prosthesis will slip as the foot leaves the ground for swing phase. The toe of the prosthesis can catch on the ground or the movement of the socket against the skin may cause abrasions (**Fig. 7.22**).

Uneven Step Length

Clients may develop the habit of taking a long prosthetic step and a short step with the unamputated leg. This is most likely a training problem. If gait training

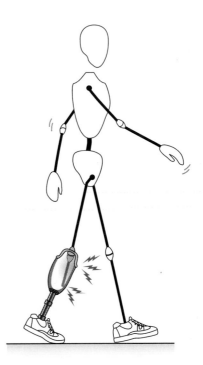

FIGURE 7.21. Terminal stance: A too long toe lever arm causes an extension moment.

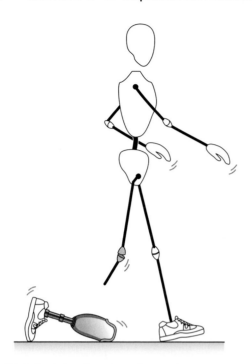

FIGURE 7.22. Swing phase: Loss of suspension.

does not focus on balance, weight shifting on and off the prosthesis, and single-leg stance, the person may not feel comfortable trusting the prosthesis through the complete stance phase. Patients may have difficulty with terminal stance and need to be taught this critical part of normal gait.

TRANSFEMORAL PROSTHETIC EVALUATION

Table 7.2 depicts the key items to check initially with a transfemoral prosthesis. In addition to the socket fit, suspension, comfort, leg length, and static alignment that are similar to the transtibial level, knee stability is an important consideration in the transfemoral limb. There are two aspects of knee control: alignment and active hip and pelvic motion. All types of knee mechanisms need to be aligned in a line or slightly posterior to a line drawn from the trochanter through the knee to the ankle axis (TKA) (see Fig. 6.20). This allows the body weight to fall anterior to the knee to create an extension moment

TABLE 7.2	**Static Transfemoral Prosthetic Checkout**	
Checkout Item	**What to Check**	**Possible Problem**
Before Donning Is the prosthesis as prescribed?	Compare to prescription and residual limb	Changes in prescribed components need to be justified
Is the inside of the socket smoothly finished?	Feel the inside of the socket	Skin abrasions
Do all components function properly?	Check particularly the knee mechanism; check stance, support knees by putting weight on them with the knee in slight flexion	Too much or too little knee resistance can create gait deviations; failure of stance support can lead to falls
Sitting Is the socket securely on the residual limb?	Pull on the socket slightly	Suspension should be maintained in all positions
Do the length of the shin and thigh correspond to the shin and thigh of the unamputated leg?	Check to see that the knees are level when the client is sitting with the knee flexed to 90 degrees	A high prosthetic knee could indicate a misaligned knee joint and lead to poor swing through
Can the client sit comfortably without burning or pinching?	Check the posterior wall; there should be a smooth and thin socket or liner layer	A sharp posterior wall can cause sciatic nerve pressure
Is the client able to lean forward and reach his or her shoes?	Check the anterior wall height when sitting	The anterior wall may impinge on the abdominal area

TABLE 7.2	Static Transfemoral Prosthetic Checkout—cont'd	
Checkout Item	What to Check	Possible Problem
Standing Does the socket fit properly and comfortably?	Ask the client if he or she is comfortable	Areas of discomfort can cause gait deviations, noncompliance with wearing the prosthesis, and skin problems
Is the knee stable when weight is placed on the prosthesis?	The knee joint is initially aligned on or just behind a line dropped from the trochanter to the knee axis (TKA); if the knee is in front of the line, it will be unstable Microprocessor and some hydraulic knees may be aligned on the TKA line	An unstable knee can lead to an insecure gait
Is the pelvis level when weight is borne evenly on both legs?	Palpate both iliac crests with the client standing with weight equally distributed on the two legs	Too long or too short a prosthesis will lead to gait deviations
Does the socket maintain good contact with the residual limb on all sides as the client shifts his or her weight?	Check the brim of the socket as the client shifts his or her weight	Too loose or tight a socket may lead to skin abrasions and discomfort
Is there an adductor roll?	Check high in the groin for excessive tissue around the medial wall	An adductor roll can be pinched between the top of the medial wall and the pubic ramus, leading to pain and an abducted gait
Is there pressure on the pubic ramus?	Ask the client	Pain can lead to an abducted gait

on initial contact. If the knee axis is on or anterior to the line, the body weight will fall behind the knee, creating a flexion or unstable moment (see Chapter 6). Alignment may vary slightly with different types of knee mechanisms. It is important for the client to have a stable knee during stance phase yet be able to flex the knee smoothly in terminal stance to initiate swing phase. Mechanical swing phase knee mechanisms additionally require the patient to extend the residual limb against the posterior wall of the prosthesis to maintain the knee in extension from heel strike to midstance. The extent of this motion varies with the type of knee mechanisms; microprocessor knees swing and stance phase hydraulic components function better with active hip and pelvis motion but have mechanisms that control knee stability even if the knee is not fully extended at initial contact. As described in Chapter 6, microprocessor knees actually allow initial knee flexion simulating normal gait. It is important for the therapist to understand the proper alignment and characteristics of each client's knee mechanism. Close communication with the prosthetist and regular review of the manufacturer's description of specific knee mechanisms is a valuable activity for therapists.

TRANSFEMORAL GAIT ANALYSIS

Normal Transfemoral Gait

Initial Contact to Midstance, Lateral View

Knee function and knee control varies with the type of knee mechanism in the prosthesis. If the patient is fitted with other than a microprocessor knee, generally, the knee is in extension from heel contact to midstance as the foot descends smoothly to the floor and the weight of the body progresses easily to a balanced point over the support leg. The pelvis moves forward and slightly lateral to achieve this position.

If the patient is fitted with a microprocessor knee, the prosthetic knee will approximate normal knee function with slight knee flexion from heel contact to mid-stance.

Midstance, Anterior View

The individual exhibits good medial lateral stability and balance on the prosthesis as the contralateral foot is picked up for swing phase. The width of the gait base should not exceed 5 cm. There may be a slight pelvic drop, not more than 5 degrees and no more than 2.5 cm of lateral trunk bending depending on the length and fleshiness of the residual limb.

Midstance to Toe Off, Lateral View

There is smooth heel rise as the weight is brought forward over the prosthetic forefoot. The hip extends without lumbar lordosis, and the knee begins to flex as the toe leaves the ground.

Swing Phase, Lateral View

The foot leaves the ground and the prosthetic knee bends smoothly. The hip and knee flex as the prosthetic leg swings forward in the line of progression. Heel rise is adequate for the prosthetic toe to clear the floor but is not excessive. The shank swings smoothly and quietly forward, and the knee is extended just prior to the next heel contact. The stride length is equal on both sides.

Transfemoral Gait Deviations

Initial Contact to Midstance, Lateral View

Knee Instability

Knee instability is the major problem that can occur from initial contact to midstance (**Fig. 7.23**).

Microprocessor knees are designed for slight flexion at initial contact. For all other knee mechanisms, even those with a stumble factor, making initial contact with the knee in extension will lead to a more secure gait pattern.

Causes of knee instability in other than microprocessor knees include the following:

1. If the knee axis is placed anterior to the TKA line, the line of body weight falls behind the knee creating a flexion moment. The knee can be malaligned if the socket is placed too far anterior (long heel lever arm).

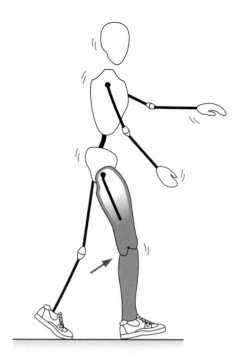

FIGURE 7.23. Heel contact to midstance: Knee instability.

2. Knee instability can also be caused by lack of adequate socket flexion limiting the client's active hip extension and forward motion of the pelvis.
3. Heel support that is too hard and does not accept body weight may also create a flexion moment at heel strike.
4. A severe hip flexion contracture not accommodated in the socket makes it difficult for the client to control the knee.

Knee instability with the microprocessor may be caused by the patient creating a flexion moment by putting pressure on the toe of the prosthesis inadvertently. While mechanical failures can occur, they are rare.

Foot Slap

If the forefoot descends too rapidly, it will make a slapping sound as it hits the floor (**Fig. 7.24**). This may be caused by plantar flexion resistance that is too soft or a heel lever arm that is too short. The client may also be driving the prosthesis into the walking surface too forcibly to assure extension of the knee. It is not a frequent problem.

Foot External Rotation

In the transition from initial contact to foot flat, the foot should remain in the line of progression.

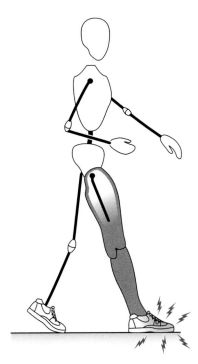

FIGURE 7.24. Heel contact to midstance: Foot slap.

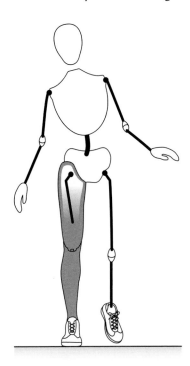

FIGURE 7.25. Midstance: Lateral trunk bending to prosthetic side.

Obvious foot external rotation at this point may be caused by

1. Foot that is aligned in too much external rotation
2. A socket that is too loose or that has been improperly donned
3. Excessive soft tissue in the residual limb with an intimate fitting socket

Midstance, Anterior-Posterior View

Lateral Trunk Bending

Most individuals walking with a transfemoral prosthesis exhibit some lateral bending from the midline to the prosthetic side because the prosthesis cannot fully compensate for loss of skeletal fixation to the ground (**Fig. 7.25**). Excessive bending may have several causes:

1. A socket or lateral wall not adducted adequately may cause this.
2. A prosthesis that is too short will cause a hip drop at midstance along with lateral trunk bending.
3. If the medial wall of the socket is too high, the individual may bend laterally to avoid pressure on the pubic ramus.

4. The client may not have adequate balance to properly shift the weight over the prosthesis or may have a very short residual limb that fails to provide a sufficient lever arm for the pelvis.
5. The client may have weak abductors on the prosthetic side and be unable to control the body weight over the prosthesis.
6. This gait deviation may also be seen if the client has a painful residual limb.

Abducted Gait

An abducted gait is characterized by a gait base that is wider than 5 cm at midstance (**Fig. 7.26**). Causes include the following:

1. A prosthesis that is too long
2. A high medial wall that causes the client to hold the prosthesis away to avoid ramus pressure
3. An abduction contracture
4. Inadequate gait training or poor gait habit

Extensive Trunk Extension

The client creates an active lumbar lordosis during stance phase if the following occurs (**Fig. 7.27**):

1. Insufficient initial socket flexion leads the client to extend the lumbar spine to obtain hip

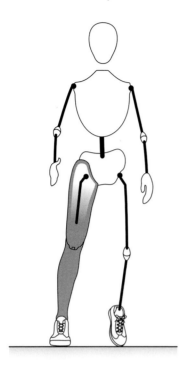

FIGURE 7.26. Midstance: Abducted gait.

extension and bring the pelvis over the support point.

2. The client may have a flexion contracture that cannot be accommodated prosthetically.
3. The client may have weak hip extensors and or weak abdominals.

Terminal Stance (Preswing), Lateral View

Drop Off

As with the transtibial prosthesis, there is a sudden downward movement of the trunk as anterior support is lost prematurely (**Fig. 7.28**). The main reason is usually a short toe lever arm. It is an unstable deviation, as it may cause the knee to buckle prematurely.

Inadequate Heel Off

If the client does not feel secure allowing the body weight to shift forward over the toe of the prosthesis, the heel may not come off the floor until the whole foot is brought forward. This deviation is associated with uneven steps discussed below.

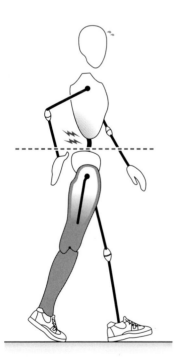

FIGURE 7.27. Midstance to toe off: Lumber lordosis.

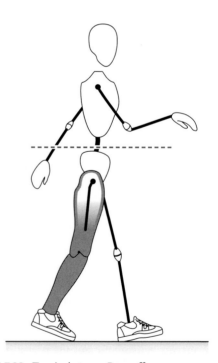

FIGURE 7.28. Terminal stance: Drop off.

Delayed Knee Flexion

If the client does not properly shift his or her weight over the forefoot and toes and reach forward with the unamputated leg, the client will not activate the knee flexion mechanism. This is particularly true with hydraulic and microprocessor knee mechanisms.

Swing Phase, Anterior-Posterior View

Circumducted Gait

During a circumducted gait, the prosthesis swings laterally in an arc-like manner during swing phase. Causes include the following:

1. The prosthesis may be too long.
2. The mechanical knee may have too much alignment stability or resistance in the knee, making it difficult to bend the knee in swing.
3. The client may lack confidence and not flex the prosthetic knee.
4. The stance phase control knee may not be functioning properly.

Vaulting

The client rises on the toe of the sound foot to swing the prosthesis through with little knee flexion. Some individuals use this maneuver temporarily to walk rapidly. Unwanted or continuous vaulting may be caused by

1. A prosthesis that is too long
2. Inadequate socket suspension
3. Excessive stability in the alignment or some limitation of knee flexion
4. Inadequate training

Medial or Lateral Whips

Whips are best observed when the client walks away from the observer (**Fig. 7.29**). A medial whip is present when the heel travels medially on initial flexion at the beginning of swing phase; a lateral whip exists when the heel moves laterally. Prosthetically, whips are always related to alignment of the knee mechanism:

1. Medial whips result from excessive external rotation of the prosthetic knee.
2. Lateral whips result from excessive internal rotation of the prosthetic knee.

Other causes may include a socket that is too tight, thus reflecting residual limb rotation or the client may

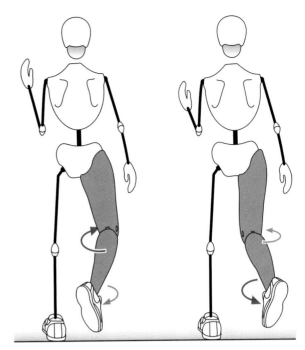

FIGURE 7.29. Swing phase: (Left) medial heel whip; (Right) lateral heel whip.

have donned the prosthesis in internal or external rotation.

Throughout the Gait Cycle: Uneven Arm Swing and Uneven Steps

These two deviations go together. The arm on the prosthetic side is held close to the body and the individual takes steps of unequal duration and length with a short stance phase on prosthesis. The major cause is poor or inadequate training and fear of putting weight on the prosthesis.

Case Study Activities

1. Design a prosthetic training program for each client. What do you already know how to do, and what do you need to learn?
2. Compare and contrast the prosthetic training program for an individual fitted with a transtibial prosthesis and someone fitted with a transfemoral prosthesis.
3. What parts of the training program are appropriately delegated to a physical therapist assistant?

DONNING THE PROSTHESIS

Proper prosthetic donning is one of the first things to be learned. Teaching proper donning involves showing the client the appropriate reference points between the residual limb and the socket and learning the correct feel of the prosthesis.

Socket Interfaces

Gel Liners

Today, most individuals use a gel liner as the socket interface. Gel liners fit directly over the residual limb, fit closely, and come several centimeters above the knee. Liners come in various shapes, sizes, and thicknesses (Chapter 6). The therapist must know the type of liner and any special donning strategies needed for that particular liner. Generally, the patient dons the liner by rolling it down, fitting the distal end of the residual limb directly into the distal end of the liner, then rolling the liner smoothly over the residual limb (see Fig. 7.9). Clients should be taught to avoid pulling on the top of the liner. There should be no space distally between the end of the residual limb and the end of the liner. The residual limb should be clean and dry, and except in special instances, nothing should be applied to the skin before applying the liner. Once again, close therapist prosthetist contact is necessary for the therapist to know the specific characteristics of the liner. Sometimes this information is available on the Web site of the manufacturer.

Residual Limb Socks

Some prostheses are worn with cotton or wool socks rather than a gel liner. The socks function as the socket interface and are applied similarly to the gel liner. The patient needs to learn that the distal sock seam must run parallel to the incision line in a medial–lateral direction to avoid placing the thicker seam over the distal end of the tibia. Care must be taken that the sock is smooth and wrinkle free. If the client is using a sleeve suspension, the sleeve must come at least 2 inches higher than the top of the socks to properly suspend the prosthesis. Socks come in different thicknesses or plys. A thin cotton sock is considered to be one ply; wool socks are made in either three or five plys.

Some clients may choose to wear a thin nylon sheath under the liner or sock to reduce skin friction during ambulation. There are other sheaths available for individuals with sensitive skin or dermatological conditions (Chapter 6).

Limb Shrinkage

As the residual limb shrinks, cotton or wool socks are added between the liner and the socket. If the liner incorporates a shuttlelock pin, the sock must have a hole in the bottom to allow the pin to come through. Care must be taken that no lint, thread, or piece of sock remains around the pin, or it is likely to jam the mechanism, making it hard to remove. One-ply socks are added as the residual limb gets smaller. When the individual is wearing three one-ply socks, he or she can substitute a three-ply wool sock. By the time the individual needs a total of 10 to 15 plys, it is time to replace the socket. The physical therapist or physical therapist assistant teaches the client how to adjust socks as the residual limb becomes smaller.

Transtibial Prosthesis

The transtibial prosthesis is usually donned sitting. Once the liner has been applied, it is a simple matter to place the limb in the socket (**Fig. 7.30**). The patellar bar is a good reference point for the client. If the prosthesis fits snugly, the person may have to stand to get the residual limb properly in the socket. When wearing a suction prosthesis, the person stands after donning to expel any remaining air. The suspension sleeve is rolled up, making sure that at least 3 or 4 cm of sleeve is in contact with skin. The shuttlelock system requires that the individual fits the pin carefully into the receptacle and then stands to push

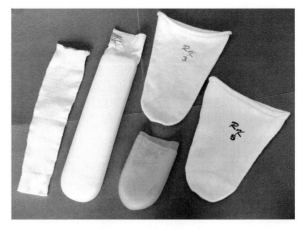

FIGURE 7.30. Residual limb socks and sheaths.

the limb well into the socket until the lock is heard to click into place. The limb is removed by pushing the small button built into the medial socket wall.

Transfemoral Prosthesis

When the client dons the ischial containment socket, care must be taken to ensure that the socket is not rotated internally or externally. The lateral wall and foot position are guides to proper donning. There are transfemoral sockets that can be donned sitting and some that require standing. New suction liners can now be put on with the client sitting, only standing to expel residual air. Physical therapists working with amputees need to learn the variety of configurations to properly reinforce proper donning with the patient. The therapist can check that the ischial containment socket has been donned properly by palpating the ischial tuberosity within the socket and palpating the pubic ramus to ensure that there is not excessive pressure on the medial wall.

The suction socket must fit intimately to maintain suction. In most situations, the patient "pulls" himself or herself into the socket by donning a special sock or a piece of stockingette. The person then puts the residual limb and sock into the socket and pulls the sock out through the valve hole as illustrated in **Figure 7.31**. While pulling the sock out, the person pumps and pushes the residual limb all the way into the socket. The process needs to be done standing and requires good balance.

Donning the quadrilateral socket is similar, and the patient can use the adductor channel at the anterior medial corner of the socket as a guide to proper donning. The therapist can check for proper fit by palpating the ischial tuberosity as it sits on the posterior wall as well as the adductor longus in the channel. There should not be excessive pressure on the pubic ramus in this socket either. In both sockets, palpating the ischial tuberosity is easier if the patient leans forward a little bit initially to allow access to the area, and then places his or her weight in the prosthesis.

PROSTHETIC TRAINING

The major goal of prosthetic rehabilitation is for the client to attain a smooth, energy-efficient gait that allows the individual to perform activities of daily living and participate in desired employment and recreational activities. Prosthetic ambulation is a skilled psychomotor activity, and the client must learn to adapt well-developed patterns of movements to new situations. They must learn new feedback mechanisms, and the higher is the level of amputation, the more complex the tasks.

Factors that contribute to a smooth, energy-efficient gait include the ability to

- Accept the weight of the body on each leg
- Balance on one foot in single-limb support
- Advance each limb forward and prepare for the next step
- Adapt to environmental demands

Traditional prosthetic training has focused on breaking down the gait cycle into small steps and teaching each step. However, normal gait is an integrated activity that may not be learned most efficiently through the practice of each part. Dennis and McKeough[14] developed a taxonomy of motor tasks based on the work of Gentile[15] that describes environmental conditions involved in regaining independent function. The taxonomy is easily applicable to the clinical setting and provides a reference point for organizing and sequencing gait training.

Figure 7.32 is a schematic representation of the Dennis and McKeough taxonomy as a two-dimensional grid. One dimension (the horizontal axis of the grid) represents desired outcomes, progressing from simple goals requiring body stability (eg, sitting or standing) to more demanding goals requiring transporting the body through space and time (eg, walking). Both classes of outcomes—body stability and body in motion—are subdivided into two classifications: goals that do not require manipulation (eg, sitting while someone combs the client's hair) and those that do (eg, reaching for an object). The result is four categories of goals ranged along the horizontal axis and progressing from simple on the left to more demanding on the right. Similarly, the vertical axis of the grid represents variables in environment, with the less demanding environmental situations at the top and the more demanding at the bottom. The two primary categories in the environmental dimension are closed and open. A closed environment, for example, a room with furniture but no people, is one that does not change during the performance of the desired goal. An open environment, for instance, a room with a dog moving around, is one that changes during the task performance.

Again, each major category is further subdivided into two variables: in one there is no change in the environment between trials (eg, the space remains the same each time the client attempts the activity); in the other, more difficult variable, the environment changes between trials (eg, furniture is moved closer together, the dog runs around the room). As with the horizontal axis, the categories on the vertical axis are arranged in order of increasing difficulty, the simplest at the top and the most challenging on the bottom. Each of the 16 cells on the resulting grid represents a separate level of task or goal difficulty, with the simplest in the upper left and the most difficult in the lower right.

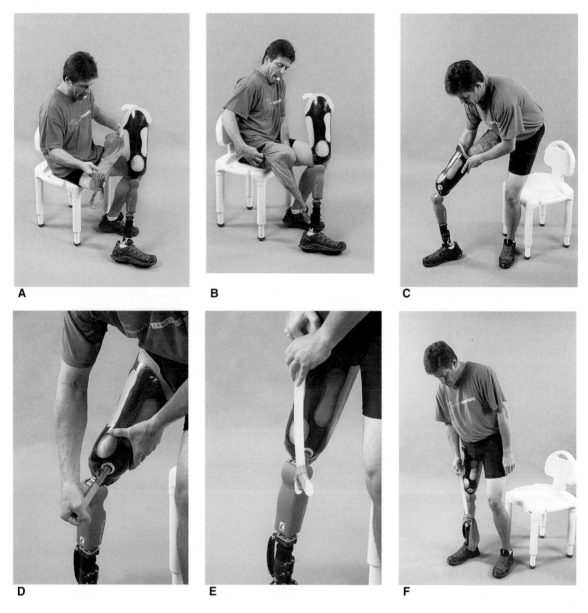

FIGURE 7.31. Donning the suction transfemoral prosthesis: **(A)** The donning sock has a tab at the end to make it easier to pull through the valve hole. **(B)** The sock is put on the residual limb, making sure it is brought all the way to the hip. **(C)** Standing, the patient pushes the end of the sock through the valve hole. **(D)** Pulling the sock out through the valve hole pulls the residual limb into the socket. **(E)** A tool provides leverage to pull the sock out. **(F)** The sock must be completely removed. **(G)** The valve is replaced securely and all air is expelled. **(H)** The completed prosthesis.

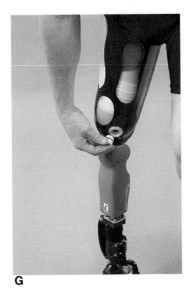
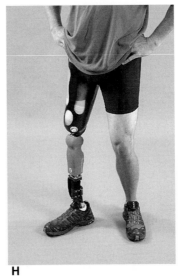

G   H

FIGURE 7.31. CONT'D

		Without Manipulation	With Manipulation	Without Manipulation	With Manipulation
C L O S E D E N V I R O N M E N T	**Without Intertrial Variability**	Body is stable, arms and legs are still, the task does not change, the environment is fixed in time & space.	Body is stable, task does not change, environment is fixed in time & space, arms or legs are moving.	Body is moving, limbs moving in relation to movement task, task does not change, environment is fixed in time & space.	Body is moving, arms or legs moving independently of task, environment is fixed in time & space.
	With Intertrial Variability	As above but task changes require slight modification in motor plan from trial to trial.	As above but task changes require slight modification of motor plan from trial to trial.	As above but task changes require slight modification of motor plan from trial to trial.	As above but task changes require slight modification of motor plan from trial to trial.
O P E N E N V I R O N M E N T	**Without Intertrial Variability**	Body is stable, arms & legs are still, task is fixed, environment is changing in time and space.	Body is stable, task is fixed, arms & legs are moving independently of tasks, environment is changing in time and space.	Body is moving, task is fixed, arms and legs and synchronous with task, environment is changing in time & space.	Body is moving, arms or legs moving independently of task, task is fixed, environment changing in time & space.
	With Intertrial Variability	As above, but task changes each trial.	As above, but task changes each trial.	As above but task changes each trial.	As above but task changes each trial.

FIGURE 7.32. Taxonomy of motor tasks: Dimensions of task difficulty. *(Adapted from Dennis JK, and McKeough DM: Mobility. In May BJ: Home health and rehabilitation: concepts of care. F.A. Davis, Philadelphia, 1993.)*

These concepts can guide the therapist in planning the sequence of training activities. The training program starts in a closed environment with stability then mobility activities and progresses to the more complex open environment. As success is achieved at one level, activities can be made more complex by varying the independent limb mobility or adding intertrial variability.

Teaching Prosthetic Control

Table 7.3 depicts the critical elements of a gait training program and suggested early training activities. It is critically important to the success of a prosthetic training program that the person learns to balance and integrate the prosthesis into closed environment balance activities before starting coordinated walking. Today's limited funding for rehabilitation has led many physical therapists to give the prosthetic patient a walker or other form of external support and have

the patient walk before he or she has learned how to balance, weight shift, and, particularly for someone with a transfemoral prosthesis, achieve knee control. The patient must learn to trust that the prosthesis will support his or her body weight and that the patient can control the components. A walker should never be used as part of a prosthetic training program, because the walker reinforces an asymmetrical gait pattern; interferes with the function of the prosthesis, especially the transfemoral prosthesis; and causes the patient to use excessive energy in a slow and uneven gait. The patient started using a walker or other form of external support may never be able to progress beyond this level. If only a limited time is authorized for gait training, it is better to help the person develop good bipedal and single-leg standing balance and integrate the prosthesis into goals-oriented movement patterns as he or she develops confidence that the limb will support him or her. Through these goal-oriented activities, the individual can also develop

TABLE 7.3	Critical Training Elements		
Element		Activity	Details
Stability—both legs (TT/TF) 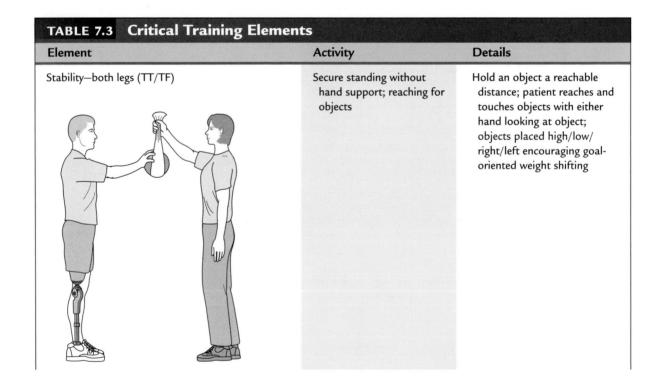		Secure standing without hand support; reaching for objects	Hold an object a reachable distance; patient reaches and touches objects with either hand looking at object; objects placed high/low/ right/left encouraging goal-oriented weight shifting

TABLE 7.3   Critical Training Elements—cont'd

Element	Activity	Details
Knee control (TF)	Secure standing without hand support; slightly bend and straighten prosthetic knee to varying degrees	Encourage patient to develop kinesthetic feel of knee position by socket pressures
Stability on prosthesis (TT/TF)	Secure standing without hand support; place 6- to 8-inch stool directly in front of patient	In a controlled manner, patient places unamputated foot on stool and back on the floor

Continued

TABLE 7.3   Critical Training Elements—cont'd

Element	Activity	Details
Stability on prosthesis (TT/TF)	Secure standing without hand support; place soccer ball in front of unamputated leg	In a controlled manner, patient kicks the ball with the unamputated foot
Prosthetic control (TT/TF)	Secure standing without hand support; place soccer ball in front of prosthesis	In a controlled manner, patient kicks the ball with the prosthetic leg

TABLE 7.3   Critical Training Elements—cont'd

Element	Activity	Details
Proprioception (TT/TF) 	Secure standing both legs on a piece of paper with a clock face drawn and without hand support	On command, patient shifts weight to 12, 3, 6, and 9 o'clock in random order; learns to recognize where prosthetic foot is in relation to weight bearing
Pelvic control (TT/TF) 	Secure standing without hand support, prosthetic leg behind unamputated leg; provide resistance to forward pelvic progression at initial contact to foot flat	Encourage patient to transfer weight smoothly with forward and slight lateral pelvic motion by providing resistance as patient brings prosthesis forward

Continued

TABLE 7.3	Critical Training Elements—cont'd	
Element	**Activity**	**Details**
Stepping with prosthesis (TT/TF)	Secure standing without hand support, step forward and back with prosthesis	Start with double-leg stance, shift weight to unamputated leg, and step forward with prosthesis; return prosthesis to position behind sound leg; emphasize knee control with TF
Stepping with sound leg (TT/TF)	Secure standing without hand support, step forward and back with unamputated leg	As above but with unamputated leg; make sure patient brings weight to forward part of foot before stepping on unamputated leg; emphasize toe off on TF to activate swing initiation

TABLE 7.3	Critical Training Elements—cont'd	
Element	Activity	Details
Side stepping; backward stepping (TT/TF) 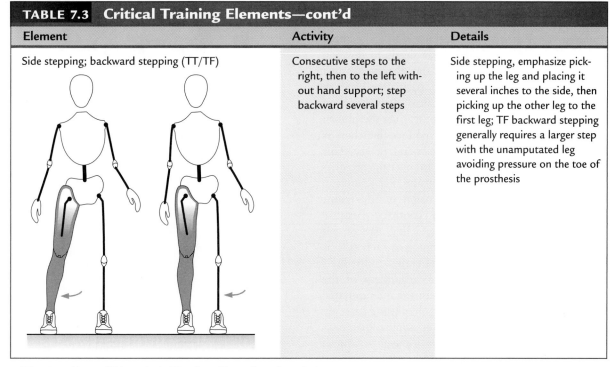	Consecutive steps to the right, then to the left without hand support; step backward several steps	Side stepping, emphasize picking up the leg and placing it several inches to the side, then picking up the other leg to the first leg; TF backward stepping generally requires a larger step with the unamputated leg avoiding pressure on the toe of the prosthesis

TT, patient with transtibial prosthesis; TF, patient with transfemoral prosthesis.

new patterns of proprioception and learn to use socket pressures to feel where the foot is in space. It is important to limit the wearing time of the prosthesis during early training and to check the residual limb often to avoid possible residual limb problems. Ideally, the patient should be seen daily or even twice daily if in an inpatient rehabilitation center. The residual limb should be wrapped after wearing to avoid rebound edema. If the patient cannot be seen daily and there is adequate supervision in the home, the person should be taught to don the prosthesis daily and perform basic balancing exercises at home in an appropriate setting. Wearing time each day is determined by the condition of the residual limb and the patient's tolerance. Usually, wear is limited to no more than 2 hours at a time and is gradually increased. The patient can put the prosthesis on in the morning and again in the afternoon until the residual limb has adjusted. Generally, by the time the person has learned good balance and is able to walk with the prosthesis, he or she can wear it safely for 6 to 8 hours a day. Very active individuals may try to stretch this gradual adjustment and sometimes develop skin abrasions that keep them out of the prosthesis for several days or a week. It may take several weeks for the active person to be able to resume sports or other strenuous activities depending on the cause of amputation and the condition of the residual limb.

Early training starts in a closed environment with simple motion problems; gradually the movement problems become more complex. The patient needs to be in a secure environment for gait training, but it is better not to use the hands for support if possible. Having the patient stand in a corner with the therapist in front provides both security and dependence on the prosthesis for support. Reaching activities as outlined in Table 7.3 can be made more complex by increasing the distance the patient has to reach and having the patient reach across his or her body to the object. Single-leg stance can also be made more difficult by using a higher stool or rolling the ball to the patient to be kicked. However, rolling the ball to the patient creates an open environment. Integrating some open environment activities such as ball catching or kicking can be a valuable training tool as can doing balance activities on a compliant surface such as a mat or foam pad.

Individuals with transtibial prostheses must learn to let their knee flex slightly from initial contact to midstance in a natural gait pattern. Similarly, individuals fitted with transfemoral prostheses with a microprocessor knee also need to let the knee flex slightly from initial contact to foot flat as the mechanism is designed to do. (A CD outlining the specifics of gait training with a microprocessor knee may be obtained from Otto Bock at www.ottobockusa.com.) The client wearing a transfemoral prosthesis needs to develop voluntary knee control early; the therapist must understand the function of the particular knee to properly teach the client knee control. Pelvic motion is an important aspect of knee control. As the person comes forward from heel contact to foot flat, there is a transverse rotation of the ipsilateral pelvis. This helps bring the body weight forward over the prosthesis and maintain the knee in extension. Pelvic motion also enhances the natural extension of the femur which also contributes to knee control.[16] Because individuals rarely walk in a straight line, part of gait training should include side stepping to each side as well as walking backward. Generally, individuals wearing transfemoral prostheses, regardless of the type of knee mechanism, lead with the unamputated leg when walking backward, to avoid putting pressure on the toe of the prosthesis and creating a knee flexion moment. In most instances it is a step-to pattern although the prosthetic foot can pass the unamputated leg as long as weight is kept on the heel or mid foot. This activity should be taught and practiced.

Clients often tend to look at the foot during initial training because they cannot feel the floor directly. A mirror helps the individual keep the head erect and focus on feeling the socket pressures change during the different parts of weight shifting (**Fig. 7.33**). Focusing on achieving the goals of an activity such as touching a ball or reaching into a cabinet also helps prevent looking at the feet. Individuals who develop skill in the early training program are most likely to develop a smooth, energy-efficient gait pattern and become functional prosthetic users. The early emphasis on balance and control of the prosthesis helps the patient develop confidence in his or her ability and has been shown to be positively related to functional prosthetic mobility. Miller and associates, in a study of the effect of balance confidence, found that individuals with less confidence in their ability restricted their activities and prosthetic use.[16] In another study, balance was found to be the only significant variable related to prosthetic mobility in a systematic review of pertinent literature.[17]

Initial Walking

When the patient has become competent in the basic activities outlined in Table 7.3, coordinated walking

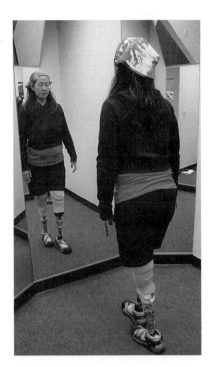

FIGURE 7.33. Training in front of a mirror reduces the tendency to look at the floor.

is the next part of training. Initial walking may take place in or out of the parallel bars but may be better outside the bars where the person can develop a coordinated and rhythmic gait pattern and use normal trunk and arm movements. Patients often tend to take a large step with the prosthesis and a small step with the unamputated leg leading to an asymmetrical gait pattern. Encourage even-sized steps from the beginning. Gailey recommends having the patient take a larger step with the sound leg and slightly smaller steps with the prosthesis to help overcome asymmetry in gait.[18] Developing even trunk rotation and arm swing is also important to an energy-efficient gait. As the patient initiates coordinated walking, the therapist can walk behind and provide stimuli to the shoulders to encourage the movement (**Fig. 7.34**). Yigiter and associates used PNF techniques with a group of traumatic transfemoral amputees to determine if this approach improved gait parameters.[19] PNF patterns were used for resisted standing balance in a variety of directions, and approximation on the prosthetic side to improve proprioception and resistance to forward pelvic motion were part of the program. The control group received a more traditional approach including weight shifting in various directions. Yigiter and associates found that both groups developed functional

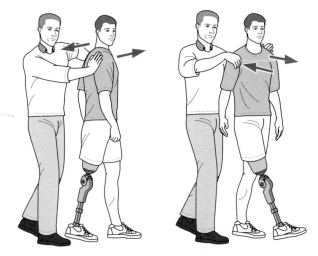

FIGURE 7.34. The therapist can facilitate proper shoulder and trunk motion in gait.

gait patterns and improved over the pretreatment measures, but the PNF group showed significantly greater improvement in most gait parameters including weight acceptance, even gait pattern, and velocity.[19] If at all possible, initial walking should be performed without ancillary support. The patient will be better able to develop a symmetrical gait pattern if not dependent on a cane or crutch.

Feedback

Throughout, the client, as an integral part of the team, needs to learn to give himself or herself feedback on the performance. Feedback includes knowledge of both performance and outcome. The client needs to be aware of his or her own performance. Feedback can be verbal, tactile, visual, or auditory, and all have a place in the therapist's toolbox. Asking the client, "How did that feel?" and "What would help you make the performance feel natural?" are helpful in drawing the patient's attention to his or her performance. Care should be taken not to talk too much. Therapists sometimes have the tendency to fill the void and talk all the time, distracting the patient from concentrating on the task. Verbal feedback should be delayed a bit to allow the patient to integrate the performance. Tactile feedback should be distinct and well timed. In addition to resistance for pelvic motion described above, tapping on the hip on the prosthetic side as the patient initiates weight bearing can be a reminder to shift the weight.

Real-time visual feedback has been found to be useful in helping clients improve gait symmetry when walking on a treadmill and seeing their performance on a computer screen.[20] In an interesting article, Dickstein and Deutsch summarized articles on the use of mental imagery in improving motor performance.[21] The use of mental imagery to improve a motor task is well known in the athletic world and has been used in the rehabilitation of patients with varied neurological problems. Although not specific to amputees, Dickstein and Deutsch found a number of studies where mental imagery improved motor performance. The article describes methods of using mental imagery with patients, and its application in the training of amputees is clear.

The military created two state-of-the-art gait laboratories to help in the rehabilitation of wounded service members. Walter Reed Medical Center developed a computerized force plate walking system to gather data on varied dimensions of the amputee's gait and compare the data to the same dimensions of normal gait. The data are used by therapists and prosthetists in the gait training program. A video camera is also used to provide feedback.[22] The laboratory is part of the advanced rehabilitation facility at Walter Reed Army Medical Center. The Center for the Intrepid is a multimillion dollar state-of-the-art rehabilitation center developed with private funds at Brooke Army Medical Center[23] (http://www.fallenheroesfund. org/About-IFHF/Fund-History/The-Center-for-the-Intrepid.aspx). The center is an advanced rehabilitation outpatient facility, and the length of stay varies according to patient needs. While receiving treatment, individuals reside in appropriate military housing nearby. The center includes all the facilities of a modern rehabilitation center plus a virtual reality laboratory as well as high-activity equipment and facilities such as a running track and climbing wall (Fig. 7.35). In the virtual reality laboratory, patients can confront a wide variety of realistic virtual environments such as city streets, beaches, elevators, and boat rides. A moving walkway will take the person through these environments and simulate the motions and changes. The computerized system provides real-time feedback, real-time gait training, and motion-capture capabilities. There are also virtual games that can be played that simulate real activities. Advanced gait analysis laboratories and video feedback are not generally available in most clinics. Cole and associates developed a clinical gait service based on a reduced data set from video and similar technologies; they incorporated biweekly sessions as part of the initial training of 18 amputees, then gave the subjects a satisfaction survey. All the patients

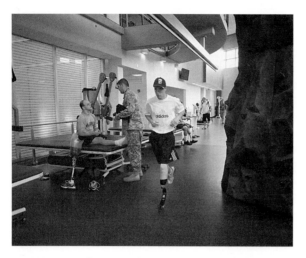

FIGURE 7.35. The Center for the Intrepid includes a running track, climbing wall, as well as regular therapeutic equipment. *(Reprinted with permission and courtesy of Susan Gaetz [susangaetz.com].)*

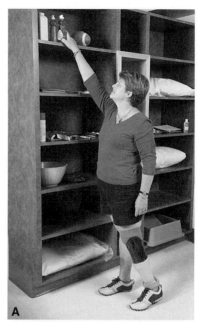

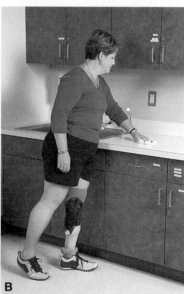

FIGURE 7.36. Prosthetic training in the home: Incorporating functional activities increases the internalization of prosthetic use.

responded positively to this additional gait analysis and feedback believing that it enhanced their gait training activities.[24]

In the home setting, incorporating everyday activities such as reaching for something on a high shelf, making a bed, or wiping a counter all encourage prosthetic weight shifting in a functional pattern (**Fig. 7.36**). Getting up and down from a chair is usually part of early gait training. Depending on the knee mechanism of the transfemoral prosthesis, the person must learn to take all the weight off the prosthesis before sitting or, with the C-Leg and some hydraulic knee systems, may be able to use the mechanism to sit with some weight on the prosthesis (**Fig. 7.37**). When teaching sitting, make sure the patient puts some pressure on the toe of the prosthesis to initiate knee flexion. Leaning slightly forward ("nose over the toes") facilitates the flexion moment.

External Support

As stated earlier, energy expenditure is a major concern and a major factor in successful prosthetic mobility. Energy expenditure is directly related to balance and gait symmetry. It is desirable to train the person for functional ambulation without external devices if at all possible. The therapist must be aware that age alone does not indicate the need for external support. Some individuals opt to use a single point or quad cane outside in the community. On occasion, crutches may be needed if the client has other medical conditions that preclude ambulating with less support. A four-point gait is usually taught unless the client needs to protect the unamputated leg from full weight bearing. A walker is usually not indicated as the terminal external support and should not be considered as an intermediate step between the parallel bars and a cane. A walker does not allow a smooth symmetrical gait, reinforces uneven steps and forward

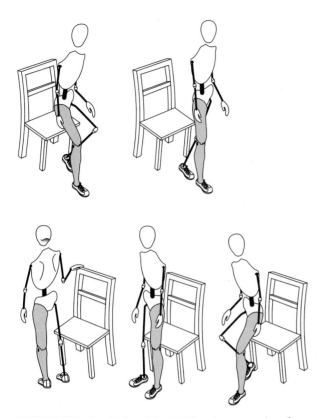

FIGURE 7.37. Prosthetic training: **(A)** learning to stand up from and **(B)** sit down on a chair is an early training activity.

trunk flexion, and eliminates the normal use of the arms. Using the walker as a shortcut to allow the client to be discharged from treatment early or to use the prosthesis at home before a good gait has been achieved leads to gait deviations and a dependency on the walker that may never be overcome. A walker should be used only if it is obvious that the individual will not be able to use the prosthesis with any other form of external support. An unstable person who can go to the bathroom independently with a walker is easier to care for at home than one who may be wheelchair dependent. In a study comparing gait efficiency of individuals using a four-point walker versus using a two-point wheeled walker, Tsai and associates found that patients used a smoother but equally safe gait with the two-point wheeled walker.[25] However, the walker should be used sparingly and only after careful evaluation of the individual's potential. All unilateral lower extremity amputees need support for times when they are not wearing a prosthesis. Many will use the same support used during the preprosthetic period.

Advanced Training

Case Study Activities

1. Design a training program for each patient which incorporates the progression from a closed to an open environment.
2. Identify at least two activities for each cell of the model that you would do in a rehabilitation center and in a home environment.

Changing the environment is an integral part of the gait training program. It is hardly functional to have the client walk only in the sheltered and simple environment of the physical therapy gym. Functional ambulation takes place in complex closed environments and in open environments. It is the physical therapist's and physical therapist assistant's responsibility to provide opportunities to practice these skills. Walking around furniture, through narrow doorways, on rugs, and around obstacles is very different from walking in the gym. Even though this is still a closed environment, it is more complex than wide pathways without obstacles. Placing obstacles on the floor to step around or over or walking in a busy hallway of the treatment center are progression activities. The home environment is also replete with opportunities for such progression. An even more complex closed environment is required by picking something up from the floor or carrying an object in one hand (**Fig. 7.38**). These activities require balance, coordination, and the ability to shift one's weight on and off the prosthesis in different body positions. It becomes an open environment activity if there are people in the room or hall. During advanced training, the client is taught to get up and down from chairs of different heights and seat resilience, especially toilet seats. An interesting obstacle course can be created using chairs, single steps, and blocks to walk around as well as different surfaces.

Steps and Ramps

Individuals wearing transtibial prostheses generally have little difficulty mastering steps and ramps once they have achieved good balance and prosthetic control. The ability to go down step over step requires fair balance but is generally achieved by most individuals whether or not they use a handrail. Going up step over

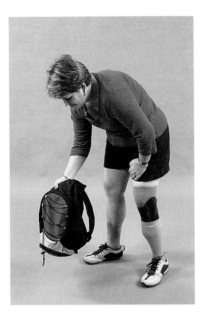

FIGURE 7.38. Learning to pick up an object from the floor requires balance and coordination.

step requires good quadriceps strength and a medium to long residual limb. Some gait adaption may be needed for steep ramps or hills depending on the type of prosthetic foot. The more limitation of dorsiflexion, the harder it is to go up a steep hill step over step. Many individuals take a long step with the prosthesis and a shorter step with the unamputated foot. Going down a steep hill again requires good quadriceps and prosthetic control but is achieved by most individuals.

The technique for going up and down stairs and ramps will again vary for an individual wearing a transfemoral prosthesis depending on the type of knee component. Until the power knees come into general use (Chapter 6), the person will have to go up steps one step at a time leading with the unamputated leg. Depending on the height of the step, some people will go up two steps with the unamputated leg and bring the prosthesis to that step level. Individuals fitted with a stance phase control knee system will have to go down steps one at a time leading with the prosthesis. All others have the potential of going down step over step, although, except for the C-Leg and some hydraulic units, it requires considerable balance. It is necessary for the individual to place the prosthetic heel only on the step to create a flexion moment in the knee as weight is brought forward, thereby allowing the knee to flex and the person to bring the unamputated leg down to the lower step. The process is quite easy with the C-Leg, because the computer program is designed to allow smooth

flexion as the person is going down steps or a ramp (**Fig.** 7.39). Many hydraulic knee systems also allow this motion, and part of the prosthetic training program is to provide opportunities for the patient to learn this control. **Table** 7.4 depicts general techniques for some advanced activities for individuals with a transfemoral prosthesis. Once good balance, prosthetic control, and gait have been achieved, most individuals will develop their own method of doing each of these activities. Whether to teach a patient how to fall can be problematic. Most older individuals will not want to try to practice, hoping never to fall. Active people, particularly those participating in sports activities, may need to practice falling to try and fall away from the prosthesis if possible. Falling, particularly on the bent knee of a transfemoral prosthesis, can lead to hip or pelvic fractures. For more advanced activities including sports activities, see Chapter 19.

Obstacle courses can be excellent methods of advanced training. Hofstad and associates studied delayed and decreased obstacle avoidance in individuals wearing one lower extremity prosthesis. Level of amputation was not indicated but electromyographic studies were taken to study responses to obstacles. Results indicated that responses to obstacles were either delayed or decreased on both limbs regardless of which limb had the prosthesis. The authors suggested that obstacle training could be useful.[26]

CARE OF THE PROSTHESIS, RESIDUAL LIMB, LINERS, AND SOCKS

Teaching the client proper care of the residual limb, the prosthesis, and how to adjust socks is an integral part of the training program. The physical therapist

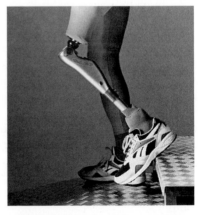

FIGURE 7.39. Person wearing C-Leg® going down stairs step over step. (*Courtesy of Otto Bock USA.*)

TABLE 7.4	Advanced Activities (Transfemoral)
Activity	**Procedure**
Sitting on the floor	Place the prosthesis about half a step behind the sound foot, keeping the weight on the sound foot. Bend from the waist and flex at the knees and hips, reaching for the floor with both arms outstretched and pivoting to the sound side. Then, gradually lower the body to the floor. This activity is one continuous movement.
Getting up from the floor	Get on the hands and knees; place the sound leg forward, well under the trunk, with the foot flat on the floor while balancing on the hands and the prosthetic knee. Then, extend the sound knee while maintaining the weight over the sound leg. Move to an erect position by pushing strongly with the sound leg and the arms, bringing the prosthesis forward when almost erect.
Kneeling	Place the sound foot ahead of the prosthetic foot, keeping the weight on the sound leg. Slowly flex the trunk, hip, and knee until the prosthetic knee can be gently placed on the floor. Clients with transfemoral limbs usually kneel on the prosthetic leg. Getting up from a kneeling position is like getting up from the floor.
Picking up an object from the floor	Place the sound foot ahead of the prosthetic foot with the body weight remaining on the sound leg. Bend forward at the waist, flexing the hips and knees until the object can be reached. Care must be taken to maintain the weight on the sound leg if wearing a mechanical knee. Some individuals like to bend sideways rather than forward, while others find it easier to keep the prosthetic knee straight and bend the sound leg until the object can be picked up.
Clearing obstacles	Face the obstacle with the sound foot slightly in front and the body weight on the prosthesis. Step over the obstacle with the sound leg, and then transfer the body weight to the sound leg. Quickly extend the prosthetic hip; forcefully flex the prosthetic hip, whipping the prosthesis forward over the obstacle. Then step forward with a normal gait pattern. An alternate method is to stand sideways to the obstacle with the sound leg closest to the obstacle. With the weight on the prosthesis, swing the sound leg over the obstacle and transfer the body weight to the sound leg. Then swing the prosthesis forward, up and over the obstacle. The C-Leg and some hydraulic unit may allow enough knee flexion to clear a small obstacles normally.

and physical therapist assistant should contact the prosthetist to learn proper care of the particular materials used in the prosthesis. Most plastic sockets and gel liners can be washed with a damp cloth and dried thoroughly. The socket and liner should be washed at night to allow plenty of drying time. Gel liners need to be laid flat or placed on the stand that may accompany the liner to dry. Under no circumstances should it be thrust into the prosthetic socket overnight. Gel liners are relatively fragile and can develop cracks or tears if not properly handled. Likewise, socks, if used, must be washed and changed daily. Wool socks require hand washing with a mild soap and flat drying. Learning to adjust socks for a shrinking residual limb or for an individual whose weight fluctuates is important. The prosthesis should be checked regularly for any mechanical problems or cracks in the socket. Although socket material and components are quite durable, an active lifestyle can create stress on

parts of the prosthesis over time. The patient must be encouraged to return to the prosthetist immediately if any signs of excessive wear are seen or a mechanical problem occurs. The patient should never attempt to repair the prosthesis himself or herself.

The residual limb needs to be treated like any other part of the body. Some people think they need special lotions or astringents for the residual limb and should be discouraged from the use of any astringent that may dry the skin. Soft, pliable skin can best tolerate the pressures of prosthetic wear. The client needs to learn to inspect the residual limb whenever the prosthesis is removed for any sign of excess pressure or developing abrasions. There are some special products available from the prosthetist for clients with excessive perspiration. On occasion, the use of antiperspirant on the residual limb is advocated before donning to help control perspiration. However, the chemicals in some antiperspirants are problematic with some gel liners; it is always advisable to consult with the prosthetist before using any lotions on the residual limb prior to donning the prosthesis. At night and after bathing, any good, nonalcoholic skin lotion will help keep the skin soft and resilient.

FACTORS AFFECTING PROSTHETIC WEAR

Residual limb problems delay prosthetic rehabilitation. Skin problems, such as dermatitis, **furuncles**, cysts, and infections, usually require avoidance of the prosthesis, care in skin hygiene, and, occasionally, medication. Soap residue left on the skin can become an irritant, and the client must be taught to rinse the residual limb, socks, socket, and liner well after washing. Skin problems are fairly common; in a 6-year retrospective study, Dudek and associates found 528 reports of skin problems among 327 subjects. Ulcers, irritations, inclusion cysts, calluses, and verrucous hyperplasia were the five most common skin problems representing 79.5% of all documented skin disorders. There was no indication to what extent the skin problems interfered with prosthetic wear.[27]

Clients with vascular disease must be alert to pressure on the residual limb from the prosthetic socket. Necrosis of distal tissue can occur even after wound healing. Individuals with diabetes who may have decreased sensation need to learn to carefully inspect the residual limb after each wearing to note any areas of redness or pressure. If some of the skin around the incision adheres to the distal end of the bone, the forces created by prosthetic wear may cause pain or abrasions and even open sores. Occasionally, skin grafts necessary for healing in some traumatic amputations may adhere to distal bone, may be insensitive, and may be the source of prosthetic pain or abrasions. Although care must be taken during the healing period to prevent adhesions by careful massage and movement of the skin around the bone, not all can be avoided. Although gel liners and the more intimate fit of the prosthetic socket make fitting such residual limbs easier, the patient must be aware of the greater risk for skin breakdown.

Occasionally, an individual wearing a gel liner with a shuttlelock system may develop a small bursa or bruised area distally. The gel liner adheres to the skin aiding in suspension, but the prosthesis pulls away from the limb a small amount on every swing phase. That pulling action may create a milking effect of

superficial issue on subcutaneous tissue, particularly in individuals who have somewhat fleshy residual limbs. The problem does not occur frequently, but the therapist must be alert to complaints of pulling or pain distally. In those instances, another type of suspension is indicated. Occasionally, bone spurs develop causing excessive pressure on the overlying skin. Children are subject to problems created by bone growth through the skin at the end of the residual limb (Chapter 9).

Pain, from whatever source, is the single biggest deterrent to prosthetic wear and the major issue of patients with amputations. In a survey of 114 individuals with lower extremity amputations, issues related to the fit of the socket were a primary concern of respondents.[28] In another study of 148 individuals who responded to a questionnaire, the presence or absence of pain in the residual limb was the most important of the factors affecting perception of the results of amputations. Other factors included the condition of the contralateral limb, the comfort and function of the prosthesis, and social issues.[29] Pain affects performance. In a study comparing individuals with chronic pain with a matched sample of subjects without pain, the individuals without pain performed better.[30] Amputee pain has been found to be quite prevalent, whether phantom limb pain, residual limb pain, or back pain.[31] In a phone survey of 914 amputees, nearly 95% reported some pain from at least one source. Although not all pain was considered intense or bothersome by the subjects, there was a significant correlation between bothersome or intense pain and depressive symptoms.[31] In another study, it was reported that transfemoral amputees were more likely to complain of back pain than transtibial amputees, and that individuals who complained of back pain were more likely to be overweight and also complain of residual limb and phantom pain. There were no differences in disc disease or degeneration between those who complained of back pain and those who did not.[32]

A neuroma is a natural sequelae of the transection of a nerve. The size and location of the neuroma is the critical issue. If the neuroma is small and situated in soft tissue well above the distal end of the residual limb, it will usually not interfere with prosthetic wear. Large superficial neuromas may be compressed between the socket wall and the bone and cause pain. Sometimes, relieving the socket wall at the site of the neuroma resolves the problem. Injecting the neuroma with an analgesic or steroid formula may be necessary, and because the relief is only temporary, this may need to be repeated several times. In more stubborn instances, surgery to excise the neuroma may be indicated. Koch and associates reported on a relatively new surgical approach that included resecting the neuroma and implanting the cut end into a vein. Twelve of the 23 patients experienced permanent cessation of pain with eight others reporting mild pain on long-term follow-up. The authors recommend further study of this technique.[33] Uygur and Sener used ultrasound to treat early neuromas in seven transtibial amputees with success. However, no further study of this technique was found.[34]

A prosthesis is, of course, a piece of mechanical equipment and as such requires regular maintenance and occasional repair. Most prosthetists schedule regular visits for recheck and maintenance. Amputee clinics schedule semiannual or annual visits for their patients who have been discharged from regular care. Such visits are important to reevaluate prosthetic fit and residual limb status and note any changes that may affect prosthetic wear and function. Patients usually need new sockets within 1 to 2 years of initial fit as the residual limb shrinks beyond adjustment. More active individuals usually need more repairs than more sedentary individuals, and the use of modular components reduces the need to replace the whole prosthesis rather than just the damaged part.[35]

LONG-TERM OUTCOMES

The goal of prosthetic rehabilitation is, of course, for the person to return to his or her premorbid level of function or higher if he or she was disabled with ulcers prior to amputation. It is not always possible for the person to return to previous employment; in many states, the Division of Vocational Rehabilitation, a state-run and partially federally funded program can help with retraining and placement. Depending on level of amputation and the extent of injury or disability, the individual may find there are barriers that impede their lifestyle. Ephraim and associates interviewed 914 community-dwelling amputees by phone to identify perceived environmental barriers related to these five domains: policies, physical/structural, work/school, attitudes/support, and services/assistance. Eighty-seven percent of those interviewed reported barriers in at least one domain, and 57% reported barriers in at least four domains.

Overall, scores were lower for individuals with cancer-related amputations and higher for those with traumatic amputations. The authors suggested that more efforts should be made to reduce perceived barriers, thereby improving long-term outcomes of amputation.[36] Dougherty surveyed 46 veterans of the Vietnam war who had been treated at the same hospital an average of 28 years after injury. The survey included a review of their medical records, questions, and the SF-36 health survey. The majority was or had been employed for more than 20 years, was or had been married, and wore their prostheses an average of 13.5 hours a day. Yet their scores on the SF-36 indicated that they perceived themselves as quite disabled.[37] MacKenzie and associates surveyed 161 patients who had undergone any level of amputation above the ankle for traumatic reasons. The survey included the Sickness Impact Profile (SIP) as well as pain; degree of independence in transfers, walking, and climbing stairs; self-selected walking speed; and the physician's satisfaction with the clinical, functional, and cosmetic recovery of the limb. The subjects were surveyed at 3, 6, 12, and 24 months after injury. There was no significant difference in SIP scores between individuals with transtibial or transfemoral amputations, although those with transtibial amputations functioned better at self-selected walking speeds and other functional outcomes. Individuals with through-the-knee amputations had lower SIP scores and did not function as well at self-selected speed. There was no information on the type of prosthesis worn, and the authors suggested that more research was needed to compare function and type of prosthesis.[38] In a study of job satisfaction in the Netherlands between 144 individuals with limb loss compared to a matched group of nonamputees, Schoppen and associates reported greater job satisfaction in the amputee group despite poorer general health. Among the areas of dissatisfaction, workplace adaptation and comorbidities were the most important.[39] Burger and Marincek[40] performed a comprehensive review of the literature and reported a wide percentage of individuals who were able to return to the same job following amputation (22% to 67%). As expected, many factors affected the ability to resume the same employment, including age, gender, and level of amputation. The authors concluded that better coordination between rehabilitation personnel, employers, insurance companies, and vocational counselors was needed.[40]

Individuals with limb loss may need several new prostheses over the years depending on age at the time of amputation. Not all patients want the latest components, as some individuals prefer the components with which they are familiar. However, when there is considerable improvement in function, prosthetists may encourage the person to try the latest components. Hafner and associates fitted 21 transfemoral amputees with the C-Leg after using a mechanical knee and found that the subjects performed significantly better on stair and hill descent, on ramps, and on level walking.[41] Amputees in need of new prostheses should be apprised of the continued improvement in technology and the new components available to them.

SUMMARY

Training the individual to regain independence in mobility with a prosthesis is a sequential program of balance and basic and advanced gait activities. It is critical for the individual to develop competence in balance, coordination, and prosthetic control before coordinated walking is instituted, and the time spent on these activities will lead to a positive outcome. The therapist must understand gait mechanics and be able to diagnose gait and balance problems to individualize the rehabilitation program. The training program demands the physical therapist and physical therapist assistant to be creative as well as have an understanding of motor skills acquisition.

KEYWORDS FOR LITERATURE SEARCH

Artificial limb

C-Leg®

CATCAM

Components

Computerized prosthesis

Prosthesis

Prosthetics

Prosthetist

REFERENCES

1. Smith DG, Granville RR: Amputee care. J Am Acad Orthop Surg 14(10):S179–S183, 2006.
2. Marzoug EA, Landham TL, Dances C, Bamji AN: Better practical evaluation for lower limb amputees. Dis & Rehab 25(18):1071–1074, 2003.
3. Gailey RS, Roach KE, Applegate EB, et al: The amputee mobility predictor: an instrument to assess determinants of the lower-limb amputee's ability to ambulate. Arch Phys Med Rehabil 83(5):613–627, 2002.
4. Miller WC, Deathe AB, Speechley M: Lower extremity prosthetic mobility: a comparison of 3 self-report scales. Arch Phys Med Rehabil 82:1432–1440, 2001.
5. Deathe AB, Miller WC: The L Test of Functional Mobility: measurement properties of a modified version of the timed "Up & Go" Test designed for people with lower-limb amputations. Phys Ther 85:626–635, 2005.
6. Fatiuk-Haight ED (ed): Proceedings: outcome measures in lower limb prosthetics. AAOP, September 7–9, 2005.
7. Puhalski EM: How are transfemoral amputees using their prosthesis in Northwestern Ontario? JPO 20:53–60, 2008.
8. Davies B, Datta D: Mobility outcomes following unilateral lower limb amputation. Prosthet Orthot Int 27:186–190, 2003.
9. Fletcher DD, Andrews KL, Buitters MA, et al: Trends in rehabilitation after amputation for geriatric patients with vascular disease: implications for future health resources allocation. Arch Phys Med Rehabil 83:1389–1393, 2002.
10. Waters RJ, Mulroy SJ: Energy expenditure of walking in individuals with lower limb amputations. In Smith DG, Michael JW, Bowker JH (eds): Atlas of amputations and limb deficiencies: surgical, prosthetic and rehabilitation principles, 3rd ed. Rosemont, IL, AAOS, 2004, pp 395–408.
11. Pinzur MS, Gold J, Schwartz D, Gross N: Energy demands for walking in dysvascular amputees as related to the level of amputation. Orthopedics 15:1033–1037, 1992.
12. Perry J: Normal gait. In Smith DG, Michael JW, Bowker JH (eds): Atlas of amputations and limb deficiencies: surgical, prosthetic and rehabilitation principles, 3rd ed. AAOS, Rosemont, IL, 2004, pp 353–366.
13. Perry J: Amputee gait. In Smith DG, Michael JW, Bowker JH (eds): Atlas of amputations and limb deficiencies: surgical, prosthetic and rehabilitation principles, 3rd ed. AAOS, Rosemont, IL, 2004, pp 367–384.
14. Dennis JK, McKeough DM: Mobility. In May BJ: Home health and rehabilitation: concepts of care. Philadelphia, F.A. Davis, 1993, pp 143–171.
15. Gentile AM: A working model of skill acquisition with application of teaching. Quest 27:3, 1972.
16. Miller WC, Deatj AB, Speechley M, Koval M: The influence of falling, fear of falling, and balance confidence on prosthetic mobility and social activity among individuals with lower extremity amputation. Arch Phys Med Rehabil 82:1238–1244, 2001.
17. van Velzen JM, Polomski W, Slootman JR, van der Woude LH, Houdijk H: Physical capacity and walking ability after lower limb amputation: a systematic review. Clin Rehabil 20(11):999–1016, 2006.
18. Gailey R: Physical therapy. In Smith DG, Michael JW, Bowker JH (eds): Atlas of amputations and limb deficiencies: surgical, prosthetic and rehabilitation principles, 3rd ed. Rosemont, IL, AAOS, 2004, pp 589–620.
19. Yigiter K, Sener G, Erbahceci F, Bayar K, Ulger OG, Akdogan S: A comparison of traditional prosthetic training versus proprioceptive neuromuscular facilitation resistive gait training with trans-femoral amputees. Prosth Orth Int 26(3):213–217, 2002.
20. Davis BL, Ortolano MC, Richards K, Redhed J, Kuznicki J, Sahgal V: Realtime visual feedback diminished energy consumption of amputee subjects during treadmill locomotion. JPO 16(2):49–54, 2004.

21. Dickstein R, Deutsch J: Motor imagery in physical therapist practice. Phys Ther 87:942–953, 2007.

22. Baker FW III: Walter Reed gait laboratory puts amputees back in step. American Press Services, U.S. Department of Defense, Defense Link News.

23. Segeday A: Virtual environments enable real recovery. BioMechanics, 2006 June.

24. Cole MJ, Durham S, Ewins D: An evaluation of patient perceptions to the value of the gait laboratory as part of the rehabilitation of primary lower limb amputees. Prosthet Orthot Int 32(1):12–22, 2008 Mar.

25. Tsai HA, Kirby RL, MacLeod DA, Graham MM: Aided gait of people with lower-limb amputations: comparison of 4-footed and 2-wheeled walker. Arch Phys Med Rehabil 84(4):584–591, 2003 Apr.

26. Hofstad CJ, Weerdesteyn V, van der Linde H, et al: Evidence for bilaterally delayed and decreased obstacle avoidance responses while walking with a lower limb prosthesis. Clin Neurophysiol 120(5):1009–1015, 2009 May.

27. Dudek NL, Marks MB, Marshall SC: Skin problems in an amputee clinic. Am J Phys Med Rehabil 85:424–429, 2006.

28. Legro MW, Reiber G, del Aguila M, et al: Issues of importance reported by persons with lower limb amputations and prostheses. J Rehabil Res Devel 36(3):155–163, 1999.

29. Matsen SL, Malchow D, Matsen FA: Correlations with patients' perspectives of the results of lower-extremity amputation. J Bone Joint Surg (Am) 82-A(8):1089–1095, 2000.

30. Rudy TE, Lieber SJ, Boston JR, Gourley LM, Baysal E: Psychosocial predictors of physical performance in disabled individuals with chronic pain. Clinic J Pain 19(1):18–30, 2003 Jan–Feb.

31. Ephraim PL, Wegener ST, MacKenzie EJ, Dillingham TR, Pezzin LE: Phantom pain, residual limb pain, and back pain in amputees: results of a national survey. Arch Phys Med Rehabil 86(10):1910–1919, 2005.

32. Kulkarni J, Gaine WJ, Buckley JG, Rankine JJ, Adams J: Chronic low back pain in traumatic lower limb amputees. Clin Rehabil 19(1):81–86, 2005 Jan.

33. Koch H, Haas F, Hubmer M, Rappl T, Scharnagl E: Treatment of painful neuroma by resection and nerve stump transplantation into a vein. Ann Plast Surg 51(1):45–50, 2003.

34. Uygur F, Sener G: Application of ultrasound in neuromas: experience with seven below-knee stumps. Physiotherapy 81(12): 758–762, 1995 Dec.

35. Nair A, Hanspal RS, Zahedi MS, Saif M, Fisher K: Analyses of prosthetic episodes in lower limb amputees. Prosthet Orthot Int 32(1):42–49, 2008.

36. Ephraim PL, MacKenzie EJ, Wegener ST, Dillingham TR, Pezzin LE: Environmental barriers experienced by amputees: the Craig Hospital Inventory of Environmental Factors-Short Form. Arch Phys Med Rehabil 87(3):328–333, 2006.

37. Dougherty PJ: Long-term follow-up of unilateral transfemoral amputees from the Vietnam war. J Trauma-Inj Infect Crit Care 54(4):718–723, 2003 Apr.

38. MacKenzie EJ, Bosse MJ, Castillo RC, et al: Functional outcomes following trauma-related lower-extremity amputation. J Bone Joint Surg Am 86-A(8):1636–1645, 2004 Aug. [See comment][erratum appears in J Bone Joint Surg Am 86-A(11):2503, 2004 Nov.]

39. Schoppen T, Boonstra A, Groothoff JW, et al: Job satisfaction and health experience of people with a lower-limb amputation in comparison with healthy colleagues. Arch Phys Med & Rehabil 83(5):628–634, 2002.

40. Burger H, Marincek C: Return to work after lower limb amputation. Disability & Rehabil 29(17):1323–1329, 2007.

41. Hafner BJ, Willingham LL, Buell NC, Allyn KJ, Smith DG: Evaluation of function, performance, and preference as transfemoral amputees transition from mechanical to microprocessor control of the prosthetic knee [erratum appears in Arch Phys Med Rehabil 88(4):544, 2007 Apr] Arch Phys Med Rehabil 88(2):207–217, 2007 Feb.

Other Levels of Amputation

OBJECTIVES

At the end of this chapter, all students are expected to:

1. Implement an intervention program designed to meet the special needs of individuals with amputations at the foot, ankle, knee, or hip disarticulation levels or with bilateral lower extremity amputations.
2. Describe the major prosthetic components and their function for the levels of amputation included in this chapter.

Physical Therapy students are expected to:

1. Determine the diagnosis for patients with levels of amputation included in this chapter.
2. Select, implement, and interpret the results of all appropriate tests and measures.
3. Design an appropriate plan of care including selecting interventions for all patients included in this chapter.

CASE STUDIES

Zach Fells, a 39-year-old high school math teacher, was in a severe motorcycle accident 2 weeks ago and had to have his right leg amputated through the knee. Mr. Fells is an active weekend athlete who is married with four children. He rides his motor bike to and from school daily. He has insurance through the county school system.

Penny Griger, a 42-year-old drugstore clerk, was recently diagnosed with a sarcoma of the upper thigh and had a left hip disarticulation amputation a week ago. She is a single mother of two small children and lives with her mother who takes care of the children while Penny is at work.

Case Study Activities

All Students

1. Functionally compare and contrast the transtibial, knee disarticulation, transfemoral, and hip disarticulation levels of amputation.

Physical Therapy Students

1. Develop a physical therapy diagnosis for each of these patients.
2. Design a preprosthetic examination and intervention program for each assuming you are seeing each at the time stated above. Assume additional information you might want to develop the intervention program.

Physical Therapist Assistant Students

1. What part of the preprosthetic intervention program would you be comfortable doing?
2. What information would you want from the physical therapist to treat each of these patients at this time?

Although the transtibial and transfemoral are the most common levels of amputation, an individual may sustain an amputation through any structure of the lower extremity. Figure 4.1 in Chapter 4 outlines the different levels of amputation. Many of the patients presented in this chapter can be treated through the postsurgical and gait training program outlined in previous chapters. Prosthetically, they may require slightly different or modified components that will be presented here. This chapter focuses on the special needs of individuals amputated at other than transtibial and transfemoral levels as well as the needs of individuals who have bilateral amputations.

AMPUTATIONS THROUGH THE FOOT

Surgical Considerations

The majority of partial foot or **transmetatarsal** amputations are performed because of infection usually related to dysvascularity and diabetes. Many individuals will lose one or more toes, a total ray, or the front part of the foot over a period of time before sustaining a transtibial or transfemoral amputation. The most common traumatic cause of partial foot amputations is related to lawnmowers or motor vehicle accidents.[1] The level of amputation is determined by tissue viability and the presence of adequate circulation in the area to allow healing.

Toe amputations are generally indicated for localized demarcated gangrene of the distal end of the toe. A single toe can be amputated through the phalanx or disarticulated at the base of the proximal phalanx. On occasion, an entire ray (toe plus metatarsal) may be removed. The **metatarsal ray resection** is indicated in some cases of congenital anomalies, gangrene secondary to frostbite, neoplasms, severe chronic infections of a single metatarsal, or a deep **subaponeurotic** foot abscess. Trauma may result in a variety of digit or partial foot amputations. Loss of the great toe or first ray will have the greatest effect on ambulation because of the loss of support in the final phase of terminal weight transfer. Physical therapists and physical therapist assistants are rarely involved with primary toe amputations, although clients with other levels of amputation may have lost one or more toes on the other side.

Transmetatarsal amputation is removal of the toes and distal ends of the metatarsals (Fig. 8.1). It is a very functional amputation for problems with toes but requires well-fitting prosthetic replacement. Foot balance is maintained because the residual limb is symmetrical in shape, and major muscle attachments are preserved. In a transmetatarsal amputation, the surgeon tries to salvage as much metatarsal length as possible for maximum function as well as bevel the ends of the metatarsals to reduce distal pressure when walking. Postoperatively, a cast may be applied to maintain the foot in a neutral alignment during healing. The selection of the transmetatarsal level of amputation among patients with vascular disease is somewhat controversial, and there are few studies on

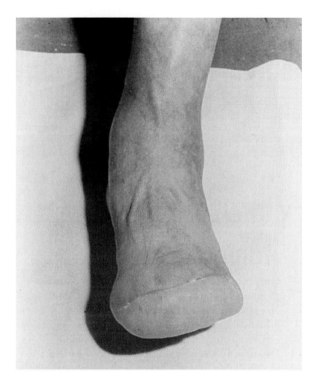

FIGURE 8.1. Transmetatarsal residual limb.

healing rates. Blume and associates reported that 69% of patients healed either initially or within a 3-month period. The major cause of nonhealing was end-stage renal disease.[2] Nguyen and associates reported a successful healing rate of 59% with 40% of the patients in his study requiring eventual transtibial amputation.[3] In both studies, patients whose transmetatarsal amputation healed showed good walking capabilities with prosthetic replacement.

There are other through the foot and ankle amputations such as the Lisfranc, a tarsometatarsal disarticulation, and the Chopart, a midtarsal disarticulation. Both were named after the surgeon who initially designed the procedures, and both are rarely used, mostly for traumatic injuries. The major concern is maintaining balance in the remaining foot to prevent deformities that will interfere with prosthetic fitting and ambulation. These patients are generally fitted with modified shoes or boots and are rarely seen in a physical therapy clinic unless the patient has other disabilities (**Fig. 8.2A,B**).

Postsurgical Care

Patients with a simple partial foot amputation may not be referred to physical therapy for postsurgical

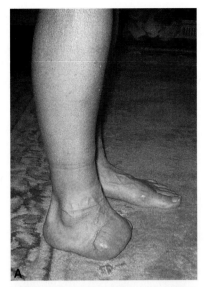

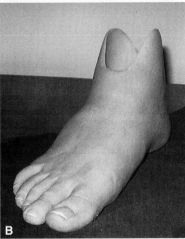

FIGURE 8.2. (A) Chopart residual limb. **(B)** Suction prosthetic foot.

care. The evaluations and interventions outlined in Chapter 5 are perfectly well applicable to this population. Generally, patients do very well, ambulating with limited weight bearing on the amputated foot until it has healed and is ready for prosthetic fitting.

Prosthetic Components

The functional effects of losing part of the foot increase with the amount of the foot that is lost. Losing even a small part of the foot, a ray or several toes, reduces the forefoot load-bearing area. Loss of the big toe and the first metatarsalphalangeal joint may limit push off in terminal stance. Loss of the

whole forefoot in a transmetatarsal amputation leads to a premature loss of support in terminal stance and the gait deviation known as "drop off" (Chapter 6). Other partial foot amputations may lead to imbalances between muscles that are still functioning and those that have lost their distal attachments. The surgeon always tries to leave a balanced foot, but in some surgeries, fusion of one or more joints of the foot may be necessary. Such fusions may reduce the ability of the foot to respond to some of the forces generated in mobility activities.

Depending on the type and extent of partial foot loss, the patient may be fitted with a shoe insert, a modified ankle–foot orthosis (AFO) or some form of prosthesis. The prosthetist makes a careful assessment to determine the amount of control over the remaining foot joints, the degree of sensitivity or insensitivity, the amount and fragility of the tissues, the vascularity of the part, and the presence or absence of any neuropathy. The variety of materials currently available gives the prosthetist many options. Whatever is designed for the patient must be comfortable to use and provide the necessary amount of both support and stabilization while not interfering with function. For example, individuals amputated at the transmetatarsal level are often provided with an individually molded shoe insert with a carbon filament sole to facilitate weight transfer on stance. A soft insert may also be needed to prevent loading at the end of the residuum.[4]

Physical Therapy Care

Most patients with a unilateral amputation through the foot are not seen by a physical therapist. Once an appropriate prosthetic replacement is fitted, these patients can ambulate as they did before the amputation and without difficulty. Physical therapists usually see these patients if they have other problems requiring physical therapy or if they have an amputation through the other limb.

ANKLE DISARTICULATION (SYMES) AMPUTATIONS

Surgical Considerations

In 1843, James Symes, an orthopedic surgeon, described an amputation through the ankle that preserved the heel pad for weight bearing. This level of amputation is used for severe foot trauma, some congenital anomalies such as severe club foot, and occasionally for individuals with wet gangrene of the forefoot. To be successful, there must be satisfactory circulation to the heel pad.[5] Throughout the surgery, the posterior tibial neurovascular structures and the fat-filled chamber of the heel pad are carefully maintained. In early days, the malleoli were generally left intact, but in 1972, Sarmiento recommended removing a small part of the distal tibia and narrowing the malleoli to allow for better socket fit (**Fig. 8.3**).[6] The heel pad needs to be closely adhered to the end of the tibia during closure, as movement between the heel pad and the end of the bone interferes with effective prosthetic fit and can cause pain. The surgeon will often fit the patient with a cast immediately after surgery to allow the heel pad to heal properly.

Postsurgical Care

Patients amputated at the **ankle disarticulation** level (Symes amputation) must avoid pressure on the limb in the early postsurgical period; pressure on the distal end of the residual limb or the incision can lead to a loose end pad (**Fig. 8.4A,B**). If the limb is not secured in a cast, the patient must be taught to move in bed or transfer without pushing or stabilizing with the

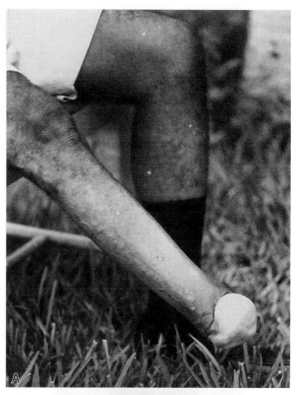

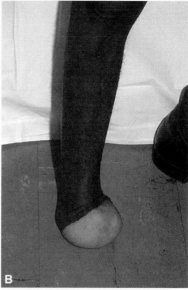

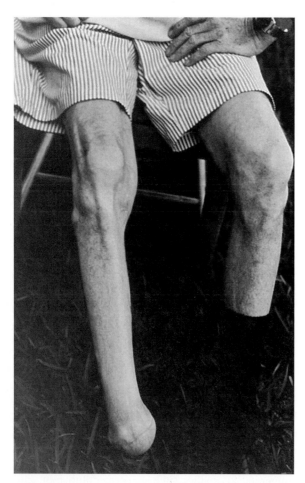

FIGURE 8.3. Modified ankle disarticulation residual limb.

FIGURE 8.4. (A) Standard ankle disarticulation residual limb. **(B)** Unstable heel pad on ankle disarticulation residual limb.

residual limb. Once there is adequate healing, the surgeon may place the limb in a walking cast and allow weight bearing. Generally, these patients do very well and require little postsurgical care unless there are complications or comorbidities.

Other than the special care of the distal end pad, the management of an individual following ankle disarticulation will be similar to that following transtibial amputation as outlined in Chapter 6.

Prosthetic Components

The ankle disarticulation is a very functional level of lower extremity amputation. The long lever arm provides for excellent prosthetic control as well as broad surfaces for distribution of stabilizing forces. The prosthesis for this level is composed of a socket and a foot with suspension built into the configuration of the socket.

Sockets

The ankle disarticulation prosthesis provides for a weight-bearing surface at the distal end as well as along the shaft of the tibia and a little at the patella tendon. It is molded over the shaft of the fibula and the medial flares of the tibia for stabilizing pressure. If the distal end is not modified as described above, the distal end with its intact malleoli will be considerably wider than other parts of the limb. To enable the prosthesis to be donned and then anchored for suspension over the malleoli, a window is cut along the medial wall of the socket. The window is covered by a panel that fits snugly into the opening and is secured by two straps (**Fig. 8.5**). The decrease in limb circumference proximal to the bulbous end enables suspension by virtue of the irregular contours of the socket. This conventional ankle disarticulation prosthesis is functional but not very cosmetic with a thick distal end and the straps. The medial window also reduces the mechanical strength of the prosthesis.

Modifying the distal end surgically by shaving the malleoli provides for a smaller distal end and allows for the construction of a closed, expandable socket (**Fig. 8.6**). The prosthesis is fabricated with a liner attached to the inner wall of the socket. The liner is made of a flexible plastic and extends from the distal end of the socket to a point where the diameter of the proximal leg equals the bulbous end distally. A space is created between the inner socket and the outer laminate, and the liner stretches as the end of the residual limb is inserted into the socket. The liner closes

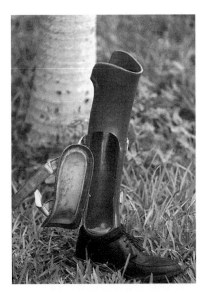

FIGURE 8.5. Standard ankle disarticulation prosthesis.

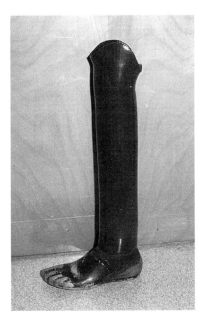

FIGURE 8.6. Ankle disarticulation prosthesis for modified ankle disarticulation.

around the length of the residuum to maintain total contact and aid in suspension.

Foot

Ankle disarticulations result in the loss of all ankle–foot movements; however, several companies make dynamic response feet particularly for the ankle disarticulation prosthesis. They provide a place within the configurations of the foot for the distal end of the residual limb.

Physical Therapy Care

An individual wearing a properly aligned ankle disarticulation prosthesis can exhibit a normal gait pattern and perform all desired functional and leisure activities with no measurable additional expenditure of energy.[7,8] Individuals with unilateral ankle disarticulations may not be referred to physical therapy following prosthetic fitting. When referred, the major role of the physical therapist is to evaluate the fit of the prosthesis and provide appropriate balance and gait training as outlined in Chapter 7.

KNEE DISARTICULATIONS

Surgical Considerations

The advantages of knee disarticulation are that it provides a long lever arm and, depending on the specifics of the surgical procedure, a weight-bearing residual limb (**Fig. 8.7**). Some of the earlier cosmetic disadvantages that included the wide distal end of the condyles and the need to set the knee axis on the prosthetic side well below that of the unamputated leg, have been somewhat mitigated by variations in surgical procedures that include reducing the breadth

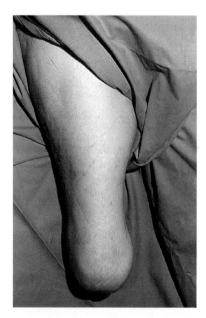

FIGURE 8.7. Knee disarticulation residual limb.

of the distal condyles and slightly reducing the overall length of the femur. Generally, the major indications for a knee disarticulation include the inability to provide an adequate transtibial residual limb because of the extent of trauma, severe knee flexion contracture beyond 45 degrees, infection of the soft tissue close to the knee joint, and some congenital deformities. To be successful at any level of amputation, the surgeon must be able to provide a soft tissue envelope of mobile muscle covered with full-thickness skin at the distal end of the bone. This level is rarely used with patients with dysvascularities, usually because even a short transtibial residual limb is more functional than a knee disarticulation. However, some surgeons advocate this level for patients who are morbidly obese and difficult to fit with the usual transtibial prosthesis or those who are marginal walkers and who may lose the other leg in the near future. Bilateral knee disarticulations provide a better sitting platform than bilateral transfemoral amputations.[9]

Postsurgical Care

Patients amputated through the knee are treated postsurgically as transfemoral amputations (Chapter 5). The longer lever arm and full muscle length lessen the potential for development of contractures. Once again, care must be taken to avoid pressure on the distal end of the residual limb. This is particularly important when the patient is moving in bed or transferring.

Prosthetic Components

Prostheses for the knee disarticulation level have the same problems as the ankle disarticulation. The larger distal end, although not as prominent as the ankle disarticulation, still must be accommodated as the patient dons the prosthesis. Additionally, the length of the residual limb mitigates against fitting some knee mechanism if the axis of the prosthetic knee is to be at the same level as the unamputated limb.

Sockets

Although attempts have been made over the years to create an end-bearing residuum, the knee disarticulation limb usually does not allow for end bearing. The knee disarticulation socket is generally configured similar to that of the transfemoral socket, with the greater length of the residuum allowing for greater distribution of weight-bearing and stabilizing forces through the soft tissues.[10] Variations in the socket are often dictated by the bulkiness of the femoral condyles and whether or not the distal end can tolerate any end bearing. Today's materials allow for the creation of a flexible socket on a carbon filament frame which is both functional and cosmetic. If the distal end is not too large, a thermoplastic or gel liner can be used on a fully closed socket (**Fig. 8.8A,B**).

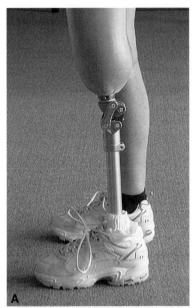

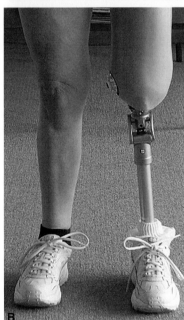

FIGURE 8.8. Knee disarticulation prosthesis: **(A)** side view and **(B)** front view.

Suspension

There are various ways the prosthesis can be suspended, again depending on the length of the residual limb and the bulkiness of the femoral condyles. In some instances, a posterior window can be cut into the socket similar to the ankle disarticulation prosthesis. Preferably, the flexible liner on a frame allows the condyles to slip through then reform to provide suspension. Suction, as described in Chapter 6, is also an option and is the use of a shuttlelock system if the femur on the amputated side is shorter than that on the unamputated side.

Knee Mechanisms

The choice of a knee mechanism is determined by the length of the residual limb in relation to the other leg. Most knee mechanisms need some room between the end of the residuum and the knee axis. If not enough room exists to allow the knee axis to be at the same level on both legs, an outside joint similar to orthotic joints may be used. Using a traditional transfemoral knee mechanism usually results in a lowered knee axis on the amputated side. If minimal, this may not cause any major problem and can be an appropriate choice for individuals with bilateral knee disarticulations. There is also a group of polycentric knee mechanisms that were designed specifically for this level, providing the patient with improved stance phase stability while not protruding during sitting.[10]

Feet

Any of the feet described in Chapter 6 can be used with a knee disarticulation prosthesis.

Physical Therapy Care

Balance and gait training for a person with a knee disarticulation is similar to that for someone wearing a transfemoral prosthesis as described in Chapter 7. Generally, the longer level arm gives the patient good control of the prosthesis for all activities. The rehabilitation program needs to start with balance and knee control, as with the transfemoral patient, then progress to ambulation and advanced activities. Individuals wearing knee disarticulation prostheses usually do not need any external support and can participate in desired leisure and work activities.

HIP DISARTICULATIONS, TRANSPELVIC AMPUTATIONS

Surgical Considerations

Amputation through the hip joint or through the pelvis is usually performed to save the life of the patient. The major causes of such amputations are a malignancy that is not amenable to limb-sparing techniques with chemotherapy and radiation, severe infection or wet gangrene in a debilitated patient, or, less frequently, severe trauma not amenable to any reconstruction. The disease process determines if the amputation is to be performed as a **hip disarticulation** or through the pelvis. The surgeon is concerned with removal of all diseased tissue while maintaining an adequate soft tissue envelope for primary closure and bony coverage (**Fig. 8.9**). The end result should provide the patient with a good soft tissue flap for comfortable sitting and pressure tolerance.[11]

Postsurgical Care

Patients with hip disarticulations or **transpelvic** have one or more drains in the surgical site and are often stressed from the surgery. Care must be taken to protect the surgical site from pressure or shear forces. The patient will not be able to lie on the amputated side and may, initially, have some difficulty sitting. While patients with a hip disarticulation may eventually be able to sit balanced with both ischia present, individuals following hemipelvectomy may require some sort of sitting platform once healing has taken place. In both instances, sitting balance is disturbed, and balance exercises, both sitting and standing, should be part of the postsurgical program. Because ambulation with crutches or a prosthesis requires considerable energy expenditure,

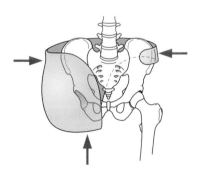

FIGURE 8.9. Hemipelvectomy residual limb showing socket outline.

a general strengthening and fitness program involving the total body is an important part of the postsurgical program. It is important for the person to be able to get up and down from the floor, sit on surfaces at various levels, and handle bathroom and bathtub activities independently. However, patients amputated for some form of cancer will undergo radiation and chemotherapy and may not have the ability to participate in a fitness program until the course of adjuvant therapy is finished. In some instances, patients amputated at the transpelvic level may incur some problems with bowel or bladder function. Generally, patients amputated at this level will need a wheelchair for general use.

These high-level amputations have a broad effect on function in all areas, including body image, sexual capabilities, and self-esteem, as discussed generally in Chapter 3. Referral to a support group or organization is often advisable.[12]

Prosthetic Components

Rejection rates for these prostheses are high, as the gait cadence is slow and much more energy consuming than even the transfemoral level. Wearers often find the prostheses heavy and uncomfortable. Hip disarticulations and transpelvic prostheses are quite similar in component and alignment. The major difference between the two levels is the amount of bone loss and the availability of bony support for weight bearing and suspension.

Sockets

Both sockets are essentially a padded plastic bucket intimately molded of lightweight material to provide support for the body weight on stance, contain all the soft tissue, and stabilize on available bony prominences.[13] Socket fit is critical and must provide comfort throughout the gait cycle as well as intimate suspension to maintain the prosthesis properly in swing phase. The patient is essentially sitting in the prosthesis with full weight taken throughout the soft tissue of residuum.

The hip disarticulation socket encloses the ischial tuberosity for weight bearing and covers the iliac crest for stability and suspension. It encircles the pelvis with an anterior slit to allow ease of donning and removal. The medial aspect is cut to provide clearance for the other leg and genitalia. Relief is provided over the anterior and posterior iliac spines.

Variations in socket construction include a lateral-opening diagonal socket and a full socket similar to the transpelvic that encloses both iliac crests for stability. The transpelvic socket is similarly made except that it must include the contralateral iliac crest for proper stabilization and suspension (**Fig. 8.10A,B**). Weight bearing is primarily on the remaining soft tissue and the contralateral ischium. Suspension comes above the iliac crest and locks onto the waist bilaterally. Care must be taken when constructing both sockets that no excess pressure exists on bony prominence or in the perineum. There is a delicate balance between having enough suspension for minimal displacement on swing and comfort in standing and sitting. Comfort, of course, is primary, but the patient needs to understand the balance and work closely with the prosthetist to attain the best possible socket fit.

Both sockets are made of lightweight thermoplastic materials inside a rigid carbon-fiber-reinforced frame. The socket is usually padded with some form of gel liner for increased comfort on weight bearing.[14]

Hip, Knee, and Foot

Both prostheses can use the same hip, knee, and foot components. Usually, a single-axis hip joint with a posterior stop is attached to the anterior distal aspect of the socket. Generally, the joint is unlocked, but, on occasion, a manual hip lock is used to provide additional stability on stance. A locked hip joint results in a slower gait with shorter steps and requires the patient to unlock the hip prior to sitting. A spring assist mechanism may be incorporated for young active clients to aid in initiating swing phase, and an elastic extension strap is used to control limb extension in swing. Any knee joint and foot can be used in these prostheses depending on the person's activity level and ability to control the weight of the prosthesis (see Chapter 6). In a small study with three patients, Chin and associates compared the energy requirements of walking at three different speeds with a hip disarticulation prosthesis fitted with a standard stance phase knee mechanism and a computerized knee joint.[15] The computerized knee reduced oxygen consumption at the higher two speeds in all three patients and at the slower speed in two of the three patients.

Physical Therapy Care

Both prostheses are biomechanically aligned to be stable from heel contact to toe off. The anterior placement of the hip joint automatically brings the body weight line anterior to the knee joint, making it stable. As weight bearing progresses from heel contact to midstance, the floor reaction forces maintain the knee in extension until terminal stance. At this point, the weight line moves posterior to the knee joint creating a flexion moment and aiding in initiating swing. Momentum and pelvic motion initiate

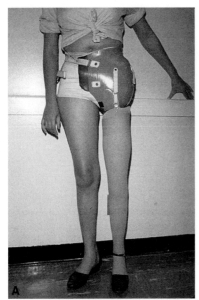
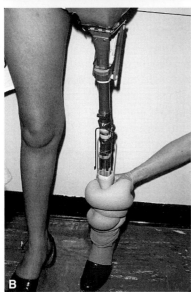

FIGURE 8.10. **(A)** Hemipelvectomy prosthesis with cosmetic cover. **(B)** Hemipelvectomy prosthesis showing elastic deceleration strap.

swing that can be aided by a spring assist in the hip joint. The extension strap limits the forward motion of the prosthesis bringing the heel back to the floor in time for the next step. Initial balance training is necessary to help the patient develop confidence in the prosthesis as well as learn to shift weight on and off the prosthesis. Training is also needed to teach the person how to initiate swing. Step length is limited by the prosthesis, but timing and continuity are necessary to develop an appropriate rhythm. The patient needs to be taught to use a continuous, rhythmic gait pattern to limit excess energy expenditures. Many individuals at this level will use some form of external support, usually a single-point cane.

The patient also needs to be taught to properly shift the weight on and off the prosthesis when sitting and getting up from a chair. If the person has a manual hip lock, he or she must unlock the hip prior to sitting. It will usually lock automatically when the person is fully standing. Going up and down stairs is limited to one step at a time leading with the unamputated leg going up and with the prosthesis going down.

Not surprisingly, walking with a hip disarticulation or transpelvic prosthesis is slow and extremely energy consuming. Living with a prosthesis at this level requires many adjustments. The person may need to remove the prosthesis to use the bathroom. Individuals with a transpelvic amputation may also have a permanent colostomy and need to make a hole in the undergarment to provide access. Many individuals, rather than use some form of a body sock, will adapt a sport or spandex garment with one leg opening sewn together. However, any garment worn between the skin and socket must be totally free of wrinkles to prevent the development of any sores. As with all amputees, weight control is most important, as weight gain puts additional stress on the remaining extremity as well as changes the fit of the socket.

Prosthetic acceptance, in the long term, is very limited at this level, and patients often find it easier to function on crutches or in a wheelchair for daily activities. Some patients will wear the prosthesis part of the day, removing it at home. Sitting is a problem for people with a transpelvic amputation and for some individuals with hip disarticulation amputations. These individuals should be fitted with a sitting socket for proper spine alignment and distribution of weight. A sitting socket, like the prosthetic socket, is made for the individual and padded to provide both support and comfort.[14]

BILATERAL AMPUTATIONS

CASE STUDIES

1. Mr. Canan, 79 years old, lost his right leg below the knee 4 years ago secondary to vascular insufficiency and diabetes. He was fitted with a prosthesis and became independent with a cane. He was a functional prosthetic user until about 8 months ago when he began to have problems with his left foot. He continued to wear his prosthesis, but he did less walking as the foot became infected. He has just had a left transtibial amputation.
2. Sgt. James McDonald lost both of his legs above the knee in Afghanistan. The 28-year-old marine was initially treated at Brooks Army Medical Center for acute care and initial rehabilitation. He is now ready for prosthetic fitting and training.

Case Study Activities

1. How would the goals and treatment program differ for Mr. Canan and Sgt. McDonald from those of individuals with unilateral amputations?
2. From the information given, what would be the desirable functional outcomes in each instance?

There are a variety of causes of bilateral amputations. Essentially, all of the causes of amputation listed in Chapter 4 may lead to the loss of one or both limbs. Recent wars have led to a number of young people with bilateral lower limb loss due to explosive devices, shrapnel, and other war-related wounds. Individuals with vascular disease who lose one limb have about a 53% chance of undergoing a major amputation in the contralateral limb within 5 years.[16] There are variations in these figures depending on the particular study, but there is general agreement that the likelihood of contralateral limb amputation at some level increases over time. The individual with bilateral amputations, whether both amputations are performed at the same time or whether there is a long time lag between amputations, presents special challenges to the rehabilitation team. Surgical considerations are the same as presented in Chapter 4 and will not be repeated here.

Postsurgical Care

As outlined in Chapter 5, postsurgical care for the person with bilateral loss of the lower limbs focuses on enhancing healing; preventing contractures; increasing strength of the remaining parts of the body, especially the trunk; and increasing mobility. Many parts of the postsurgical period will be the same; however, there are two areas where the programs will differ.

Individuals who have lost two lower extremities will need to adjust to the loss of proximal weight in sitting and bed mobility activities. Balance evaluation and retraining must be started early and become increasingly important the higher the level of amputation. Diagnosis of balance problems includes both static and dynamic balance on all types of surfaces and when moving from one surface to another. An accurate determination of the person's specific balance problems will inform the intervention activities. Care must be taken during early balance activities not to put undue stress on the recently amputated residual limb.

Upper extremity and trunk strengthening exercises are also quite important as the individual will use the arms for many transfers and bed mobility activities. Moving on a mat in all different directions helps the patient relearn how to move his or her body. Trunk strengthening is very important to help the person maintain balance in a variety of positions as well as coming to sitting from a supine position.

Wheelchair activities are an integral part of the postsurgical program; transfers on and off a variety of surfaces, getting in and out of a car, bathroom independence, and handling the wheelchair outside the home must be included. In the early postsurgical period, bed mobility will be easier if one amputation predates the second so that the healed residual limb can be used to assist in movements. If the person had been independent with a transtibial prosthesis prior to losing the second limb, he or she can often use that prosthesis to aid in transfer. Some individuals are able to ambulate short distances with the one transtibial prosthesis and crutches or a walker. Care must be taken to ensure that such ambulation can be tolerated by the residual limb, but this ability often makes it possible for the individual to get in and out of the bathroom unaided. If the individual was a unilateral transfemoral amputee prior to losing the other limb at whatever level, using the prosthesis for transfers or even limited ambulation is more difficult and is usually not attempted. The change in body weight distribution in any bilateral amputation requires some adjustment to the wheelchair to make sure it does not readily tip backward. A special amputee wheelchair with offset back wheels may be obtained, or simple weights can be taped to the forward frame of the wheelchair to perform the same function. Antitip devices can also be used on most wheelchairs, and sometimes, leaving the footrests attached may provide the necessary weight depending on the patient's size and weight. However, the footrests sometimes interfere with mobility, particularly in small houses and tight spaces. Obviously, individuals with bilateral amputations who wear prostheses some of the time need removable footrests for those times when they are sitting with the prostheses.

Prosthetic Components

The decision to fit or not to fit someone with bilateral lower extremity amputations is difficult and will generally depend on many factors. As with any amputee, the individual's mobility status prior to the second amputation and the person's general health and endurance are critical. The energy requirement for walking with two prostheses is enormous and grows exponentially with the higher levels of amputation.[17]

In general, components used with the unilateral prosthesis are also used when the person is fitted with two prostheses (Chapter 6). It is advantageous to make two new prostheses even if the individual was initially fitted as a unilateral amputee. However, this is not always financially possible. It depends on the age and condition of the first prosthesis and the availability of funding for two new limbs. The person wearing two transtibial prostheses may be a bit more stable if the feet have somewhat softer heel compression, but that, again, depends on the balance, coordination, and strength of the individual.

Ambulation with bilateral transfemoral prostheses, even with microprocessor knee mechanisms, is slow and energy demanding. There may be improved proprioception if the person is fitted with direct contact suction sockets rather than gel liners. Younger, fit individuals, particularly service personnel who lost their limbs while in the military, can be functionally fitted with today's technologically advanced prosthetic components. Many older individuals may prefer to use a wheelchair rather than attempt ambulation. It is often unwise to try to fit individuals who do not exhibit considerable strength, endurance, balance, and good range of motion of both hips. Hip flexion contractures can militate against any ability to ambulate with prostheses. All bilateral amputees will need a wheelchair for times they are not wearing their prostheses. To be functional with bilateral transfemoral prostheses, the individual should be able to ambulate step over step with no more than one cane for external support. There are some who recommend fitting an individual with bilateral transfemoral prostheses with one manual locked knee. This is rarely advisable, as it is hard to come to standing with a locked knee, and ambulation is slower and requires more energy. If the individual was particularly tall, the bilateral prostheses may be made shorter to aid in balance and control. On occasion, foot size may be changed if it is determined that either a larger or smaller foot size will aid prosthetic use. These are also foam, nonfunctional cosmetic limbs that can attach to the wheelchair for individuals who do not use functional prostheses.

Fitting an individual with bilateral transfemoral amputations initially with short prostheses also known as "shorties" or "stubbies" can be useful to help the individual develop strength and balance in the upright position. Stubbies are transfemoral prosthetic sockets set on rockers or pylons and small training prosthetic feet and are used to help the individual move around in an upright position (**Fig. 8.11**). The

sockets adhere to all prosthetic fitting principles and must be accommodating to the demands of the residual limb. Many people find stubbies cosmetically unacceptable because of the extreme reduction in height. Ambulation in stubbies obligates exaggerated trunk rotation. Short canes or crutches may be needed. Sitting in a chair and stair climbing are difficult because of the shortness of the prostheses. The limbs also protrude in front of the chair while the person is sitting because of the lack of knee joints. If the individual becomes proficient in walking with stubbies, then the question of whether to have full-length prostheses can be raised. Although the person may be very stable when walking with stubbies, the lack of height may be a source of embarrassment. Carroll and Richardson advocate the use of short prostheses in the initial care of the person with bilateral transfemoral amputations. They have developed a program starting initially with short prostheses and gradually increasing the height as the person develops the confidence, balance, and coordination to walk with articulated full-length limbs.[18]

Physical Therapy Care

Bilateral Transtibial Amputations

The basic gait-training activities for a person with bilateral transtibial prostheses are similar to those used with one prosthesis. If the individual ambulated with one prosthesis prior to losing the other limb, the process is easier. Some individuals with two prostheses will need some form of external support, especially for elevation activities; however, with good balance training, many, particularly at the transtibial level, will be able to complete all activities without external support.

Considerable time needs to be spent on balance and weight-shifting activities because the individual no longer has any direct contact with the ground. Individuals with two prostheses may use a somewhat wider base of support than those with one prosthesis, and many exhibit a tendency to roll a bit from side to side. These extraneous movements need to be minimized, but they may not be completely eliminated, particularly at the transfemoral level. The client should progress directly from the parallel bars to whatever form of external support will be used at home. A walker is again not the external support of choice. Functional outcomes are directly related to the balance, strength,

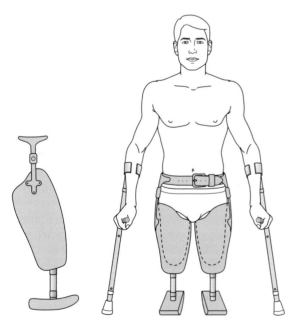

FIGURE 8.11. Stubbies.

and coordination of the patient and to the levels of amputation. Many individuals with two transtibial amputations can regain full functional independence, often without external support or with one case depending on the individual's balance and endurance. Younger, fit individuals often regain the ability to run, exercise, and participate in all aspects of a normal life (**Fig. 8.12**) (see Chapter 19). Depending on the length of the residual limbs, the types of components, and the person's strength, the person may well be able to go up and down steps one leg over the other. The amount of energy expended must not preclude participation in other activities. The higher the levels of amputation are and the more external support is needed, the less functional is the ambulation.

Bilateral Transfemoral Amputations

Gait training for individuals with bilateral transfemoral amputations, even if the individual was functional on one prosthesis before losing the other limb, is difficult and requires a very fit individual. It has been estimated that walking with two transfemoral prostheses requires about 280% more energy than that expended by a nonamputee.[18] Starting with short prostheses and transitioning to full length prostheses is time consuming. Some individuals do not want to learn initially on the short prostheses, and many struggle to learn to use the full-length limbs initially. The short prostheses, of course, do not have

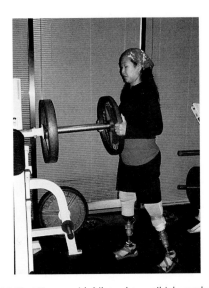

FIGURE 8.12. Woman with bilateral transtibial prostheses working out at the gym.

any knee mechanisms. As the person is gradually raised in height, the knee mechanisms are introduced as the limbs reach close to normal length. The results are not always as desired, as it takes considerable physical fitness and conditioning to become a bilateral transfemoral prosthetic user, even with today's microprocessor limbs. The individual must want to become ambulatory and be willing to spend the time and energy to succeed.[17] Peer support is another positive adjunct of the rehabilitation program. Many individuals gain considerable confidence by seeing others with similar disabilities who have succeeded and by discussing with them the realistic problems of living with a disability. As discussed in Chapter 3, organizations such as the Amputee Coalition of America can be resources for finding well-qualified peer visitors.

Many older individuals or those with limited strength and endurance need to be taught to become fully functional in a wheelchair and be provided with an appropriately fitted wheelchair.

Advanced Activities

Part of the training program for patients with bilateral amputations at any level must include all aspect of daily activities, including coping with obstacles that may be encountered in daily life such as escalators, curbs, and ramps. Individuals functioning with the short prostheses will encounter high counters or shelves in stores and must learn to adjust to those conditions. Teaching falling and getting up from the floor is important. Although every effort is made to avoid falling, falls are inevitable, particularly with an active individual. Teaching the person how to fall and how to get up again is an important part of the prosthetic training program.

SUMMARY

Although transtibial and transfemoral amputations are the most common, physical therapists and physical therapist assistants will see individuals with amputations at other levels. The special needs, prosthetic components, and management concepts related to these levels have been presented in this chapter. It is important to recognize that the higher the level of amputation and the presence of multiple amputations present unique challenges that must be met through individual diagnosis, evaluation, and treatment.

KEYWORDS FOR LITERATURE SEARCH

Bilateral amputation

Chopart amputation

Hip disarticulation

Knee disarticulation

Lisfranc amputation

Stubbies

Transmetatarsal amputation

Transpelvic amputation

REFERENCES

1. Bowker JH: Amputations and disarticulations within the foot: surgical management. In Smith DG, Michael JW, Bowker JH (eds): Atlas of amputations and limb deficiencies: surgical, prosthetic and rehabilitation principles. Rosemont, IL, AAOS, 2004, pp 429–448.
2. Blume P, Salonga C, Garbalosa J, et al: Predictors for the healing of transmetatarsal amputations: retrospective study of 91 amputations. Vascular 15(3):126–133, 2007.
3. Nguyen TH, Gordon IL, Whalen D, Wilson SE: Transmetatarsal amputation: predictors of healing. Am Surg 72(10):973–977, 2006.
4. Condie DN, Bowers R: Amputations and disarticulations within the foot: prosthetic management. In Smith DG, Michael JW, Bowker JH (eds): Atlas of amputations and limb deficiencies: surgical, prosthetic and rehabilitation principles. Rosemont, IL, AAOS, 2004, pp 449–458.
5. Bowker JH: Ankle disarticulation and variants: surgical management. In Smith DG, Michael JW, Bowker JH (eds): Atlas of amputations and limb deficiencies: surgical, prosthetic and rehabilitation principles. Rosemont, IL, AAOS, 2004, pp 459–472.
6. Sarmiento A: A modified surgical prosthetic approach to the Syme's amputation: a follow up report. Clin Orthop 85:11–15, 1972.
7. Pinzur MS: Restoration of walking ability with Syme's ankle disarticulation. Clin Orthop 361:71–75, 1999.
8. Berke GM: Ankle disarticulation and variants: prosthetic management. In Smith DG, Michael JW, Bowker JH (eds): Atlas of amputations and limb deficiencies: surgical, prosthetic and rehabilitation principles. Rosemont, IL, AAOS, 2004, pp 473–480.
9. Pinzur MS: Knee disarticulation: surgical management. In Smith DG, Michael JW, Bowker JH (eds): Atlas of amputations and limb deficiencies: surgical, prosthetic and rehabilitation principles. Rosemont, IL, AAOS, 2004, pp 517–524.
10. Cummings DR, Russ R: Knee disarticulations: prosthetic management. In Smith DG, Michael JW, Bowker JH (eds): Atlas of amputations and limb deficiencies: surgical, prosthetic and rehabilitation principles. Rosemont, IL, AAOS, 2004, pp 525–532.
11. Chansky HA: Hip disarticulation and transpelvic amputation. In Smith DG, Michael JW, Bowker JH (eds): Atlas of amputations and limb deficiencies: surgical, prosthetic and rehabilitation principles. Rosemont, IL, AAOS, 2004, pp 557–564.
12. Smith DG: Higher challenges: the hip disarticulation and transpelvic amputation levels. InMotion 15:1, 2005 Jan/Feb.
13. Shaffer E: Advances in hip disarticulation socket design. InMotion 13(5): 2003 Sept/Oct.
14. Carroll KM: Hip disarticulation and transpelvic amputation: prosthetic management. In Smith DG, Michael JW, Bowker JH (eds): Atlas of amputations and limb deficiencies: surgical, prosthetic and rehabilitation principles. Rosemont, IL, AAOS, 2004, pp 565–574.
15. Chin T, Sawamura S, Shiba R, Oyabu H: Energy expenditure during walking in amputees after disarticulation of the hip: a microprocessor-controlled swing-phase control knee versus a mechanical-controlled stance-phase control knee. J Bone and Joint Surg (British) 87:117–119, 2005.
16. Izumi Y, Satterfield K, Lee S, Harkless LB: Risk of reamputation in diabetic patients stratified by limb and level of amputation: a 10-year observation. Diabetes Care 29(3):566–570, 2006 Mar.
17. Waters RI, Mulroy SJ: Energy expenditure of walking in individuals with lower limb amputations. In Smith DG, Michael JW, Bowker JH (eds): Atlas of amputations and limb deficiencies: surgical, prosthetic and rehabilitation principles. Rosemont, IL, AAOS, 2004, pp 395–408.
18. Carroll K, Richardson R: Improving outcomes for bilateral transfemoral amputees: a graduated approach to prosthetic success. Academy Today 5(2):A-4–A-9, 2009 Mar.
19. Huang CT, Jackson JR, Moore NB, et al: Amputations: energy cost of amputation. Arch Phys Med Rehabil 60:18–24, 1979.

9

The Child With an Amputation

OBJECTIVES

At the end of this chapter, all students are expected to:

1. Classify congenital amputations according to International Standard Organization terminology.
2. Differentiate between congenital and acquired amputations in relation to
   a. The residual limb
   b. Developmental effects
   c. Rehabilitation program
3. Discuss the role of the family in working with children with amputations.
4. Develop an assessment program for a child with a unilateral amputation.
5. Develop an intervention program for a child with a unilateral amputation.

CASE STUDIES

Michael Donnagin is a 6-month-old boy brought to the clinic by his mother. Michael was born with only half a humerus on the right side and only the medial two toes on the right foot. The rest of the extremities are normal. He is an only child. His father is a loan officer at a bank, and his mother is on leave from her job as a legal secretary.

Jenny Smith, 6 years old, had a left transfemoral amputation secondary to a farm accident 4 weeks ago; an attempt was made to reattach the limb, but it failed. She was discharged from the hospital about 4 days after the amputation and has been at home with visiting physical therapy and nursing services. She is referred to an amputee clinic for evaluation and treatment. She lives with her parents and four older siblings on a moderate-size dairy farm about 60 miles from the city.

Case Study Activities

1. Classify Michael's amputations using appropriate terminology.
2. Compare and contrast acquired versus congenital amputations.
3. Determine the appropriate practice pattern(s) for each child.
4. Using the practice pattern as a guide, develop an appropriate examination plan for each child.
   a. What critical data do you need that can best be obtained through interview?
   b. What critical historical data do you need?
   c. What tests and measures would you perform today? Why?
   d. What might be the parents' concerns at this time?
   e. What information would you like to have from the parents?
5. Compare and contrast the prosthetic rehabilitation program for each of these children and an adult with a similar disability.

The habilitation of children with single or multiple limb loss is a complex, long-term process involving specialists from many disciplines with training in pediatric care. This chapter provides a brief overview of this topic, offering general guidelines for the therapist who may occasionally work with a child who has lost one limb. Most physical therapists and physical therapist assistants, knowledgeable in the prosthetic care of adults as well as normal development, can provide effective therapy to a child with one limb loss. The care of the child with multiple limb deficiencies requires considerable expertise by all members of the team, and such children should be referred to special pediatric centers for optimum care.

A child is not a miniature adult. Children have special problems related to developmental tasks, parental adjustment, and adjustment and acceptance of the artificial limb. The rehabilitation program involves the whole family, and the attitudes of the parents, other siblings, and family members have considerable influence on the adjustment of the child. Children with congenital amputations usually do not experience a sense of loss and see the prosthesis as an aid to function. If the appliance is not seen by the child as helpful, he or she may well reject it. The child with an acquired amputation, unless very young, will experience a sense of loss and need a period of adjustment, much like adults. How well the child adjusts to the loss may affect the child's attitude toward the prosthetic device.

Congenital amputations occur at a rate between 0.03 and 1 out of every 1000 live births. Approximately 58% of congenital limb deficiencies occur in the upper extremity with longitudinal hand deficiencies the most common. In the lower extremity, longitudinal toe deficiencies are reported to be the most common. Multiple limb loss has been reported to represent about 17.8% of all newborns with congenital limb loss.[1]

TERMINOLOGY

Amputations in the pediatric population are either congenital or acquired. Nomenclature for describing acquired amputations is the same as for adults as described in Chapter 4. The International Standards Organization (ISO) has developed a standardized method for describing congenital limb deficiencies; the descriptions focus on skeletal deficiencies and anatomical and radiological characteristics and are translatable in many languages.[2] Deficiencies are described as either transverse or longitudinal. In a transverse deficiency, the skeletal portion of the limb has developed normally but no following skeletal element exists. For example, a child with a normal shoulder joint and a small part of a humerus but no other part of the arm would be described as "transverse, upper arm, upper third" (**Fig. 9.1**). In a longitudinal deficiency, there is a partial or complete loss of one or more skeletal elements within the long axis on the bone. For example, a child born without a fibula and with only part of the foot would be listed as "total longitudinal deficiency of the fibula and

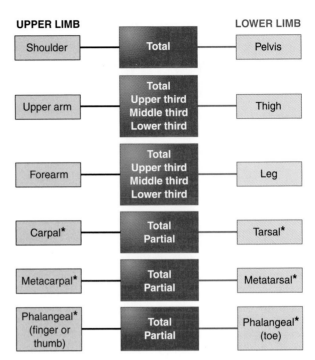

FIGURE 9.1. International Standards Organization (ISO) designation of levels of transverse deficiencies of upper and lower limbs. Note that the skeletal elements marked with an asterisk are used as adjectives in describing transverse deficiencies (eg, transverse carpal total deficiency). A total absence of the shoulder or hemipelvis (and all distal elements) is a transverse deficiency. If only a portion of the shoulder or hemipelvis is absent, the deficiency is of the longitudinal type. (*From ISO Standard 8548-1, 1989.*)

absence of the first, second, and third rays of the foot" (**Fig. 9.2**). Longitudinal deficiencies of the upper extremity are depicted in **Figure 9.3**.

Congenital amputations are the result of a prenatal or birth defect and may vary in configurations. There may be a vestigial component attached to a proximal part, digits may not be separated, and individuals may sustain multiple limb deficiencies or anomalies. An innovative and creative approach to surgical interventions and fitting is used by members of the child limb deficiency clinics.

SURGICAL INTERVENTIONS

Congenital Deformities

The aim of amputation surgery in children, if performed, is to produce a limb that is adequate for a prosthesis and that will remain adequate throughout the growth period and adulthood. Among children with congenital absence of a limb, amputation surgery is usually done to provide the child with a

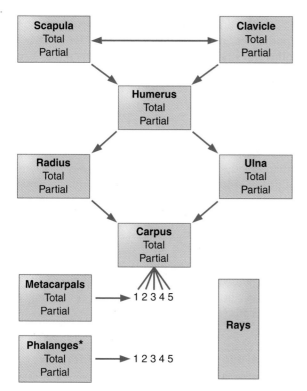

FIGURE 9.2. Description of longitudinal deficiencies of the upper limb using the International Standards Organization (ISO) system. The asterisk indicates that the digits of the hand are sometimes referred to by name: 1, thumb; 2, index; 3, middle; 4, ring; 5, little (or small). For the purpose of this classification, such naming is deprecated because it is not equally applicable to the foot. *(From ISO Standard 8548-1, 1989.)*

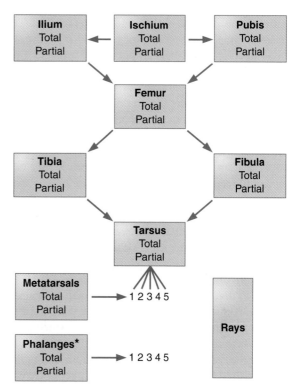

FIGURE 9.3. Description of longitudinal deficiencies of the lower limb using the International Standards Organization (ISO) system. The asterisk indicates the great toe, or hallux. *(From ISO Standard 8548-1, 1989.)*

residual limb that can be fitted with a prosthesis. Whenever possible, surgery is delayed to allow as much bone growth as possible. Prostheses can be adapted to a great variety of congenital deformities, allowing the child to perform relatively normal bipedal or bimanual activities. Surgery, whenever performed, should create a pain-free weight-bearing, stable an adequately sensate limb, near-normal gait, maximum bone growth, and satisfactory cosmetic appearance. Amputation for cosmetic reasons alone is usually delayed until the child is old enough to share in the decision.

Upper Extremity

Reconstructive surgery is frequently used to improve congenital deformities. Function and then cosmesis are the primary concerns. The surgeon must consider bone loss and incompletely developed muscles and ligaments that may affect joint function. In the upper extremity, reconstructive surgery plays a major role in the management of children with longitudinal upper arm or forearm deficiencies that result in nonfunctional hands, polydactyly, or other deformities. New techniques and technology have provided the surgeon with many tools to provide the child with a functional hand, and physical therapists and physical therapist assistants working in these centers will need advanced training to function effectively. Surgical reconstruction may be performed in infants to allow for normal development in manual tasks. Surgeon, prosthetist, and therapists work closely together, and children are monitored closely throughout the developmental stages.

Lower Extremity

In the lower extremity, reconstructive surgery is often delayed to allow for the greatest amount of bone growth possible. Maintenance of long bone growth plates allows for the greatest development of limb length. Individuals with short proximal skeletal pieces may eventually develop a usable residual limb. Severe deformities that interfere with early fitting or with function require early surgical intervention. The surgeon considers overall function and related muscular development. It is important to prevent progressive deformities that may occur as a result of muscle and nerve imbalances. Surgery to increase bone length using the Ilizarov technique can be successfully performed to provide the child with a functional residual limb. **Ilizarov's technique** is based on the principle of distraction osteogenesis (*osteo* for bone, *genesis* for formation). The theory is that new bone will form between surfaces that are pulled apart gradually in a controlled manner.[3] However, bone-lengthening procedures can take many months during which the child is not weight bearing on the extremity. There are other possible complications from bone-lengthening procedures including infections and proximal joint contractures.[4,5] In a case report, Villarruel[6] discussed a special temporary prosthesis that was fabricated to allow the patient to walk with the external fixator in place during the bone consolidation process. The Ilizarov procedure has been used for many years with both congenital and acquired amputations. As in the upper extremity, surgeons have many options to improve the function of children with congenital limb deficiencies, and such children need to be treated in specialized pediatric centers.

Acquired Amputations

Trauma is the major cause of acquired amputations in children, with power machines the most likely cause. Despite improvements in lawnmower safety, lawnmower injuries continue to be a contributing factor in amputation in children.[7] Surgical approaches for children are somewhat different than those for adults. Consideration must be given to protecting the growth plates in the bones whenever possible. Because children heal better than adults, some procedures that conserve limb length, such as split thickness skin grafts, may be successful.[8] Whenever possible, reconstructive surgery is considered over amputation, but the type and amount of damage may dictate surgical procedure.

The second most likely cause of amputation in children is malignant tumors. In recent years, the success of tumor resection and reconstructive surgery has dramatically decreased the need for amputation with equal survival rates. However, once again, reconstructive surgery may require multiple procedures over many months and may lead to complications.

Nagarajans and associates reviewed all major surgical approaches and illustrated the need for long-term follow-up studies to provide better data on the effects of various approaches.[9] Surgery is followed by chemotherapy and sometimes radiation. In surgery, all malignant tissue is removed with wide surgical margins. Reconstruction may take several forms depending on the parts involved. A custom **endoprosthetic device** may be inserted, allograft or **autograft** reconstruction may be performed, or a combination of procedures may be utilized. **Rotationplasty** may be used for tumors of the distal femur or proximal tibia (**Fig. 9.4**). In a rotationplasty, the tumor and knee joint are totally removed, and the lower segment is turned and reattached with nerve structures intact. After healing, the ankle joint functions as a knee component allowing the use of a transtibial prosthesis. This procedure may also be used with some congenital deformities.

COMPLICATIONS OF SURGERY

Terminal Bony Overgrowth

Bony overgrowth at the end of the residual limb is a common complication of amputation in children. Bones most frequently involved include the tibia/fibula, humerus, and sometimes the femur. Because proximal growth plates are intact, the bone continues to grow, and the child will complain of pain on weight bearing at the end of the residual limb and may have evidence of inflammation. On occasion, small spicules of bone may protrude through the skin. Bony overgrowth is reported to occur in as little as 4% or as much as 35% of patients.[8] Various modifications to the amputation process have been tried with some success, but bony overgrowth continues to be a problem. Repeated surgical resection of bony overgrowth can lead to scarring of the residual limb as well as shorten it over time. Depending on the amount of overgrowth, various prosthetic adjustments can be made to relieve pressure distally, delaying the need for surgery as long as possible. Parents need to be taught to take complaints of distal pain seriously and inspect the child's residual limb carefully to recognize early signs of overgrowth.

Adventitious Bursae

These bursae may develop in the soft tissue over an area of terminal overgrowth. They may be treated by

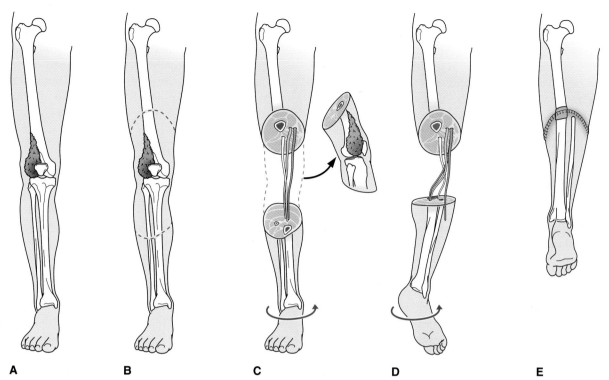

A   **B**   **C**   **D**   **E**

FIGURE 9.4. A rotationplasty reconstruction for malignant bone tumors of the distal femur. Following this procedure, with an appropriate prosthesis, the ankle joint serves the function of the removed knee joint. **(A)** Preoperative status (distal femoral sarcoma). **(B)** Skin incision. **(C)** Resected specimen with remaining limb and intact neuromuscular structures. **(D)** Rotation component of procedure. **(E)** Resultant limb after osteosynthesis and repair of soft tissues. *(Adapted from Atlas of amputations and limb deficiencies, American Academy of Orthopaedic Surgeons, Figure 7, p 845.)*

steroid injection, socket modification, or aspiration, but permanent relief usually necessitates surgical excision of the bursae and underlying bone.

Scarring of the Residual Limb

Residual limb scarring can be a problem with children as well as adults. Scarring from trauma, from repeated surgeries, or from other causes can interfere with prosthetic fitting. Although children have more resilient tissues and heal faster than adults, scarring in weight-bearing areas may necessitate adjustments in prosthetic design and fitting. On rare occasions, surgical reconstruction may be necessary to remove scars that cannot be accommodated prosthetically.

PSYCHOLOGICAL CONSIDERATIONS

Working with children with a disability involves working with the whole family. Although children with limb deficiencies and amputations have been described as generally showing good adjustment, loss of one or more limbs, whether congenital or acquired, is emotionally challenging for all involved.[10]

Today's prenatal technology makes it possible for parents to know well ahead of birth that the fetus has one or more limb deficiencies. Psychologists debate the benefits and limitations of advanced knowledge. In a small study of parents of children with a variety of congenital problems, mothers who had known of the deformities prior to birth reported significantly greater burden than mothers who had not known.[11] The authors warn that the sample was too small for generalization. Generally, the limited studies suggest that there is little difference in adaptation between children with congenital limb deficiencies and those with acquired limb loss. Other factors have much greater influence on the child's adjustment to the disability.

Not surprisingly, studies indicate that parental response and actions greatly influence the child's response to the disability. Marital discord increases anxiety and lowers the child's self-esteem.[12] Other factors such as parent and family response to the disability, peer responses, cultural considerations, cause of the amputation, and age at acquired amputation are also influences on adaptation to disability.

Providing information to the parents and caregivers early, explaining the medical situation, treatment options, and possible prognosis, is important in helping the family adjust to the birth of a limb-deficient child. Parents should be encouraged to ask questions and to share their concerns and feelings openly and with acceptance. Support, through counseling, support groups, or other means should continue throughout the child's development and growth. The child born without one or more limbs will not realize that he or she is different from others for a number of years. Support for both the child and family will be needed during these changing times. Adolescence can be particularly difficult, for both the child with a congenital handicap as well as the one with an acquired amputation. Peer pressure can lead the child to discard an upper extremity prosthesis as well as lose self-esteem and withdraw from interactions.

Box 9.1 lists a series of activities important to help children and family adjust to a disability. Physical therapists and physical therapist assistants need to be aware that the level of distress and degree of adjustment are not directly related to the severity of the disability, and that distress can change over time as family dynamics and child development occur. Parents and children may question why a congenital disability occurred. Because most congenital limb deficiencies have no known causes, the lack of an answer can increase the family's feelings of loss of control. Research indicates that coping with stressors created by situations over which we do not have any control can be the most devastating. Families want to find meaning in the events that shape their lives. This, of course, may also occur with acquired amputations. Providing the child and parents with some control, some involvement in decision making is helpful.

Physical therapists and physical therapist assistants working with children and families should be aware of the community resources available for support and assistance. The Association of Children's Prosthetic-Orthotic Clinics (www.acpoc.org) has numerous resources, publishes a newsletter, and can provide guidance to families and health-care providers.

PROSTHETIC CONSIDERATIONS

Prosthetic components are presented in Chapter 7, and many manufacturers provide the same components in smaller sizes for children. Prosthetic adaptations are often necessary for infants and young children, especially those born with longitudinal congenital deformities associated with weakened musculature, unstable joints, and limb length differences. Prosthetists working with children have many challenges. A child may have a unique skeletal configuration, such as a foot attached to the end of the femur which needs to be maintained during growth or that may act as a substitute hand. Children need to be active and have prosthetic components durable enough for active sports and yet padded enough to prevent injuries to themselves or others. As children grow, the fit of the prosthesis changes and needs adaptation. Compared to adults who add socks as the residual limb shrinks, children may initially be fitted with more socks than necessary to allow for growth and sock removal. Children may not have the same weight-bearing or stabilizing surfaces in the residual limb, although the advent of gel liners has enhanced the prosthetist's ability to fit deformed or scarred residual limbs. When selecting prosthetic components, the team needs to consider all aspects of the child's life; the ideal component may be too heavy or too large for the child or the child may not be ready for the complexity of the device. Often the prosthesis is left cosmetically unfinished, particularly in the lower extremity, to allow for frequent alignment changes as the child develops. The great variety of orthopedic reconstructive surgeries, including the rotationplasty discussed above, also require special prosthetic considerations.[13] The prosthetist is often the team member who has the closest ongoing contact with the child and the family, as a growing child requires frequent adjustments and changes in the prosthesis. The prosthetist plays an important role in helping educate the patient and the family in the use and care of the prosthesis. Close communication between the therapist and prosthetist helps ensure good continuity in the treatment program.

BOX 9.1	Helping Parents and Children Cope

- Provide information
- Accept fears and concerns
- Use active listening
- Involve in decision making
- Foster child independence
- Refer to support groups
- Refer to mental health professional (if indicated)

Lower Extremity

The goal of prosthetic replacement in the lower extremity is to facilitate normal development of crawling, kneeling, standing, and running. Whenever possible, the child with a congenital amputation is fitted as he or she starts crawling and pulling to stand. The great variety of possible congenital deformities requires very individualized prosthetic replacements. Sockets are contoured to support weakened structures, and functional appendages are used in congenital amputations. The "step in" prosthesis is used following rotationplasty when the ankle is substituted for the knee joint (**Fig. 9.5**). As the child gains in range of plantar flexion, function improves.

Socket design for both acquired and congenital amputations must account for differences in pressure tolerance and strength of residual bone in children as compared to adults. Sometimes others areas of support need to be included, such as the use of a thigh corset in a young child with a short transtibial residual limb. Gel liners have been useful in protecting

sensitive tissue from shear forces created by walking and running. Suspension is sometimes difficult because of limited limb length, body fat, and the use of diapers. Lightweight belts and suspension sleeves are available for children for both transtibial and transfemoral prostheses. Suction suspension is generally not used with young children because rapid growth leads to frequent loss of suspension.[14] There are a great variety of prosthetic components fabricated in children's size and weight. There are small, yet strong articulating knee joints for toddlers as well as articulating ankles. Children adapt to a lower extremity prosthesis fairly easily, and even young children can learn to control a knee mechanism almost automatically.

As the child grows, changes in prosthetic design are often needed to meet structural as well as functional maturation. If the child has lost the distal epiphyses of the residual limb, the limb will not grow at the same rate as the unamputated limb. What started as a long residual limb in a young child can be a very short residual limb by adolescence. Disarticulation is often a very functional level for the child. It maintains all the growth plates, avoids the problem of bony overgrowth, and provides for excellent suspension and prosthetic control.[14]

Upper Extremity

Prosthetic replacement for upper extremity loss is more complex than that for lower extremity loss and is briefly reviewed in Chapter 10. As in the lower extremity, not all terminal devices are available for children, but there are devices specifically made for children. Children with congenital loss or deformities of the hand or upper extremity are fitted early to facilitate bilateral hand activities. Once again, the goal is to foster normal development to the extent possible. Prosthetic acceptance is more of a problem in the upper than the lower extremity. The upper extremity prosthesis is not as responsive to the variety of complex hand functions necessary for daily life, and the appliance is not as easily covered by clothing as a lower extremity prosthesis. In a large multicenter study, Wagner and associates found that lack of function was the primary reason for prosthetic rejection. The respondents to the questionnaire stated they could function as well without the prosthesis. Discomfort was the second most stated reason for discontinuing wear, and cosmesis was the third.[15] The survey included only children with unilateral limb

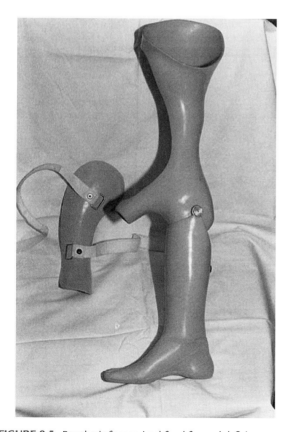

FIGURE 9.5. Prosthesis for proximal focal femoral deficiency.

loss; children with bilateral upper extremity loss may become more dependent on prostheses for function. There have also been studies indicating that children fitted before 2 years of age accepted the prosthesis better than those fitted later.[16]

Passive prostheses are fitted on infants and very young children, usually a lightweight socket with a padded nonfunctioning terminal device that allows bilateral grasping, crawling, and early reaching. An active terminal device is not used until the child can follow simple directions and begins to place objects in the passive device, usually around 2 years of age or later. There do not appear to be general guidelines for the use of **myoelectric prostheses**. Cost is always an issue, but some centers fit very young children with myoelectric limbs, and others wait until the child has shown the ability to use a body-powered device on a full-time basis.[16] There are a variety of terminal devices that can be used with children; very young children will need a lighter device with less resistance to opening than older children. Children are generally fitted with a hook rather than a hand as the hook is more versatile and durable.

THERAPY

The physical therapist is as much a teacher for the family and child as a direct caregiver. Range-of-motion and strengthening exercises need to be integrated into daily life, incorporating prosthetic function and noting changing needs becomes a part of the family's routine. The physical or occupational therapist or assistant working with a young child must be cognizant of normal development to incorporate appropriate activities in the therapy routine. Early intervention is valuable, particularly with children with congenital limb loss and deformities. The first year of life is the foundation for development, and parents must be guided to learn an appropriately structured program.[17] Parents need to be involved in the development and structure of the home program and prosthetic training activities. Therapy needs to be fun for the child and incorporate play activities that facilitate desired movements and motions. As the child grows, participation in sports and recreational activities is important. Participation in sports can help with self-esteem and a sense of accomplishment. Throughout the growth period, the therapy program is aimed at helping the child learn and perform age-appropriate activities.

SUMMARY

Children with congenital or acquired amputations present special needs and generally require a team of experts knowledgeable in this field. Physical therapists and physical therapist assistants working in pediatric centers may encounter a juvenile amputee on occasion and need to determine whether or not the child needs referral to a special center. This chapter is designed to help the therapist make that determination and to provide adequate care for the child who may not need a special center.

KEYWORDS FOR LITERATURE SEARCH

Bone overgrowth

Child amputee

Congenital limb deficiency

Ilizarov technique

Rotationplasty

REFERENCES

1. Fisk JR, Smith DG: The limb deficient child. In Smith DF, Michael JW, Bowker JH (eds): Atlas of amputations and limb deficiencies: surgical, prosthetic, and rehabilitation principles. Rosemont, IL, AAOS, 2004, pp 773–778.
2. Fisk JR: Terminology in pediatric limb deficiency. In Smith DF, Michael JW, Bowker JH (eds): Atlas of amputations and limb deficiencies: surgical, prosthetic, and rehabilitation principles. Rosemont, IL, AAOS, 2004, pp 779–782.
3. Taber's Cyclopedica Medical Dictionary (18th edition). F A Davis, Co, Philadelphia, 1997, pp 963.
4. Barker KL, Shortt N, Simpson HR: Predicting loss of knee flexion during limb lengthening using inherent muscle strength. J Pediatr Orthop, Part B 15(6):404–407, 2006.
5. Antoci V, Ono CM, Antoci V Jr, Ransy EM: Bone strengthening in children: how to predict the complication rate and complexity. J Pediatr Orthop 26(5):534–640, 2006.
6. Villarruel G: Temporary prosthetic fitting over tibial lengthening device: JPO 15:113–117, 2003.
7. Vollman D, Khosla K, Shields BJ, Beeghly BC, Bonsu B, Smith GL: Lawn mower-related injuries to children. J Trauma 59(3):724–728, 2005 Sep.
8. Dormann JP, Erol B, Nelson CB: Acquired amputations in children. In Smith DF, Michael JW, Bowker JH (eds): Atlas of amputations and limb deficiencies: surgical, prosthetic, and rehabilitation principles. Rosemont, IL, AAOS, 2004, pp 841–852.
9. Nagarajan R, Neglia JP, Clohisy D, Robison LL: Limb salvage and amputation in survivors of pediatric lower-extremity bone tumors: what are the long-term implications? J Clin Oncol 20(22):4493–4501, 2002.

10. Kahle AL: Psychological issues in pediatric limb deficiency. In Smith DF, Michael JW, Bowker JH (eds): Atlas of amputations and limb deficiencies: surgical, prosthetic, and rehabilitation principles. Rosemont, IL, AAOS, 2004, pp 801–812.

11. Hunsfeld JA, Rempels A, Passchier J, Hazelbrook JW, Tibboel D: Brief report: parental burden and grief one year after the birth of a child with congenital anomaly. J Pediatr Psychol 24:520–525, 1999.

12. Trute B, Hiebert-Murphy D: Family adjustment to childhood developmental disability: a measure of parent appraisal of family impact. J Pediatr Psychol 27:271–280, 2002.

13. Cummings DR: General prosthetic considerations. In Smith DF, Michael JW, Bowker JH (eds): Atlas of amputations and limb deficiencies: surgical, prosthetic, and rehabilitation principles. Rosemont, IL, AAOS, 2004, pp 789–800.

14. Dorman JP, Erol B, Nelson CB: Acquired amputations in children. In Smith DF, Michael JW, Bowker JH (eds): Atlas of amputations and limb deficiencies: surgical, prosthetic, and rehabilitation principles. Rosemont, IL, AAOS, 2004, pp 841–852.

15. Wagner LV, Bagley AM, James MA: Reasons for prosthetic rejection by children with unilateral congenital transverse forearm total deficiency. JPO 19:51–54, 2007.

16. Patton JG: Occupational therapy. In Smith DF, Michael JW, Bowker JH (eds): Atlas of amputations and limb deficiencies: surgical, prosthetic, and rehabilitation principles. Rosemont, IL, AAOS, 2004, pp 813–830.

17. Coulter-O'Berry C: Physical therapy. In Smith DF, Michael JW, Bowker JH (eds): Atlas of amputations and limb deficiencies: surgical, prosthetic, and rehabilitation principles. Rosemont, IL, AAOS, American 2004, pp 831–840.

10

OBJECTIVES

At the end of this chapter, all students are expected to:

1. Describe the major causes of upper limb amputations.
2. Briefly describe upper-limb amputation surgery.
3. Recognize the function of major upper extremity components.

Physical Therapy students are expected to:

1. Establish a physical therapy diagnosis for a simulated upper limb amputee.
   a. Determine what information is necessary to establish a diagnosis.
   b. Design a plan of intervention based upon the diagnosis.
2. Describe the major components of an upper extremity training program.

Physical Therapist Assistant students are expected to:

1. Participate in implementing a program of intervention.
2. Determine what guidance is needed from the supervising physical therapist.

CASE STUDIES

Hector Rodriguez, a 41-year-old carpenter, sustained a left long transradial amputation when the safety cover broke off the band saw he was operating. Attempts to reattach the hand were unsuccessful. He is referred to physical therapy 24 hours after amputation. He has an immediate postoperative cast on his lower arm anchored just above the olecranon.

    Laura Tyler, a 27-year-old Air Force helicopter pilot, lost her right arm at the transhumeral level secondary to a helicopter crash in Florida. During surgery, an **angulation osteotomy** was performed,

and the residual limb was casted with a figure-eight suspension to maintain the cast in position.

Case Study Activities

1. What data would be needed for each of these patients to establish an appropriate physical therapy diagnosis?
2. What kind of emotional response and questions can you anticipate from each person?
3. What are the critical elements of the postsurgical program for each of these individuals?

The majority of upper limb amputees are treated by occupational therapists. However, on occasion, an upper limb amputee may be referred to a physical therapist when no occupational therapist is available. The purpose of this chapter is to provide a brief overview of upper extremity amputations and rehabilitation. Physical therapists involved with upper extremity amputees should refer to more detailed sources and consider taking continuing education courses in this area.

Upper limb amputations are a small percentage of the total amputations performed in the United States but a majority of amputations performed for trauma.[1] Physical therapists and physical therapist assistants may not treat many individuals with upper limb loss; however, they need to understand the basic concepts for those occasions when they treat an individual with such an amputation. An upper extremity amputation has a major impact on the individual's physical, social, vocational, and emotional life. In some ways, it can be more devastating than a lower extremity amputation. **Figure 10.1** outlines the major levels of upper extremity amputation.

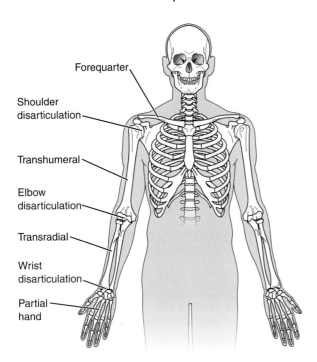

Forequarter

Shoulder
disarticulation

Transhumeral

Elbow
disarticulation

Transradial

Wrist
disarticulation

Partial
hand

FIGURE 10.1. Upper extremity amputation levels.

Amputations can occur at every level from the loss of a phalanx to the loss of the entire upper limb. Trauma of all kinds is the major cause of acquired upper extremity amputations in children and adults. Trauma may include motor vehicle accidents, lawnmower or other machine-driven causes, electrical or other burns, as well as war-related injuries and a great variety of other trauma. On occasion, the amputation is secondary to severe trauma that does not respond to limb reconstruction surgery or reattachment surgery. The second major cause of upper extremity amputation is a tumor that is not amenable to removal. Rarely is an upper limb amputated because of vascular insufficiency.

SURGERY

The basic principles of amputation surgery outlined in Chapter 4 are as applicable to the upper as to the lower extremity:

- Maintain as much length as possible.
- Create a pliable, painless, and nonadherent scar in an appropriate location.
- Stabilize severed muscles through myodesis or myoplasty.
- Resect nerves to prevent painful neuromas.
- Maximize wound healing and a functional residual limb.

Hand, Partial Hand, Digits

Most partial hand and digit amputations are treated with either replantation or reconstruction surgery. Limb replantation through microsurgery has developed greatly in the past 40 years and has become fairly common for the loss of one or more digits. There are indications and contraindications to digit replantation, and the final decision to amputate and reconstruct or reattach rests with the surgeon. It is reported that survival approaches 90% with functional outcomes reported from 30% to 50%.[2] Hand replantation has also become more common if more complex; the process requires great patient compliance. In a study of 24 consecutive replantations, Lanzetta and associates reported that all patients eventually attained protective sensation and 12 attained two-point discrimination. The level of function was not discussed.[3] Hand and digit rehabilitation is a specialized field and beyond the scope of this text.

Transradial and Wrist Disarticulation

Transradial is probably the most common level of upper extremity amputation. Wrist disarticulation, a functional level that maintains some degree of pronation and supination, is somewhat more difficult to fit prosthetically because the length of the residual limb fitted with prosthesis and terminal device makes the amputated arm longer than the unamputated arm. Often, much of the residual pronation and supination is lost in the socket fit.[4] Equal-length flaps are generally used in the transradial amputation with the incision situated in a soft tissue envelope created at the distal end of the residual limb. After surgery, unless there is the possibility of infection, the residual limb is generally placed in an immediate postoperative cast to be activated prosthetically as soon after surgery as possible. Some surgeons prefer to use elastic wrap initially but fit with a temporary prosthesis as soon as possible. The postoperative cast greatly reduces edema and pain. It can also be equipped with a **terminal device** and **harnessing** to allow the patient to adapt to prosthetic function early.[5]

Transhumeral, Elbow Disarticulation, Shoulder Disarticulation

Once again, length preservation is important, although there is controversy among surgeons over the advantages and disadvantages of a long transhumeral amputation versus an elbow disarticulation. In adults, the elbow disarticulation often results in an uncosmetic prosthesis making the long transhumeral level a better choice. In children, the elbow disarticulation is preferred to eliminate the bony overgrowth that occurs after transhumeral amputation (Chapter 9). As with the lower extremity, the higher the level, the greater extent of dysfunction and the more difficulty in suspension and harnessing.

Shoulder disarticulations present many surgical options depending on the extent of injury and remaining tissue. The higher the level of amputation, the greater is the loss of normal body symmetry and balance. The loss of the weight of the arm results in an elevation of the shoulder on the amputated side that is often not compensated by the lighter weight of the prosthesis. Amputations through the shoulder can lead to the development of a scoliosis. These postural changes must be addressed in the postsurgical period.[6]

POSTOPERATIVE CARE

The goals of the postsurgical period for the upper extremity amputee are similar to those for the lower extremity amputee:

- Enhance residual limb healing.
- Prevent contractures and muscle weakness of adjacent areas.
- Maintain or regain independence in functional activities.
- Prepare for definitive prosthetic fitting.
  - Shrink and shape the residual limb.
  - Determine possible myoelectric control sites.
- Prevent postural deformities.
- Facilitate emotional adjustment.

Data Gathering

The type and extent of data gathering that can be achieved immediately after surgery will, of course, depend on the extent of injury and the individual's physiological response to the trauma and surgery. **Box 10.1** outlines the basic data to be gathered to make an appropriate physical therapy diagnosis and develop a plan of care. Generally, although not uniformly, the residual limb will have been placed in an immediate postsurgical cast that may limit motion of the most proximal joint. As in the lower extremity, the rigid dressing helps prevent postoperative edema and reduce postoperative pain.

The physical therapy diagnosis will focus on activities of daily living, particularly those involving bilateral

---

BOX 10.1 | Postsurgical Data

History
- Vocational
- Leisure activities
- Handedness

General Systems Review
Postsurgical Status
- Cardiovascular
- Respiratory
- Whether OOB (out of bed)
- Infection

Pain
- Incisional
- Phantom

Functional Status
- Bed mobility, transfers
- Self-care
  - Dressing, bathing, and so forth

Gross Range of Motion and Strength
- Unamputated extremity including scapula (grossly for comparison)

Specific Measurement
- Transradial
  - All shoulder motions including scapular depression
  - Elbow movements once incisional healing occurs.
- Transhumeral
  - All scapular motions
  - Shoulder motions once incisional healing occurs

Cognition/Emotion

---

hand activities. If the amputated extremity was the dominant side, data gathering and diagnosis will focus on developing dexterity in the remaining upper extremity. The importance of our hands and arms in everyday life is such that the loss of an arm may create major emotional problems. The Amputee Coalition of America (www.amputee-coalition.org), with its nationwide chapters, is a good resource for peer visitors.

Plan of Care

The earlier that a patient can be fitted with a functional terminal device and learn to use it, the more likely the patient will become a functional prosthetic user.[4]

Whether or not the person has been fitted with a cast, the plan of care must include[7]:

- Range-of-motion (ROM) and strengthening exercises for the adjacent joints and muscles.
  - Range and strength in pronation and supination is important for the transradial amputee even though some motion is lost in the socket.
  - Full range of motion in the shoulder and elbow facilitate grooming and prosthetic function.
  - Strengthening exercises for the shoulder should include scapular as well as glenohumeral motions.
- ROM and strengthening exercises for the shoulder on the amputated side to prevent postural changes.
- Residual limb bandaging if not casted.
  - As in the lower extremity, figure-eight bandaging is taught. Circular bandaging should always be avoided. Depending on the size of the extremity, 2- or 3-inch wide bandages are used. The transradial bandage is anchored above the elbow while the transhumeral bandage must be anchored with a loop around the opposite axilla. The bandage should cross in the back as it loops around the unamputated axilla. Shrinkers can also be used once the sutures have been removed.
- Independence in self-care and lifestyle activities, preferably with a temporary **body-powered** prosthesis or with the remaining upper extremity and necessary adapted devices. Part of this training may include helping the individual change dominance if the previously dominant arm was amputated. Bilateral upper extremity amputees present special challenges and are best treated in centers with expertise in their needs.
- Preparation for definitive prosthetic fitting.
  - Part of the preparation is myoelectric site testing. A **myotester** is a device used to determine the electric potential generated by various muscles in the residual limb and assist in selecting sites for myoelectric controls. Advanced training is required to use this equipment, and often, the therapist and prosthetist work together to determine the best sites.[7] Electrodes usually involve the flexors and extensors; the patient needs to learn how to contract one muscle group isometrically while maintaining relaxation of the antagonists.
  - Shoulder ROM exercises preparatory to body control motions. Depending on the level of amputation, the patient will need good strength and full ROM in the residual limb to properly

control and position the upper limb for full activities. The motions include the following:
  - Scapular abduction and humeral flexion to open the terminal device.
  - Chest expansion especially for transhumeral and higher-level amputees.
  - Shoulder depression, extension, and abduction that operate the elbow flexion lock of the body-powered transhumeral prosthesis.
  - Elbow flexion and extension to position the transradial terminal device and reach for objects in different locations.
  - Forearm pronation and supination for the wrist disarticulation and long transradial amputee to help position the terminal device.[7]
- The patient needs to understand the function and limitations of currently available prosthetic replacements. A trip to the prosthetic shop to view and handle the various components is often helpful as are visits by peer visitors. Upper extremity loss can be emotionally more devastating than lower extremity loss, and the patient will need appropriate counseling.

CASE STUDIES

Both patients are ready for definitive prosthetic fitting. Mr. Rodriguez had a harness and terminal device attached to the postoperative cast for 2 weeks, while Captain Tyler wore a postoperative cast for only 3 weeks.

Case Study Activities

1. Compare and contrast the mechanisms of body-powered versus myoelectric-powered prostheses.
2. Which type of powering would be most appropriate for each patient?

PROSTHETIC COMPONENTS

Acceptance of the upper extremity prosthesis is generally lower than the lower extremity prosthesis. The longer a patient is without a prosthesis, the more he or she will learn to function one handed, using the residual limb for object stabilization as needed. The higher is the level of amputation, the heavier is the prosthesis. Bilateral upper extremity amputees, however, generally become prosthetic wearers because of their limitations without limbs. Prosthetic components for the upper extremity have improved dramatically over the years, with considerable improvement in socket fit and hand function. However, to date, the terminal device lacks one important function—sensation. The person can only feel what he or she is holding or picking up by looking at the object or by the pressure generated by the terminal device grip and translated into the socket pressure. Some individuals become very adept at holding all types of objects, from an ice cream cone to a hammer, with just the right amount of pressure. Others find the lack of sensation difficult to overcome and may use the prosthesis only for dress occasions.

The upper extremity prosthesis basically consists of a socket, a method of suspension, a power source, plus elbow and shoulder joints depending on level of amputation. There are two basic types of upper extremity prostheses: body powered and myoelectric.

Body-Powered Prostheses

Body-powered prostheses have been in use for many centuries and may still be the most common in use today.[8] Essentially, a body-powered prosthesis uses body movements, harnessed with control straps and cables, to operate the **terminal device**. Body-powered controls are mechanically simple, low in cost, and highly reliable. However, they also limit the range in which the person can operate the terminal device and may restrict some motions of the unamputated side. The amputee may have to exaggerate body movements to operate the terminal device, and fine control is not available. Body-powered devices are generally not as cosmetic as myoelectric prostheses.

Terminal Devices

Figure 10.2 depicts a variety of hooks, and **Figure 10.3** illustrates a variety of hands. The terminal device may be a hook or a hand. Often, patients are

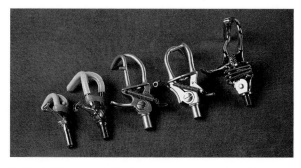

FIGURE 10.2. Assorted hooks. *(Courtesy of Otto Bock HealthCare US.)*

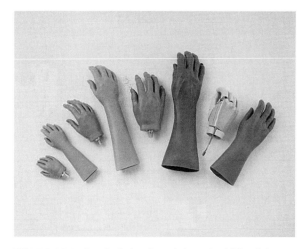

FIGURE 10.3. Prosthetic hands and gloves in child, adolescent, and adult sizes.

fitted with both a hook and a hand. The hook is more durable, but the hand is more natural looking. **Table 10.1** describes the various classes of terminal devices. Within each class, there are a great variety of devices, each with its own advantages and limitations. Hooks are usually made of aluminum alloy and are coated on the inside to enhance gripping. Hands, for body-powered prostheses, do not provide good graded prehension; the rubberized, skin-toned glove that covers the hand can also impede motion. The prosthetist is the most knowledgeable about these devices and must be involved in the selection of components for each person.

Body-powered devices may be either **voluntary opening** (VO) or **voluntary closing** (VC). The VO, the most common, requires the amputee to use body force to open the device to the size required for the object. Once the device is closed around the object, force is exerted by rubber bands around the end of the device. In body-powered prostheses, the amputee can control the closing force by maintaining pressure on the cable that opens the device. In that manner, the amputee can limit the force expended in closing around a fragile object or allow full force to strongly hold an object. Voluntary closing devices are generally open when the amputee is relaxed and are closed by the pressure the person places on the cables.

Suspension and Control

Body-powered prostheses are suspended through a closely fitting socket and through the properly fitted harness that controls the terminal device and, if necessary, the elbow joint. The transradial prosthesis uses a

TABLE 10.1	Terminal Devices		
Terminal Device	**Description**	**Use/Advantage**	**Limitations**
Passive mitt	Soft, flexible, mitten-shaped device covered with skin-tone rubberized material	For infants to initially develop bilateral activities; for sports to prevent injury	No active controls; cover can tear and become soiled
Passive hand	Lightweight hand-shaped device with bendable or spring-loaded fingers for static grasp	Can hold an object placed within the hand and looks natural; lightweight; some have special tool holders	No active controls; cover can tear and become soiled
Prehensive hand	Artificial hand provides thumb and two-finger function to grasp an object; may be voluntary opening or voluntary closing	For body-powered and myoelectric prostheses; great variety of hand designs, some using all fingers; natural skin-tone cover	Cover is fragile, tears and stains easily, and may limit force that can be applied to an object
Prehensive hooks	Voluntary-opening (VO) or voluntary-closing device that comes in many shapes for different functions; rubber bands provide force in VO hooks	Most commonly used terminal device that comes in all sizes; hooks are coated to help hold and grasp; usually made of aluminum alloy; some provide graded prehension	Not very cosmetic; may not meet all needs
Child Amputee Prosthetic Project (CAPP)	Unique voluntary-opening device, initially developed for children, with large gripping surface	Requires little body power but provides large gripping surface	Unique shape unlike hand or hook
Myoelectric devices	May be hook or hand; powered by electric motor at end of socket	Power may be proportional or direct; great variety of shapes and speeds	May be more difficult to learn controls

figure-eight harness that loops around the nonamputated axilla (**Fig. 10.4**). The terminal device is operated by the cable that attaches to the **tricep pad** around the elbow to the terminal device. The patient opens the terminal device through flexion of the humerus (**Fig. 10.5**). There are other variations for individual situations. The harness must fit comfortably and snugly, and the cable must be the proper length and be carefully attached for optimum terminal device function.[9]

The transhumeral prosthesis is similarly suspended (**Fig. 10.6**), and a dual cable system is used to operate the elbow lock and the terminal device (**Fig. 10.7**). In this situation, the person must first bend and lock the elbow and then operate the terminal device.

Other Components

Socket interfaces for body-powered prostheses are similar to those for lower extremity amputees. Gel or silicone liners may be used, while some patients prefer to use a thin cotton sock. All upper extremity prostheses are fitted with a wrist unit that enables the patient to pre-position the terminal device for optimum function. The wrist unit allows easy changing of terminal

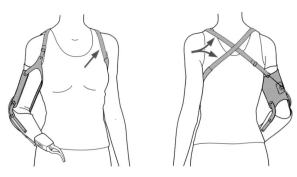

FIGURE 10.4. Figure-eight harness for transradial amputee.

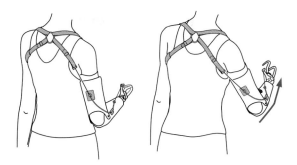

FIGURE 10.5. Humeral flexion operates terminal device.

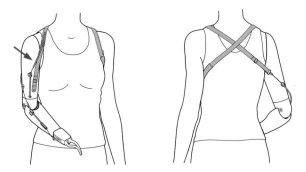

FIGURE 10.6. Transhumeral suspension system.

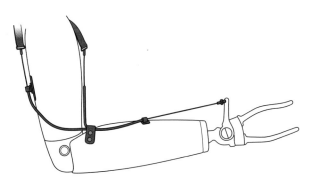

FIGURE 10.7. Dual cable system to operate elbow lock and terminal device.

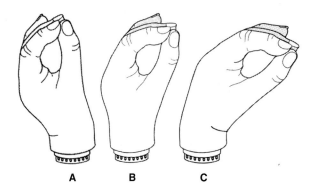

FIGURE 10.8. Three-position wrist unit: **(A)** extension, **(B)** neutral, and **(C)** flexion. *(Courtesy of Motion Control, Inc.)*

the elbow to allow positioning of the terminal device in a wide range of motions. These components are used with both body-powered and myoelectric limbs.

Myoelectric Prostheses

Myoelectric prostheses have also been in use for many years. Essentially, one or more electrodes are implanted in the prosthetic socket in the correct position for the selected muscles. The patient contracts the muscle and sends a signal to a myoelectric controller that operates off a small battery located at the distal end of the socket. In this manner, the patient uses one muscle to open the terminal device and another to close it. In patients with transhumeral or higher-level amputation, additional controls may be provided either by different muscle sites or other methods. The miniaturization of batteries and computer chips has greatly enhanced the variations of function and power sources.

Terminal Device

Terminal devices for myoelectric prostheses come in a variety of forms that may or may not look like the human hand. Regardless of shape, the hands are usually electrically powered devices with one degree of freedom which bring two or three surfaces together to grasp objects. The fingers are usually slightly flexed with the gripping surface, either rubberized glove or prehension surface, coated with a material to enhance grip and avoid slippage. Prehension forces tend to duplicate the range of human force, although there are some devices capable of higher prehension. The width of the opening varies somewhat with the different devices and ranges from 7 to 10 cm. The speed of response varies with the terminal device,

devices as well as rotation to simulate pronation and supination. Some include a flexion component, particularly for bilateral amputees, to allow the terminal device to be brought close to the body (**Fig. 10.8**).

Transhumeral and higher-level amputees also have an elbow unit to allow for flexion and extension of the forearm and terminal device. Elbow units lock in position throughout the range of flexion to allow terminal device use in any position.[8] Transhumeral and higher prostheses also incorporate a rotator just above and more recent developments have emphasized both increased speed of response and a quieter motor. Adult hands usually come in two or three different sizes to accommodate most individuals. Several also come in pediatric sizes. The hands vary in individual characteristics, but most allow the user to control opening, closing, and prehension force. Most also have a locking mechanism that will hold the fingers in the last position when the battery is off. This allows the user to relax the muscles when just holding an object. Wrist flexion units may be incorporated in the hand mechanism (**Fig. 10.9**).[10] Microprocessor systems for the upper extremity function similarly to the lower extremity as reflex control. For example, if the computer senses that the object being held is beginning to slip, the computer will automatically increase the gripping force. The automatic and reflex controls are designed for operation with minimum conscious thought to ease the stress of controlling the prosthesis.[11]

Most hands do not use all five fingers, but there is one hand on the market that does. The I-Limb®, allows all five fingers to bend at the same time. It also provides for changes in thumb position for side gripping and allows the index finger to extend individually (**Fig. 10.10**). Full five-finger grip is advantageous for gripping various-sized objects, but no research could be found on the advantages and disadvantages of this particular design.

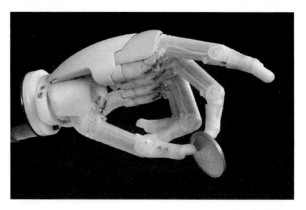

FIGURE 10.10. The I-Limb®, a computer-adjusted myoelectric prosthesis. *(Courtesy of Touch Bionics.)*

Suspension

Myoelectric prostheses do not require the figure-eight harness for suspension. There are several methods of suspending the transradial prosthesis:

- Supracondylar suspension that molds over the humeral condyle with intimate socket fit
- External sleeve suspension similar to that used in the transtibial prosthesis
- Shuttlelock or lanyard locking system similar to that used in lower extremity prostheses

There are advantages and disadvantages to each of these methods of suspension; selection is dictated in part by the length and contour of the residual limb and patient preference. All systems limit elbow motion to some degree.[4]

At the transhumeral level, the sockets can be suspended by the traditional harness without the control cables or by suction using a valve at the end of the socket and a lightweight sleeve. The latter requires stable limb volume but provides for a comfortable fit and good shoulder range of motion. A myoelectric transhumeral prosthesis, such as the Utah Arm 3®, can be both cosmetic and functional with combined elbow and terminal device function computer adjusted to the individual (**Fig. 10.11A,B**).

There are advantages and limitations to both body-powered and myoelectric devices. Myoelectric prostheses eliminate the need of the harness around the upper body which many patients find irritating and cumbersome. For some, the myoelectric limb is cosmetically more like the human limb. However, studies have shown that while the myoelectric grip is usually stronger than the body-powered grip, response time is slower. Additionally, the myoelectric

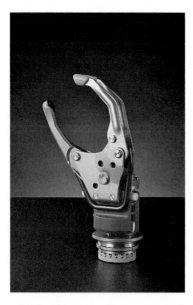

FIGURE 10.9. The SensorHand® myoelectrically controlled prosthesis. *(Courtesy of Otto Bock HealthCare US.)*

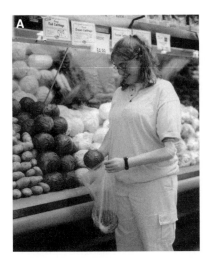

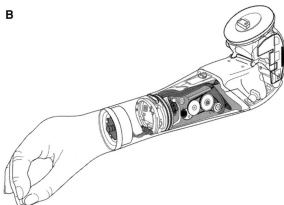

FIGURE 10.11. (A) The Utah Arm 3®, a computer-adjusted myoelectric prosthesis. **(B)** Schematic of the Utah Arm 3 showing battery pack. *(Courtesy of Motion Control, Inc.)*

components are not as durable and do not lend themselves to use in dirty environments. Some individuals like to have both types of prostheses.[4]

Research and Developments

Research is continuing in improving both the cosmesis and the function of the prosthetic hand. New developments incorporate the use of multiple control options to allow the patient to use the terminal device with greater ease and speed. Precision of grip in the wide range of positions necessary for daily life is a continuing challenge, and computerized terminal devices are being developed to reduce the need to concentrate on the controls. Although some research incorporates the five-fingered hand, there is some thought that the current forceps type of grip is more durable. Electronics and

computer-driven total arms are being developed for higher-level amputees as well.

There has been little research into implantable sensors that would provide better neural feedback for more selective and fine control of the terminal device. There is also some research trying to provide some sensory feedback to the user, although the small population of appropriate patients has limited such activities. Overall, the limited number of upper extremity amputees as compared to lower extremity patients has limited both research and development of new components in these areas.[10]

Acceptance/Rejection

Upper extremity amputees abandon prosthetic wear at a greater rate than do lower limb amputees. In a survey of articles published in the last 25 years, Biddiss and Chau found that 45% of children fitted with body-powered prostheses and 35% of children fitted with myoelectric limbs stopped using them. In the adult population, the rejection rates were 26% and 23%, respectively.[12] In another study of patients who had been treated at one rehabilitation center, it was reported that up to 33.75% of patients rejected their prostheses, and many who continued to wear them did not find them useful for daily activities or work. They wore the prosthesis mostly for cosmetic occasions.[13] Investigating factors affecting prosthetic wear, Biddiss and Chau reported that length between amputation and fitting appeared to be a critical factor. Patients fitted within 2 years of birth or 6 months of acquired amputation were more likely to use the prosthesis than those fitted later.[14] It was stated that fitting within 30 days of amputation is the most beneficial. Most of the authors agreed that today's prostheses need to be improved for comfort and function to gain greater acceptance.

PROSTHETIC TRAINING

Upper extremity prosthetic training requires a more detailed understanding of upper extremity function than is provided in this text. Briefly, the steps to prosthetic training include

- Check out prosthetic fit.
- Teach donning, doffing, and care of the prosthesis.
- Provide basic controls training.
- Provide functional use training.

Basic checkout of the upper extremity prosthesis includes checking the residual limb before and after wearing as well as making sure the socket fits comfortably and the controls are working properly. The prosthetist makes sure the cables of the body-powered limb are the correct length and are correctly placed and that the electrodes and chips of the myoelectric device operate as required. In a voluntary opening body-powered terminal device, the length of the cable should allow the hook to be comfortably closed when the arm is in the rest position. However, the cable should be tight enough so that only minimum body movement is needed to activate the terminal device. During early training, the prosthesis should be worn for only 30 minutes to an hour at a time, several times a day. The wearing time is gradually increased until the residual limb has acclimated to the pressures.[7]

Donning and Doffing

The body-powered prosthesis with a figure-eight harness can be donned like a pullover sweater. The liner or sock is slipped over the residual limb, and then, with the unamputated hand holding the distal end of the prosthesis overhead, the person slips the axillary loop over the unamputated arm and then slips the residual limb into the socket. The procedure is reversed to remove the prosthesis. If desired, the prosthesis can also be donned as a coat with the socket donned first.

The myoelectric prosthesis is worn without a sock; it is donned similarly to the traditional suction transfemoral socket. A pull sock or special sleeve is slipped over the residual limb with the distal end of the sock pulled out through a hole in the socket. The residual limb is drawn snugly into the socket, and suction is created. Doffing requires gently tugging on the distal part of the prosthesis until it is off the forearm. The upper extremity socket is cared for like the lower extremity socket except that batteries and electrical components must be off when the prosthesis is being donned or not worn. The lower part of the socket and terminal device must not be immersed in water.

Basic Control Training

Basic control training involves teaching the amputee how to control each part of the prosthesis either manually with the unamputated arm or with the controls of either the body-powered or myoelectric prosthesis. Each step should be taught individually before

putting them together in a goal-oriented training program.

■ Positioning the terminal device: The terminal device opening needs to be rotated much like we turn our hand depending on the task to be accomplished. Unilateral amputees position the terminal device manually with the other hand; bilateral amputees must push the device against a fixed object.
■ Rotating the elbow joint: Rotating the elbow to properly position the terminal device anywhere in an arc around the body is done manually with the other hand.
■ Using the wrist flexion unit: The wrist flexion unit is usually controlled by applying pressure on a button in the unit.
■ Opening and closing the terminal device: Whether using body-powered or myoelectric controls, the patient must learn to control opening and closing the terminal device in all sorts of positions, including in front of the body, out to the side, over the head, and all ranges in between. Through practice, the patient eventually learns to sense the right amount of muscle contraction necessary to operate the terminal device for different tasks.

Function Use Training

To be useful, the person must be able to use the prosthesis to carry out normal activities of everyday life, such as opening a jar, tying one's shoes, cutting meat, and so forth. The prosthesis generally becomes the helping hand regardless of previous dominance. When cutting meat, for example, the prosthesis holds the fork while the actual cutting is done with the unamputated hand. Functional use training starts with simple tasks and builds to the more complex (**Fig. 10.12**). The tasks selected should be functional for the particular person and should be sequenced to provide opportunities for success. The higher is the level of amputation, the more complex is the training. Teaching bilateral upper extremity amputees requires specialized training in upper extremity prosthetics and rehabilitation.

Functional use training incorporates a variety of objects to be manipulated, such as moving pegs in a peg board, hammering nails in a board using the prosthesis to hold the nail, lifting a glass or cup to the

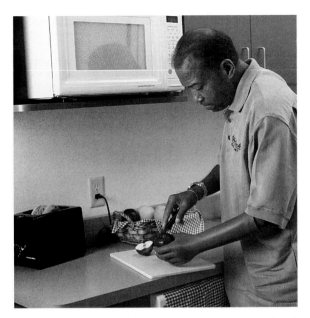

FIGURE 10.12. Using the prosthesis as an assisting hand. *(Courtesy of Motion Control, Inc.)*

KEYWORDS FOR LITERATURE SEARCH

Control training

Myoelectric prostheses

Partial hand amputation

Transhumeral amputation

Transradial amputation

Upper extremity prosthesis

Wrist disarticulation

mouth, picking up something fragile such as an egg, or picking up something heavy such as a tool. In recent years, virtual reality and the use of **haptic** devices have been used to provide a wide variety of sensory feedback through the terminal device.[15] Although relatively new, improved training benefits have been reported.

Vocational Training

Most upper extremity amputees are within working age and may or may not be able to return to their previous occupation. Consideration of vocational retraining needs to be considered early in the rehabilitation program and appropriate referral made.

SUMMARY

Physical therapists do not often treat upper limb amputees other than in the postsurgical period. Physical therapists who find themselves working regularly with this population need to take continuing education courses to become proficient in this area. As in the lower extremity, prosthetic components are constantly changing; current information can be obtained through the websites of manufacturers and from local prosthetists. A good general website is www.oandp.com.

REFERENCES

1. National Limb Loss Fact Sheet (www.amputee_coalition.org), 2008.
2. Ouellette EA: Partial hand amputation: surgical management. In Smith DG, Michael JW, Bowker JH (eds): Atlas of amputations and limb deficiencies: surgical, prosthetic, and rehabilitation principles, 3rd ed. Rosemont, IL, AAOS, 2004, pp 197–208.
3. Lanzetta M, Petruzzo P, Margreiter R, et al: The International Registry on Hand and Composite Tissue Transplantation. Transplantation 79(9):1210–1214, 2005.
4. Brenner CD: Wrist disarticulation and transradial amputation: prosthetic management. In Smith DG, Michael JW, Bowker JH (eds): Atlas of amputations and limb deficiencies: surgical, prosthetic, and rehabilitation principles, 3rd ed. Rosemont, IL, AAOS, 2004, pp 223–230.
5. Owens P, Ouellette EA: Wrist disarticulation and transradial amputation: surgical management. In Smith DG, Michael JW, Bowker JH (eds): Atlas of amputations and limb deficiencies: surgical, prosthetic, and rehabilitation principles, 3rd ed. Rosemont, IL, AAOS, 2004, pp 219–222.
6. Smith DG: Amputations about the shoulder: surgical management. In Smith DG, Michael JW, Bowker JH (eds): Atlas of amputations and limb deficiencies: surgical, prosthetic, and rehabilitation principles, 3rd ed. Rosemont, IL, AAOS, 2004, pp 251–262.
7. Atkins DJ: Prosthetic training (upper extremity). In Smith DG, Michael JW, Bowker JH (eds): Atlas of amputations and limb deficiencies: surgical, prosthetic, and rehabilitation principles, 3rd ed. Rosemont, IL, AAOS, 2004, pp 275–284.
8. Fryer CM, Stark GE Jr, Michaels JW: Body-powered components. In Smith DG, Michael JW, Bowker JH (eds): Atlas of amputations and limb deficiencies: surgical, prosthetic, and rehabilitation principles, 3rd ed. Rosemont, IL, AAOS, 2004, pp 117–130.
9. Fryer CM, Michaels JW: Harnessing and controls for body-powered devices. In Smith DG, Michael JW, Bowker JH (eds): Atlas of amputations and limb deficiencies: surgical, prosthetic, and rehabilitation principles, 3rd ed. Rosemont, IL, AAOS, 2004, pp 131–144.
10. Dietl H: New developments in upper limb prosthetics. In Smith DG, Michael JW, Bowker JH (eds): Atlas of amputations and limb deficiencies: surgical, prosthetic, and rehabilitation principles, 3rd ed. Rosemont, IL, AAOS, 2004, pp 343–351.

11. Childress DS, Weir RF: Control of limb prostheses. In Smith DG, Michael JW, Bowker JH (eds): Atlas of amputations and limb deficiencies: surgical, prosthetic, and rehabilitation principles, 3rd ed. Rosemont, IL, AAOS, 2004, 173–196.

12. Biddiss EA, Chau TT: Upper limb prosthesis use and abandonment: a survey of the last 25 years. Prosthet Orthot Int 31(3):236–257, 2007.

13. Datta D, Selvarajah K, Davey N: Functional outcome of patients with proximal upper limb deficiency-acquired and congenital. Clin Rehabil 18(2):172–177, 2004.

14. Biddiss EA, Chau TT: Multivariate prediction of upper limb prosthesis acceptance or rejection. Am J Phys Med Rehabil 86:977–987, 2007.

15. Kayyali R, Alamri A, Eid M, et al: Occupational therapist evaluation of haptic motor rehabilitation. Proceedings of the 29th Annual International Conference of the IEEE EMBS. August 2007.

Orthoses

11

Examinations for Orthotic Prescription and Checkout

OBJECTIVES

At the end of this chapter, all students are expected to:

1. Describe and discuss the relationships among impairments of body structure and function, functional activity limitations, and participation restrictions.
2. Recognize functional activity limitations and participation restrictions that may be improved with orthotic, ambulatory, or assistive devices.

Physical Therapy students are expected to:

1. Describe the components of and perform a client preorthotic prescription examination to develop functional goals, orthotic goals, and an orthotic prescription.
2. Evaluate preorthotic prescription examination findings to identify client impairments, functional activity limitations, and participation restrictions that may improve with the prescription of an orthosis.
3. Describe the role of functional assessment, biomechanical analysis of function, and gait analysis in determining an orthotic prescription for a client.
4. Select appropriate functional status or outcome instruments to measure the effectiveness of an orthotic device in improving client function.
5. Describe the process and components of an orthotic checkout examination, evaluate the findings, and develop an appropriate plan of action.

CASE STUDIES

Harry Green is a 67-year-old man who suffered a thrombotic cerebral vascular accident (stroke) with right hemiparesis. Mr. Green's case is described in Chapter 2.

Anne O'Callahan is a 55-year-old woman who has right knee pain that is interfering with her ability to stand, walk, and climb steps. Using the numerical rating scale to assess her pain, she rates her pain as 6/10 on standing 30 min or more. She is only able to do steps when absolutely necessary using a step-to pattern, while keeping her right knee extended. Anne is a second-grade teacher and needs to spend much time on her feet. She received a diagnosis of right knee tibiofemoral osteoarthritis (OA) about 10 years ago but does not have OA in any other joints. She attributes her right knee OA to multiple injuries to her right leg that she suffered in an automobile accident when she was 35 years old. Recent x-rays show medial compartment OA. She has had episodes of right knee pain in the past, which were related to overuse and were relieved by limiting activity and taking anti-inflammatory medication. This current episode of knee pain has lasted 2 months, and it is not improving. She visited an orthopedic surgeon who administered hyaluronic acid viscosupplementation injections, with no significant improvement, and suggested that she is not a candidate for osteochondral transplant procedures. It is now October, and Anne does not want to consider any surgical approaches until all else has failed or at least until the school year is completed. Anne's body mass index (BMI) is 22. Her right knee ROM is 5° to 100° and demonstrates a 25° varus deformity. She had walked regularly for exercise prior to this current episode of knee pain but has discontinued due to swelling and increased knee pain after walking distances longer than two blocks. In order to continue to manage her classroom of second graders, Anne must be able to stand continuously for at least 1 hour, climb two flights of steps twice per day at school, and walk at a speed of at least 3 mph for a distance of three blocks.

Luis Sanchez is a 12-year-old boy with cerebral palsy and mild to moderate spastic diplegia. Luis has received physical therapy intervention and supervision since he was 3 years old. During elementary school, he attended public school and participated in the regular classroom for about one-half of the day and spent the rest of the day in a special education classroom. He is now in middle school and this year is participating in regular classes, full time. This requires that he change classrooms each period. Although Luis demonstrates some gait abnormalities and asymmetries, he had been safe and functional without orthoses or ambulatory aids. However, since he has to do more walking in crowded spaces than previously, he is having difficulty with fatigue and tripping and has fallen several times. The falls are associated with excessive knee flexion during stance and insufficient swing phase knee flexion to consistently clear his feet from the ground. In order to be independent in his school building, Luis must be able to walk at a speed of 3 mph while changing classes in crowded hallways. Although there is an elevator available at one end of the school, moving around the building is easier if he can negotiate two flights of steps at least twice per day at school. He must be able to walk up to 0.25 mile to change classes (one end of the building to the other).

Case Study Activities

All Students:

1. Identify and discuss the client's impairments, functional activity limitations, participation restrictions, and the relationships among them.
2. Identify those impairments, functional problems, and participation restrictions that may improve with an orthotic device, ambulatory aid, or assisted device.

Physical Therapy Students:

1. Discuss the advantages and disadvantages for the client of using an orthotic device, ambulatory aid, or other assistive device.
2. Write functional goals for prescription of an orthotic device, if one is indicated for the client.
3. Describe the examination process and components that you would use to gather the data necessary to develop an appropriate orthotic prescription for the client.
4. Describe the functional assessments that you would include in your preorthotic prescription examination of the client.
5. Describe the methods you would use to determine if a prescribed and delivered orthosis is acceptable and effective in improving client function. Be specific.

EXAMINATION PROCEDURES FOR ORTHOTIC APPLICATIONS

Although some orthoses can be selected similarly to the way in which an assistive device or ambulatory aid is chosen ("pick it and try it"), most orthoses require careful individual design and prescription to insure maximum benefit and the best outcome. Selecting orthoses based on the client's pathology (eg, stroke, osteoarthritis, cerebral palsy) using the "one design fits all" approach may improve his or her function but often does not yield the most effective solution. Because an orthosis applies forces to a part of the wearer's body, the most effective orthosis is the one that applies forces in a way that minimizes the specific impairments that contribute to the individual's particular functional problems. Two clients may be similar in pathology and have the same functional problems, but each may have different impairments that require different orthotic solutions to achieve the best outcome. For example, imagine two individuals who both exhibit hemiplegia caused by a stroke which causes difficulty with step initiation and foot clearance during gait. One patient has excessive extensor tone, a stiff knee, and plantarflexion spasticity, while the other demonstrates flexor tone, excessive knee flexion, and a flaccid ankle. Although their pathologies and functional problems are the same, their specific impairments differ; thus the same orthosis will not be optimal for both individuals. Thus, in order to develop the most effective and practical orthotic solution for each individual, practitioners must carefully examine and evaluate each client in order to determine the following:

■ Is an orthosis likely to be helpful and improve function?
■ If the previous is true, what specific type of orthosis will be most effective and efficient?
■ Are other interventions necessary to achieve maximum function?

In order to gather the information necessary to answer these questions and develop an appropriate orthotic prescription, practitioners must perform systematic and methodical examinations to identify the client's functional abilities, activity limitations, and participation restrictions, as well the specific impairments that contribute to the client's functional problems. This is called a **preorthotic prescription examination**, and the process is diagrammed in **Figure 11.1**.

Once an appliance has been prescribed and manufactured, the prescribing practitioner must evaluate the device to determine if it has been manufactured as prescribed and if the product is acceptable for the client to wear and use. This process of examination of the orthosis and the client wearing the orthosis is termed an **orthotic checkout examination**. An

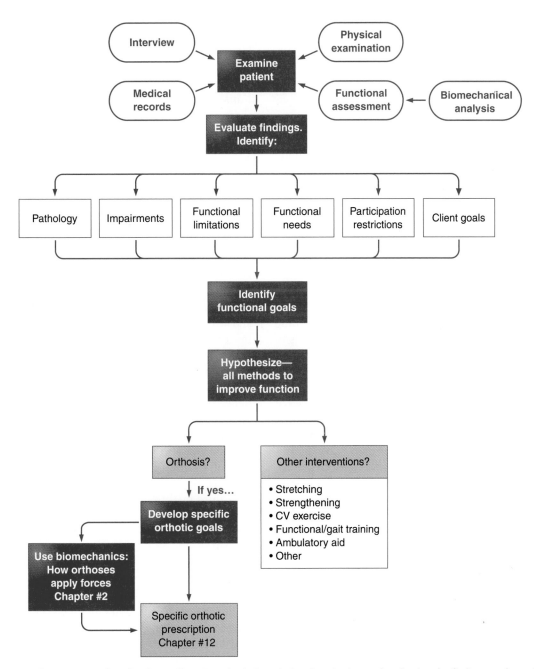

FIGURE 11.1. The processes of performing a client Preorthotic Prescription Examination and evaluating the findings to determine an orthotic prescription.

orthotic checkout should be performed on all new appliances before the client begins to use and train with the new device. A checkout examination should also be performed on an older orthosis to determine the cause of any new problem that develops or if a wearer plans to resume using an appliance that has not been worn for some time.

It is assumed that the reader of this textbook is familiar and has some experience with the general processes of client examination; therefore, this chapter adapts the general patient examination process and focuses on the specific examination methods required to

■ Perform a preorthotic prescription examination of a client to develop an orthotic prescription.
■ Determine the effectiveness of an appliance in improving function.
■ Perform a checkout examination of an orthotic appliance to evaluate its fit, function, comfort, and cosmesis.

CLIENT EXAMINATION: PREORTHOTIC PRESCRIPTION ASSESSMENTS

Assessment of Function

The primary purpose of an orthotic device is to improve function. Thus, the first step in determining the most appropriate appliance for an individual is to identify the client's functional activity limitations and participation restrictions as well as his or her functional needs and goals. Function is traditionally categorized as basic activities of daily living (eg, personal hygiene, dressing, bathing, eating), instrumental activities of daily living (eg, using the telephone, preparing meals, shopping, light and heavy housekeeping, managing money), and mobility both around the house as well as within the community beyond walking distance.

There are a variety of ways to discover information about a client's functional abilities and limitations as well as his or her functional needs and goals. These include

■ Client interview
■ Self-report functional status surveys
■ Direct observation of performance

The first approach should always be to ask the client during an *interview* what activities he or she is unable to do or has difficulty doing independently and what activities are necessary or desired. *Functional status surveys* are also used in conjunction with interview to gather this information. These surveys are usually self-report questionnaires on which clients rate their ability to perform various functional tasks. A large number of these instruments are available, and clinicians must choose carefully to gather meaningful information. Some are designed specifically for groups of people with a specific pathology or condition. For example, the WOMAC (Western Ontario McMaster Universities Osteoarthritis Index) is designed for individuals with osteoarthritis of the hip or knee.[1] Others are generic and can be used to assess functional status in individuals regardless of the cause of their limitations (eg, the Barthel Index and the Functional Independence Measure).[2,3] More functional status instruments can be located by performing a literature search using the keywords and search terms for literature searches listed at the end of this chapter.

The Orthotics and Prosthetics Users' Survey (OPUS) is an outcome measurement instrument designed specifically for users of prosthetic or orthotic devices.[4] The OPUS has four parts in which individuals who use prostheses or orthoses self-assess upper or lower extremity functional status, health-related quality of life, and their satisfaction with the device and with the service provided. On the functional status component, users rate their ability to perform selected activities from 1 (very easy) to 5 (cannot perform) and indicate if they perform the activity with or without the appliance. **Box 11.1** provides example items from selected components of the OPUS. In addition to helping practitioners identify the specific functional problems and needs of their clients, these instruments also are used to document progress or lack of progress during functional training with an orthosis.

A third method to identify functional problems is *direct observation* of the client performing selected functional activities. While observing the activity, practitioners make qualitative and quantitative assessments. Qualitatively, clinicians observe the methods used by the client to perform the activity and identify for remediation those that are ineffective, inefficient, or unsafe. Quantitatively, clinicians time how long it takes a client to complete an activity or how long the client can continue to perform the activity before fatigue or another limiting factor causes him or her to stop. Alternatively, clinicians can count

BOX 11.1 | **Sample Items From the Orthotic and Prosthetic Users' Survey (OPUS) Northwestern University, 2001[4]**

Lower Extremity Functional Measure (20 total items)

Clients self-rate the difficulty of each task from 1 (very easy) to 5 (cannot perform activity).

- Get up from the toilet
- Dress lower body
- Get up from the floor
- Stand one-half hour
- Run one block

Health-Related Quality of Life Measure (23 total items)

Clients respond to items that ask "how much..." using a scale from 1 (not at all) to 5 (extremely) and respond to items that ask "how often...," using a scale from 1 (all the time) to 5 (none of the time).

- How much do you keep to yourself to avoid reactions to the use of your orthosis/prosthesis?
- How much does your physical condition restrict your ability to do paid work?
- How much have you felt so down in the dumps...during the past week?
- How often during the last week did you feel worn out?

the number of times the client can repeat an activity in a given time period.

To assess functional mobility, there are a variety of *timed walk tests* that are valid, reliable, responsive, and recommended for use with clients using prosthetic or orthotic devices.[3] The *Timed Up and Go* (TUG) test requires the client to start in a seated position in a standard chair, arise, walk 3 meters (10 feet), turn, and return to the chair and sit down.[2] An advantage of the TUG is that it includes getting up and down from a chair and turning, which are activities that may challenge balance. Thus, the TUG may reveal functional mobility deficits that may not be apparent when observing straight, level surface walking alone. Other timed walking tests specify either a particular walking distance or a specific walking time. Commonly used formats for short distance walking are timed 10- or 20-meter walks.[5] Several versions of tests that measure the distance walked during a fixed time period are also used. The most commonly used formats are the *two-, six-, or 12-min walk tests*.[6,7,8]

Functional improvements typically correlate with the ability to perform a task in less time. Thus, when appraising function, it is important to consider not only the client's ability to perform a task, but also how much time is required to complete it. If performance of a functional activity requires too much time or energy, it may be impractical for the individual to do the activity independently. In this case, an orthosis that reduces the time or energy requirement may be indicated. For example, in the United States, most city traffic lights require an individual to walk at a speed of about 2.7 mph or faster in order to cross the street before the light changes. An individual who is able to walk without orthotic or ambulatory aids, but walks very slowly, may be more functional and safer using an orthotic device or ambulatory aid, if it increases walking speed or reduces the energy expended.

When a necessary functional activity is limited, the next step in the examination process is to perform a **biomechanical analysis** of the individual while attempting the activity. The purpose of the biomechanical analysis is to ascertain the impairments that restrict the individual's ability to perform a particular functional task. Biomechanical analysis requires the practitioner to methodically observe the client performing the functional activity, break the activity into component parts, compare the movements in each component to "normal" or effective movement, and identify the impairments that may limit the individual's function or make it inefficient. When the functional problems focus on ambulation, a gait analysis is necessary to identify specific gait impairments (Chapter 2). Examples of **impairments, functional activity limitations, participation restrictions**, and the relationships among them are presented in **Figure 11.2**, using the *International Classification of Functioning, Disability, and Health* (ICF).[9] Practitioners can use this classification system to identify, categorize, and determine associations among an individual's specific problems. Organizing the client's problems (impairments of body structure and function, functional activity limitations, and participation restrictions) in this conceptual framework helps practitioners develop clear, functionally oriented, and specific orthotic goals that are necessary to guide the orthotic prescription process. Those interested in learning more about this classification system can perform a literature search using the keywords listed at the end of this chapter. The process of developing specific orthotic goals as

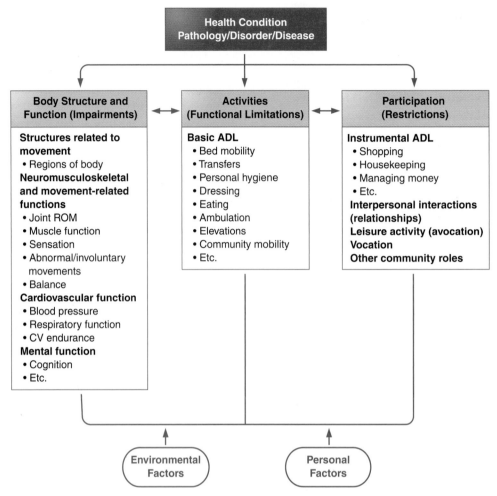

FIGURE 11.2. The International Classification of Functioning, Disability, and Health (World Health Organization, 2001) provides a useful framework to understand associations among impairments, functional activity limitation, and participation restrictions.

the basis for developing an orthotic prescription is discussed in Chapter 12.

Assessments of Impairments

To confirm that the client has the impairments suspected based upon the functional and biomechanical analyses, practitioners must perform a **pre-orthotic prescription clinical examination** of the patient. This clinical examination is performed prior to developing an orthotic prescription and includes the following:

■ Physical assessment of the specific region of the body that may require an orthosis
■ General assessment of the client's ability to function, use, and manage a device safely, effectively, and efficiently

The physical assessment includes relevant aspects of musculoskeletal, neurological, integumentary, and cardiovascular/pulmonary examinations. The general assessment provides an overview appraisal of psychological and cognitive factors that affect orthotic usage. **Box 11.2** outlines relevant components of the pre-orthotic prescription examination.

Musculoskeletal Examination

The musculoskeletal examination includes assessment of the involved limb or limbs for which fitting with an orthosis is under consideration as well as of the noninvolved limbs and trunk. If lower extremity impairments affect ambulation, ambulatory aids may be required that place significant demands on the upper extremities. Examination of the upper extremities, trunk, and the better-functioning lower

BOX 11.2 | Preorthotic Prescription Clinical Examination

Musculoskeletal Examination
- Joint mobility (passive range of motion)
- Joint stability (ligaments, capsule, articular surfaces)
- Deformities or alignment abnormalities
- Limb length
- Motor function
  - Selective muscle control
  - Muscle strength and endurance
  - Coordination

Neurological Examination
- Sensation (touch, pain, proprioception, kinesthesia)
- Reflexes
- Muscle tonicity, involuntary spasms
- Vision
- Balance

Integumentary Examination
- Wounds, scars
- Skin integrity and quality

Cardiovascular/Pulmonary Examination
- Limb edema
- Clinical signs of peripheral vascular disease
- Cardiovascular/pulmonary endurance, ability to tolerate energy demands of activity
- Aerobic capacity, fitness
- Heart rate, blood pressure, respiratory rate response to performing functional activities

Psychological and Cognitive Screening
- Ability to understand and carry out directions
- Ability and willingness to adhere to procedures necessary for safe orthotic use
- Motivation to achieve functional goals

---

limb allows the clinician to select the most appropriate ambulatory aid and may also help to determine the specific type of orthosis that will be most effective for the client. Examination of hand strength and dexterity is also important, regardless of where the orthosis will be worn. Hand strength and dexterity are required to independently **don** (put on) and **doff** (take off) an appliance. When hand function is impaired, accommodations must be made in the orthotic design to facilitate donning and doffing.

Poor muscle control, limited joint motion, and joint instability are common reasons why an individual may need an orthosis. However, alignment abnormalities and deformities are also important considerations. Deformities that are fixed or structural should be accommodated or supported by an orthosis; orthotic correction of these deformities is not possible and may actually cause additional injury. If a deformity is flexible or nonfixed, an orthosis designed to apply corrective forces may be used effectively. For example, a fixed or bony deformity of the foot producing an inversion-type (varus) deformity must be accommodated, balanced, or supported. Attempts to apply orthotic forces to correct it will increase pressure where the forces are applied, producing pain and possibly skin breakdown. If the same deformity is flexible, corrective orthotic forces may be effective with an appropriately designed and fitted appliance.

Neurological Examination

A neurological examination is also included in the preorthotic prescription assessment, even for clients who do not have a primary neurological disorder. Components of a neurological exam that have implications for orthotic prescription include sensation, reflexes, muscle tonicity, vision, and balance. Sensation may be impaired in a variety of conditions, including both central and peripheral nervous system disorders. When pain sensation is impaired, individuals are more susceptible to skin breakdown or ulceration. When an orthosis is worn over an area of impaired sensation, the client must be instructed to carefully check the skin and orthotic fit daily. An orthosis prescribed for a client with poor pain sensation must include design modifications that minimize the risk of high pressure over bony prominences and at the orthosis–limb interfaces.

Impaired proprioception or kinesthesia (sense of position or movement sense, respectively) may also affect orthotic prescription. Individuals with impaired position or movement sense may require bracing even if the motor function present does not require bracing. For example, an individual who is able to actively dorsiflex and evert his or her ankle but lacks ankle proprioception may not consistently initiate stance phase with a heel strike and may overturn (excessively invert) the ankle during stance. This individual may require an ankle–foot orthosis for safety, even though the muscular ability to control the ankle is unimpaired.

Muscle hypertonicity, hyperactive reflexes, or involuntary muscle spasms, which are present in some patients with upper motor neuron disorders, pose additional problems for orthotic prescription. Muscle hypertonicity may fluctuate and is influenced by environmental circumstances. Thus, the need for an orthosis or the type of orthosis required may vary depending on the severity of the spasms or hypertonicity under various conditions at different times. For example, stressful activities or those that require faster movements may increase abnormal muscle contractions that interfere with function or safety. When hypertonicity is mild, no or minimal orthotic control may be required. However, at other times, when the hyperactive muscle contractions are more severe, a more rigid or restrictive orthosis may be needed. In these cases, the practitioner recommending the orthosis must observe the client under many different circumstances on numerous occasions to insure that the appliance prescribed strikes the best balance between restricting unwanted movements and enabling safe functional mobility.

The ability of the client to maintain balance also affects the orthotic prescription. Balance is the ability of an individual to maintain equilibrium and is influenced by somatosensory, vestibular, and visual function. Impairments in any of these systems may result in balance loss and falls. An orthosis to improve stability may be prescribed to enhance safety during functional activities. During the preorthotic clinical examination, therapists must assess balance under a variety of static and dynamic conditions that simulate the functional demands of the patient. Movement and distractions such as turning and carrying things may reduce an individual's ability to maintain balance and must be included when assessing balance to determine the need for appliances.

Integumentary Examination

The skin where an orthosis will be applied must be examined prior to developing an orthotic prescription. Except for orthoses that have direct skeletal attachments, the skin provides the interface between the wearer's body and the orthosis. Because orthoses are designed to apply forces, the ability of the skin and subjacent tissues to tolerate mechanical loading is an important consideration. Molded total contact orthoses have large surface areas of contact with the skin. Because they apply their forces over a larger area, the pressure is lower (force application per unit surface area) as compared to those that apply the same amount of force but with less surface area of contact (see Chapter 2 to review pressure). Thus, total contact orthoses are often prescribed to minimize surface contact pressure. Other methods to minimize orthotic pressure on the skin include the use of orthotic relief areas that shift loads away from pressure-sensitive areas to those that are more pressure tolerant and the use of compliant or resilient materials to provide cushioning.

When examining clients' skin, it is important to observe any wounds, healed wounds, or scars, as these are less tolerant of force application and may require special accommodation in the orthosis. The skin of the elderly and those with inflammatory arthritis, such as rheumatoid arthritis, is typically atrophic (thin) and less tolerant of pressure and may require special orthotic accommodations to reduce pressure and shear forces.

The nature of the subcutaneous tissue also affects the ability of the skin to tolerate orthotic loading. Skin that lies directly over bony prominences, such as the malleoli, is more pressure sensitive and susceptible to skin breakdown and requires orthotic accommodation. Skin that has subjacent muscle and connective tissue is more pressure tolerant, better able to dissipate orthotic force applications, and less susceptible to breakdown. Orthoses should be designed to apply their forces to pressure-tolerant areas.

Cardiovascular and Pulmonary Examination

Cardiovascular and pulmonary assessments that are included in the preorthotic prescription examination evaluate limb edema, clinical signs of peripheral vascular disease, and cardiovascular and pulmonary endurance. Some of the effects of peripheral vascular disease (PVD) have significant implications for orthotic design. For example, impaired cardiac function and peripheral circulation may produce edema in the limbs. Edema, particularly fluctuating or unstable edema, poses significant problems for orthotic fit. When fluctuating edema is present, the limb may change dimension from day to day, or even within one day, causing an orthosis to be "too big" at one time and "too small" at another. The fluctuating dimension of a limb may lead to abnormal limb movement within the orthosis and skin breakdown. Other conditions, such as kidney disease, that also produce extremity edema also require caution when prescribing an orthosis. Total-contact molded orthoses may be inappropriate for clients with fluctuating edema in the braced limb. PVD also affects the quality of the skin, making it more susceptible to breakdown in response to mechanical irritations. Additionally, if a wound occurs due to orthotic irritation of the skin, it may heal more slowly when PVD is present. Orthotic prescriptions for clients with these diagnoses should include accommodations to prevent inadvertent detrimental skin complications from orthotic use.

Assessment of clients' cardiovascular and pulmonary endurance or ability to respond to exercise and activity also provides valuable information needed to develop an appropriate orthotic prescription. Impairments that alter the usual walking pattern increase the amount of energy expended during walking.[10] Typically, impaired individuals accommodate for the increased energy expenditure by walking more slowly.[11] Walking with some orthoses, although functionally beneficial, may actually increase the energy expenditure of mobility, as in some patients with spinal cord injury.[12] However, others (eg, individuals with hemiplegia) use less energy to walk when using an orthosis than when without one.[13] Regardless of the specific impairment present, it is important to understand an individual's ability to respond physiologically to the increased energy demands of functional activities and walking caused by the combination of pathology, impairment, and having to use abnormal movement patterns during function.

Using the Client Examination Findings

The findings gathered from the functional assessments and preorthotic prescription clinical examinations are used to answer the three questions originally posed in the beginning of this chapter:

- Is an orthosis likely to improve function? If yes,
  - Which functions can be improved by the orthosis?
  - How much do you expect each function to improve?
  - Will there be any negative effects of orthotic use?
  - Will the benefits of orthotic use outweigh any negative effects?
- Which specific orthosis will be most effective and efficient?
  - Which impairments should be addressed in the orthotic prescription?
  - How should the orthosis apply forces to accomplish the desired effect?

- Are other interventions needed, either with the orthosis or instead of an orthosis, to help the client achieve maximum function?
  - Which interventions might be useful to maximize function? For example,
    - Therapeutic exercise—stretching, strengthening, exercise to improve cardiovascular endurance, and so forth
    - Ambulatory aids and gait training
    - Assisted devices and functional training

If, after evaluating the examination findings, it is decided that an orthosis is indicated, the next step, as in selecting any type of intervention, is to develop specific functional goals followed by the development of specific goals for the orthosis. **Figure 11.3** demonstrates the application of this problem-solving process (presented in Fig. 11.1) for Anne O'Callahan, one of the case study patients presented at the beginning of this chapter. The process of developing a specific orthotic goal and the prescription to accomplish the goal is discussed in Chapter 12.

EXAMINATION OF THE ORTHOSIS AND CLIENT: THE CHECKOUT

The purpose of an orthotic checkout is to examine the appliance prescribed and delivered to a client to determine if it is acceptable for wear in terms of fit, function, comfort, and cosmesis. If problems are identified, the professional performing the checkout evaluation must communicate and work with the orthotist who made the appliance and the patient to achieve a successful resolution to the problems. The checkout procedure is complete when the client can begin to wear and use the device to work toward achieving the functional goals identified at the beginning of the prescription process. An orthotic checkout is performed on all new appliances before the client begins to use and train with the new device. A checkout is also performed on an older appliance to determine the cause of new problems reported by the wearer or if a wearer plans to resume using an appliance that has not been worn for some time.

An overview of the components and process of an orthotic checkout examination is provided in **Box 11.3.** Checkout items relevant to specific types of orthoses are discussed in subsequent chapters on orthotic applications for specific regions of the body. However, regardless of the specific type of orthosis, an

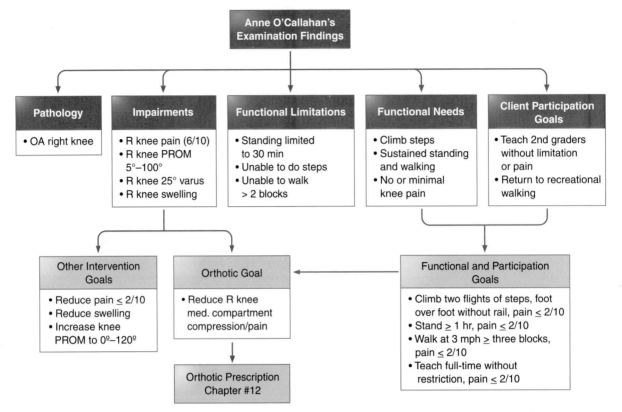

FIGURE 11.3. The Preorthotic Prescription Examination process for Anne O'Callahan, a client case presented at the beginning of this chapter. The general examination process is outlined in Figure 11.1.

orthotic checkout examination and evaluation includes five parts:

- Examination of the orthosis (off the client)
- Cursory reexamination of the client's physical status
- Examination of the orthosis on the client—static
- Examination of the orthosis on the client—dynamic
- Examination of the skin after sustained orthotic wear

First, the appliance is examined separately from its wearer to insure that it has been made as prescribed and with good workmanship. Second, if the examiner has not seen the client since measurements for the orthosis were taken, a cursory client reexamination is performed to insure that there have been no changes in the client's anatomy or impairments that might affect the fit or function of the appliance. It is particularly important to verify that the client's body weight and the girth of the body part on which the orthosis will be worn have not changed significantly. Joint range of motion is reassessed to insure that no contractures have developed since fitting.

In the third component of an orthotic checkout, the practitioner assesses the fit and function of the device on the wearer under static conditions. First, the practitioner applies the appliance to the client and checks the fit and comfort under static conditions, such as sitting, standing, and any other static position in which the client will wear the orthosis. Once the practitioner verifies that the appliance can be applied properly and fits well, the client is taught to don the orthosis. Static fit and comfort are rechecked after the client has applied the orthosis. Rechecking fit and function insures that the client is able to properly apply the orthosis either independently or, if needed, with the help of someone who will be available to provide assistance at home. The skin is checked for signs of excessive pressure or potential irritation. The client is also instructed in how to remove the orthosis properly and examine the skin for signs of excessive pressure.

The fourth component of the checkout is the dynamic assessment. This is the phase in which the client begins to use the orthosis functionally. If the

BOX 11.3 | Components and Process of an Orthotic Checkout Examination

1. *Examination of the orthosis (off client)*
   - Does it meet the specifications of the prescription?
   - Is workmanship acceptable?
   - If it is a lower extremity appliance, is the shoe appropriate for the orthosis?
2. *Cursory reexamination of the client*
   - Has the client changed since the orthosis was prescribed or measured?
     - Body weight?
     - Limb girth (circumference, volume)?
     - Joint range of motion?
3. *Examination of the orthosis on the client—static conditions*
   - Put the orthosis on the client and examine fit. If it is a lower extremity device, examine fit while the client is sitting and standing. For all wearers, assess fit in all positions in which the orthosis is worn or used.
     - Is it comfortable?
     - If there are articulating orthotic joints, are they aligned appropriately with the anatomical joints?
     - Are there areas of excessive pressure?
     - In standing, is alignment appropriate in the sagittal, frontal, and transverse planes?
     - Is the client stable in standing? Is static balance acceptable?
   - Teach the client to don and doff the appliance. Recheck fit and comfort after client self-application of the appliance.
4. *Examination of the orthosis on the client—dynamic conditions*
   - Is the orthosis stable during use and movement? Does the orthosis move or migrate on the body?
   - Does the orthosis function as prescribed?
   - Does the orthosis achieve its goals?
   - Is there any excessive pressure or skin irritation during or after movement?
   - Does the client demonstrate gait or functional usage abnormalities that require training?
   - Is there anything that requires appliance revision by the orthotist?
   - Is the client satisfied with the orthosis?
5. *After wearing the appliance for at least 30 min, remove and recheck skin*
   - Are there signs of skin irritation, excessive pressure, or poor fit?
   - Prescribe a schedule to progressively increase wearing time.

client has never used an orthosis before, the clinician may also need to provide some training in the use of the device. It is important that the appliance is stable on the client during functional usage and that it functions as desired and achieves the orthotic goals for which it was prescribed. Fit is reassessed after usage, as the appliance may migrate during usage causing excessive skin pressure or irritation. Most often, even when the orthosis fits and functions well, clients require additional training to use the device effectively and efficiently and to achieve maximum benefit.

In the fifth and final step in the checkout process, the client must wear the device for at least 30 continuous minutes in the clinic before leaving with the orthosis. The fit and function of the appliance and the skin are rechecked after sustained wearing time to insure that all possible problems are identified and resolved prior to sending the client home to begin orthotic use. New wearers are provided with a progressive schedule to gradually increase wearing time. By gradually increasing the orthotic wearing time each day, minor issues with skin or joint irritation can be avoided, and adjustment to orthotic usage is

smoother. Clients must also be taught to perform daily checks of the orthosis and their skin to insure that the device continues to function properly and to identify and report any problems that might develop early when solutions are relatively easy.

SUMMARY

There are two types of orthotic examinations. The first is a preorthotic prescription examination of the client to determine if an orthosis is needed to improve function. If yes, the examination findings are used to develop a specific orthotic prescription. This client examination must include a functional assessment, biomechanical analysis of the functional tasks that are difficult, as well as a clinical examination to identify the client's specific impairments. Based on these examination findings, specific functional and orthotic goals are established and are the basis for the specific orthotic prescription.

The second type of orthotic examination is a checkout examination of the appliance and the wearer. Once the orthosis is prescribed, manufactured, and delivered, the practitioner must perform an orthotic checkout examination of the appliance alone and on its user to insure proper orthotic fit, function, comfort, and cosmesis. Clients should not wear or use their orthoses until proper fit and function have been verified through the checkout procedures.

KEYWORDS FOR LITERATURE SEARCH

Functional Status Surveys

Database searches: Combine these terms with a term for a condition of interest (eg, osteoarthritis, cerebral palsy) using the Boolean term "AND".

Functional status

Health status

Measurement development

Outcome assessment (health care)

Psychometric properties

Physical disability

Quality of life

KEYWORDS, SEARCH TERMS, AND LINKS

International Classification of Functioning, Disability, and Health (World Health Organization, 2001)

Disabled persons/classification

International Classification of Function

World Confederation for Physical Therapy (www.wcpt.org; select Global Health/ICF)

World Health Organization/Family of International Classifications/International Classification of Functioning, Disability, and Health (ICF) (www.who/int/classifications/icf/en)

REFERENCES

1. Bellamy N, Buchanan WW, Goldsmith CH, Campbell J, Stitt LW: Validation study of WOMAC: a health status instrument for measuring clinically important patient relevant outcomes to antirheumatic drug therapy in patients with osteoarthritis of the hip or knee. J Rheumatol 15:1835–1840, 1988.
2. Finch E, Brooks D, Stratford P, et al.: Physical rehabilitation outcome measures. Baltimore, Lippincott Williams & Wilkins, 2002.
3. Condie E, Scott H, Treweek S: Lower limb prosthetic outcome measures: a review of the literature, 1995 to 2005. JPO 18(1S):13–31, 2006.
4. Heinemann AW, Bode RK, O'Reilly C: Development and measurement properties of the orthotics and prosthetics users' survey: a comprehensive set of clinical outcome instruments. Prosthet Orthot Int 27:191–206, 2003.
5. Leerar PJ: Concurrent validity of distance-walks and timed-walks in the well-elderly. J Geriatric Phys Ther 25:3–7, 2002.
6. Butland RJ, Pang J, Gross ER, Woodcock AA, Geddes DM: Two-, six-, and 12-minute walking tests in respiratory disease. BMJ 284:1607–1608, 1982.
7. Enright PL, McBurnie MA, Bittner V, et al.: The 6-min walk test: a quick measure of functional status in elderly adults. Chest 123:387–398, 2003.
8. Solway S, Brooks D, Lacasse Y, Thomas S: A qualitative systematic overview of the measurement properties of functional walk tests used in cardiorespiratory domain. Chest 119: 256–270, 2001.
9. Jette AM: Toward a common language of function, disability, and health. Phys Ther 86:726–734, 2006.
10. Waters RL, Mulroy S: The energy expenditure of normal and pathological gait. Gait Posture 9:207–231, 1999.
11. Zamparo P, Francescato MP, De Luca G, Lovati L, di Prampero PE: The energy cost of level walking in patients with hemiplegia. Scand J Med Sci Sports 5:348–352, 1995.
12. Brissot R, Gallien P, Le Bot MP, et al: Clinical experience with functional electrical stimulation-assisted gait with Parastep in spinal cord-injured patients. Spine 25:501–508, 2000.
13. Danielsson A, Sunnerhagen KS: Energy expenditure in stroke subjects walking with a carbon composite ankle foot orthosis. J Rehabil Med 36:165–168, 2004.

12

Designing and Prescribing Orthoses

OBJECTIVES

At the end of this chapter, all students are expected to:

1. Use biomechanical orthotic terminology appropriately.
2. Discuss the materials and processes used by orthotists to fabricate orthoses.
3. Describe the process by which an orthoses is obtained for a client.

Physical Therapy students are expected to:

1. Develop orthotic goals to address a client's impairments and functional limitations identified during preorthotic prescription examinations.
2. Design an orthosis using biomechanical principles of orthotic force application (as discussed in Chapter 2) to achieve the orthotic goals.
3. Collaborate with physician, orthotist, other health-care providers, and the client to prescribe an orthosis to achieve the orthotic goals and improve client function.

CASE STUDIES

Harry Green is a 67-year-old African American retired widower who suffered a thrombotic cerebral vascular accident (stroke) with right hemiparesis. Mr. Green's case is described in Chapter 2.

Anne O'Callahan is a 55-year-old second grade teacher who has right knee pain and osteoarthritis that is interfering with her ability to stand, walk, and climb steps. Ms. O'Callahan's case is described in Chapter 11.

Luis Sanchez is an 11-year-old middle school student with cerebral palsy and spastic diplegia. Luis's case is described in Chapter 11.

Case Study Activities

All Students:

1. Identify the impairments and functional problems that may be improved with an orthosis, ambulatory aid, or assisted device. Suggest ambulatory aids or assistive devices that may improve the client's function.
2. Identify and discuss various patient factors that will influence orthotic prescription in addition to the specific need or purpose for the orthosis (eg, body size and weight, activity level).
3. Discuss ways that you can improve client acceptance of the appliance and adherence to using the orthosis during functional activities.

Physical Therapy Students:

1. List and describe functional goals for each client. Which functional goals will require that the patient be fit with an orthosis in order to achieve the goal? Provide justification for your decisions.
2. Describe and discuss the type of orthosis that you would recommend. Write specific goals for the orthosis. Relate each orthotic goal to the patient's impairments.
3. Describe the biomechanical methods of orthotic force application that you would select to achieve the orthotic goals that you identified for the client. That is, do you want to use methods to
   a. Limit or prevent unwanted or abnormal movement?
   b. Assist insufficient movement?
4. Use biomechanical terminology to name the orthosis that you recommend for the client.
5. Discuss the types of orthoses and the different materials that could be used to fabricate the orthosis prescribed for the client. Discuss advantages and disadvantages of the different types of orthoses that could be used to accomplish the orthotic goals.

DEVELOPING AN ORTHOTIC PRESCRIPTION

Orthoses should improve the quality of daily life by improving or maintaining an individual's ability to perform functional activities. An orthosis has a favorable effect on a client's ability to function when it makes tasks possible to perform that are not possible without it or when it makes functional activities less difficult, more consistent, safer, or more efficient (requiring less energy). To insure that the best and most effective orthosis is prescribed, practitioners must employ a stepwise process of clinical decision making that leads to an orthosis that is specifically designed for each client. The framework of this

process, outlined in **Figure** 12.1, includes the following sequence of clinical decisions:

1. Evaluate the preorthotic examination findings to identify the client's impairments, functional activity limitations, and participation restrictions (Chapter 11).
2. Develop functional goals for the client that can be achieved by using an appropriate orthosis.
3. Develop specific goals for the orthosis (based on the client's impairments) to guide the prescription of the orthosis.
4. Design an orthosis that applies the forces necessary to achieve the orthotic goals.
5. Prescribe an orthosis that enables the client to achieve the desired functional outcome.

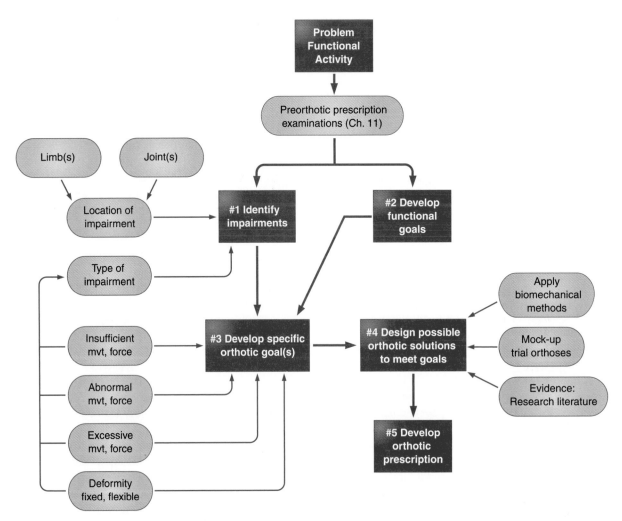

FIGURE 12.1. Overview of the process used by clinicians to develop an orthotic prescription (ovals, sources of information; rectangles, clinical decisions to develop orthotic prescription; mvt, movement).

Evaluate Preorthotic Prescription Examination Findings

Before specific orthotic goals are established, the clinician must evaluate the preorthotic prescription examination findings to identify the impairments that the orthosis must address to produce the desired improvement in function. This examination process is discussed in Chapter 11. Through observation and biomechanical analysis of the client's problem functional activities, practitioners must identify the specific location and nature of the impairments that cause the functional problems. Limitations of functional activities may be caused by impairments, such as

- Insufficient limb or joint movements
- Abnormal (and deleterious) limb or joint movements
- Excessive limb or joint movements
- Limb or joint deformity (fixed or flexible)

Qualifying the specific location and nature of the client's impairments allows clinicians to develop specific intervention and orthotic goals that correspond directly to the impairments identified (see Fig. 12.1).

Develop Goals for the Orthosis

Like all interventions (treatments), an orthosis requires clear, specific goals. Goals also provide the benchmarks by which the success of the appliance is judged. A successful and effective orthosis accomplishes its goal(s) during functional activities, while producing minimal negative side effects. Thus, it is important to develop functional goals as well as specific goals for the orthosis prior to developing the orthotic prescription for the client. Orthotic goals are grouped into four general categories:

- To *assist* joint movement when *joint movement is insufficient*
- To *stabilize* a joint by stopping or limiting motion when *joint movement is excessive, abnormal, or unwanted*
- To *protect* a joint or skeletal component from *excessive, unwanted, or deleterious loading or forces* that may cause pain or injury
- To assist in the management of *joint or skeletal deformities*
  - To *prevent* the development of deformity
  - To *accommodate,* balance, or support existing fixed deformities
  - To *correct* existing flexible deformities that interfere with function

An example using this systematic process to develop orthotic goals from functional observations and biomechanical analyses is demonstrated in **Figure 12.2** for a client who reports multiple falls. Gait analysis of the client walking reveals the following impairments:

- Insufficient ankle dorsiflexion during swing
- Insufficient plantarflexion during terminal stance (push off)
- Excessive hip adduction, knee flexion, and foot pronation during stance

A specific goal is developed for each impairment that contributes to the functional problem, and interventions are selected to address each goal. Note that a combination of interventions including an orthosis, an ambulatory/assistive device, as well as other interventions, such as exercise and training, are used together to produce the most effective and practical functional result. Attempting to design an orthosis that addresses all the client's impairments would be cumbersome, inefficient, and, most likely, impractical.

Design a Biomechanical Orthosis

After specific goals have been established for the orthosis, practitioners must design an orthosis that applies forces to the client to achieve the goals. The various ways in which appliances apply forces are described in Chapter 2 on biomechanics. A summary of these methods of orthotic force application is presented in **Box 12.1**. However, readers are encouraged to review the section in Chapter 2 called: "Biomechanical Principles: Applications in Prosthetic and Orthotic Design and Function." To design effective and practical orthoses, practitioners must have a sound working knowledge and understanding of these biomechanical principles and how they interact with clients and their impairments and pathologies.

A variety of biomechanical methods can be employed in an orthosis to produce or control forces. Thus, deciding which device to select or how to design an orthosis for a particular client can be confusing and difficult. Clearly stated orthotic goals can be used by clinicians to guide the selection or prescription of appropriate appliances. For example, the orthotic goals listed previously in this chapter fall into two broad categories:

- Goals to stabilize or protect joints by stopping or limiting unwanted movement
- Goals to facilitate or assist insufficient joint movements

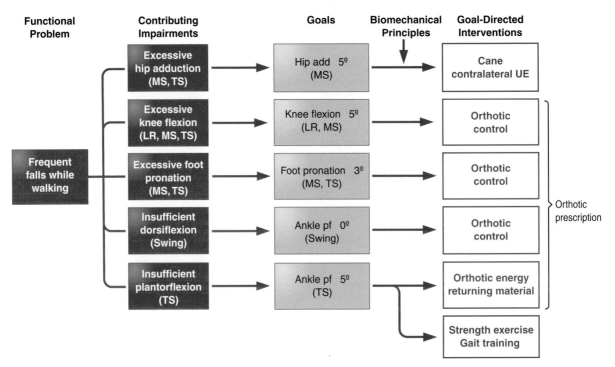

FIGURE 12.2.   An example of the systematic process to develop orthotic goals and goal-directed interventions to improve function. (MS, midstance; TS, terminal stance; LR, loading response; pf = plantarflexion; UE = upper extremity)

| BOX 12.1 | Biomechanical Principles for Orthotic Design and Function |

Methods of Force Application to *Produce Movement* (substitute for or assist insufficient joint movement)

- Select orthotic materials, components, or designs that store and release energy.
- Design the orthosis to manipulate the ground reaction force vector (GRFV) or line of gravity (LoG) to produce movement.
- Use functional electrical stimulation to substitute for weak or paralyzed muscles.
- Use an external power source.

Methods of Force Application to *Limit, Control, or Stop Movement* (restrict or stop abnormal or excessive joint movement)

- Use three- or four-point counterforce systems or force couples.
- Select orthotic materials, components, and designs that enhance rigidity across joints or dampen or slow movement.
- Design the orthosis to manipulate the GRFV or LoG to stop or restrain unwanted movement.

If the orthotic goal for a client is to stabilize or protect a joint, choose a biomechanical method that limits or controls motion. However, if the goal is to assist or substitute for insufficient movement, choose from the methods that produce or facilitate motion (see Box 12.1). If more than one equally effective biomechanical method is available to achieve the goal, clinicians must consider additional factors to choose the best solution for a particular client. Some of these factors are summarized in **Box 12.2**. The use of these factors to guide selection of the best biomechanical method to achieve an orthotic goal is illustrated for the client complaining of frequent falls described in Figure 12.2. One of the impairments contributing to this individual's falls is excessive knee flexion during the stance phase of gait. Thus, a goal is to design an orthosis that will prevent this unwanted, excessive motion during stance (**Fig. 12.3A**). Two different biomechanical methods can be used to achieve this goal:

- A three-point counterforce system to limit or prevent knee flexion (**Fig. 12.3B**)
- Manipulation of the ground reaction force vector (GRFV) to produce an extension moment at the knee (**Fig. 12.3C**)

BOX 12.2 | **Factors to Consider When Choosing Biomechanical Methods to Accomplish Orthotic Goals**

When more than one biomechanical design will accomplish a goal, consider the following factors to choose the best method for a specific client:

■ Choose the method that provides the least control that is effective, as determined by client physical factors, such as

    ■ The number of joints in a limb that require orthotic control

    ■ Muscle strength and available range of motion at the involved and adjacent joints

    ■ The presence of abnormal muscle tone or involuntary muscle contractions

    ■ The size and weight of the client

■ Choose a method that interferes the least with normal movement patterns at the involved and adjacent joints during functional activities.

■ Choose a method that minimizes the energy cost of performing functional activities with the orthosis.

■ Choose a method that applies forces as close to or at the joint(s) at which the impairments causing the problem are located.

■ Look for negative side effects of the orthosis at one joint on other joints or regions of the body. Choose the method that minimizes these negative side effects on other joints or body regions.

■ Look for negative effects of an orthosis designed to improve one functional activity on other activities. Choose the design that maximizes all functions and minimizes negative effects on any function.

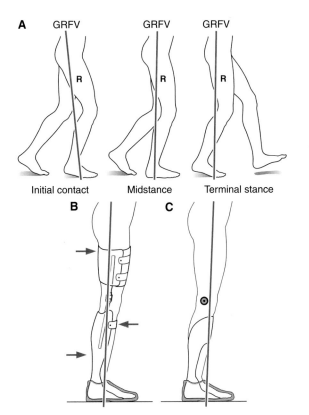

FIGURE 12.3. (A) A client demonstrates excessive knee flexion during stance phase. Two methods to limit excessive knee flexion with an orthosis include **(B)** a three-point counterforce system or **(C)** manipulation of the ground reaction force vector so it passes anterior to the knee joint axis.

Although both methods effectively prevent excessive knee flexion, practitioners must also consider potential negative effects of orthoses and their impact on overall function. In this case, the orthosis with the three-point counterforce system and lock extends above the knee and eliminates knee flexion during swing as well as stance phase (Fig. 12.3B). This requires the client to alter how he or she advances the limb and clears the foot during swing phase by using "hip hiking" or contralateral trunk lean and ipsilateral circumduction. Both of these methods require alteration of normal movement patterns during gait, decreased efficiency, and increased energy expenditure.[1,2,3] The alternative orthosis manipulates the GRFV to produce an extension moment at the knee without locking it in an extended position (Fig. 12.3C). This solution provides the necessary stance phase knee extension moment but allows the client to flex his or her knee during swing. The latter orthosis permits a more normal gait pattern that is more efficient. In this case, although both biomechanical methods effectively accomplish the desired orthotic goal, the ground reaction orthosis promotes a more normal and efficient movement pattern and is thus preferred.

Because most orthoses are designed to achieve more than one goal, this process is repeated to determine the most appropriate biomechanical solution for each goal. Clinicians must insure that the various biomechanical methods used to achieve each of an orthotic device's goals are complementary and do not result in the prescription of an impractical or cumbersome appliance. One way to do this is to use temporary or trial appliances that are commercially available and can be adjusted to apply the desired forces. Another way is to fabricate a "mock-up" device that applies the desired biomechanical control but uses less expensive splinting or casting materials, elastic bandage, or tape (**Fig. 12.4**). Although these devices may not be safe for use outside of the clinical setting, they allow clinicians to observe and evaluate if the proposed orthotic solution for a functional problem is effective and practical. If the trial, temporary, or mock-up device shows that function is improved with a particular orthotic design, a definitive appliance using this design can be developed with confidence.

Develop the Orthotic Prescription

Developing the prescription for a definitive (permanent or long-lasting and durable) orthosis requires a thorough knowledge and understanding of the various types of orthoses, materials, methods, and components available for manufacturing an appliance. The most effective orthosis for an individual may be a very simple device or it may be quite complex. Therapists

involved in securing orthoses for clients must be knowledgeable about the range of devices, materials, and components available and guide the client to or through the appropriate process. The most effective appliance may be a simple, prefabricated, "over-the counter" device that is purchased from a medical supplier, or it may be a custom-fit and individually manufactured device fabricated by an orthotist. Orthotists are certified and in some states are also licensed professionals who are trained in the fabrication and fitting of orthotic devices and are knowledgeable and skilled with conventional as well as the newest orthotic materials, components, and technologies (**Box 12.3**). Licensed orthotists are required to secure an order to fabricate custom devices from an authorized healthcare provider.[4] However, the recommendation derived from the collaboration of the *orthotic rehabilitation*

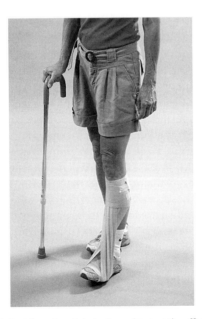

FIGURE 12.4. A "mock-up" device is used to test the effectiveness of an orthotic application prior to prescribing a definitive orthosis. The elastic bandage provides a dorsiflexion assist force to evaluate the effect of a possible orthosis on gait.

BOX 12.3	To Learn More About Orthotists and the Orthotic Profession

- **American Academy of Orthotists and Prosthetists**
  1331 H Street, NW, Suite 501
  Washington, DC 20005
  Phone: 202-380-3663
  www.oandp.org
- **American Board for Certification in Orthotics, Prosthetics, and Pedorthics**
  333 John Carlyle Street, Suite 210
  Alexandria, VA 22314
  Phone: 703-836-7114
  www.abcop.org
- **National Association for the Advancement of Orthotics and Prosthetics**
  1501 M Street, NW, 7th Floor
  Washington, DC 20005
  Phone: 202-624-0064
  www.naaop.org
- **National Commission on Orthotic and Prosthetic Education**
  330 John Carlyle Street, Suite 200
  Alexandria, VA 22314
  Phone: 703-836-7114
  www.ncope.org
- **Association of Children's Prosthetic and Orthotic Clinics**
  6300 N River Road, Suite 727
  Rosemont, IL 60018
  Phone: 847-698-1637
  www.acpoc.org

team members, which includes the client along with his or her physician, physical or occupational therapists, and orthotist, usually leads to the best prescription, particularly with complex, changing, or progressive conditions. Other professionals such as a social worker or psychologist may also contribute valuable insights to assist in developing the most effective and practical appliance to meet the client's needs and produce the best outcome. In addition to the client's functional and biomechanical needs, other factors must be considered when developing the orthotic prescription, including the client's preferences and financial resources.[5,6] Information included in the orthotic prescription is outlined in **Box 12.4.**

Orthotic Classifications

To participate in the prescription process, practitioners must understand the classifications and terminology used to describe orthotic devices. Some terms with specific orthotic definitions are listed in **Box 12.5.** As this terminology implies, there is a wide range of orthotic appliances, and to make it more complicated, many terms are defined differently by different people. In this text, an **orthosis** is defined as an externally applied device that applies forces to the body to achieve therapeutic goals, including correction, support, or compensation for impairments related to neuromusculoskeletal disorders or acquired conditions. Orthotic devices are classified and described using three methods:

- By method of manufacture
- By biomechanical terminology
- By the types of materials or components used in the device

Orthotic devices are broadly classified according to the method by which they are manufactured as custom-made or prefabricated orthoses. **Custom-made orthoses** are manufactured and fit by an orthotist for a specific individual. The process involves taking individual measurements or making a model from a cast or computer scan of the client.

BOX 12.4 | Information Included in an Orthotic Prescription

Client's name and identifying information
Date of prescription
Pathology diagnoses
Impairments that affect function
Functional goal(s) for the orthosis
Specific orthotic goals (specific location and type):
- To assist insufficient motion (_____)
  - For example: to assist right ankle dorsiflexion during swing phase
- To limit or stop excessive, deleterious motion (_____)
  - For example: to prevent excessive right knee flexion (buckling) during stance phase
- To protect or stabilize (_____)
- To prevent, balance, correct deformity (_____)
  - For example: to balance/support right fixed forefoot varus of 8°
Name of orthosis, using biomechanical terminology:
- Location—limb(s), joint(s)
- Type of orthotic control—free, assist, resist, stop, variable stop, hold, lock, deweighting (joint unloading)
Precautions (client factors that will affect specific orthosis prescription):
Justification—describe the need for the appliance, including an explanation of how the orthosis will enhance or maintain the client's functional abilities
Recommended by:

BOX 12.5 | Terminology With Specific Orthotic Definitions[4]

- A **custom-fabricated and -fitted orthosis** is an orthosis or pedorthic device that is fabricated to original measurements or a model of a particular client for use by only that individual to meet a specific prescription.
- A **custom-fitted orthosis** is a prefabricated orthosis or pedorthic device that is sized or modified for use by a particular client to meet a prescription.
- An **"off-the-shelf" orthosis** is a prefabricated orthosis that is sized or modified for use by a client in accordance with a prescription but does not require substantial clinical judgment or substantive alteration for appropriate use.
- An **"over-the-counter" appliance** is a prefabricated, mass-produced device that is prepackaged and requires no professional advice or judgment in either size selection or use, such as fabric or elastic supports, corsets, generic arch supports, and elastic hose.
- **Pedorthic devices** include therapeutic footwear and foot orthoses for use at the ankle or below, as well as modified footwear made for therapeutic purposes. Nontherapeutic shoe inserts or inlays and accommodative footwear are not included.

This "one-of-a-kind" appliance is then individually fit and modified for the client. **Prefabricated orthoses** are not manufactured for a particular individual but are usually mass produced for the general population using typical sizing for "average" individuals (eg, right or left; women's or men's; small, medium, large). Some prefabricated "off-the-shelf" appliances can be modified to better fit a particular individual; however, the client with deformity or atypical anatomy is often difficult to fit comfortably and effectively with a prefabricated device. Many prefabricated devices are much less expensive than custom-made appliances and are useful as trial or temporary devices to determine the usefulness of an orthosis in improving function.

Orthotic Terminology

The use of standardized and clear nomenclature to refer to specific orthoses is necessary for effective communication among rehabilitation professionals working with a client, as well as insurance payers. For many years, orthoses were referred to by using proper names, or eponyms, usually based on the name of the designer of the device or the city or facility where it was developed. Examples of orthoses often referred to by using *eponymous terminology* include the Klenzak short leg brace, Craig-Scott long leg braces, and the Milwaukee spinal brace. A problem with using eponyms to name orthoses is that the names are not precise. Because these names do not include standardized criteria or orthotic componentry, different practitioners and payers often had differing concepts of what was included in a device and what it could achieve. As a result, a new system of orthotic nomenclature was developed in the 1970s that is based on biomechanical terminology.[7] *Biomechanical terminology*, which is most commonly used today, has two components. First, the name lists the major joints enclosed within the orthosis, and the joints are referred to in an acronym formed from the first letter of each contained joint's name. **Box 12.6** lists the orthotic acronyms typically used for upper and lower extremity and spinal orthoses. The second component of the biomechanical name describes the type of control exerted by the orthosis on the enclosed joints. These control terms are listed and defined in **Box 12.7**. By using this terminology, clinicians can clearly communicate the biomechanical requirements and characteristics of an orthosis prescribed for a particular client. For example, the biomechanical terminology that names the orthosis drawn in **Figure 12.5** is an AFO (ankle–foot orthosis) with dorsiflexion assist and plantarflexion resist. The

BOX 12.6	**Biomechanical Orthotic Terminology: Acronym Designations for Upper Extremity, Lower Extremity, and Spinal Orthoses**

Lower Extremity Orthoses

FO	Foot orthosis
SMO	Supramalleolar orthosis
AO	Ankle orthosis
AFO	Ankle–foot orthosis
KAFO	Knee–ankle–foot orthosis
KO	Knee orthosis
HKAFO	Hip–knee–ankle–foot orthosis
LS-HKAFO	Hip–knee–ankle–foot orthosis with lumbosacral support

Upper Extremity Orthoses

HdO	Hand orthoses
WHO	Wrist–hand orthosis
EWHO	Elbow–wrist–hand orthosis
EO	Elbow orthosis
SEWHO	Shoulder–elbow–wrist–hand orthosis

Spinal Orthoses

SIO	Sacroiliac orthosis
LSO	Lumbosacral orthosis
TLSO	Thoracolumbosacral orthosis
CTLSO	Cervical thoracolumbosacral orthosis
CTO	Cervicothoracic orthosis
CO	Cervical orthosis

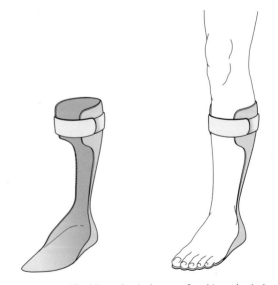

FIGURE 12.5. The biomechanical name for this orthosis is an ankle–foot orthosis (AFO) with dorsiflexion assist and plantar flexion resist. It is also called a posterior leaf spring (PLS) AFO.

BOX 12.7	Biomechanical Orthotic Terminology: Terms to Describe the Control Exerted by the Orthosis on the Enclosed Joints
Free	No control is exerted, and the joint is free to move in a designated plane.
Assist	Assists motion by applying an external force to increase the range, velocity, or force of a desired motion (eg, a spring, elastic band, motor, pneumatic force, muscle electrical stimulation).
Resist	Resists unwanted motion by applying a force to decrease the velocity or force of an undesirable movement.
Stop	Stop or limit motion at a joint. The prescription must indicate the specific motion to be stopped and when the stop is to occur in the range of motion (ROM) (eg, an AFO with a plantarflexion stop at 0°. This orthosis allows the ankle to plantarflex only to neutral or 0°.)
Hold	Controls and eliminates all motion at a joint in all planes. The prescription must indicate the specific joint position for the hold (eg, AFO to hold the ankle at 5° dorsiflexion [df] and subtalor neutral). When the hold is at the ankle, it is often described as a solid ankle orthosis (eg, AFO-SA at 5° df).

Additional Descriptors

Variable	May be used with the terms *stop, resist,* or *assist* to indicate the need for an adjustable system, with the desired ROM specified (eg, a KO with a variable stop set at 90° flexion stop and –20° extension stop).
Lock	An optional mechanism that when engaged or "on" holds or locks the joint in a fixed position. When the lock is disengaged, movement is permitted.
Deweighting: Weight-Relieving	An orthotic design that reduces axial loading through part of a limb. The prescription includes the amount of loading to be carried by the orthosis as a percent of normal limb loading (eg, AFO to reduce axial loading of the calcaneous 15%).

name makes it clear where the device is located and how it acts during function.

Types of Orthoses

Because various types of orthotic materials and components are available, more than one orthosis can be designed to correctly meet the requirements of a biomechanically named orthosis. For example, **Figure 12.6** depicts three different orthoses that correctly carry

the same biomechanical name. Although each orthosis uses the same method of exerting control, the differences among them are in the materials and components used to achieve that control. Thus, a third way to classify orthotic devices is by the materials and components used in fabrication. Using this classification method, orthoses are termed as follows:

■ **Conventional orthoses** are made primarily from metal components and leather.

Biomechanical terminology

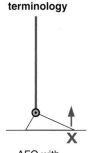

AFO with pf* stop

*pf = plantar flexion

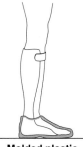

Conventional
• Metal uprights
• Leather cuff
• Attaches to shoe
• Space between leg and upright accomodates edema

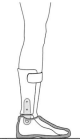

Molded plastic
• Plastic one-piece shell
• No moving parts
• Total contact
• Fits into shoe (can change shoes)

Articulating hybrid
• Plastic molded calf shell and shoe insert
• Articulating ankle joint
• Can change shoes

FIGURE 12.6. Three different orthoses are presented that offer the same biomechanical control. The orthosis that best meets the client's needs is chosen by considering the advantages and disadvantages of the various materials and components, client-specific factors, and anticipated orthotic usage.

■ **Molded orthoses** are made from **thermosetting plastics**, **thermoplastics**, and **composite** materials.

■ **Hybrid orthoses** are hinged or articulated and commonly use a combination of conventional and molded componentry.

There are advantages and disadvantages to all materials; thus, when the biomechanical control requirements of an orthosis are determined, clinicians must decide which materials and components will best serve the specific needs of the individual client. Because the materials, components, and fabrication technologies are constantly changing, decisions concerning specific materials and componentry are usually best made by the orthotist who will manufacture the appliance. Orthotic components and their advantages and disadvantages are described in subsequent chapters that present orthotic solutions for impairments in specific body regions and joints.

Box 12.8 summarizes the three classification methods used to describe orthotic devices. Use of terminology from these classification systems helps clinicians select orthoses to match the specific needs and goals of their clients, describe the devices accurately, and communicate clearly with others. The use of this classification terminology to name the three biomechanically similar orthoses depicted in Figure 12.6 illustrates how this terminology facilitates clear and effective communication. All three are custom-made orthoses. Thus, the term "custom made" is followed by the individual name for each appliance:

■ Conventional double-upright AFO with pf (plantarflexion) stop
■ Molded AFO (sometimes labeled mAFO) with pf stop
■ Articulating (hinged) hybrid AFO with pf stop

Evidence-Based Orthotic Prescription

Although orthoses are mechanical interventions designed to primarily affect a wearer's musculoskeletal system, the effectiveness of an orthosis in improving an individual's functional abilities is also impacted by neuromuscular control, cardiovascular/pulmonary function, as well as complex interactions among many personal and environmental factors. Thus, recommending a particular orthosis on the basis of biomechanical

---

BOX 12.8 | Classification Methods for Orthotic Devices

Classification by Method of Manufacture
■ Custom manufactured
  ■ Local manufacturing
  ■ Central manufacturing
■ Prefabricated
  ■ With custom fit ("off the shelf")
  ■ Without individual fitting ("over the counter")

Classification by Biomechanical Terminology
■ Acronym made from the names of the joints enclosed by the orthosis
■ Type of biomechanical control exerted by the orthosis on the limb and joints (eg, free, assist, resist, stop, hold; lock, variable stop, axial deweighting or unloading)

Classification by Types of Materials and Components Used in Fabrication
■ Conventional: Primary components and materials:
  ■ Metal uprights and components
  ■ Uprights attached directly to shoe for most lower extremity devices

  ■ Leather cuffs; cloth, canvas, or elastic parts
  ■ Made from measurements taken from the involved limb
■ Molded: Primary components and materials:
  ■ Thermoplastics, thermosetting plastics, reinforced plastics, and composite materials
  ■ Manufactured over custom mold of client
  ■ Usually total contact design
  ■ Usually made of one piece without moving parts or joints
  ■ Has a shoe insert that slides into shoe without attaching for most lower extremity devices
■ Hybrid: Composed of both molded and conventional materials:
  ■ Limb cuffs, shells, and shoe insert are usually molded
  ■ Usually has articulations (hinged, moving joints) that include some nonmolded and conventional componentry

principles alone can be misleading and may not produce the best orthotic prescription. In addition to knowledge, clinical examination findings, experience, and recognition of the client's goals and preferences, effective clinical decision making regarding orthotic prescription requires practitioners to consider the best available information about orthotic effectiveness from up-to-date relevant research.

To find the research relevant to making an orthotic recommendation for a particular client, practitioners can access both primary and secondary sources. Primary sources are research articles in which the author presents the findings of an original study. To find pertinent studies relevant to a particular client, practitioners can search electronic databases using keywords descriptive of the intervention (orthotic device) and characteristics of the client. The Keywords for Literature Search section at the end of this chapter presents example search domains, keywords, or medical subject headings (MeSH terms) that can be used to focus a database search to find applicable research studies. Secondary sources include integrative review articles, systematic reviews, and meta-analyses. Well-done systematic reviews are particularly useful sources of evidence, as they gather and appraise the quality of relevant studies and synthesize the findings to answer a clinical question. **Box 12.9** lists electronic databases that clinicians can use to find relevant, current research literature and systematic reviews to guide clinical decision making concerning orthotic prescriptions.

GETTING FROM THE PRESCRIPTION TO THE ORTHOSIS

There are many different ways to obtain an orthosis once it is prescribed. "Off-the-shelf" and "over-the-counter" appliances are typically ordered from medical suppliers. If significant modification or individual fitting is expected, this is typically done by an orthotist. Thus, in these cases, ordering from the supplier is usually done by the orthotist. When little or no adjustments are needed or the device is a trial or temporary appliance, the orthosis may be ordered and fit by a therapist working with the client.

Custom-made orthoses are manufactured for a specific individual by orthotists or orthotic technicians. This requires selection of the most appropriate materials and components to achieve the orthotic and functional goals for the specific client. Many factors, in addition to the prescription requirements, influence the selection of orthotic materials, including individual client factors as well as how and in what environment the orthosis will be used. For example, a heavy, tall adult who is very active and intends to use the orthosis

---

BOX 12.9 | Electronic Databases to Locate Relevant Research Studies

Database Name	Access
Medline (National Library of Medicine)	Library access
Ovid (A platform to access medical databases)	Library access; subscription www.ovid.com (www.gateway.ovid.com for subscribed users)
Pubmed (National Library of Medicine)	www.ncbi.nlm.nih.gov/entrez
CINAHL (Cumulative Index of Nursing and Allied Health Literature)	Library access; subscription www.cinahl.com
Google Scholar	www.scholar.google.com
Hooked on Evidence (American Physical Therapy Association)	APTA members; www.apta.org
Open Door (American Physical Therapy Association): portal to databases—Proquest, Cochrane, CINAHL, etc	APTA members; www.apta.org
Cochrane Database of Systematic Reviews (EBM Reviews)	www.thecochranelibrary.com
ACP Journal Club and Evidence Based Medicine	www.acpjc.org (subscription required)
PEDro (The Physiotherapy Evidence Database)	ww.pedro.fhs.usyd.edu.au/index.html

in all types of indoor and outdoor environments requires an orthosis that is very strong, durable, and made from fatigue-resistant materials. A small child who is only able to walk indoors requires an orthosis that is less strong but lightweight. Thus, even when the prescription requirements are the same, different individuals may require different types of orthoses to optimize their function. Orthotists typically have the best and most current knowledge of components, materials, and material properties and thus usually choose the orthotic materials, components, and fabrication methods. Other practitioners who work with clients using orthoses, however, must be familiar with the various orthotic materials and components in order to understand appropriate orthotic uses and limitations. An in-depth discussion of specific materials used to fabricate orthoses is beyond the scope of this text; however, important material properties and the most commonly used orthotic materials are reviewed.[8]

Orthotic Materials and Their Properties

The materials commonly used in today's orthotic devices include metals; materials such as leather, canvas, and synthetic and elastic fabrics; thermoplastics; thermosetting plastics; thermoplastic and thermosetting composites; foamed plastics; and elastomers. These materials present a wide range of mechanical properties, which makes each suited to particular orthotic applications. For example, some foamed plastics are quite soft and resilient and thus provide cushioning that decreases pressure, while metal and some plastics are hard and stiff and are used where resistance to large forces is required. To understand the use of specific materials for particular orthotic applications, clinicians need a good understanding of the materials' mechanical properties. Selected material properties that are important for understanding orthotic applications are listed and defined in **Box 12.10**.

BOX 12.10 | Important Mechanical Properties of Orthotic Materials

Strength	The maximum external load or force that a material can sustain or support before breaking. Orthoses are commonly subjected to compressive, tensile, and bending forces.
Brittleness	Materials that when loaded do not deform (change in shape) before breaking are called brittle.
Ductility	Materials that yield or deform in response to loading prior to breaking are called ductile.
Stiffness	The amount of deformation (eg, bending or compression) that occurs when a material is loaded. Materials that do not deform very much in response to loading are very stiff; those that deform a lot in response to loading are not very stiff.
Elasticity	The ability of materials that deform in response to loading to return to their original dimensions when unloaded. Materials that can return to their predeformed size and shape have good elastic *memory*. Elastic materials are also described as *resilient*.
Plasticity	The ability of materials that deform in response to loading to retain the deformation (elongation or compression) even after the deforming force has been removed.
Viscoelasticity	The ability of materials to demonstrate both elasticity and plasticity when deformed in response to loading. **Compression set** is a measurement of the ratio of the elastic to viscous (plastic) components of an elastomer's response to a given compression load. Materials with "high compression set" do not recover from deformation during unloading, which clinically is often called "bottoming out." Materials with "low compression set" have a more elastic response and recover from their deformations.
Hardness	A material's resistance to permanent indentation in response to a compression load. The measure of a material's hardness is referred to as its **durometer** (Shore durometer), which is a number from 0 to 100. High-durometer materials are very hard; low-durometer materials are soft or compliant.
Density	A material's weight per unit volume. Because weight is an important factor in determining the energy cost of orthotic use, materials that are lightweight but strong are most desirable.
Durability or fatigue resistance	The ability of a material to withstand cyclic loading without breaking or deforming significantly.
Corrosion resistance	The degree to which a material is able to resist degradation in response to exposure to chemicals. In orthotic materials, exposure to water, perspiration, and urine pose risks of degradation that will undermine the material properties.

In addition to materials' inherent mechanical properties, certain *physical characteristics* of the materials also affect how they behave in an orthosis. Both the thickness and the shape of the material used in an appliance affect device function. For example, for a given thermoplastic material used in an orthosis, increasing its *thickness* also increases its rigidity, as well as the weight and bulk of the resulting orthosis. The *shape* of the material is also important. For example, the strength of a molded thermoplastic orthosis is increased by including corrugations (an added curved shape), rolled edges, or reinforcements in highly stressed areas (**Fig. 12.7**). Orthoses shaped with acute angles are more likely to break than those with obtuse angles. Thus, orthoses are more susceptible to breakage at sites of nicks and scratches than in smooth areas.

The most common materials used in today's orthotic devices are summarized with typical applications.

Metals

Most metals used in orthotic devices are alloys, such as steel, aluminum, and titanium. Metals are used in conventional orthotic componentry such as uprights, articulating (hinged) joints, and fixed and variable locks. *Stainless steel* (iron, nickel, and chromium) is stronger and stiffer but also heavier than most other materials. Orthoses that include stainless steel components are strong but quite heavy and thus also result in high energy expenditure during function. Aluminum, alloyed with copper, manganese, and other elements, is much lighter (about one third as much as a comparable amount of

steel) and easier to work with, but it is also less strong and less stiff when compared to steel. These properties may make aluminum components unsatisfactory for lower extremity orthoses for large, heavy individuals. However, in other applications in which the orthosis is subjected to lower stresses, aluminum may be sufficiently strong and more desirable due to its lighter weight. Components made of aluminum, however, are more susceptible to fatigue failure. Titanium alloys are very strong, lightweight, and corrosion resistant but are very expensive and more difficult to work with. Titanium is used in some orthotic joints but is found more frequently in preformed prosthetic componentry than in orthotic applications.

Leather and Fabric

Although leather has been used for decades in conventional orthotic devices mostly to cover and pad metal bands, as cuffs, and as straps and belts, it is infrequently used in orthoses today. Plastics are typically used today to form cuffs and bands. Straps and belts are often made of *cotton/synthetic webbing* rather than leather. Pull-on sleeves, aprons, or other soft goods used to attach or secure orthotic components to the body are made of *synthetic fabrics* or neoprene. Neoprene is a synthetic rubber material that may be backed with nylon fabric. It is flexible, conforms to the body, and is resilient. The noncoated surface grips the skin and may be used to hold an orthosis in place and prevent slippage or appliance migration.

Plastics

Plastics are carbon-containing organic materials that began to be used commonly in orthotic applications in the 1970s. This revolutionized orthotic prescription because the newly developed plastics offered materials that were strong and lightweight and were fabricated by molding over a positive model of the client's limb. This allowed orthoses to be fit intimately to the client with total contact, which increased their ability to exert effective control with less weight and bulk. Plastics are synthetic materials made from raw chemical materials called monomers (one chemical unit), such as ethylene or propylene. When monomers are reacted together, they polymerize to form long chains of repeating units called polymers, such as polyethylene or polypropylene. There are many different

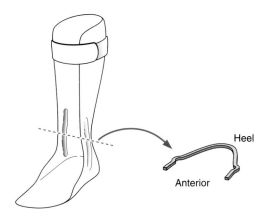

FIGURE 12.7. An ankle–foot orthosis designed with corrugations increases strength at the high-stress ankle area. A cross section through the orthotic shell at the level of the corrugations demonstrates the increased curved shape that contributes to improved orthotic strength.

types of plastics or polymers, which provide a wide range of materials with an equally wide range of mechanical properties that match virtually every orthotic need. As a group, plastics are relatively strong; lightweight; easy to shape, mold, or adjust; corrosion resistant; and easy to clean. There are two major categories of plastics: thermoplastics and thermosetting plastics. Both types of plastics can be reinforced with fibers such as glass and carbon (graphite) to form plastic composites that have greater load-bearing capability and ability to store and release energy.

Thermoplastics

Thermoplastics are materials that are solid at room temperature but become malleable when heated. These plastics are purchased as sheets and heated for molding to form an orthosis. Once molded, thermoplastic materials can be reheated to reshape or modify the appliance. There are two types of thermoplastics. Most *low-temperature thermoplastics* become malleable at 150° to 175°F and can be molded directly on the client's body. *High-temperature thermoplastics* require processing temperatures in the general range of 300° to 400°F and must be molded over a positive model of the client's limb. Although easier and quicker to form, orthoses made from low-temperature materials are less strong and thus are useful only for upper extremity devices, such as hand or wrist splints, or lower limb appliances for small children. Thermoplastic lower extremity and spinal orthoses for adults are usually constructed from high-temperature materials. Another advantage of low-temperature materials is that they can be heated in a warm water bath, such as an electric fry pan, and cut with scissors. High-temperature materials, however, require skilled technicians and special ovens and equipment to heat and form into orthoses by molding over plaster models of the body.

Foamed Thermoplastics

Foamed thermoplastics are formed by forcing nitrogen or some other gas into the plastic during heating. These materials are resilient, offering varying degrees of softness or cushioning. Foamed thermoplastics are *open-cell* or *closed-cell* materials, depending on whether the "cells" formed by the gas bubbles are connected (open cell) or remain separated from one another (closed cell). Important properties of these materials that help to determine appropriate orthotic applications are *durometer* and *compression set* (see Box 12.10). Some of these foamed materials will mold and conform to the shape of the body part under loading (weight bearing), while others do not. Foamed thermoplastics are frequently used in the fabrication of foot orthoses, as padding on hard thermoplastic appliances and in certain cervical orthoses. Closed-cell foams do not absorb moisture such as perspiration; however, open-cell resilient materials do and thus may require coverings to prevent absorption of perspiration that will cause the material to deteriorate.

Elastomers

Elastomers are noncellular, but resilient, thermoplastics that are able to stretch and deform at room temperature. They are often termed viscoelastic materials because they exhibit both elastic and plastic characteristics. Due to their ability to absorb and dissipate loads, they are used in shock-absorbing shoe inserts and antivibration gloves.

Table 12.1 presents a list and description of some of the commonly used thermoplastics, their characteristics, and typical orthotic applications.

Thermosetting Plastics

Thermosetting plastics or resins, like thermoplastics, are also synthetic organic polymers. However, they differ from thermoplastics in that once polymerization takes place and the material cures or hardens, the material cannot be made malleable again by reheating. Thus, orthoses made from thermosetting plastics, or thermosets, cannot be modified by heating once they have been formed. Adjustments can only be made by grinding or cutting to remove material. The thermosets most commonly used in orthotic applications are polyester and epoxy. These resins are liquid at room temperature. When mixed with a promoter and catalyst, they cross-link or cure at room temperature into permanent form. Thermosets can be formed in molds or on positive models. However, in orthotic application, they are often impregnated into a base material, such as nylon or Dacron fabrics, fiberglass, or Kevlar (aramid), to form laminates. Although thermosetting plastics are very hard, they have poor impact resistance. Thus, orthoses that require toughness (resistance to fracture) are better made from thermoplastic materials.

TABLE 12.1	Commonly Used Thermoplastics in Orthoses[8,9]	
Generic Name (Brand Name)	**Characteristics**	**Orthotic Applications**
High-Temperature Thermoplastics Polyethylene	Flexible and easy to vacuum form; not as strong as some other materials; types: low density, high density, ultra high density (strongest)	Ankle-foot orthoses (AFOs), spinal orthoses, some upper limb orthoses
Polypropylene	Durable, stronger, and stiffer; more difficult to form and mold	Rigid AFOs, floor reaction orthoses, knee-ankle-foot orthoses (KAFOs)
Copolymer	Blend of polyethylene and polypropylene; more fracture resistant and durable	Orthoses requiring some flexibility and durability
Ionomer of polythene and metallic acrylates (Syrlyn)	Transparent, tough, durable, and easily formed	Upper and lower extremity orthotics; spiral and hemispiral AFOs
Low-Temperature Thermoplastics Transpoly isoprene (Orthoplast; Ezeform)	Rubbery thermoplastic that is easy to form directly on client, molds easily and adheres to self	Hand and upper extremity (UE) splints; protective splints for sports medicine
Polycaprolactone (Polyform)	A more rigid low-temperature material, drapes more easily	Hand and UE splints, trunk orthoses
Foamed Thermoplastics Polyethylene foam (Plastizote, Pelite, Aliplast)	Closed cell structure; resilient, lightweight; comes in various durometers; moldable, some mold under pressure without heat	Foot orthoses and shoe inserts, accommodative footwear, padding on rigid orthoses
Ethylene vinyl acetate (EVA) plus polyethylene (PE) foam (Nickelplast)	Denser and stronger than PE foam alone, resists "bottoming out," good shock-absorbing capabilities, moldable with heating	Base for semirigid foot orthosis, posting material
Polyurethane foam (Poron, PPT)	Open-cell foam, low compression set, effective as shock absorber and minimizes shear when next to skin, nonmoldable	Shoe inserts or inlays
Elastomers Polyurethane thermoset (Sorbothane, Viscolas)	Low compression set, good plastic memory; absorbs and dissipates shock and vibration; resilient	Shoe inserts/inlays, vibration gloves and grips

Silicone (Silipos®, Niagara Falls, NY 14304) is a thermosetting polymer composed of silicon with carbon, hydrogen, and oxygen. Silicone is flexible, nonstick, repels water, and is permeable to oxygen. It is useful in orthotic applications as a padding material to relieve pressure over sensitive structures such as bony prominences or scars as well as for a growing number of other applications.

Composite Materials

Composite materials are formed from the combination of a plastic with one or more additives so that the resultant composite material has special properties not possessed by the plastic alone. In industry, many different additives are used in making composites for specific purposes. Typical composite materials used in orthotic applications are either thermoplastics or thermosets to which glass, carbon (graphite), or aramid (Kevlar®, E.I. du Pont de Nemours and Co., Wilmington, DE 19898) fibers have been added to improve strength. Plastic composites have a high strength-to-weight ratio. Thus, orthoses made from composite materials can be very thin, yet very strong and durable. Many of the orthoses that are designed to store and release energy take advantage of this property of carbon fiber–reinforced plastic composites.

ORTHOTIC FABRICATION METHODS

Just as there are many different types of materials used in the construction of orthoses, there are also a variety of methods of fabricating and obtaining an orthosis for a client. Orthoses and orthotic componentry are either mass produced or custom made. *Mass-produced appliances* are manufactured in various sizes and selected for an individual client by measurements. A device obtained by ordering from a supplier is adjusted to fit the client if needed by an orthotist or other practitioner. *Custom-made devices* are manufactured for a specific individual either from linear and circumferential measurements or from a model made of the part of the body where the orthosis will be worn. Conventional orthoses are typically constructed from metal factory-made componentry that is bent and assembled by an orthotist to meet specific client measurements. Orthoses made from plastic and composite materials are usually formed over a **positive cast** or three-dimensional model of the part of the client's body to be braced. The orthosis made from this model is either manufactured locally or is sent to a central manufacturing site, which services a large number of orthotic practices.

After developing the orthotic prescription, the traditional process of obtaining the custom-made orthosis for the client includes

1. Taking linear and circumferential measurements of the region of the body to be braced, as well as recording height and weight
2. Making a **negative cast** (mold or impression) of the part of the client's body where the orthosis will be worn

3. Making a positive cast or model from the negative mold
4. Modifying the positive cast to provide relief for pressure-sensitive areas and to incorporate the required orthotic control
5. Forming the orthosis over the modified positive model by vacuum-forming or some other method
6. Removing the molded orthosis from the positive cast, finishing the appliance, and adding strapping as required
7. Fitting the finished appliance to the client and making adjustments as necessary

One of the most important steps in this process is making the **negative cast** or impression, because the final product is only as good as the negative cast is accurate. This is traditionally accomplished by wrapping a thin layer of plaster or some other type of casting bandage (eg, fiberglass) around the body part, allowing it to harden, and then removing it to be used as the mold for the positive cast or model. Alternatively, *computer-assisted design and computer-assisted manufacturing (CAD-CAM)* techniques are used. With this technology, a digitization device, such as an optical-laser scanner or a surface-contacting stylus, is used to record the surface contours of the body. This "digital negative impression" is then fed into computer software, modified electronically, and used to direct milling machinery to fabricate either a positive model or the orthotic device. CAD-CAM technology is particularly useful when central manufacturing facilities are used, because digital negative molds can be sent and stored electronically more easily than physical plaster positive models. However, whether traditional manual methods or CAD-CAM technology are used in manufacturing, the device must be fit and usually adjusted to the client by a skilled orthotist and a checkout examination of the orthosis and its wearer (Chapter 11) performed by the therapist prior to the beginning of training.

SHOES FOR ORTHOTIC DEVICES

Shoes are an important component of a lower extremity orthosis, even when not directly attached to the orthosis. The types and characteristics of shoes that are important for specific types of lower extremity orthoses are discussed in Chapter 13 and subsequent chapters. Practitioners are reminded to consider the specific shoe requirements and modifications that are needed to maximize function when making an orthotic prescription. Clients must be instructed in the specific shoe requirements for a particular orthosis and how to insure proper shoe fit with the orthosis. A properly prescribed, manufactured, and fitted lower extremity orthosis cannot function optimally unless it is used with a well-fitting shoe, which has the necessary characteristics.

SUMMARY

Orthoses are external appliances designed to apply forces to the body to improve function by

- Assisting movement when joint motion is insufficient
- Stabilizing a joint when joint movement is excessive or abnormal
- Protecting a joint or skeletal segment
- Helping in the management of joint or skeletal deformity by preventing, supporting, or correcting them

Orthotic prescriptions are developed by a team of individuals including the client and healthcare practitioners who are knowledgeable about the client's functional needs and current orthotic componentry, including orthotist, physician, and therapists. Orthotic prescriptions are developed to achieve specific orthotic goals by applying biomechanical principles through orthotic design and material and component selection. Other factors that affect orthotic prescription include the anticipated duration of orthotic use, the environments in which the orthosis will be used, the overall physical capabilities of the client, and the financial resources available to pay for the device.

Although orthoses were referred to by eponyms or proper names for many years, biomechanical terminology is currently the preferred method of naming orthotic devices. Biomechanical terminology includes two components:

- An acronym composed of the first letter of the names of the joints enclosed within the orthosis
- Designated words that describe the type and location of the mechanical control exerted by the orthosis on the braced body part

In addition to a biomechanical name, orthoses are classified according to the method of manufacture and the types of materials and components used.

Various materials and components are used in contemporary orthoses, including metal, fabrics, plastics, composites, as well as other materials. The selection of materials for construction of a particular orthosis depends on the specific orthotic goals, the biomechanical design, and the material properties required to achieve the goals. Material properties to consider include the weight, strength, durability, fatigue resistance, flexibility, elasticity, plasticity, and corrosion resistance, to name a few.

Many factors influence how the prescribed orthosis is obtained for the client. The orthosis may be prefabricated or custom made and fit. Construction methods include manual measurement and casting and manual construction of the device, computer-assisted design (CAD) with computer-assisted manufacture (CAM), or a combination of techniques.

KEYWORDS FOR LITERATURE SEARCH

Select keywords from relevant domains and search by combining the appropriate keywords with the Boolean term "AND". This list is not intended to be exhaustive but to provide readers with ideas for selecting search terms.

Search Domains	Keywords, MeSh Terms
Intervention	Orthotic device
Conditions—general (examples only)	Nervous system disease
	Neuromuscular disease
	Musculoskeletal disease
Conditions—specific (examples only)	Cerebral vascular accident; stroke
	Hemiplegia
	Cerebral palsy
	Spinal cord injury
	Anterior cruciate ligament tear
	Patellofemoral pain syndrome
	Osteoarthritis
	Rheumatoid arthritis
Age	Infant
	Child
	Adolescent
	Aged
	Frail elderly
Activities; Outcomes	Activities of daily living
	Walking; gait
	Stair climbing
	Exercise
	Physical fitness
	Energy expenditure
	Work
	Automobile driving

REFERENCES

1. Waters RL, Campbell J, Thomas L, et al: Energy cost of walking in lower-extremity plaster casts. JBJS 64:896–899, 1982.
2. Mattsson E, Brostrom L-A: The increase in energy cost of walking with an immobilized knee or an unstable ankle. Scand J Rehab Med 22:51–53, 1990.
3. Kaufman KR, Irby SE, Mathewson JW, et al: Energy-efficient knee-ankle foot orthosis: a case study. J Prosthet Orthot 8:79–85, 1996.
4. American Board for Certification of Orthotics and Prosthetics, Inc.: Model orthotics, prosthetics, and pedorthics practice act. www.abcop.org/Assets/PDF/ABCModelLicensureBill.pdf; accessed 7/01/08.
5. Vinvi P, Gargiulo P: Poor compliance with ankle-foot-orthoses in Charcot-Marie-Tooth disease. Eur J Phys Rehabil Med 44:27–31, 2008.
6. Skaggs D, Oda J, Lerman L, et al.: Insurance status and delay in orthotic treatment in children. J Pediatr Orthop 27:94–97, 2007.
7. Harris EE: A new orthotic terminology: a guide to its use for prescription and fee schedules. Orthot Prosthet 27:6–9, 1973.
8. Lunsford TR: Strength and materials. In Goldberg B, Hsu JD (eds): Atlas of orthoses and assistive devices, 3rd ed. St. Louis, Mosby, 1997, pp 15–66.
9. Edelstein JE, Bruckner, J: Orthotics: a comprehensive clinical approach. Thorofare, NJ, Slack, 2002.

13

Shoes and Orthoses for Foot Impairments

OBJECTIVES

At the end of this chapter, all students are expected to:

1. Describe the types of shoes, shoe modifications, and foot orthoses and their functions.
2. Describe the components of shoes, shoe modifications, and foot orthoses.
3. Describe the proper fit of shoes, shoe modifications, and foot orthoses.

Physical Therapy students are expected to:

1. Determine the need for specialized shoes, shoe modifications, or foot orthoses for a client.
   a. Evaluate relevant client examination findings to diagnose impairments that may be improved by specialized shoes, shoe modifications, or foot orthoses.
2. Develop appropriate goals for specialized shoes, shoe modifications, or foot orthoses.
3. Describe the biomechanical methods employed in therapeutic shoes, shoe modifications, or foot orthoses to achieve the goals.
4. Develop and execute a search strategy to identify research evidence for the uses and effectiveness of therapeutic shoes, shoe modifications, and foot orthoses.
5. Recommend shoes, shoe modifications, or foot orthoses as part of a plan of care for individuals with impairments of the foot.
6. Evaluate shoes, shoes with modifications, and foot orthoses for fit, function, comfort, and cosmesis.

CASE STUDIES

Tim Higgins is a 24-year-old man with bilateral foot pain during any sustained walking or standing longer than 30 min. He was diagnosed as a teenager with flexible flat feet, which made it impossible for him to play high school sports. He recently graduated from college and is employed as a civil engineer, which requires him to do considerable walking over all types of outdoor terrain to monitor work sites and projects. Despite wearing expensive, supportive boots with arch support inserts, Tim's foot pain has gotten worse, is now present all the time, and is making it difficult to get through his workdays. Examination findings are presented in **Box 13.1**.

Michael Ferris is a 55-year-old man with a diagnosis of non-insulin-dependent type II diabetes mellitus, who is a chief financial officer for a large insurance company. He lives in Philadelphia and commutes by train daily to New York City to work and thus spends much time sitting and eating fast food in busy train stations. At a company-required annual physical examination, it was discovered that he has developed diabetic neuropathy bilaterally. Selected examination findings are presented in **Box 13.2**.

Janice Simmons is a 63-year-old woman who sustained a left transtibial amputation for gangrene of her left foot. Her case is described in Chapters 4, 5, 6, and 7. She has been walking independently with a prosthesis for about 6 months and returns to Vascular Clinic for a recheck. She is wearing extra-depth shoes. Results of her vascular evaluation are outlined in **Box 13.3**.

Case Study Activities

All Students:

1. Describe the biomechanical principles that explain how the footwear or orthosis will improve client function.

2. Describe how a specialized shoe, shoe modification, or foot orthosis affects each person's gait.
3. If a foot orthosis is recommended, describe the shoes that the client should wear with the orthosis to achieve comfort and a good functional outcome.

Physical Therapy Students:

1. Describe the impairments that contribute to each client's functional limitations and participation restrictions.
2. Develop specific goals for footwear or foot orthoses.
3. Develop a plan of care for each person.
   a. What appliance (if any) would you prescribe? (use appropriate terminology)
   b. What other interventions would you advise?

BOX 13.1 | Clinical Findings for Tim Higgins

General
■ Tim is 5' 11" and weighs 165 pounds. All findings reported below are bilateral and symmetrical.

Posture Assessment: In self-selected, usual standing position,
■ Leg lengths are equal
■ Mildly excessive genu valgus and recurvatum
■ Foot position:
   ■ Toe out is 20°
   ■ Calcanei are in 20° of valgus
   ■ Navicular tubercles are 1 cm from the floor and well below the Feiss line

Lower Extremity Musculoskeletal Assessment (non-weight-bearing)
■ Passive ROM is normal, except that he has only 5° dorsiflexion.
■ Strength in both legs is 5/5, except posterior tibialis and peroneus longus muscle strength is 4/5. He is able to perform a maximum of 10 unilateral heel raises with discomfort.
■ Ligamentous stability: All joints are grossly stable but are somewhat hypermobile or hyperflexible.
■ Foot position in subtalar neutral is 10° hindfoot varus, 10° forefoot varus.
■ Foot pain is reported after 20 to 30 minutes of weight-bearing, 6/10; rest pain, 4/10; no night pain is reported.

BOX 13.2 | Clinical Findings for Michael Ferris

General: Mr. Ferris is 6 feet tall and weighs 300 lbs. He wears leather, oxford men's dress shoes with leather soles and heels most of the time. When he is relaxing at home, he wears moccasins.

Vascular:
■ Both lower extremities are cool to touch and hairless from mid-calf down.
■ Pedal pulses are 1+ bilaterally (2+ is normal).

Physical:
■ Fungal infections of the toenails are seen on both feet.
■ Passive ROM of both feet is normal except for ankle dorsiflexion, which is 45° to 0° bilaterally.
■ Flexible claw toe deformities (caused by muscle weakness and imbalance due to peripheral neuropathy) are seen with callusing over dorsum of the IP joints.
■ Lacks protective sensation on the plantar surfaces of both hallux and metatarsal heads I, II, and IV bilaterally. Protective sensation is present under the heel and on the dorsum of the foot. (Tested with the 5.07 [10 gm] Semmes-Weinstein monofilament.)
■ Proximal to his feet sensation is normal.
■ Leg strength is grossly 4/5, but his muscle endurance is poor. (Muscle strength grades drop a half grade after 10 repetitions and a full grade after 20 repetitions.)

SHOES

Shoes traditionally have been designed to protect the feet from injuries and inclement weather, and to support the feet during activities. Over the years, shoes have become a fashion statement and often do not effectively serve the other functions. Improper shoes can cause problems such as blisters, calluses, ulcers, and deformity as well as more serious injuries to the lower extremities. Shoes are also important to the function of any lower extremity orthosis, particularly those that include componentry at the foot and ankle and either attach to or fit into shoes. Improper footwear can undermine the desired effect of an appropriately prescribed orthosis as well as produce additional problems. Therapeutic

BOX 13.3	Vascular Findings for Janice Simmons

Observation:

- Skin is dry and somewhat flaky
- Slight clubbing of nails
- No hair below the knee
- Hammer toes of digits II to V
- Hallux valgus
- No ulcers or skin breakdowns
- Shoes are worn, especially at the heel

Clinical Data:

- ABI is 0.8
- Dorsalis pedis artery nonpalpable
- Posterior tibial artery is +1
- Sensation on dorsum of foot up to midshin (tested with 10 gm Semmes-Weinstein filament)
- No sensation on the medial border of the foot or dorsum of the toes (10 gm SW filament)
- Decreased sensation on the plantar surface of the foot (10 gm SW filament) with callous formation evident under the head of the first metatarsal

footwear are specialized shoes that have special features designed to:

- Enhance shock absorption.
- Reduce shear stresses on the foot.
- Accommodate and support foot deformities.
- Accommodate or relieve pressure-sensitive areas.

- Accommodate shoe inserts and other orthotic devices that are worn inside the shoe.

Shoe modifications are made by adding materials to a shoe, either internally or externally, to achieve specific therapeutic goals. These are discussed subsequently in this chapter. Physical therapists need a basic understanding of shoes and shoe modifications to treat patients with foot dysfunction and to recommend suitable shoes for use with lower extremity orthotic devices.

Types of Shoes

Shoes are composed of three general parts:

1. The upper (the part of the shoe over the dorsum of the foot)
2. The sole
3. Reinforcements

These shoe parts may be put together in a variety of ways to form seven main types (or styles) of shoes that are drawn in **Figure 13.1**.[1] *Oxfords* are low-top shoes with laces to hold the shoe on the foot. *Boots* have high quarters that extend over the malleoli. *Pumps* are slip-on, low-cut shoes, usually without straps or ties, with low or high heels. *Mules* are backless shoes, with or without a strap. Due to their characteristics, oxfords and boots, constructed as athletic or nonathletic shoes, are most commonly used effectively with orthoses. They are also the most common shoe type adapted or

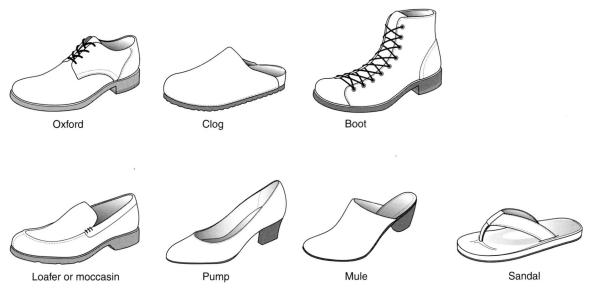

Oxford   Clog   Boot

Loafer or moccasin   Pump   Mule   Sandal

FIGURE 13.1. Basic shoe types or styles. The oxford (athletic or nonathletic) and boot styles are most appropriate for use with orthoses, because they provide necessary stability and are more effective in securing the orthosis to the foot.

modified for clients with foot impairments. Although contemporary orthoses can be made from materials that are thin and strong and can fit into many shoe styles, moccasins, mules, and pumps rarely provide the support or stability necessary to either securely hold the foot onto the orthosis or allow for modifications.

Regardless of style, shoes are constructed over a **last**, which is a real or virtual model or "statue" of a foot.[1] The shoe last determines the shoe size and shape. Unfortunately, different shoe manufacturers, and even different shoes manufactured by the same company, do not use standardized shoe lasts for sizing. This often creates problems for patients, who must try on many shoes with or without an orthosis before finding ones that fit and function well. Accommodation of an orthosis that fits into the shoe may require the wearer to use a wider shoe. Selecting a longer shoe to accommodate the orthosis often causes problems with fit on the uninvolved side and may also lead to tripping. Practitioners must know the types of shoes currently available that are appropriate for particular orthoses or refer orthotic clients to **pedorthists**, professionals who fit and dispense foot orthoses, shoes, and shoe modifications according to prescription.[2] Individuals with dysvascular foot problems may require evaluation by a podiatrist or a specialized foot clinic for prescription of appropriate shoes.

The *last* for a typical shoe simulates the shape of the normal weight-bearing foot. It typically has a greater inward curvature on the medial side of the foot with the forefoot portion angled medially to the heel by about 7°. Other lasts are also available and are often used for specific therapeutic purposes. These are shown in **Figure 13.2** and include

- *Straight*
- *Inflare*
- *Outflare*

A straight last shoe is one that has little curvature and when bisected from the heel, has equal right and left halves. A shoe with an inflare last has a forefoot that curves medially from the heel more than typical shoes. An outflare shoe curves laterally. Inflare or outflare shoes may be used to accommodate foot deformities or, in young children, to provide corrective forces.

Parts of a Shoe

The parts of shoes are drawn and labeled in **Figure 13.3** for both athletic and nonathletic shoe types.[1,3] Their characteristics and implications for shoe selection with specific orthotic applications are discussed below.

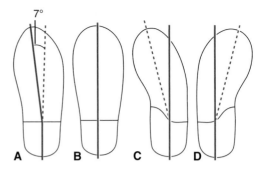

FIGURE 13.2. The shoe last determines the size and shape of the shoe. Shoe lasts (drawn for a right shoe) include **(A)** normal, **(B)** straight, **(C)** inflare, and **(D)** outflare.

The Upper

The *upper* is the part of the shoe that covers the dorsum, the sides, and the back of the foot. The characteristics of the upper that are most important to consider include

- Shoe depth
- Toe box height and width
- Height of the quarters
- Throat style
- Type of closure
- Features that contribute to hindfoot stability, such as counters and rearfoot stabilizers
- The material from which the upper is constructed

The *depth of the shoe* is determined by the shoe last as well as the type of insole. Removing the insoles from shoes with removable inserts provides extra room that may be sufficient to accommodate some foot deformities, therapeutic foot orthoses, or orthotic foot plates. For appliances that require more space, extra-depth shoes may be needed. *Extra-depth shoes* are specially manufactured shoes that have an additional quarter inch of depth throughout the shoe and provide wearers with two ¼-inch inserts.

The *height of the toe box* is another important consideration, particularly for individuals with deformities such as hammertoes and claw toes. Individuals with diabetic neuropathy and arthritis often develop these toe deformities, which make them more susceptible to painful callusing and ulceration on the dorsum and distal end of the toes (**Fig. 13.4**). In addition to the toe box height, the toe region of the shoe should have adequate length and width. The toe region should be approximately ½ inch longer than the longest toe in weight-bearing, and the width must accommodate the widest part of the foot, which is

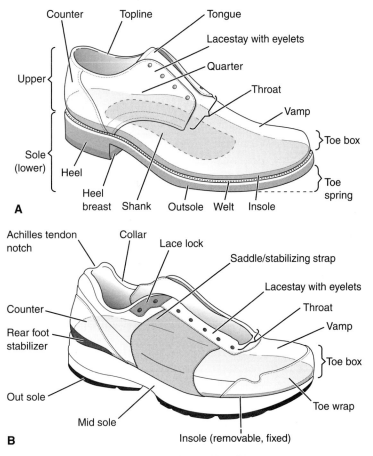

FIGURE 13.3. The terminology for the parts of (A) nonathletic and (B) athletic footware.

usually at the level of the metatarsal heads. When the shoe insert or foot plate of an orthosis wraps around the medial and lateral sides of the foot, a shoe with sufficient space to contain the appliance and the foot without exerting excessive pressure is required (**Fig. 13.5**). This may be more difficult for clients with hallux valgus and bunions, which increase the width of the forefoot. For these individuals, shoes made from a bunion last that provides additional width may be necessary. Straight last shoes also usually have more width in the metatarsal region.

The height of the **quarters** (sides and back of the shoe upper) in a low-top shoe terminates just distal to the malleoli (see Fig. 13.1). Low-top shoes are usually sufficient for most orthotic applications. High-top shoes, or boots, extend over the malleoli and provide additional stability to the rearfoot and are particularly useful in controlling unwanted medial–lateral instability. In some clients with foot drop without significant spasticity, shoes with high quarters that extend above the malleoli may be sufficient to stabilize the ankle

without an orthosis. However, high-top shoes may also cause increased pressure in areas with diminished sensation.

Shoes require an opening that allows the foot to enter easily. Some shoes simply "slip-on" and do not have any particular method of closure to secure the shoe to the foot. These shoes are generally not suitable for use with orthoses or for various foot deformities. Laces (preferably with four to five pairs of eyelets) or multiple wide straps are the best methods of securing the shoe to the foot or orthosis. They also provide the greatest range of adjustability to accommodate changes in foot girth that occur in clients with fluctuating lower limb edema. Clients with impaired hand function who are unable to tie laces can use various adaptations or replace the laces with straps that close with velcro™ pressure-sensitive tape.

The **throat** is the portion of the shoe where the foot enters and where the shoe closure attaches to the quarters (see Fig. 13.3). Three basic throat styles are

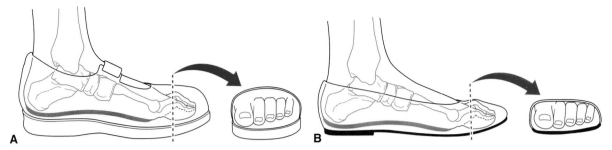

FIGURE 13.4. Adequate toe box height is an important shoe feature for clients with toe deformities (hammertoes or claw toes) or who use in-shoe orthoses. One shoe **(A)** adequately accommodates the orthosis and the toes, and the other **(B)** is inadequate.

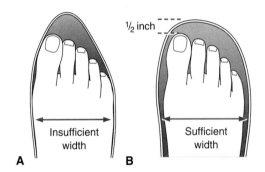

FIGURE 13.5. The toe box region must provide adequate length and width so that excessive pressure is not exerted on the foot/orthosis unit within the shoe. The shape of the toe region should match the natural anatomical shape of the weight-bearing foot. The toe box region drawn in **(B)** is appropriate.

distinguished by the design of the anterior margin of the quarters where they meet the vamp (**Fig. 13.6**):

- Blucher
- Bal or Balmoral
- "Open-to-the-toe" (surgical)[3]

Shoes with the **Blucher** throat style are preferred for use with most orthoses because they provide greater adjustability for changes in foot volume and produce a large opening, making it easier for the client to don and doff the shoe. In the Blucher style, the tongue is an extension of the vamp, and the anterior edges of the quarters are free to open and fold back during donning and doffing of the shoe. In shoes with a *Bal* throat style, the tongue is a separate piece of material sewn to the vamp and quarters. In addition, the anterior edges of the quarters are connected together, making the opening for the foot smaller and less adjustable. In the "*open-to-the-toe*" (surgical) throat style, the quarters and the tongue extend all the way to the toe of the shoe. Thus, when the shoe is unlaced, the quarters and tongue can be folded back

so that the foot can be placed flat on the insole of the shoe. This type of opening may be required for clients with severe spasticity, rigid deformities, healing ulcers or wounds, or orthoses with very rigid ankle–foot componentry.

There are several locations in the upper where *reinforcements* may be added to strengthen the shoe in areas of anticipated high stress (see Fig. 13.3). Additional stiffer material may be added to the *toe box* to protect the toes. For example, manual laborers wear boots in which the toe box has a steel reinforcement. A reinforcement added to the quarters to support the medial longitudinal arch is called a *saddle* or *arch bandage*.[1] A **counter** is a reinforcement of the posterior aspect of the quarters that cups the heel and stabilizes the hindfoot. The medial and lateral counters usually extend anteriorly to the end of the heel. However, the medial counter often extends further anterior to support the medial longitudinal arch. This long medial counter may help to support the midfoot in a client with excessive pronation. Many running and athletic shoes have an additional rigid rearfoot stabilizer added to the outside of the counters that reinforces them and provides additional assistance for stabilization of the hindfoot during high-impact activities. These additional reinforcements present in many "regular" shoes may be beneficial and contribute to the effectiveness of an orthosis in improving function.

The upper can be made from a variety of materials ranging from stiff or soft natural leathers to lightweight synthetic fabrics. The upper material must be durable but must also be soft enough to form to the foot and appliance without exerting excessive pressure on the foot. The upper material must be "breathable" and allow moisture to escape. Many contemporary orthotic appliances are made of thermoplastics, which are not breathable and cause foot sweating. Excessive moisture may cause the skin to become

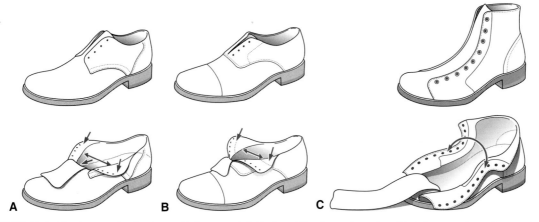

FIGURE 13.6. The throat styles for shoes with laces are **(A)** Blucher, **(B)** Bal or Balmoral, and **(C)** "open-to-the-toe" or surgical. Blucher shoes are preferred for use with most orthoses because they are easier to don and doff with an appliance and offer greater adaptability to accommodate foot volume changes.

macerated, leading to skin tears or wounds. The use of an appropriate cotton sock or cloth lining to wick perspiration away from the skin may also help with this problem. Clients with significant foot deformities may require shoes with elastic or moldable uppers to avoid excessive pressure on the dorsum of the foot.

The Sole

The *sole* of the shoe is the material to which the upper attaches and is located under the foot. The parts of the sole include (see Fig. 13.3).

- Outsole
- Welt
- Midsole
- Insole
- Heel
- Shank

The *outsole* is the material that contacts the ground. Some features of outsole materials which affect shoe selection for specific orthotic applications include durability, flexibility, weight, resilience, and ability to provide traction. The outsole often adds considerable weight to a shoe. A very heavy shoe, coupled with a heavy orthotic device, may increase the energy cost of walking. Thus, the lightest shoe that meets the client's functional needs is most desirable. The flexibility of the soling material is also an important consideration. A sole must be flexible and facilitate the "toe break" or toe extension that occurs in late stance phase and is required for a smooth roll-over transition to swing phase. Orthoses that are very rigid should be worn with shoes that have resilient

(compressible) soles that offer good shock absorption capability. The sole must also provide traction, particularly in early stance phase, to prevent slipping. However, for individuals who have difficulty with limb advancement, smooth soles are more appropriate; shoes with textured bottoms may catch on the floor and possibly cause stumbles or falls.

The *insole* or *sock liner* is the part of the sole that lies in contact with the plantar surface of the foot. These may be made of thin, flat, paper-like materials or molded or unmolded thermoplastics. Insoles or sock liners that are removable are usually desired in shoes that are worn with orthotic devices that fit into the shoe. Removing the sock liner that comes with the shoe provides more space inside the shoe to accommodate a therapeutic insert.

Midsoles, located between the insole and outsole, are most often present in athletic shoes. They are usually made of foamed polymers and serve to increase shock absorption and improve foot stability. A **shank** is a longitudinal reinforcement of the midportion of a nonathletic shoe. It is typically made of spring steel or carbon fiber and is placed between the insole and outsole. A shank typically extends from the heel to the metatarsal heads and determines where the sole flexes during late stance phase for toe extension and roll-over into swing phase. A shoe that will be fastened to a conventional double upright orthosis using a stirrup attachment requires a steel shank, so that the orthotic stirrup can be riveted securely to the shoe through its steel shank.

The *heel* is the shoe component that is added to the outsole, usually directly under the anatomical heel (calcaneus). Characteristics of heels that can dramatically affect function include their height, size, as well as resilience or ability to compress. The significance of the size of the heel is obvious: small heels contact the floor with a small area and thus can contribute to balance loss by reducing the size of the base of support. Small heels also offer little surface area for traction. The second factor to consider when selecting a shoe for use with an orthosis is the resilience or compressibility of the heel. Orthoses that restrict ankle movement should be worn with shoes that have resilient heels that compress at heel strike, absorb the impact of loading, and facilitate a smooth transition to foot flat. Shoes with very stiff or hard heels, when worn with very rigid orthoses, may produce early stance phase knee instability or buckling. The third heel characteristic to consider when selecting a shoe is its height. Researchers studying the effect of heel height on function report that as heel height increases, more weight is shifted onto the forefoot and metatarsal heads. This redistribution of weight-bearing may aggravate symptoms in individuals with metatarsalgia, hammertoes, or bunions.[4,5] Another study reports that healthy individuals wearing 2½ inch heels expend more muscular effort to maintain balance than when wearing low-heeled shoes.[6] Therefore, shoes with low, broad heels that compress and absorb shock are usually recommended for use with most lower extremity orthoses and most prostheses. This type of heel minimizes stress on the metatarsal heads and maximizes heel stability.

Heel height also affects the function of foot or ankle–foot orthoses (AFOs) as well as prostheses.

Prosthetists and orthotists usually request clients to provide a new shoe that is used to guide appliance alignment during the manufacture process. Although contemporary prostheses and orthoses can be worn with different shoes, most appliances are aligned to be worn with shoes of a particular heel height. Clients must understand that all shoes worn with a particular orthosis or prosthesis, especially an appliance with a rigid ankle, must have the same (or at least similar) heel height. Wearing a shoe with a significantly different heel height affects the position of the knee and may have significant consequences for function and safety. Wearing a lower heeled shoe may produce knee hyperextension and other gait deviations, while a higher heeled shoe is likely to produce excessive stance phase knee flexion (**Fig. 13.7**). This does not apply to prostheses fitted with an adjustable ankle component (see Chapter 6).

Shoe Construction

The type of shoe construction also affects the functional characteristics of the shoe. Shoe construction refers to the method by which the upper portion of the shoe is attached to the sole. **Figure 13.8** shows the most common methods of shoe construction (lasting), which include slip lasting, board lasting, and combination lasting.[1,3] A *slip-lasted* shoe is constructed by wrapping the upper material around the dorsum of the foot (last) and sewing it together under the foot. This is attached to the soling material, and a sock liner is used rather than an insole board. When the sock liner is removed from a slip-lasted shoe, the

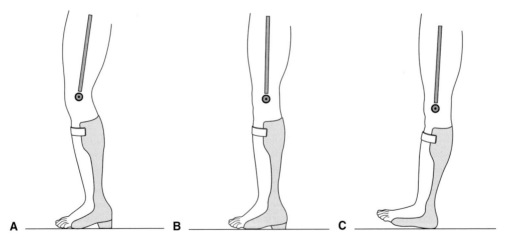

FIGURE 13.7. The effect of shoe heel height on the knee when wearing a solid ankle orthosis. The orthosis was manufactured to be worn with the shoe in (**B**). The same orthosis worn with a shoe with a higher heel (**A**) tilts the leg forward, producing excessive stance phase knee flexion and possible instability. Using the same orthosis with a lower heel (**C**) produces knee hyperextension.

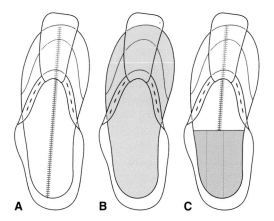

FIGURE 13.8. Shoe construction methods include **(A)** slip lasting, **(B)** board lasting, and **(C)** combination lasting.

seam or stitching that connects the right and left sides of the upper material under the foot is seen. Shoes made with this construction are usually flexible and lightweight.

A *board-lasted* shoe is made by stretching the upper material over the last. The underflaps of the upper are glued to an insole board, midsole components are added, and finally, the outsole is glued to the underside. Shoes made with this construction are less flexible and offer more stability to the foot. Board-lasted shoes with a steel shank in the midfoot region are usually required for attachment of the stirrup of a conventional double upright metal orthosis. A *welt* (see Fig. 13.3) is a strip of leather, rubber, or plastic that is stitched to the upper and insole of a shoe, as an attachment point for the sole. Selecting a shoe with a sole that is attached by using a welt is desirable when a conventional metal orthosis will be attached.

More than one construction technique can be used in the production of a shoe. Many shoes, especially athletic shoes, are board lasted in the rearfoot for more stability and slip lasted in the forefoot when flexibility is desired.

Shoe Modifications

Additional materials or modifications can be added to shoes, either internally or externally, to accomplish specific therapeutic goals. Often the same therapeutic goal can be achieved with either an internal or external modification. Foot orthoses provide additional options to achieve the goals. However, combinations of foot orthoses and shoe modifications often offer the best solutions for clients with multiple foot impairments.

Types of Shoe Modifications: Internal or External

Internal modifications are made by adding materials directly to the insole board of a shoe or by using a shoe insert as a base for the modification. In this text, shoe inserts refer to over-the-counter mass-produced appliances that are purchased in retail stores without prescription. Internal modifications that are attached to the insole board are usually preformed materials made of orthopedic felt or thermoplastic materials that are positioned in the shoe and secured in place with self-adhesive backing. These modifications cannot be moved easily from shoe to shoe, while shoe inserts can be taken out and used in different shoes. Internal modifications are typically used to provide cushioning and shock absorption, to relieve pressure-sensitive structures, or to balance small leg length discrepancies. Because these internal modifications do not permanently alter the shoe and are relatively inexpensive to purchase, they can be used as trial devices to evaluate the effectiveness of a proposed orthotic solution to a patient problem. Although they are less durable, if effective, they can be replaced with more definitive, longer-lasting appliances.

External modifications are added to the outsole by a pedorthist or a shoe repair person. Because they are attached to the outsole, they are permanent and cannot be moved from shoe to shoe. Materials added externally on the outsole or heel are subject to wear and tear and thus require periodic replacement. External modifications are typically used to balance leg length discrepancies, relieve pressure-sensitive areas on the plantar aspect of the foot, or shift the center of pressure on the weight-bearing foot. Some commonly used shoe modifications, most of which can be applied internally or externally, are presented below.

Lifts to Balance Leg Length Discrepancies

Leg length discrepancies up to 3/8 inch can be balanced with internally placed heel wedges or three-quarter-length inserts. Internal lifts do not extend under the metatarsal heads, because they may make the shoe too tight. Discrepancies that require larger lifts must be applied to the outsole, either as a heel or heel and sole lift.

Heel Wedges

Heel wedges are used to address rearfoot problems, such as fixed or functional hindfoot varus, valgus, or equinus deformities (**Fig. 13.9**). For example, a *lateral heel wedge* can be used to apply a corrective force to a flexible hindfoot varus to shift the center of pressure medially during weight-bearing. However, a *medial wedge* is used to support or balance a fixed hindfoot varus, minimizing the need for compensations at other joints. An equinus deformity that contributes to a painful foot condition, such as tendinitis, may be accommodated with a temporary heel wedge to minimize stress on the inflamed tissues. The size of the heel wedge should be the minimum effective amount. Wedges are commonly measured by the degree of the angle (apex) of the wedge (eg, 2° or 4°) or the height at the widest portion (eg, 1/8", ¼" or 3 mm, 6 mm). If the wedge is too high, the foot will slip down the slope of the wedge causing the modification to lose its effectiveness.

Other Heel Modifications

Other heel modifications include variations in the shape of the heel breast (anterior edge of the heel), the resilience or compressibility of the heel, and the addition of flares or offsets (**Fig. 13.10**). A *Thomas heel* is one in which the anterior edge or breast is curved and extends further anterior on the medial side to provide additional support to the sustentaculum tali and the posterior portion of the medial longitudinal arch in a pronating foot. A *reverse Thomas heel* is curved and extends further anterior on the lateral side.

A *SACH* (solid ankle cushion heel, taken from prosthetic foot terminology) or *plantarflexion heel* incorporates a wedge of softer or more resilient material into the posterior part of the heel to cushion the impact of limb loading during heel strike. This softer, more compliant heel may also facilitate foot flat by simulating the effect of plantarflexion. This is a desirable feature for a shoe that is used with an orthosis that restricts plantarflexion.

Heel flares increase the width of the heel on either the medial (heel *inflare*) or lateral (heel *outflare*) sides, thus increasing the size of the foot's base of support. Heel flares also provide additional hindfoot stabilization for clients with rearfoot varus or valgus deformities. For example, an outflare heel may help to prevent unwanted calcaneal inversion. An *offset heel* is also used to manage hindfoot varus or valgus alignment problems. Like the flared heel, the offset heel extends the heel width either medially or laterally, providing a broader base of support. However, in addition, the offset extends proximally and provides reinforcement or buttressing to the heel counter. This heel modification is alternatively termed an external counter or buttress. Heel offsets are often used in combination with other shoe modifications. For example, a shoe modification prescribed for a client with a fixed rearfoot varus deformity might include a medial heel wedge and a lateral offset heel. This combination of modifications supports the fixed varus deformity and provides additional lateral reinforcement to prevent unwanted inversion injuries.

Pressure Relief Additions

Another type of shoe modification is designed to reduce pressure on pressure-sensitive structures by shifting weight-bearing loads away from pressure-sensitive areas onto pressure-tolerant areas or structures. This type of shoe modification is called a pressure **relief pad** or simply a **relief**. For example, in the hindfoot, the calcaneal tubercle (the proximal attachment site for the plantar fascia) on the plantar surface of the heel is often painful in patients with plantar fasciitis. A heel insert or wedge with either a cut-out (void) or an area filled with a soft, more compliant material placed under the calcaneal tubercle can reduce pressure and thus relieve the painful structure. This modification is termed a heel wedge with a calcaneal tubercle relief (Fig. 13.10, G).

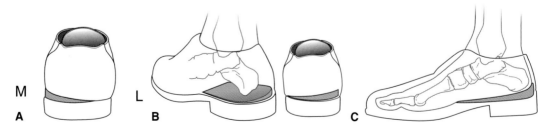

FIGURE 13.9. Heel wedges are applied externally **(A)** or internally **(B,C)**. Medial **(A)** or lateral heel wedges are used to balance or correct hindfoot varus or valgus deformities. Heel wedges **(C)** are also used to balance leg length discrepancies, accommodate equinus deformity, or produce a small flexion moment of the knee.

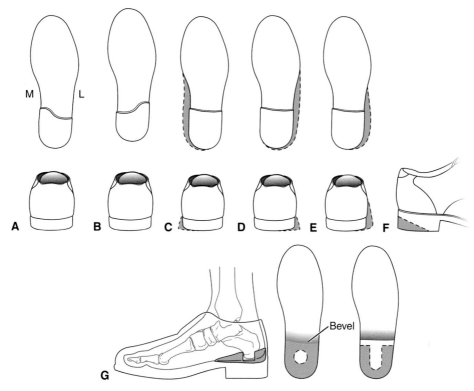

FIGURE 13.10. Heel modifications applied to a right shoe: **(A)** Thomas heel; **(B)** reverse Thomas heel; **(C)** medial outflare; **(D)** lateral outflare; **(E)** lateral offset; **(F)** solid ankle cushioned heel (SACH), cushion, or plantarflexion heel; and **(G)** insert with calcaneal tubercle relief (M = medial, L = lateral).

Forefoot Shoe Modifications

Although forefoot shoe modifications can be added either inside the shoe or to the outsole, they are most often applied internally, either by attachment directly to the insole board or via a shoe insert. Shoe modifications for the forefoot include medial or lateral wedges as well as pads of various shapes designed and positioned to relieve pressure-sensitive and painful foot structures **(Fig. 13.11)**. Medial or lateral forefoot wedges are used to support or balance forefoot structural deformities such as forefoot varus or valgus, respectively.

Relief pads are commonly used to reduce pressure on the metatarsal heads or other structures. When designed to relieve prominent or painful metatarsal heads, these pads are usually called metatarsal pads, or met pads. To be effective, however, careful placement of these pads is imperative. Metatarsal relief pads are not positioned under the painful metatarsal head but are placed just proximal to the head under the metatarsal shafts. When placement is done correctly, the metatarsal pad off-loads (relieves) the metatarsal head and shifts weight-bearing onto the pressure-tolerant metatarsal shafts.

Forefoot modifications added externally to the outsole are metatarsal bars and rocker soles **(Fig. 13.12)**. A *metatarsal bar* is intended to perform the same task as the internally applied metatarsal relief pad. It reduces plantar pressure on the metatarsal heads by adding a wedge of firm material across the sole of the shoe just proximal to the metatarsal heads. Although identical in function, externally applied metatarsal bars are rarely used today because they detract from the appearance or cosmesis of the shoe, may cause tripping, and require frequent replacement.

Rocker Soles

A **rocker sole** is a curved external shoe modification that allows the foot to roll from heel strike to toe-off without requiring the foot to bend. Rocker soles are used to

■ Reduce pressure on the metatarsal heads
■ Simulate or substitute for ankle plantar/dorsiflexion or toe extension during the stance phase

There are different types of rocker soles, ranging from those that involve the entire sole of the shoe to

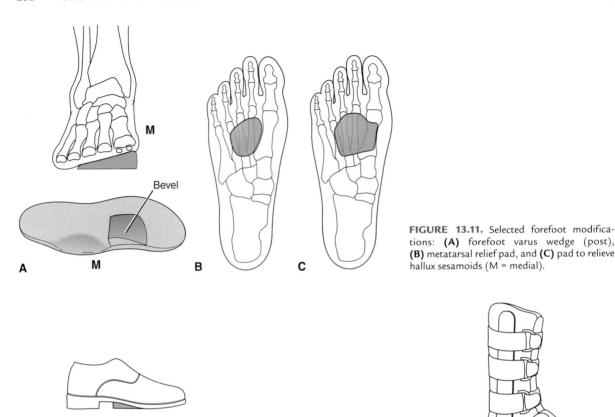

FIGURE 13.11. Selected forefoot modifications: **(A)** forefoot varus wedge (post), **(B)** metatarsal relief pad, and **(C)** pad to relieve hallux sesamoids (M = medial).

FIGURE 13.12. Sole modifications: **(A)** a metatarsal bar is positioned proximal to the metatarsal heads to reduce pressure, **(B)** forefoot and hindfoot rockers, **(C)** forefoot rocker, **(D)** a walking boot or Cam walker that immobilizes the ankle and provides a rocker sole to substitute for restricted ankle and foot movements.

those with only rearfoot or forefoot rockers (see Fig. 13.12). A forefoot rocker placed just posterior to the metatarsal heads will reduce metatarsal head pressure.[7,8] Forefoot rockers are also used to simulate toe extension during late stance phase when a rigid sole is used for immobilization. A heel or posterior rocker substitutes for plantar flexion during the loading response. Cast shoes or walking boots that immobilize the ankle often have a rocker sole to facilitate smoother roll-over and forward propulsion during stance phase. Rocker soles are also commonly used as part of specially designed shoes to minimize plantar pressures under the metatarsal heads.

FOOT ORTHOSES

Foot orthoses are custom-made and custom-fit or modified prefabricated appliances designed to apply forces to an individual's foot to improve function.

There are many different types of foot orthoses available; thus, selection of the most appropriate appliance requires the practitioner to identify specific therapeutic goals for the orthosis before making a recommendation. Specific goals for foot orthoses are listed in Box 13.4. The general process used to diagnose impairments, develop specific orthotic goals, and prescribe an appliance that can achieve them is described in Chapters 1, 11, 12, and 20. However, practitioners who recommend foot orthoses must also consider additional factors, including

- The size and weight of the patient
- How and where the client intends to use the device
- The source of abnormal forces or loads that contribute to the patient's complaints

In addition to the specific goal for a foot orthosis, the size and weight of the client as well as the client's intended usage for the device must be considered

BOX 13.4 | **Therapeutic Goals for Foot Orthoses**

■ Provide cushioning to improve shock absorption.
■ Provide relief for pressure-sensitive plantar structures.
■ Reduce shearing forces on the foot.
■ Balance or support the joints of the foot in a neutral position and protect them from abnormal or excessive compensatory stresses during function.
■ Limit or restrict excessive or abnormal movements.
■ Correct flexible deformity.
■ Accommodate and support a fixed deformity.

when selecting a foot orthosis. For example, even with the same orthotic goal, the foot orthosis that is successful for a 6-foot, 180-pound individual who wants to use the appliance during running will need to be different from the device for a 80-pound individual who will only use the device to walk short distances. An effective orthosis for the larger, more active individual needs to withstand and produce greater forces. However, this device is likely to be too rigid and may actually impair function if given to the lighter, less active client.

The source of the abnormal forces causing a client's complaints also impacts the orthotic selection process. Generally, orthotic forces are most effective when applied at or near the source of the problem. For example, consider two clients who report the same complaint: painful and excessive pronation throughout stance phase during walking. One client has structural foot deformities with normal biomechanical function at the hip and knee joints. The other client has structurally normal feet but has significant weakness at the knees and hips, resulting in compensatory and abnormal joint postures in the feet (**Fig. 13.13**). The first client will benefit from foot orthoses that support or balance the structural foot abnormalities. The second client requires interventions to address the impairments at the hips and knees. Foot orthoses to support the feet of the second client will most likely be both ineffective and painful.

Types of Foot Orthoses

Foot orthoses are divided into two broad categories based on function: accommodative orthoses and functional (biomechanical) orthoses. **Accommodative orthoses** are designed to provide protection or relief to particular areas or structures of the foot. They are used

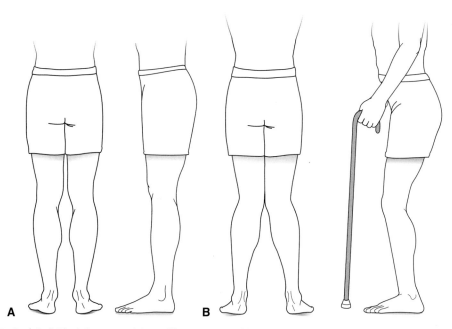

FIGURE 13.13. Both individuals have complaints of foot pain caused by excessive subtalar pronation. **(A)** This individual has structural alignment abnormalities in his feet that produce compensatory excessive pronation, but there are no impairments at the hips and knees. **(B)** This individual's feet are structurally normal, but there are impairments at the hips and knees.

to reduce plantar pressure and improve shock absorption, reduce shearing forces on the plantar aspect of the foot, and relieve painful or pressure-sensitive structures. They are prescribed for clients with impaired plantar sensation, such as those with diabetic or other types of neuropathies. Accommodative devices are also useful for those with significant rigid or fixed deformities, such as those that occur in clients with arthritis.

Functional orthoses are designed to control and support the subtalor joint, rearfoot, and forefoot and influence the biomechanical functioning of the foot during activities such as walking and running. Functional orthoses usually include wedges or posts that support the forefoot or rearfoot to prevent abnormal compensatory movements at joints within the foot or at adjacent joints proximal to the foot.

Foot orthoses are further classified by the physical properties of the materials from which they are constructed as soft, semirigid, or rigid devices.[9] Accommodative orthoses are typically soft appliances made from soft, low **durometer** materials (see Table 12.1) such as foamed thermoplastics. Examples of foamed thermoplastic materials that are used in soft orthoses are listed in **Table 13.1**. Although some accommodative orthoses are nonmolded, flat shoe inserts, most are molded to the client's foot to provide total contact between the foot and the appliance. This is particularly important when reduction of plantar pressures and relief of pressure-sensitive bony prominences, such as the metatarsal heads, is a goal. Total contact soft orthoses are usually constructed from multiple layers of different materials, in which each layer has a particular function.[10] **Figure 13.14**

TABLE 13.1	Foot Orthoses: Goals and Examples of Materials Commonly Used to Achieve Them		
Type of Orthosis	**Part of FO**	**Goal**	**Example Materials**
Functional— semirigid	Top cover or sock liner	Conform to foot; cushion	Aliplast® #10; Plastazote®— soft; Spenco®, PPT®, Poron®
	Base	Support foot and joints	Aliplast XPE; Aliplast—firm; Plastazote—firm; Suborthelen (polyethylene)
	Posts	Wedge supports for parts of foot	Nickelplast; Plastazote—firm
	Forefoot extension	Provide softness under fore-foot with ¾-length FO	PPT, Poron
Functional—rigid		Support foot; prevent compensatory movements	Acrylics, polypropylene, carbon graphite–reinforced materials
Accommodative— soft, molded	Top cover or sock liner	Conform to foot; cushion	Plastazote—soft
	Base	Support foot; absorb shock	Plastazote—medium durometer
	Additions/reliefs	Relieve pressure-sensitive areas	Plastazote—medium durometer
Accommodative— soft, nonmolded		Cushion; absorb shock	PPT, Poron, Spenco; Sorbothane®, Viscolas®

Aliplast, Nickelplast: Alimed Inc, Dedham, Massachusetts; Plastazote: Bakelite Xylonite Limited, London, United Kingdom; Poron: Rogers Corporation, Woodstock, Connecticut; PPT (Professional Protective Technology), Langer Inc., Deer Park, New York; Sorbothane: Sorbothane, Inc., Kent, Ohio; Spenco: Spenco Medical Corporation, Waco, Texas; Viscolas: Viscolas, Inc., Soddy Daisy, Tennessee.

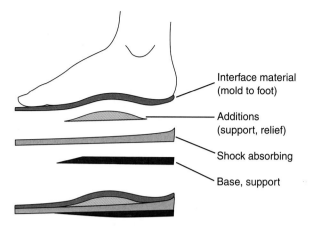

FIGURE 13.14. An accommodative foot orthosis may have multiple layers, each made from a different thermoplastic material with different properties. Softer durometer materials are used next to the foot, and a firmer material forms the base.

Interface material (mold to foot)

Additions (support, relief)

Shock absorbing

Base, support

BOX 13.5	Shoe Requirements for Use With Soft, Accommodative Orthoses
■ Shoe depth	Shoes with removable inserts or extra-depth shoes; must have sufficient space to accommodate the insert and the foot without exerting excessive pressure anywhere on the foot
■ Toe box height	High toe box is required to ensure there is sufficient space to accommodate the metatarsal relief mound
■ Toe box width	Sufficient width to accommodate any wrap-around orthotic material on the medial or lateral sides of the ball of the foot
■ Throat style and closure method	Sufficient ability to open the throat for easy donning and doffing; closure method that allows adjustability to accommodate the appliance (Blucher style)
■ Low heel height	Low heel height, usually not greater than 1 to 1.5 in.; increased heel height shifts weight onto MT heads
■ Upper material	Should be soft (moldable) and breathable
■ Sole material	Resilient to facilitate shock absorption

demonstrates how a multilayer, soft orthosis might be constructed. Different materials are selected for each layer by matching their physical properties to the specific purpose of each layer. Because these soft, accommodative orthoses include multiple layers, they are often thicker than usual shoe inserts and must be worn with shoes that provide sufficient space for the insert plus the foot without exerting excessive pressure on the foot. As a result, clients require specific instruction on the characteristics of shoes that are appropriate to wear with these orthoses. Shoe requirements for this type of soft, accommodative orthosis are listed in **Box 13.5**.

Functional orthoses are usually semirigid or rigid appliances. Because these orthoses are biomechanically designed to affect function and minimize unwanted compensatory motions, they require materials that are able to support the parts of the foot during weight-bearing without becoming compressed. Because semirigid and rigid appliances are always molded devices, they can also be designed to provide relief for pressure-sensitive areas, such as the metatarsal heads. Semirigid orthoses, like soft appliances, are usually composed of at least two layers of different materials (**Fig. 13.15**). The base layer holds and supports the joints of the foot during weight-bearing. Additional wedges of material, called posts, can be added to the orthotic base in specified areas of the hindfoot or forefoot. When abnormal structural foot alignment is present, these wedges are used to support the joints of the foot in positions where they can function more normally. Posts along with a supportive orthotic base material prevent or minimize unwanted compensatory

joint motions that can abnormally stress joints' soft tissue limiters, causing pain. Additional materials may be added to the top of the orthosis to provide a comfortable interface with the foot.

Rigid foot orthoses are usually fabricated from a single, thin layer of material that achieves all the purposes

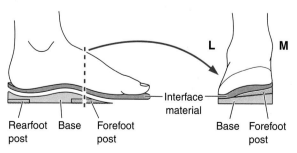

FIGURE 13.15. A semirigid functional foot orthosis is molded to the plantar surface of the foot and has at least two layers, each made of a different material.

Rearfoot post   Base   Forefoot post

L   M

Interface material

Base   Forefoot post

described for the multiple layers of a semirigid device. In order to achieve all the goals in one thin layer, the material used must be very rigid. Because rigid orthoses are very thin, they can fit into more types of shoes, which is desirable to many individuals. However, rigid appliances also have disadvantages. Because they are more rigid than any other type of foot orthosis, they "give" or yield less during use and are often uncomfortable for many wearers. Adjustments cannot be made easily or effectively after they have been formed, and their rigidity makes them more susceptible to fractures that cannot be repaired. Thus, semirigid orthoses are the most commonly selected appliances to achieve biomechanical or functional goals. Table 13.1 summarizes the types, goals, and examples of materials commonly used in many contemporary foot orthoses. More information on the properties of the materials listed is available in Table 12.1.

Parts and Features of a Foot Orthosis

The parts of a foot orthosis are diagrammed and labeled in **Figure 13.16**. The major components include the following:

- *Top cover* or *sock liner*, which interfaces with the foot
- *Base,* which provides the structural support for the orthosis
- *Relief additions,* which reduce pressure on pressure-sensitive areas by transferring loads to more tolerant locations
- Rearfoot or forefoot *posts* or *wedges*

The *orthotic base* is designed to support the foot without interfering with normal gait. The *length of the base* is an important feature of an orthosis that can affect the gait pattern of the wearer and thus must be carefully considered during the prescription process. The length of an orthosis is described as

- Three-quarter length when the orthotic base ends just proximal to the metatarsal heads
- Sulcus length when the orthosis extends under the metatarsals but ends at the sulcus between the ball of the foot and the toes
- Full length when the device extends the full length of the foot (heel to the distal end of the toes)

Most functional orthoses are three-quarter length, because an appliance of this length does not interfere with the toe extension required for a normal, smooth "roll-over" during terminal stance. Because most accommodative appliances are designed to relieve and cushion the metatarsal heads, these devices are usually full length. However, they usually do not affect the gait pattern of the wearer, because they are flexible and do not restrict joint movements. Rigid appliances cannot be longer than three-quarter length, because a longer rigid orthosis would prevent toe extension and drastically alter gait during terminal stance. Rigid or semirigid three-quarter length orthoses may have a forefoot extension constructed from a thin, resilient, but flexible material that provides comfort under the metatarsal heads without interfering with late stance roll-over. These orthotic lengths are drawn in **Figure 13.17**.

Posts are wedges of material added to the orthotic base to balance or support a fixed deformity or to correct a flexible one. For example, when a fixed foot deformity is present, foot pain may occur during weight-bearing activities because the deformity causes some joints to function atypically to compensate for the abnormal position. A post is added to a foot orthosis to support and accommodate the deformity, minimize the need for compensation, and allow the joints of the foot to move around their neutral positions during weight-bearing activities despite the deformity (**Fig. 13.18**).

Posting is also used to apply corrective forces when flexible deformities are present. For example, an individual with a fixed hindfoot varus deformity requires a post affixed under the medial side of the calcaneus to support the deformity and minimize the need for compensatory movements or positions. However, another client with a flexible hindfoot varus deformity may benefit from a laterally positioned heel wedge. For this client, the lateral rearfoot post provides a medially directed corrective force to improve the positioning of flexible foot deformity during weight-bearing activities,

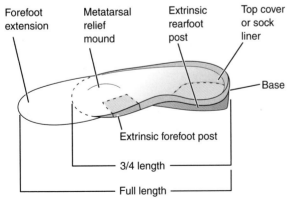

FIGURE 13.16. Parts of a foot orthosis with extrinsic posting. Not all orthoses have all the parts labeled. Medial wedges are termed varus posts; valgus posts are laterally placed wedges.

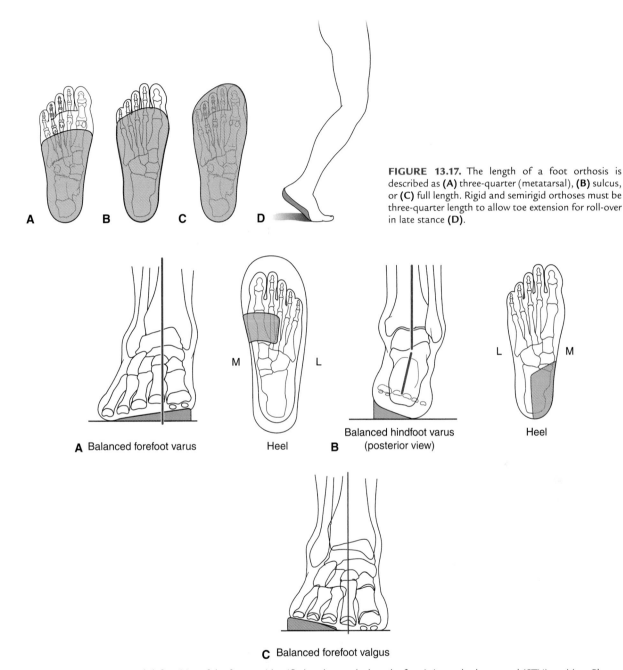

FIGURE 13.17. The length of a foot orthosis is described as **(A)** three-quarter (metatarsal), **(B)** sulcus, or **(C)** full length. Rigid and semirigid orthoses must be three-quarter length to allow toe extension for roll-over in late stance **(D)**.

FIGURE 13.18. Structural deformities of the foot are identified and named when the foot is in a subtalar neutral (STN) position. Plantar support or balancing orthoses are posted to "bring the floor up" to balance the foot and minimize compensatory movements. Forefoot varus **(A)** and valgus **(C)** deformities are balanced with posting applied to the medial or lateral forefoot, respectively. Rearfoot varus **(B)** is balanced with a medial rearfoot post.

improving gait and function. This example demonstrates that the prescription of orthotic posting requires an in-depth understanding of foot biomechanics and function, because the incorrect use of posting may be harmful and increase foot pain or dysfunction.

Posts are named according their location on the orthotic base. For example, medial rearfoot and forefoot posts are applied to the medial side of the foot (with the apex of the wedge angle near the midline of the foot). Lateral posts are applied to the lateral side of the foot. When wedges are used to support or balance structural varus or valgus deformities in the foot, the post is also named by the deformity it supports. Thus, a medial wedge applied under the calcaneus to balance a rearfoot varus deformity is called both a medial rearfoot post and a rearfoot (or hindfoot) varus post. Likewise, a lateral forefoot post used to balance a fixed forefoot valgus deformity is also called a forefoot valgus post (see **Fig. 13.18**).

Posts are also described as intrinsic or extrinsic based on the method of incorporating the post into the orthotic base. *Extrinsic posts* are wedges of material that are added to the orthotic base, usually on the inferior (floor) surface. Because the post is added to the outside of the base, adjustments can be made after the orthosis is delivered to the client, and the post can be replaced as needed due to wear. A disadvantage of extrinsic posting is that the post makes the orthosis thicker and thus limits the type of shoe into which it can fit comfortably and effectively. With *intrinsically posted* orthoses, the wedging is accomplished by modifying the negative (real or virtual) cast over which the orthotic base is manufactured. Thus, the intrinsic post is part of the orthotic base, and no additional material is required. As a result, this type of posting can only be incorporated into rigid orthoses. An advantage of intrinsic posting is that the orthosis is quite thin and can fit into many types of shoes without modification. A disadvantage, however, is that adjustments cannot be made easily to the finished intrinsically posted orthosis.

The prescription of a biomechanical foot orthosis requires evaluation of the findings of a lower quarter biomechanical examination. Readers who are unfamiliar with the lower quarter biomechanical assessment and the processes to identify alignment abnormalities can review this material in most textbooks that present methods for the musculoskeletal examination of the foot and lower limb.[11,12,13]

Functional Foot Orthoses: Mechanisms of Orthotic Control

Foot orthoses meet the diverse goals and needs of different clients by employing various biomechanical methods. The most common biomechanical methods used in foot orthoses include

- Balancing deformities with plantar supports
- Applying three-point counterforces or force couples

Foot Orthoses That Balance Foot Deformities With Plantar Supports

These orthoses are designed to provide plantar support to maintain a desired foot position and prevent stressful compensatory movements. Appropriate footwear is required to hold the foot on top of the appliance. Shoes worn with this type of orthosis must have strong counters to stabilize the calcaneus on the orthosis. Shoes must also provide sufficient support over the dorsum of the forefoot to prevent unwanted transverse plane movement of the foot on the orthosis. Simple plantar support or balancing orthoses can only be used with clients whose feet have ligamentous stability and do not have muscle imbalance deformities.[14] Although these plantar support or balancing appliances have been reported to be effective in reducing the pain that accompanies many foot conditions, how they achieve this effect is not clear. It had been widely proposed that this type of orthosis functions biomechanically and improves symptoms by reducing abnormal or excessive impact forces or joint motion.[15,16,17] More recent studies, however, suggest that the kinematic changes associated with this type of foot orthosis are too small to achieve clinical relevance or explain symptom reductions.[18,19,20] Current research suggests alternative explanations for the improvements in foot symptoms seen with these orthoses.[21] Clinicians interested in learning more about the putative mechanisms by which foot orthoses produce clinical effects should review the current research literature. The Keywords for Literature Search section at the end of this chapter provides search terms to help interested readers find relevant research regarding the effects of foot orthoses. This section also provides search terms to identify research evidence for best practices for prescribing foot orthoses for individuals with specific foot conditions or complaints.

Foot Orthoses With Three-Point Counterforces

When clients' foot impairments include ligamentous instability, significant muscle imbalance, or tendon insufficiency and tendinopathy, plantar support or balancing foot orthoses are not effective. Effective orthoses for these impairments must apply force couples or three-point counterforces to control abnormal forces in the frontal and transverse planes. Conditions that often require this type of foot orthosis include *adult acquired flatfoot* and *flexible flatfoot in children*. Several foot orthoses are designed to provide the required forces.

The *UCBL* (University of California Biomechanics Laboratory) *orthosis* is a rigid foot orthosis custom constructed from polypropylene. It was originally developed for use with children to address postsurgical correction of congenital deformities.[22] The UCBL foot orthosis is designed to correct hindfoot valgus and limit subtalar joint motion, thus preventing abnormal hindfoot frontal plane eversion and forefoot abduction. To achieve these goals, the UCBL must wrap around the medial and lateral sides of the foot in addition to providing plantar support and medial hindfoot posting. It is typically a three-quarter (metatarsal) length appliance, but it can also extend to the sulcus (**Fig. 13.19**). Although it wraps around the medial and lateral sides of the foot, its proximal trimlines are always inferior to the malleoli. This design provides a three-point counterforce system and a force couple to control calcaneal eversion in the frontal plane and a second three-point counterforce system to restrain forefoot abduction in the transverse plane (**Fig. 13.20**). For effective forefoot control, the orthotic material must wrap around the medial and lateral sides of the metatarsals, ending just proximal to the metatarsal heads.[23] To be effective, the UCBL orthosis applies high forces over a relatively small surface area. Thus, although the appliance is effective, clients often cannot tolerate the high pressures exerted by this rigid orthosis.

The *supramalleolar foot orthosis (SMO)* is an alternative that, like the UCBL, also corrects the valgus positioning of the hindfoot and restrains excessive movement at the subtalar joint. This orthosis extends proximally over the medial and lateral malleoli but does not interfere with dorsiflexion and plantarflexion. In addition, the medial and lateral trimlines of the foot plate may extend over the dorsum of the foot,

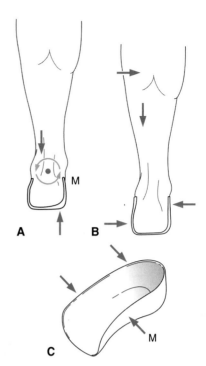

FIGURE 13.20. The University of California Biomechanics Laboratory (UCBL) foot orthosis exerts control at the subtalar joint via a force couple (**A**) and three-point counterforces to restrain calcaneal eversion (**B**). A second counterforce system (**C**) restricts forefoot abduction.

making the appliance circumferential around the instep of the foot with firm, but flexible material, usually plastic (**Fig. 13.21**). Like the UCBL foot orthosis, this appliance is effective in controlling valgus and hyperpronation, but it is more comfortable for most clients. The design of the SMO also provides the force couple and three-point counterforce systems described for the UCBL foot orthosis, as well as a counterforce system that restrains midfoot pronation and forefoot supination (**Fig. 13.21**).

If the SMO is insufficient to adequately and comfortably control the foot, an AFO is required. Two common AFO designs are the *DAFO®* (Dynamic AFO, Cascade Prosthetics and Orthotics, Bellingham, Washington) and the *Arizona AFO* (**Fig. 13.22**). The DAFO® design has a firm but flexible posterior calf "strut" that is typically used with children. The Arizona AFO is typically used with clients who have adult acquired flatfoot with significant tibialis posterior muscle/tendon insufficiency and often painful osteoarthritis as well. It is worn inside the client's footwear and is constructed from polypropylene and leather that fits circumferentially over the foot and ankle providing flexible but total containment.[14,23]

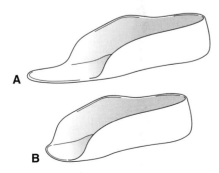

FIGURE 13.19. A University of California Biomechanics Laboratory (UCBL) foot orthosis is designed to correct hindfoot valgus, restrict subtalar joint movement, and prevent forefoot abduction. A UCBL orthosis can be sulcus length (**A**) or three-quarter length (**B**).

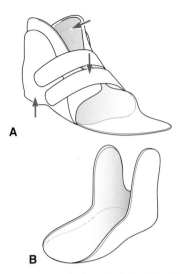

FIGURE 13.21. A supramalleolar orthosis (SMO) stabilizes the calcaneus and limits subtalar joint motion and forefoot abduction similarly to the UCBL. It also limits midfoot pronation and supination (**A**). The trimlines extend above the malleoli to limit calcaneal frontal plane motion without restricting ankle sagittal plane movement (**B**).

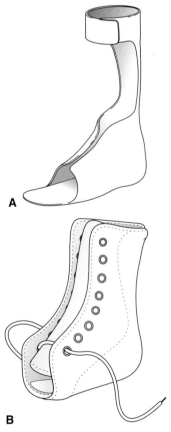

FIGURE 13.22. When foot orthoses are insufficient to control pes planus, ankle–foot orthoses (AFOs) are required. The DAFO® (**A**) is used in children with flexible flat feet. The Arizona AFO (**B**) is used with adult acquired flat foot.

SPECIAL PEDIATRIC FOOT ORTHOSES

Three specialized foot orthoses used with nonambulatory children are the Denis Browne abduction bar, the dynamic foot abduction orthosis, and the hinged shoe or Bebax bootie (Alimed, Dedham, Massachusetts). The Denis Browne abduction bar and the dynamic foot abduction orthosis are similar and are both used as part of the treatment for congenital talipes equinovarus (CTEV) or clubfoot. The hinged shoe is used to correct congenital metatarsus adductus (varus).

CTEV is a congenital deformity of the foot which includes equinovarus, supination, and metatarsus adductus. Treatment usually begins within a week of birth and requires months of manual manipulations to sequentially correct the deformity with serial casting. When the correction is completed, it must be maintained with an orthosis worn, at first, 23 hours per day and then only during sleep, until age 4.[24,25] A *Denis Browne splint* consists of a bar between the child's feet, which connects to the sole of high-top, straight last shoes with a special attachment that allows the practitioner to externally rotate the foot (**Fig. 13.23**). The abduction bar is usually the width of the child's shoulders, and the involved foot is positioned in about 70° of external rotation. The *dynamic foot abduction orthosis* is a modification of the Denis Browne splint that allows the child to move the legs reciprocally and independently to facilitate crawling. It also has a quick-release abduction bar to facilitate dressing and diaper changes without having to remove the whole brace, as well as a special mechanism as part of the shoe attachment to prevent plantarflexion. The abduction bar is attached to custom-molded plastic AFOs with soft liners that are designed to minimize skin irritations.[26] In the past, correction of other pediatric lower limb rotational deformities that originate in the femur or tibia had been attempted by using abduction foot splints. However, these orthoses are not successful in correcting deformities that originate proximal to the foot.[27]

Metatarsus adductus (varus) is a condition in which the forefoot is adducted with respect to the hindfoot. Although this condition can be acquired later in life as a muscle imbalance deformity, when it occurs as a congenital deformity in a developmentally normal child, it can be corrected with serial casting or a *hinged shoe* (Bebax bootie). A hinged shoe has a triaxial joint between separate forefoot and hindfoot parts of the shoe which allows a practitioner to make gradual progressive adjustments in all three planes

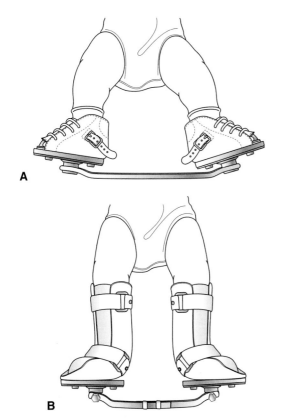

A

B

FIGURE 13.23. The Denis Browne splint **(A)** and the Dynamic foot abduction orthosis **(B)** are used to maintain corrections achieved in children with congenital club foot.

(Fig. 13.24). These shoes offer a method to normalize positioning between the forefoot and hindfoot in pre-ambulatory children.

SPECIAL SHOES AND ORTHOSES FOR INDIVIDUALS WITH DIABETES

Physical therapists and physical therapist assistants see many patients whose feet have decreased or absent sensation. This problem is associated with a number of

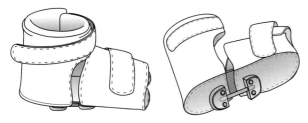

FIGURE 13.24. Hinged shoes (Bebax bootie) have an adjustable multidirectional hinge between separate forefoot and hindfoot portions of the shoe.

conditions, including atherosclerosis with diabetes, peripheral neuropathy, spinal cord injury, and spina bifida. Neuropathy is a common complication of diabetes mellitus.[28] About 60% to 70% of people with diabetes have mild to severe forms of nervous system damage, including peripheral neuropathy, and about 30% of people with diabetes age 40 years and older have impaired sensation in their feet.[28] In fact, the lifetime risk of a person with diabetes developing a foot ulcer may be as high as 25%.[29] Diabetic peripheral neuropathy impairs the motor and sensory function of the involved peripheral nerves. Impaired motor function can produce muscle imbalance deformities of the foot, which increase pressure under the metatarsal heads. Sensation acts as a protection against injury; individuals who have lost **protective sensation** due to neuropathy are likely to develop ulcers from small injuries and repetitive microtrauma. The most common cause for the development of diabetic ulcers is excessive plantar pressure in the presence of sensory neuropathy and foot deformity.[30] The most common site of ulceration is the plantar surface of the metatarsal heads. Other risk factors that also contribute to the development of diabetic foot ulcers are listed in Box 13.6.[29]

Ill-fitting shoes may contribute to the development of foot ulcers in susceptible individuals with diabetes.[31] One hundred individuals with diabetes attending a routine vascular clinic were examined for proper shoe

BOX 13.6	Risk Factors for the Development of Diabetic Foot Ulcers[29]

- Previous foot ulcer
- Peripheral neuropathy (sensory, motor, autonomic)
  - Loss of protective sensation
  - Foot deformity caused by muscle weakness and imbalances
  - Autonomic neuropathy causing dry, cracked skin
- Foot deformities (of any type)
- Partial foot amputation; amputation of contralateral lower limb
- Peripheral vascular disease
- Visual impairments (causing trauma)
- Diabetic nephropathy (causing edema, neuropathy)
- Poor glycemic control
- Cigarette smoking

fit. Only 24% had properly fitted shoes for sitting, and only 20% had the correct size for standing.[31] In another study by the Veteran's Administration, almost 75% of veterans with diabetes were wearing improperly sized shoes.[32] Patients may wear shoes that are too tight if they do not feel the extra pressure, or shoes that are too loose, believing they are reducing foot pressure, while they are actually increasing the micro trauma to the foot by slipping in the shoe during walking. The problem is compounded by the lack of consistent shoe sizes and limited availability of half sizes. Physical therapists working with individuals with diabetes should teach their patients to determine proper shoe size particularly for standing and walking. Patients should be encouraged to wear well-fitting shoes at all times and avoid walking with loose slippers, socks, or even the "booties" given to patients in the hospital.

Patient education and regular foot examination are a routine part of foot care for patients with diabetes. Foot ulceration may be prevented by proper self-care and inspection. **Box 13.7** outlines basic foot examination and principles of self-care that all patients with diabetes or vascular impairments should follow. Fitting the patient with proper shoes early can be a deterrent to the development of foot ulcers. Patients who receive Medicare Part B and whose need is certified by a physician can obtain extra-depth shoes with molded inserts once each calendar year. Some patients are not aware of this availability, and those who do not have Medicare or insurance that covers therapeutic shoes may find these shoes too expensive. Patients with atherosclerosis, particularly those with diabetes, should be seen regularly by their physician or in a specialized clinic.[30]

Therapeutic Footwear to Prevent Plantar Ulcers

The therapeutic footwear most commonly recommended for individuals with diabetes is extra-depth or depth inlay shoes. In addition to providing extra depth, these shoes typically include additional features to protect the feet and are listed in Box 13.5. These shoes provide additional space to accommodate special shoe inserts or foot orthoses that reduce pressure under the metatarsal heads. Foot orthoses or shoe inserts that are effective in reducing peak plantar pressure under the metatarsal heads are total contact inserts with specialized modifications to further reduce metatarsal head pressures.[33,34] One effective pressure-relieving modification is a medial arch build-up with a metatarsal head relief pad.[30,35] An alternative is a specially made total contact insert with multiple small removable cylindrical plugs made from a softer material which are inserted in the orthosis in the area of highest peak pressure.[36] Individuals whose foot deformities make it impossible to fit appropriately with extra-depth therapeutic shoes may require custom-molded shoes made from an individually made shoe last or three-dimensional replica of the individual's foot. The custom shoe provides a total contact fit over all surfaces of the individual's foot, including any individually required modifications to further relieve areas that are more susceptible to ulceration.

Using a cane in the contralateral hand may effectively reduce plantar pressures, particularly on the lateral side of the foot.[37,38] The use of crutches enables an individual to totally unload one limb or partially unload both limbs. However, using crutches, particularly while performing usual daily activities, may be difficult and may cause falls in individuals who also have balance issues.[38]

Orthotic Interventions for Plantar Ulcers

Despite preventative interventions, foot ulcers are a common complication of diabetes and other conditions with lower limb insensitivity. Although the use of certain types of casts and orthotic devices plays a role in the treatment of these wounds, the overall medical management of foot ulcers is beyond the scope of this textbook. To find more about the current medical management of diabetic foot ulcers, use the keywords and search terms listed at the end of the chapter.

BOX 13.7 | Guidelines for Foot and Leg Care for Patients With Diabetes

- ■ Check feet daily, morning and night
  - ■ Use mirror to check bottom of feet
- ■ Keep feet and legs clean and dry
  - ■ Wear clean socks daily
- ■ Apply water-absorbing lotion to dry skin regularly
  - ■ Keep lotions away from skin between the toes
- ■ Wear appropriately sized and supportive shoes
- ■ Do not walk barefoot or in open shoes
- ■ Trim nails straight across
  - ■ Obtain professional help for problem nails or if poor vision makes this task unsafe
- ■ Exercise feet and ankles to maintain strength and range of motion (ROM)
- ■ See foot care professional regularly to assess protective sensation

The goal of an orthotic intervention in the management of plantar ulcers is to **off-load** or relieve pressure and shear forces from the wound area. A variety of methods have been used to off-load plantar foot wounds, including bedrest, wheelchairs, crutches, total contact casting, removable walkers, and half-shoes and therapeutic shoes.[39,40] Theoretically, the use of bedrest or wheelchair or crutch ambulation should be effective methods of off-loading. The effectiveness of these methods, however, is diminished because they are rarely adhered to by patients. Additionally, they may create other problems due to the negative effects of bedrest and immobility. Although crutches and walkers effectively unload the foot, many patients with diabetic neuropathy may not have sufficient upper body strength, balance, and endurance to use them safely. The primary methods of off-loading that allow ambulation and protected weight-bearing include total contact casts, removable walking boots, half shoes, and healing shoes.[39,40]

The Total Contact Cast (TCC) is considered the "gold standard" of effective treatment of plantar ulceration in an insensitive foot.[41,42] TCCs reduce or eliminate pressure and shear on plantar ulcers while allowing the patient to remain active. Total contact casts facilitate wound healing by

- Immobilizing and protecting the wound
- Preventing edema
- Reducing pressure on the wound by its molded total contact design
- Reducing shear forces by immobilizing the joints of the foot and ankle[41–44]

Because the cast is not removable, patient compliance is ensured 24 hours per day. However, TCCs also have disadvantages: the cast must be removed and reapplied weekly by a specially trained and skilled practitioner; it must be kept dry at all times, making bathing difficult; and, many physicians do not like that the wound cannot be inspected and redressed daily.[44]

An alternative to the TCC is a removable walking boot or removable walker (RW). A RW is a padded removable AFO that immobilizes the ankle, has a rocker sole, and includes a pressure-relieving insole. It is prefabricated in different sizes and is reusable. A client with a healing plantar ulcer wears the RW when walking but can remove and reapply it daily for wound inspection and treatment as well as for bathing (**Fig. 13.25**). Various types or designs of RWs are available from different manufacturers. Some RWs are reported to be nearly as effective in reducing plantar pressures as TCCs.[45–47] Adherence to off-loading and wound protection methods may be compromised by some patients who remove their RW for ambulation in spite of instructions to use the device during all weight-bearing activities.

Another type of removable walker is a CROW, or Charcot Restraint Orthotic Walker (**Fig. 13.26**). This custom-molded, fully padded device is a combination of an AFO and a custom walking boot that was developed for diabetic patients with **Charcot neuroarthropathy**.[48] The CROW is a bivalved or clamshell appliance that fully encloses the foot and leg in molded polypropylene or copolymer, immobilizes the ankle and foot wound, and has a rocker bot-

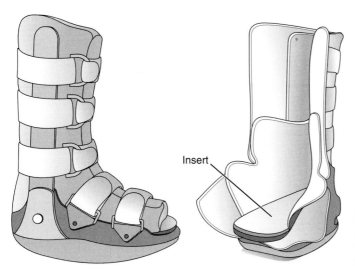

Insert

FIGURE 13.25. A removable walker (RW) or walking boot is a prefabricated orthosis that provides off-loading to the plantar surface of the foot for treatment of plantar ulcers. RWs immobilize the ankle and have a rocker sole and a pressure-relieving insert.

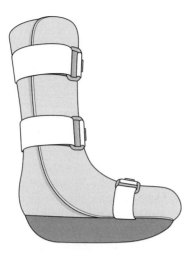

FIGURE 13.26. Charcot Restraint Orthotic Walker (CROW) is used to treat plantar ulcers in individuals with Charcot neuroarthropathy.

tom sole to prevent shear. It is worn continuously but can be removed for wound care, bathing, and sleep. Because of the rocker bottom, it usually requires the application of a lift to the contralateral shoe to minimize leg length discrepancy.

Another treatment option for off-loading the forefoot is the half shoe. A half shoe has a wedged sole that ends proximal to the metatarsal heads (**Fig. 13.27**). The wedged half sole places the ankle in a small amount of dorsiflexion that theoretically relieves metatarsal head pressure by eliminating push-off or propulsion during late stance phase. Despite this proposed mechanism, half shoes are not as effective as either TCCs or RWs in reducing plantar pressures or in facilitating healing of existing ulcers.[42,45,46] Additionally, patients with diabetic neuropathy and plantar ulcers often have heel cord contractures, which may make it difficult to achieve proper fit and safe function when wearing half shoes with dorsi-

flexed soles. Patients usually require ambulatory aids to ensure safety when walking with half shoes.

Healing shoes or sandals or postoperative shoes are often recommended as a transition from the off-loading devices to therapeutic footwear, which is worn after the ulcer is healed to prevent reulceration.[42] They are not recommended for use while a wound is still healing. Healing shoes or sandals may be custom-made or prefabricated in various sizes. They are constructed from plastazote or similar materials of various durometers that are custom molded to the client's foot. These shoes have a removable pressure-relieving insole that interfaces with the plantar surface of the foot. Most also have a rocker outer sole to minimize plantar shear forces. A variety of designs are available, and clinicians must carefully evaluate the features of commercially available healing shoes to ensure that the shoe meets the individual needs of each patient. Examples of healing shoes and sandals are shown in **Figure 13.28**.

The care of the diabetic foot, construction of individualized insoles and special shoes, has become a specialty of its own, and detailed study is beyond the scope of this text. Individualized pressure gradients can be computer developed, as are the special insoles to reduce plantar stress for each person.[49] The effectiveness of pressure-relieving total contact inserts is discussed in this chapter under the heading, Therapeutic Footwear to Prevent Plantar Ulcers. Despite evidence for their effectiveness, the problem of client acceptance of special inserts or shoes

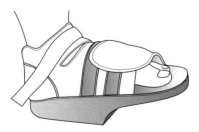

FIGURE 13.27. Half shoes may be used to off-load a forefoot ulcer. A lift may be required on the contralateral shoe to avoid leg length discrepancy.

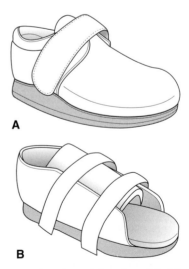

FIGURE 13.28. Healing shoes **(A)** and sandals **(B)** are made of moldable materials and include removable and replaceable pressure-relieving insoles.

remains.[50] Therapeutic shoes come in limited styles and colors and are often not aesthetically pleasing to clients. To facilitate client acceptance and use of appropriate footwear, health professionals should investigate patient preferences more thoroughly when prescribing therapeutic shoes.

A GUIDE FOR PRESCRIPTION OF SHOE MODIFICATIONS AND FOOT ORTHOSES

The process of developing an orthotic prescription is described in Chapter 12. Specific prescriptions for shoes and foot orthoses are developed through the process of identifying the impairments, establishing specific goals related to the impairments, and designing a biomechanical device to apply the forces required to achieve the goals. Practitioners who contribute to developing orthotic prescriptions must also consider client performance while using a trial or temporary foot appliance as well as evidence for appliance effectiveness as reported in current research literature. The Keywords for Literature Search section at the end of this chapter provides search terms to help clinicians identify relevant research reports. **Table 13.2** and Figure 14.21 summarize guidelines for prescription of shoe modifications and foot orthoses for common foot impairments.

THE CHECKOUT EXAMINATION FOR SHOES, SHOE MODIFICATIONS, AND FOOT ORTHOSES

When a new therapeutic shoe, shoe with prescribed modification, or foot orthosis is received, a therapist must conduct an orthotic checkout examination of the client, the device, and the client wearing the device during function. This procedure is discussed in Chapter 11. The purpose of the checkout is to ensure that the device has been manufactured as prescribed and that its fit, function, comfort, and cosmesis are acceptable. Some specific features that should be inspected in a shoe or foot orthosis are listed in **Box 13.8**. The orthotist or pedorthist, therapist, and patient must work together to resolve any problems in any of these areas. When it is determined that the device is satisfactory, the therapist must review the orthotic goals and ensure that they are achieved or implement a training program to accomplish them. Particularly for new orthosis wearers, this requires

BOX 13.8	Specific Items to Include in the Checkout Examination of Therapeutic Shoes and Foot Orthoses

- Evaluate shoe/insert fit at time of day when feet are largest (late in day or after being on feet)
- Evaluate both feet for fit individually (feet may not be same size)
- Length of shoe: about 1 cm longer than longest toe in standing
- Width of shoe: widest part of shoe's forefoot region matches the widest part of the foot in standing
- Toe break: the distance from the heel to the first and fifth metatarsal heads matches the distance from the heel of the shoe to the shoe's toe break
- Toe box height: sufficient height to avoid pressure on the dorsum of toes
- Ability to accommodate changes in foot girth (ability to tighten or loosen closure)
- Foot does not slide in shoe during walking (shear)
- Heel does not piston during walking; heel is well stabilized by counters
- If shoe modifications are present:
  - Shoe is stable on ground in weight-bearing
  - Modification achieves its goal
  - Foot is stable in shoe, does not rock or shift
- If foot orthosis is used in the shoe:
  - Insert fits snugly into shoe and is stable (does not rock)
  - Insert does not slip or slide in shoe during walking
  - Shoe fit described above is adequate with orthosis in place in shoe
  - Heel of shoe fits contours of heel of foot; heel adequately seated in shoe with orthosis in place

patient instruction in proper methods of donning, doffing, and caring for the orthosis, as well as guidelines for appropriate footwear for use with the device. Functional training may also be necessary, including gait training, as well as other types of functional activities, such as steps, negotiating all types of indoor and outdoor surfaces, ramps, and getting up and down from the floor. If running and other higher-level functions are appropriate for the client, these should be included as well. Asking patients to identify functional activities that are important to or difficult for them helps clinicians individualize training and focus on relevant functional skills.

TABLE 13.2	Guide to Prescription of Shoe Modifications and Foot Orthoses	
Impairment	**Shoes/Shoe Modification**	**Foot Orthosis**
Metatarsal head pain	• Metatarsal (MT) bar • Metatarsal pad • Rocker sole	• Soft insert (nonmolded) • $3/4$-length molded insert with MT head relief
Painful bunion (Hallux abductovalgus)	• Wide or straight last shoe • Bunion last shoe	
Painful calcaneal tubercle (plantar fasciitis)	• Cushion heel • Longitudinal medial arch support	• Molded insert with calcaneal tubercle relief • Posting to prevent compensatory pronation
Painful claw toes, hammer toes	• High toe box • MT pad	
Unstable heel	• Medial or lateral heel flares ± buttressing • Firm medial or lateral heel counters	• Heel posting to balance hindfoot and prevent compensatory movement
Hyperpronation	• Long medial counter • Thomas heel	• Heel or forefoot medial/varus posting to prevent compensation
Insufficient ankle plantarflexion for early stance	• Resilient or SACH-type heel • Heel rocker	
Insufficient ankle dorsiflexion or toe extension for late stance	• Forefoot rocker	
Leg length discrepancy	• Heel or sole lift	• Heel wedge

SUMMARY

Orthotic devices used to address problems of the foot include shoes, shoe modifications, foot orthoses, and AFOs. Foot orthoses are classified by function as accommodative or functional (biomechanical). They are also classified according to the materials used in their construction as soft, semirigid, or rigid. The components of shoes, therapeutic shoes, and shoe modifications and their applications are also discussed.

Selection of the best shoe or orthosis for a particular client relies on the findings of the preorthotic patient examination (Chapter 11), including a functional and biomechanical assessment. Based on these findings, specific orthotic goals are established, including functional and impairment-based goals (Chapter 12). An appropriate shoe, shoe modification, or orthosis is prescribed by choosing componentry to apply forces to achieve the goals. Methods by which the orthotic designs and components described in this chapter apply forces to limit unwanted movements are discussed in Chapter 2 and include plantar support forces to balance deformity, three-point counterforces, and force couples.

When a new shoe or orthosis is received by a client, the therapist must perform a checkout examination to ensure proper fit, function, comfort, and cosmesis. In addition, therapists must provide functional training in donning and doffing the device as well as required care or maintenance of the device. Patient training and instruction are required to ensure that the functional goals established when the prescription was made are achieved.

KEYWORDS FOR LITERATURE SEARCHS

For each search topic, choose relevant terms from each domain and search using the Boolean term "AND."

Search Topic: What Are the Effects of Foot Orthoses?

Intervention: Foot Orthoses
Foot + Orthoses
Orthotic devices

Effect
Foot
Kinetics
Kinematics
Electromyography
Muscle activity
Running mechanics
Joint coupling patterns
Proprioception
Balance

Search Topic: What Foot Orthoses Are Most Effective for Individuals with Particular Conditions?

Intervention: Foot Orthoses
Foot orthoses
Orthotic device + foot

Conditions:
Pronation
Plantar fasciitis
Achilles tendonitis
Patellofemoral pain syndrome
Cavus foot
Posterior tibial tendon dysfunction
Adult acquired flatfoot
Running/knee injuries, leg injuries, ankle injuries
Athletic injuries/running, knee injuries, leg injuries, ankle injuries

Search Topic: How Are Diabetic Foot Ulcers Managed Medically?

Diabetic foot/complications, drug therapy, surgery, therapy
Foot ulcer/etiology, therapy, prevention and control

Search Topic: What Type of Shoes and Shoe Inserts Are Most Effective for Individuals with Particular Conditions?

Intervention: Shoes and shoe inserts
Shoes
Orthotic devices + foot

Conditions:
Running/knee injuries, leg injuries, ankle injuries
Diabetic foot/complications, therapy
Diabetic neuropathy/complications
Foot injuries
Foot ulcers/prevention and control, therapy
Osteoarthritis + foot/knee osteoarthritis
Diabetes mellitus
Diabetes mellitus, type I
Diabetes mellitus, type 2

REFERENCES

1. McPoil TG: Footwear. Phys Ther 68:57–65, 1988.
2. Janisse DJ, Janisse EJ: Pedorthic and orthotic management of the diabetic foot. Foot Ankle Clin N Am 11:717–734, 2006.
3. Frey C: Shoes. In Goldberg B, Hsu JD (eds): Atlas of orthoses and assistive devices, 3rd ed. St. Louis, Mosby, 1997, pp 225–239.
4. Corrigan JP, Moore DP, Stephens MM: Effect of heel height on forefoot loading. Foot Ankle 14:148–152, 1993.
5. Gastwirth BW, O'Brien TD, Nelson RM, et al: An electrodynographic study of foot function in shoes of varying heel heights. J Am Podiatr Med Assoc 81:463–472, 1991.
6. Franklin ME, Chong RKY: Balance control during positive heel incline. Neurology Report 23:194, 1999.
7. Nawoczenski DA, Birke JA, Coleman WC: Effect of rocker sole design on plantar forefoot pressures. J Am Pod Med Assoc 78:455–460, 1988.
8. Posema K, Burm PET, Zande ME, et al: Primary metatarsalgia: the influence of a custom moulded insole and a rocker bar on plantar pressure. Prosthet Orthot Int 22:35–44, 1998.
9. Lockard MA: Foot orthoses. Phys Ther 68:66–73, 1988.
10. Chambers RB, Elftman N: Orthotic management of the neropathic and dysvascular patient. In Goldberg B, Hsu JD (eds): Atlas of orthoses and assistive devices, 3rd ed. St. Louis, Mosby, 1997, 427–453.
11. Wooden MJ: Biomechanical evaluation for functional orthotics. In Donnatelli RA (ed): The biomechanics of the foot and ankle, 2nd ed. Philadelphia, F.A. Davis, 1996, pp 168–183.

12. Fromherz WA: Examination. In Hunt GC, McPoil TG (eds): Physical therapy of the foot and ankle, 2nd ed. New York, Churchill Livingstone, 1995, pp 81–113.

13. Magee DJ: Orthopedic physical assessment, 4th ed. Philadelphia, Saunders, 2002, pp 765–845.

14. Richie DH: A new approach to adult-acquired flatfoot. Podiatry Today 17:32–46, 2004.

15. Bates BT, Dufek JS, Davis HP: Foot orthotic devices to modify selected aspects of lower extremity mechanics. Am J Sports Med 7:338–342, 1979.

16. Johanson MA, Donatelli R, Wooden MJ, et al: Effects of three different posting methods on controlling abnormal subtalar pronation. Phys Ther 74:149–161, 1994.

17. Rodgers MM, Leveau BF: Effectiveness of foot orthotic devices used to modify pronation in runners. J Orthop Sports Phys Ther 4:86–90, 1982.

18. Ferber R, McClay I, Dorsey WS: Effect of foot orthotics on rearfoot and tibia joint coupling patterns and variability. J Biomech 38:477–483, 2005.

19. Nester CJ, van der Linden ML, Bowker P: Effect of foot orthoses on the kinematics and kinetics of normal walking gait. Gait Posture 17:180–187, 2003.

20. Zammit GV, Payne CB: Relationship between positive clinical outcomes of foot orthotic treatment and changes in rearfoot kinematics. J Am Pod Med Assoc 97:207–212, 2007.

21. Murley GS, Bird AR: The effect of three levels of foot orthotic wedging on the surface electromyographic activity of selected lower limb muscles during gait. Clin Biomech 21:1074–1080, 2006.

22. Noll KH: The use of orthotic devices in adult acquired flatfoot deformity. Foot Ankle Clinics 6:25–36, 2001.

23. Logue JD: Advances in orthotics and bracing. Foot Ankle Clinics 12:215–232, 2007.

24. Morcuende JA, Dolan LA, Dietz FR, Ponseti IV: Radial reduction in the rate of extensive corrective surgery for clubfoot using the Ponseti method. Pediatrics 113:376–380, 2004.

25. Abdelgawad AA, Lehman WB, van Bosse H et al: Treatment of idiopathic clubfoot using the Ponseti method: minimum 2-year follow-up. J Ped Orthop 16:98–105, 2007.

26. Chen RC, Gordon JE, Luhmann SJ, et al: A new dynamic foot abduction orthosis for clubfoot treatment. J Ped Orthop 27:522–528, 2007.

27. Sass P, Hassan G: Lower extremity abnormalities in children. Am Family Physician 68:1–8, 2003.

28. The 2007 National Diabetes Fact Sheet, American Diabetes Association, 1701 North Beauregard Street, Alexandria, VA 223111: www.diabetes.org/, accessed 5/6/2010.

29. Boulton AJM, Armstrong DG, Albert SF, et al: Comprehensive foot examination and risk assessment. Diabetes Care 31:1679–1685, 2008.

30. Mueller MJ, Lott DJ, Hastings MK, et al: Efficacy and mechanism of orthotic devices to unload metatarsal heads in people with diabetes and a history of plantar ulcers. Phys Ther 86:833–842, 2006.

31. Harrison SJ, Cochrane L, Abboud RJ, Leese GP: Do patients with diabetes wear shoes of the correct size? Int J Clin Pract 61(11):1900–1904, 2007.

32. Nixon BP, Armstrong DG, Wendell C, et al: Do US veterans wear appropriately sized shoes? The Veterans Affairs shoe size selection study. J Am Pod Med Assoc 96(4):290–292, 2006.

33. Lott DJ, Hastings MK, Commean, PK, et al: Effect of footwear and orthotic devices on stress reduction and soft tissue strain of the neuropathic foot. Clin Biomech 22:352–359, 2007.

34. Zequera M, Stephan S, Paul J: Effectiveness of moulded insoles in reducing plantar pressure in diabetic patients. Annual International Conference of the IEEE Engineering in Medicine and Biology Society, 2007, pp 4671–4674.

35. Guldemond NA, Leffers P, Schaper NC, et al: The effects of insole configurations on forefoot plantar pressure and walking convenience in diabetic patients with neuropathic feet. Clin Biomech 22:81–87, 2007.

36. Actis RL, Ventura LB, Lott DJ, et al: Multi-plug insole design to reduce peak plantar pressure on the diabetic foot during walking. Med Biol Eng Comput 46:363–371, 2008.

37. Wertsch JJ, Loftsgaarden JD, Harris GF, et al: Plantar pressure with contralateral versus ipsilateral cane use [abstract]. Arch Phys Med Rehabil 71:772, 1990.

38. Kwon O-Y, Meuller M: Walking patterns used to reduce forefoot plantar pressures in people with diabetic neuropathies. Phys Ther 81:828–835, 2001.

39. Wu SC, Armstrong D: The role of activity, adherence, and offloading on the healing of diabetic foot wounds. Plastic & Reconstructive Surg 117(Suppl):248S–253S, 2006 June.

40. Bolton JM: Pressure and the diabetic foot: clinical science and offloading techniques. Am J Surg 187(Suppl):17S–24S, 2004.

41. Mueller MJ, Diamond JE, Sinacore DR, et al: Total contact casting for diabetic plantar ulcers: controlled clinical trial. Diabetes Care 12:384–388, 1989.

42. Armstrong DG, Nguyen HC, Lavery LA, et al: Off-loading the diabetic foot wound: a randomized clinical trial. Diabetes Care 24:1019–1021, 2001.

43. Rather HM, Boulton JM: Pathogenesis of foot ulcers and the need for offloading. Horm Metab Res 37(Suppl 1):61–68, 2005.

44. Sinacore DR: Total contact casting for diabetic neuropathic ulcers. Phys Ther 76:296–301, 1996.

45. Lavery LA, Vela SA, Davery DC, et al: Reducing dynamic foot pressures in high-risk diabetic subjects with foot ulcerations: a comparison of treatments. Diabetes Care 19:818–821, 1996.

46. Fleischli JG, Lavery LA, Vela SA, et al: Comparison of strategies for reducing pressure at the site of neuropathic ulcers. J Am Pod Med Assoc 87:466–472, 1997.

47. Armstrong DG, Lavery LA, Wu S, et al: Evaluation of removable and irremovable cast walkers in the healing of diabetic foot wounds: a randomized controlled trial. Diabetes Care 28:551–554, 2005.

48. Morgan JM, Biehl WC, Wagner FW: Management of neuropathic arthropathy with the charcot restraint orthotic walker. Clin Orthop 296:58–63, 1993.

49. Mueller MJ: Application of plantar pressure assessment in footwear and insert design. J Orthop Sports Phys Ther 29:747–755, 1999.

50. Johnson M, Newton P, Goyder E: Patient and professional perspectives on prescribed therapeutic footwear for people with diabetes: a vignette study. Patient Educ Counseling 64:167–172, 2006.

14

Orthoses for Ankle Impairments

OBJECTIVES

At the end of this chapter, all students are expected to:

1. Describe the types (categories) and functions of ankle–foot orthoses.
2. Identify and describe the parts of ankle–foot orthoses, including the materials and componentry used.
3. Discuss applications for ankle–foot orthoses to improve function.

Physical Therapy students are expected to:

1. Determine the need for ankle–foot orthoses for a client based on examination findings.
   a. Evaluate client examination findings, including preorthotic prescription examination, lower quarter biomechanical assessment, and functional and gait analyses to diagnose impairments that may be improved by an ankle–foot orthosis.
2. Develop appropriate goals for ankle–foot orthoses.
3. Describe the biomechanical methods employed in ankle–foot orthoses to achieve the orthotic goals.
4. Develop and execute a search strategy to identify research evidence for the effects and effectiveness of ankle–foot orthoses and to identify best practices for orthotic prescription.
5. Recommend ankle–foot orthoses as part of a plan of care for individuals with impairments of the foot and ankle to optimize function.
6. Recommend shoes with appropriate characteristics for use with specific ankle–foot orthoses.
7. Examine and evaluate ankle–foot orthoses for acceptable fit, function, comfort, and cosmesis.

CASE STUDIES

Harry Green is a 67-year-old African American widower who suffered a thrombotic cerebral vascular accident (stroke) that produced right hemiparesis. Mr. Green's case and clinical findings are described in Chapter 2.

Adam Pressman is an 18-year-old high school student who fell and landed outside the pit while practicing pole vaulting, fracturing his L4 vertebra. He was evacuated by helicopter to a trauma center and had surgery to stabilize the spine. After months of rehabilitation, he has recovered all his lower limb function, except bilateral ankle strength in dorsiflexion and eversion, which remain poor (2/5), and plantarflexion, which is fair (3+/5), but exhibits poor muscle endurance. His sensation and muscle tone are normal, and he does not experience any abnormal muscle spasms. His lower extremity range of motion (ROM) is full and pain free for all joints. Although he is able to walk, he has bilateral foot drop, which causes him to walk with a slow, steppage gait.

Malika Miller is a 30-year-old high school teacher with a chronic problem with her left ankle. She played soccer during high school and college and sustained several left lateral ankle sprains during that time. She responded typically to usual treatment, missing some games, but generally returned to play without impairment. This season she began coaching the girls' soccer team where she teaches. Four months ago while demonstrating some plays to the team, she resprained the ankle. She again received usual care and initially had her usual response. She received physical therapy for 3 weeks and was discharged with a home program 2 months ago. Currently she has full, pain-free passive ROM, and muscle strength on manual muscle testing is 5/5. However, she still is unable to run "normally," experiences swelling at the end of the day even if only walking, and, in general, feels "like it isn't right." Ligament stress testing shows she has moderate tibiotalar instability compared to the right side, mild to moderate impairment of left ankle proprioception, as well as dynamic balance deficit. She is dissatisfied with her current functional level and wants to return to amateur competitive play in soccer as well as coaching.

Case Study Activities

All Students

1. For each client, identify and discuss the functional problems that may be improved with an ankle–foot orthosis.
2. If an ankle-foot orthosis is prescribed, discuss the effects it might have on each client's gait.
3. Identify advantages and disadvantages of using an orthosis for each client.
4. Describe biomechanically how an ankle–foot orthosis will affect each client's impairments and improve function.

Physical Therapy Students:

1. Identify and describe the impairments that contribute to each client's functional limitations.
2. Develop specific orthotic goals for each client.
3. Develop an orthotic prescription to achieve the best outcome and functional improvement for each client.
4. Develop a physical therapy plan of care for each client, which includes an orthosis, if appropriate, as well as other physical therapy interventions. How will you determine and measure the effectiveness of the appliance and the overall functional outcome?
5. Using biomechanical terminology, name the orthosis that you recommend for each client.
6. Describe the type of orthosis and the componentry that will achieve the orthotic goals in the appliance that you recommend.
7. Recommend the type of shoes that the client should wear with the prescribed orthosis. Explain why the characteristics of the recommended shoes are required.

ANKLE ORTHOSES

Ankle orthoses (AOs) are appliances that affect movement at the ankle or subtalar joints but do not affect the joints of the foot. AOs are most frequently used in the management of musculoskeletal disorders of the ankle, particularly acute and chronic ankle sprains or instability. The most common type of ankle sprain occurs in inversion and plantarflexion, which injures the lateral collateral ligaments of the ankle. For acute sprains, an orthosis is used to protect the injured ligaments and promote healing by limiting inversion without restricting dorsi- and plantarflexion. These appliances are also used by individuals with chronic ankle instability and recurring sprains due to ligamentous incompetence. Two basic types of AOs are used for these applications: stirrup orthoses and lace-up or gauntlet orthoses.[1,2] Both of these types of appliances are prefabricated, over-the-counter devices that are fit according to shoe size. Both are worn inside footwear and require shoes with firm counters to stabilize the calcaneus.

Stirrup-Type Ankle Orthoses

Stirrup AOs are composed of rigid plastic struts that cover the malleoli and the medial and lateral sides of the lower one-third of the leg (**Fig. 14.1**). These struts are connected under the foot by a strap, heel cup, or foot plate. In some models, the medial and lateral struts are articulated at the ankle joint. The struts are lined with gel or prefilled air cells (Aircast Air-Stirrup, Summit, New Jersey) to provide comfortable total contact and compression that assists in reducing edema. Those with a simple strap under the foot to connect the medial and lateral struts restrict inversion and eversion with little effect on plantar- or dorsiflexion. The heel cup and footplate types of connectors provide greater restriction of movement in the joints of the hindfoot. Those with ankle articulations (joints) attempt to provide maximum stabilization to the joints of the hindfoot without restricting ankle plantar- or dorsiflexion.

Lace Up–Type Ankle Orthoses

Lace-up (gauntlet) AOs are typically made of fabric or vinyl; fit into a shoe; and encase the midfoot, subtalar

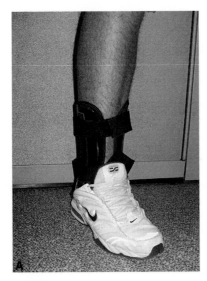

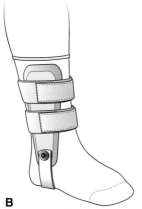

FIGURE 14.1. Stirrup-type ankle orthoses stabilize the calcaneus. They consist of medial and lateral padded struts that restrict frontal plane movements (inversion, eversion) without limiting dorsi- and plantarflexion. Both unarticulated **(A)** and articulated **(B)** styles are available.

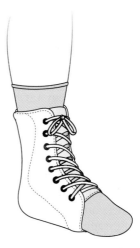

FIGURE 14.2. Lace-up (gauntlet) ankle orthoses restrict motion of the calcaneus and subtalar joint in the frontal plane but also provide some limitation of dorsi- and plantarflexion.

joint, and tibiotalar joint (**Fig. 14.2**). They have a front-lacing system to provide a snug fit, and many styles have additional Velcro straps or reinforcements to further restrain inversion. However, because they are circumferential, they may also place some limitation on dorsi- and plantarflexion ROM. Some lace-up devices also have U-shaped reinforcements around the malleoli to provide additional support to the ankle as well as compression to minimize edema. Studies that report on the effectiveness and efficacy of various types of AOs are available.[1,2] Orthotic selections for an individual with a particular ankle disorder and impairments should be made based on evidence of best practice as reported in the research literature. Keywords and

search terms that can be used to identify relevant current research findings to guide the prescription of AOs for individuals with acute and chronic ankle injuries are found at the end of the chapter.

ANKLE–FOOT ORTHOSES

Impairments that affect both the ankle and the foot may be improved by an ankle–foot orthosis (AFO). Many different types of AFOs are available, each with different designs that address different problems. AFOs are broadly classified by the types of materials and components used in their fabrication as conventional, molded, or hybrid orthoses (see Box 12.8). Specific terminology used to describe AFOs, as well as other types of orthoses, can be reviewed in Chapter 12 (see Boxes 12.5, 12.6, and 12.7).

Because AFOs contain the joints of the foot and ankle, it is not surprising that these appliances are used to affect the position and movements of these joints. However, although AFOs do not extend across the knee joint, some are designed to influence positioning, movement, and function at proximal joints, including the knee, hip, and trunk. AFOs that affect proximal joints that are not enclosed within the orthosis are termed ground reaction or floor reaction AFOs (**GR-AFO** or FR-AFO) because they exert control on nonbraced joints by manipulating the location of the ground reaction force vector (GRFV) with respect to the proximal joints. The effect of the GRFV on joint movement is reviewed in Chapter 2 on biomechanics (Methods of Force Application to Produce Movement: Designs That Manipulate the Ground Reaction Force Vector or Line of Gravity).

This chapter describes the various types of materials and componentry used in constructing AFOs. However, before prescribing an AFO for an individual with a particular problem or selecting the components of the AFO, practitioners must determine clear functional and specific orthotic goals based on functional and biomechanical assessments of the client. The pre-orthotic client examination and the orthotic prescription process are outlined in Figures 11.1 and 12.1, respectively. Readers are encouraged to review these processes prior to reading this chapter on AFO componentry and prescription.

AFOs, like most orthoses, are biomechanical interventions that achieve goals by applying forces to facilitate or restrain joint movement. The various ways in which they apply forces are described in Chapter 2 on biomechanics, and a summary of these methods of orthotic force application is outlined in Box 12.1. To be effective, clinicians who work with clients who use or may benefit from AFOs must have a sound working knowledge and understanding of these biomechanical principles and how they interact with clients, their impairments, and pathologies to improve function.

Conventional Ankle–Foot Orthotic Components

Conventional orthoses are made primarily of metal parts covered in and padded with leather, fabric, or plastic materials. For many years, these were the only types of orthotic components available. However, since the 1970s, molded plastics and, more recently, composite materials are used more commonly in AFO prescriptions. The conventional metal componentry discussed in this section is more often used today along with molded orthotic parts to form hybrid, articulated (hinged) appliances. The various types of metals used in orthotic componentry are described in Chapter 12. Although metal components are very strong and durable, they are usually heavier than those made of plastic or composite materials. Metals that are strong and lightweight are usually very expensive and may be more difficult to work with. When choosing materials to construct an orthosis, orthotists must consider componentry weight. Because heavier appliances usually require their wearers to expend more energy during functional activity, components that have sufficient strength and durability but are also lightweight are preferred.

Shoes, Shoe Attachments, and Basic Components

The shoe is an integral part of any lower extremity orthosis, but it is particularly important to the function of a conventional orthosis. In a conventional orthosis, the shoe is physically attached to the brace and must be able to contribute the necessary forces to achieve its biomechanical goal. Thus, the shoe must have strong counters to stabilize the calcaneus. It must also provide good support for the midfoot and a stable attachment point for the orthosis. A steel or carbon fiber shank in the midsole is required to provide a stable shoe-orthosis attachment (see Fig. 13.3). A properly prescribed orthosis attached to an inadequate shoe is ineffective.

Figure 14.3 depicts the basic components of a conventional double upright AFO. The conventional AFO typically has medial and lateral metal *uprights* that extend from the ankle joint to the *calf band*, which is usually located about 1 in. inferior to the fibular head. Occasionally an orthosis may have only one upright, but this makes the appliance significantly weaker, although also lighter in weight. The uprights connect to the shoe by way of a stirrup. A *stirrup* is a U-shaped piece of metal (usually steel) that is riveted to the shank of the shoe at a point that is just anterior to the calcaneus. This stirrup attachment is permanent, and the wearer cannot move the orthosis to any other shoe on a day-to-day basis. However, the orthotist can replace the shoe on the orthosis if it wears out. The superior ends of the U-shaped stirrup form the *orthotic ankle joint* where they articulate with the medial and lateral uprights. The calf band is a metal posterior connection between the superior aspects of the medial and lateral uprights. It is usually padded and covered in a leather *calf cuff*. The anterior portion of the cuff provides a closure, usually Velcro strapping, which secures the appliance to the leg.

Ankle Joints and Orthotic Joint Controls

The mechanical ankle joint is formed by the articulation between the stirrup and the uprights. If the orthosis user is expected to move the ankle while wearing the appliance, the mechanical ankle joint axis must be aligned with the axis of the anatomical joint (denoted by a line that passes through the apices of the malleoli). **Figure 14.4** demonstrates the alignment of the mechanical and anatomical ankle axes in

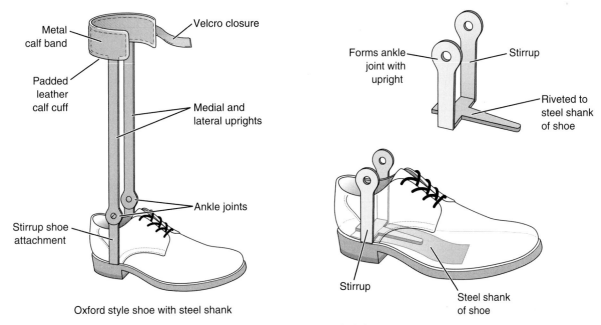

FIGURE 14.3. The parts of a conventional ankle–foot orthosis and the attached shoe.

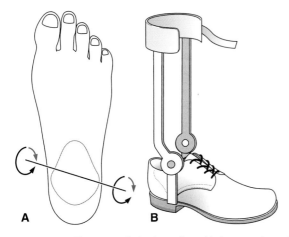

FIGURE 14.4. The anatomical axis at the ankle is approximated by a line that passes through the apices of the malleoli. (A) The medial upright of a conventional AFO curves anteriorly to align the orthotic ankle axis with the anatomical axis (B).

a conventional double upright AFO. If axis alignment is not achieved, unwanted motion between the brace and limb occurs during joint movement which may produce skin irritation, pain, or even joint deformity. The importance of alignment between mechanical and anatomical axes is discussed in Chapter 2 on biomechanics (Biomechanical Factors That Affect the Appliance–User Interface, Alignment Between the Appliance and the User's Anatomy).

The two basic types of orthotic ankle control mechanisms are stops and ankle assists. **Ankle stops** restrict ankle motion to a predetermined joint ROM. An ankle stop is named according to the motion that it restricts. Thus, an ankle joint with a plantarflexion stop is designed to limit or stop plantarflexion. A commonly prescribed ankle joint has a neutral or 0° plantarflexion stop, which limits plantarflexion beyond 0° (**Fig. 14.5**). A dorsiflexion stop restricts dorsiflexion ROM.

An **ankle assist** is a mechanism that produces force to aid a designated joint motion. In conventional orthoses, the most commonly used assisting mechanism is a dorsiflexion assist that functions during swing phase to substitute for weak or paralyzed dorsiflexor muscles. The mechanism that provides the assist is a spring that is compressed during plantarflexion and recoils when released (**Fig. 14.6**). Springs do not produce enough force to provide a practical plantarflexion assist during gait; thus, conventional plantarflexion assists are not used. A double-adjustable ankle mechanism that has two channels is also available (**Fig. 14.7**). One channel is located anterior to the joint axis, and the other is posterior to the axis. When the posterior channel contains a spring, it provides dorsiflexion assist. The anterior channel usually contains a peg (or pin) that provides a dorsiflexion stop. A peg can also be

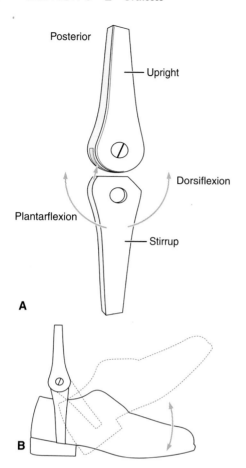

A

B

FIGURE 14.5. A conventional orthotic ankle joint with a plantarflexion stop at 0°. **(A)** The stirrup is cut to contact the upright in the joint when the ankle reaches 0° during plantarflexion. **(B)** The stirrup in the orthosis is cut to allow plantarflexion to 0°, but it does not restrict dorsiflexion.

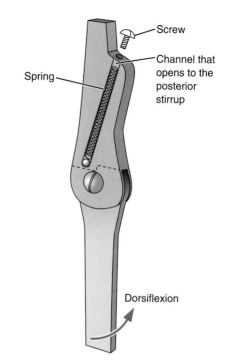

FIGURE 14.6. An ankle joint with a dorsiflexion assist has a channel containing a spring that is compressed during plantarflexion (weight acceptance) and recoils during swing phase. A screw on top of the channel is loosened or tightened to adjust the strength of the assist. An older name for this mechanism is a single channel Klenzak brace.

inserted into the posterior channel (with or without spring) to provide a plantarflexion stop. Screws placed on top of the channels are used to make adjustments to the assists or stops.

Conventional orthotic ankle joints are **single-axis joints**. This means the joint has only one mechanical axis which allows movement only in the sagittal plane. Because there are no other mechanical axes, some control of frontal plane movement (inversion and eversion) is inherent in these joints. However, for clients with significant unwanted pronation (eversion) or supination (inversion) of the foot, additional components are required to achieve effective frontal plane control. A varus (inversion) or valgus (eversion) **control strap (T-strap)** is attached to the lateral or medial side of the shoe, respectively. It is then fastened around the opposite brace upright to deter

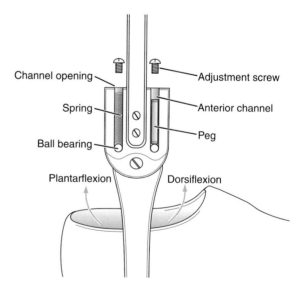

FIGURE 14.7. A double adjustable ankle joint provides a mechanism to create dorsiflexion assist as well as dorsi- and plantarflexion stops. This mechanism is also called a double channel Klenzak or a bichannel adjustable ankle lock (BiCAAL). The peg in the anterior channel produces a dorsiflexion stop.

the unwanted frontal plane movement of the foot (**Fig. 14.8**). Although effective and usually comfortable, these straps make it difficult to don and doff the appliance independently, particularly when the client has only one functional hand.

Molded Ankle–Foot Orthoses

Molded orthoses are usually constructed as one piece of material without moving articulations. They are fabricated from high-temperature thermoplastics, thermosetting resins, or thermoplastic composite materials containing strengthening agents such as carbon or glass fibers. These materials are discussed in Chapter 12, and their material or physical properties are integral to the functioning of the appliances in which they are used. Readers are encouraged to review these materials and their properties prior to studying specific orthotic applications (see Box 12.10 and Table 12.1). These molded appliances may be custom molded to a particular individual or prefabricated and custom fitted as a definitive or permanent device. Simple prefabricated molded orthoses are also sold from catalogs and used by clinicians as temporary or training devices during

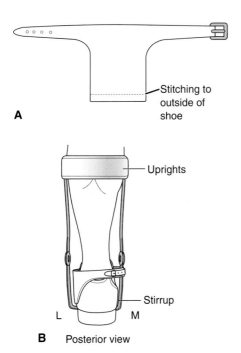

FIGURE 14.8. (A) A varus or valgus control strap (T-strap) is added to an orthosis to limit hindfoot movement in the frontal plane. **(B)** When stitched to the lateral side of the shoe and buckled around the medial upright, it provides control of inversion. A valgus control strap attaches to the medial side of the shoe and fastens around the lateral upright (M, medial; L, lateral).

rehabilitation to help determine a particular client's specific orthotic needs.

Types of Molded Ankle–Foot Orthoses

Although molded appliances are usually made as one piece, their designs vary and are created to apply forces in particular ways to achieve specific mechanical goals. For example, if a three-point counterforce system is required, the orthotic design must provide the method by which the necessary forces are applied to the limb (see Fig. 2.10). **Figure 14.9** presents four typically used configurations or types of molded AFOs:

- Posterior calf shell
- Spiral, full or hemi-spiral
- Anterior ground or floor reaction
- Anterior toe-off

Despite the various shapes and configurations, particular features of all of the devices are referred to using specific terminology. Much of the terminology used to identify the parts of molded appliances is derived from the posterior shell-type orthosis, which is labeled in **Figure 14.10**.

Despite their differences, all these molded AFOs are "total contact." Unlike conventional braces with metal uprights that do not touch the skin, total-contact molded appliances are in direct contact with the limb. This total-contact design reduces point pressure by distributing the applied forces over a larger surface area. Those appliances with greater surface area of contact between the orthosis and the limb apply lower pressures. All molded appliances, however, may also include relief additions (build-up areas) or concavities to reduce pressure on sensitive structures, such as bony prominences, and distribute forces onto pressure-tolerant areas. Areas that may require additional pressure relief include the tibial crest and tubercle, the malleoli, the navicular tubercle, and the metatarsal heads.

Because total-contact appliances fit very intimately on the limb, practitioners must take precautions to minimize skin irritation at the skin–orthosis interface. Clients with fluctuating edema, insensitivity, and wounds or scars near trimlines present special challenges to orthotic fitting and may make use of a total-contact appliance inappropriate until the issue is resolved.

Posterior Calf Shell Ankle–Foot Orthoses

Posterior calf shell AFOs, although similar in design, vary significantly in rigidity and the amount of resistance or

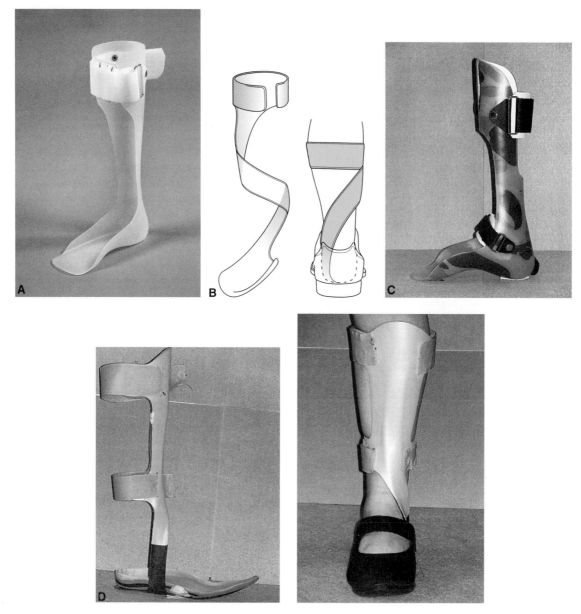

FIGURE 14.9. Common types of molded ankle–foot orthoses include **(A)** posterior calf shell, **(B)** full spiral and hemispiral, **(C)** anterior ground (floor) reaction, and **(D)** anterior toe-off.

assistance they offer to ankle motion. Rigidity is determined by the type, thickness, and shape of the material as well as by the location of the orthotic ankle trimlines. In general, the farther anterior the medial and lateral trimlines extend and the more of the limb that is enclosed in the orthosis, the more rigidly the appliance resists motion (see Fig. 2.14).[3] When the ankle trimlines are located an inch or more behind the apices (widest portion) of the malleoli, the orthotic ankle is

more flexible and supports the foot during swing phase but has little effect on the ankle during stance (see Fig. 14.14). This type of flexible orthosis is called a **posterior leaf spring orthosis** (AFO-PLS) and is appropriate for those who need dorsiflexion assist during swing phase but have little or no frontal plane imbalance (varus or valgus) or need for stance phase control. To control excessive supination or pronation in clients who only require swing phase dorsiflexion

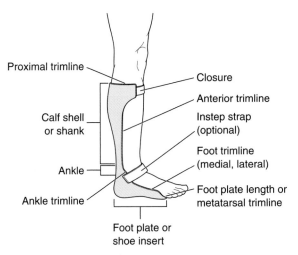

FIGURE 14.10. Terminology used to describe the features of a molded ankle–foot orthosis. Specific features of the foot plate are identified using the same terminology as that used for foot orthoses.

assist, a modification to the lateral trimline, called a flange, can be added to the calf shell without moving the entire trimline anteriorly (**Fig. 14.11**). The flange is an anterior extension of the shell located just proximal to the malleolus. A medial flange provides contact for a three-point counterforce system to control excessive pronation, while the lateral flange controls excessive supination. The flanges provide frontal plane stabilization to prevent varus or valgus hindfoot positioning in a semirigid AFO-PLS.

Ankle trimlines that extend to or anterior to the apices of the malleoli produce an orthotic ankle that

does not permit any movement. These orthoses are called **solid ankle AFOs** (AFO-SA). AFO-SAs are very strong and stable and may be necessary when significant deforming forces, such as spasticity, are present in the foot and ankle or when the orthotic goal is to affect the knee by manipulating the GRFV during stance phase. For example, an individual who demonstrates deleterious knee hyperextension during stance phase can be fit with an AFO-SA, which is fixed in a few degrees of ankle dorsiflexion (**Fig. 14.12**). Because closed-chain knee hyperextension requires the ankle to plantarflex, the dorsiflexed AFO-SA, by preventing plantarflexion, also prevents knee hyperextension. Clients who use this type of orthosis to limit knee hyperextension must have sufficient quadriceps strength to prevent knee buckling. This concept is discussed in more detail in Chapter 2 on biomechanics (Methods of Force Application to Limit, Control, or Prevent Movement; Designs That Manipulate the GRFV or LoG).

Despite the benefits of the high level of stability offered by these solid ankle appliances, they also present consequences that may have a negative effect on the client's ability to function efficiently. For example, an AFO-SA that blocks dorsiflexion makes rising from a chair, ascending ramps, squatting, and

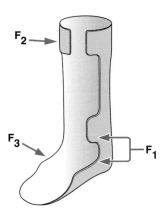

FIGURE 14.11. The medial flange on this right semirigid molded ankle–foot orthosis contributes to the middle force of a three-point counterforce system to control excessive pronation. The flange is located in the lower one-third of the leg above the ankle.

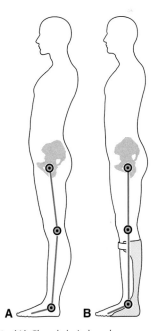

FIGURE 14.12. (A) Closed chain knee hyperextension requires the ankle to plantarflex. **(B)** A rigid solid ankle ankle–foot orthosis that fixes the ankle in dorsiflexion prevents knee hyperextension.

descending steps using a foot-over-foot pattern more difficult (**Fig. 14.13**). Blocking plantarflexion makes it difficult to descend ramps and eliminates active push-off for limb propulsion during gait, which produces gait abnormalities during limb advancement. Clinicians must consider the possible negative effects on function of a particular orthotic feature, as well as its benefits, when selecting an appliance for a client.[4,5,6]

In addition to the very flexible (AFO-PLS) and very rigid (AFO-SA) AFOs, many semirigid appliances are available. A variety of configurations are

commonly used, and others are individually designed to meet specific biomechanical needs of particular clients. **Figure 14.14** depicts some commonly used posterior shell designs that offer a range in orthotic rigidity. The material in the ankle region of semirigid posterior shell AFOs is particularly susceptible to buckling or bowing due to the high loads applied to this region during mid to late stance (**Fig. 14.15**). This bowing occurs during stance when the ankle dorsiflexes as the tibia rotates forward to advance the body over the weight-bearing limb. Various methods

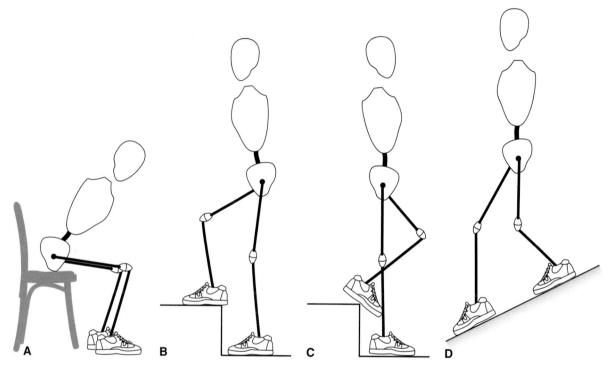

FIGURE 14.13. A solid ankle ankle–foot orthosis prevents the dorsi- and plantarflexion ankle movements necessary to perform many functional activities efficiently.

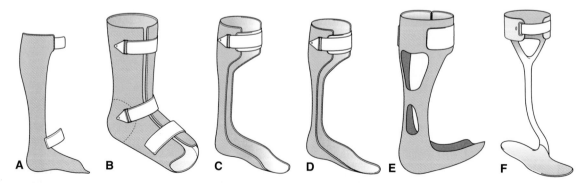

FIGURE 14.14. Various configurations of posterior calf shell molded ankle–foot orthoses that offer a range of rigidity: **(A)** solid ankle with trimline anterior to malleolus; **(B)** circumferential (most rigid); **(C,D,E)** posterior leaf springs; and **(F)** posterior carbon fiber.

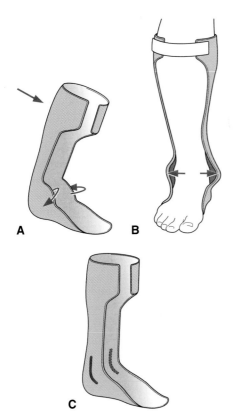

FIGURE 14.15. The ankle region of a posterior shell molded AFO sustains high stress during late stance **(A)** that can cause the plastic to buckle or bow **(B)**. One method to strengthen the ankle region is to incorporate carbon fiber composite reinforcements **(C)**.

are employed to add strength to the ankle region without increasing the overall rigidity or bulkiness of the appliance. Strength in the ankle region is increased by including corrugations or an additional curved shape in the material at the ankle (see Fig. 12.7), rolled edges, or added reinforcement materials in the highly stressed areas. Reinforcements are often added at the ankle region as boomerang-shaped pieces of graphite or carbon fiber composite material (Fig. 14.15). An optional instep strap (see Fig. 14.10) may also be added to assist in stabilizing the ankle in the orthosis or to reinforce the middle force of the three-point counterforce systems acting at the ankle.

Traditionally, the recommended height of the calf shell is as high as possible to maximize the effect of leverage on force production without interfering with the common peroneal nerve as it rounds the fibular head. Thus, the traditional height is approximately one inch inferior to the fibular head. However, in instances when maximum force is not required, lower calf shells are used effectively. Lower calf shells are appropriate for young children who are lighter in weight and do not require maximum forces. Shells that terminate inferior to the bulk of the gastrocnemius muscle bellies are also used effectively in specially designed AFOs to reduce pain or control motion and bony alignment in patients with arthritis of the ankle or subtalar joints.[7,8]

Anterior Floor Reaction Ankle–Foot Orthoses

The anterior floor (ground) reaction orthosis (anterior GR-AFO or FR-AFO) is a special type of AFO used by clients who need orthotic control at both the ankle and the knee. The design prevents the knee from collapsing into flexion during stance by restricting ankle motion. This type of orthosis is particularly useful for clients who have quadriceps weakness that causes knee buckling or those who have excessive stance phase flexion, such as occurs in crouch gait. Because closed-chain knee flexion requires the ankle to dorsiflex, an orthosis that holds the ankle at neutral or slight plantarflexion with a dorsiflexion stop prevents knee flexion. Limiting the forward rotation of the tibia by restricting dorsiflexion during stance maintains the ground reaction force vector anterior to the knee joint axis and produces a knee extension moment (see Figs. 2.6 and 12.3). To achieve this goal at the knee, the AFO must supply a proximal anterior contact area to participate in the three-point counterforce system necessary to stop dorsiflexion (**Fig. 14.16**). These orthoses are usually constructed from molded plastic or composite materials with a slightly plantarflexed solid ankle. However, clients who are able to perform active dorsiflexion during swing may have an GR-AFO with an articulated ankle with a dorsiflexion stop but unrestricted plantarflexion. Because solid ankle AFOs affect the forward motion of the tibia during stance, they also interfere with the smooth progression of the body over the weight-bearing limb. To make weight acceptance and stance phase rollover smoother, shoe modifications are needed. A compressible or resilient heel softens heel strike and weight acceptance when an orthosis has a plantarflexion stop (see Fig. 13.10F). A rocker sole on the shoe facilitates smooth forward movement of the body during mid and terminal stance by substituting for restricted ankle and foot movements (see Fig. 13.12B,C).

Spiral Ankle–Foot Orthoses

The spiral AFO was one of the first types of orthoses fabricated from thermoplastic materials.[9] The spiral design provides mild to moderate control of the foot

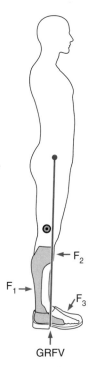

GRFV

FIGURE 14.16. An anterior ground reaction ankle–foot orthosis is designed to provide three-point counterforces at the ankle to stop dorsiflexion. The dorsiflexion stop keeps the ground reaction force vector anterior to the knee to produce a knee extension moment.

and ankle but does not interfere with the normal plantar- and dorsiflexion that occurs during the gait cycle and is necessary for the smooth progression of the body over the weight-bearing limb. The thermoplastic materials that were originally used to construct these orthoses proved to be either too brittle, leading to material fatigue and fracture, or too flexible to be effective. Newer laminated composite materials that are more fatigue resistant and can withstand repetitive loading without breaking have rekindled interest in these designs.[10] The full spiral orthosis begins on the medial side of the foot at the foot plate and makes a full 360° spiral around the leg, ending on the medial side at the calf band (see Fig. 14.9). The hemispiral appliance originates from the lateral side of the foot plate, spirals only 180° around the leg, and terminates on the medial side at the calf band. The hemispiral AFO offers more rigidity and resists a flexible varus hindfoot deformity. The advantage of the spiral AFO is that it acts like a spring, uncoiling somewhat during early stance (weight acceptance) to allow plantarflexion. While unloaded during swing phase, it returns to its neutral position and prevents foot drop. The increased use of carbon fiber or Kevlar

composite materials in spiral orthoses has increased the applications for this type of orthosis.

Anterior Shell Toe-off Ankle–Foot Orthoses

Anterior shell **toe-off AFOs** have developed due to the increased availability and use of carbon fiber and other types of composite materials in orthotic devices (see Fig. 14.9). Composites are very lightweight, strong, and fatigue resistant and have the ability to store and return energy (see Fig. 2.13). Because of their ability to store energy when deformed and release it when unloaded, they are referred to as dynamic response orthoses, and their design follows that of dynamic response prosthetic feet (see Fig. 2.12). Although a variety of configurations are available, an important benefit of this anterior design is its ability to provide dorsiflexion resistance during mid to late stance, which is returned to assist plantarflexion and propulsion as the limb is unloaded at toe-off. Because composite materials are very strong, these orthoses are quite thin and not at all bulky, and they provide considerable strength and force. There is some evidence that another possible benefit of these orthoses may be a reduction in the energy cost of walking, although studies that compare the effects of these orthoses to those of other appliances have not been published at the time that this chapter was written.[11]

Molded Foot Plates

Both molded and hybrid orthoses attach to their wearers by a molded foot plate that fits into the shoe and is secured to the foot by the shoe closure. The foot plate has features similar to those of foot orthoses (described in Chapter 13). The heel cup is molded to and stabilizes the calcaneus and may have intrinsic posting. The orthotic arch usually matches the anatomy of the foot, but a relief or built-up area may be present under the metatarsal shafts to relieve the metatarsal heads. If the orthosis is designed to provide a three-point counterforce system to control unwanted foot movements in the transverse plane (foot ab- or adduction), the foot plate must have returns, or sides, that wrap around the medial and lateral aspects of the metatarsal shafts. The typical foot plate does not extend onto the dorsum of the foot.

As in foot orthoses, the length of the AFO foot plate may vary from three-quarter (metatarsal) length to full length (see Fig. 13.17). For normal toe extension and toe-break during terminal stance, a three-quarter length foot plate is required. A rigid, full-length foot plate interferes with toe extension, delays knee flexion during terminal stance, and increases late stance knee stability (prevention of knee buckling). Thus, it may be prescribed with an anterior floor reaction orthosis to maximize stance phase knee extension moments. A full-length foot plate may also improve the effectiveness of orthoses worn by individuals with hypertonicity of the plantarflexor muscles.[12] However, when a full-length foot plate is used, a shoe with a rocker sole is required to substitute for the restricted foot movements and to facilitate roll-over. At the other extreme, a very short foot plate is used in a specially designed AFO to reduce pain and limit ankle motion in persons with ankle or subtalar joint arthritis.[7,8] This very short foot plate extends only to the distal end of the heel fat pad.

The foot plates of some orthoses used with clients with upper motor neuron disorders and hypertonicity may have special moldings, or shapes, which are purported to reduce spasticity in the limb.[13] AFOs with these specially shaped foot plates are termed *tone-reducing* ATOs (TRAFO). These foot plates are full length and many wrap around the dorsum of the foot. The heel cup is intimately molded to stabilize the calcaneus, and the plantar aspect that interfaces with the foot includes specific reliefs (depressions) and bumps (built-up areas) that are precisely located to decrease and increase pressure, respectively, on particular areas of the foot.[14,15] These special features include built-up areas (raises) under the medial and lateral longitudinal arches, transverse metatarsal arch, and toes and recessed or relief areas under the metatarsal heads and the calcaneal fat pads.[14] The therapeutic intent of these features is to provide prolonged stretch to the ankle plantarflexors and long toe flexors, provide constant pressure to the tendons of the toe flexors, inhibit reflexes evoked by tactile stimulation, and improve the recruitment and sequence of muscle activity.[16] The effectiveness of this foot plate design in affecting muscle activity is not clear.[17]

Hybrid, Hinged, or Articulated Ankle–Foot Orthoses

Hybrid, hinged, or articulated **AFOs** are composed of a calf component that is separate from but articulates with a foot plate, both of which are typically constructed from molded materials. The articulations or joints that connect the two parts are made of metal, plastic polymers, or composite materials. The metal joints used in these appliances may be the same or similar in design to the single-axis ankle joints used in conventional double upright AFOs, including various types of stops and assists. Plastic and composite joints include those with a true axis of rotation, such as simple overlap joints or Oklahoma joints, as well as nonarticulating and axisless joints, termed flexure joints (**Fig. 14.17**). Metal joints that contain mechanisms that provide dorsi- or plantarflexion stops or variable controls are commercially available; however, simple pin or strap devices attached between the posterior aspects of the calf component and foot plate are also used to restrict plantar- or dorsiflexion, respectively (**Fig. 14.18**). Hinged AFOs are often selected to allow free or unrestricted movement in the sagittal plane; however, single-axis mechanical joints inherently limit movement in the frontal and transverse planes.

Hinged AFOs are prescribed when solid ankle AFOs provide too much rigidity and movement restraint that negatively affects functional performance in activities such as gait, stair climbing, and rising from a chair (see Fig. 14.13).[18] Negative consequences of solid ankle appliances are described for particular patient populations, particularly children with spastic diplegic cerebral palsy, and include multiplanar compensations at the pelvis and trunk.[19,20] Hinged AFOs improve function in individuals by controlling moderate subtalar joint instability, correctable ankle equinus, or knee hyperextension. They also decrease the time and energy expenditure required to perform certain functional activities.[21,22]

Axial Deweighting or Weight-Relieving Ankle–Foot Orthoses

A special type of AFO to reduce axial loads on the distal part of the leg and foot during weight-bearing was first developed in the 1960s by Augusto Sarmiento as a fracture brace for distal tibial fractures.[23] Applying the principles of patellar tendon bearing developed in the 1950s for transtibial prosthetic sockets, he developed an orthosis to partially unweight the distal tibia, ankle, and foot by transferring some of the weight-bearing load onto an orthosis. This orthosis is called a patellar tendon–bearing orthosis (PTB-AFO). The original **PTB-AFO** had a proximal shell that was contoured like the brim of a PTB prosthetic socket and was attached to brace uprights. Subsequent research revealed that the orthotic features most responsible for the partial

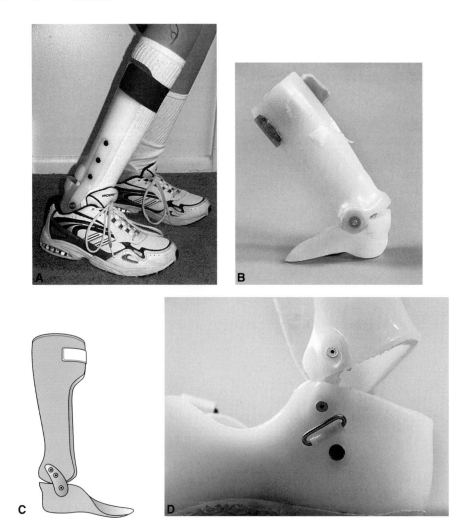

FIGURE 14.17. **(A)** A hinged (articulated) AFO can be constructed with various plastic or metal articulations. Examples include the following: **(B)** single-axis overlap joint, **(C)** Oklahoma joint, and **(D)** flexible axisless flexure (Tamarak or Gillette) joint.

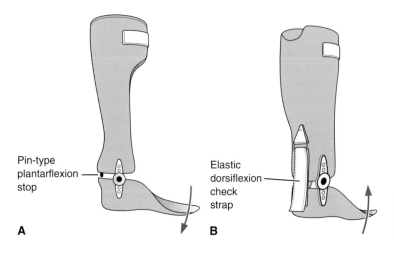

Pin-type plantarflexion stop

Elastic dorsiflexion check strap

A   **B**

FIGURE 14.18. **(A)** A hinged (articulated) ankle–foot orthosis (AFO) has a pin-type plantarflexion stop. **(B)** An adjustable elastic check strap controls dorsiflexion in an articulated AFO.

unloading of the ankle and foot are circumferential containment and restriction of ankle motion rather than the PTB shape of the proximal brim.[24] Thus current weight-relieving AFOs or fracture braces (for the distal tibia) include circumferential lace-up or molded plastic calf containment components that undercut and support the cone-shaped contour of the distal calf musculature to transfer weight away from the foot and ankle and onto the orthosis. Although the biomechanics of tibial unloading are the same, molded plastic as well as hybrid versions of this AFO are available (Fig. 14.19).

FUNCTIONAL ELECTRICAL STIMULATION

Functional electrical stimulation (FES) was first introduced by Liberson in the 1960s as an alternative to traditional orthoses for clients with foot drop and a normally functioning peroneal nerve.[25] Current commercially available FES orthoses provide transcutaneous stimulation to the common peroneal nerve as it passes posterior to the fibular head. With proper electrode positioning, balanced contraction of the anterior tibialis and peroneal muscles occurs, resulting in dorsiflexion without excessive inversion or eversion. Nerve stimulation using a single-channel battery-operated electrical stimulator

is triggered during gait by a programmable tilt sensor that measures the orientation of the leg with respect to the vertical. The tilt sensor along with stimulator and electrodes is located in a molded cuff placed around the proximal leg (Fig. 14.20). When the leg is tilted posteriorly during terminal stance, stimulation begins, and it ends when the leg is tilted anteriorly for heel strike.[26] Instead of tilt sensors, the stimulator can also be controlled by force sensors worn under the foot to detect heel-off and heel strike.[27] For appropriately selected clients with swing phase dropped foot, this device can improve the speed and reduce the energy cost of walking. Although most of the research conducted with these devices investigates their effects in clients with dropped foot due to a stroke, they can also be used by patients with incomplete spinal cord injury or other impairments of the central nervous system. Individuals with plantarflexion contracture, stance phase knee or ankle instability, obesity, or excessive soft tissue over the peroneal nerve or severe hypertonicity are not good candidates for these devices. In addition to the orthotic benefits, there is some evidence that FES orthoses can have a positive therapeutic or carryover effect on gait in stroke patients, potentially stimulating some degree of motor recovery and improved gait function without orthotic stimulation.[28]

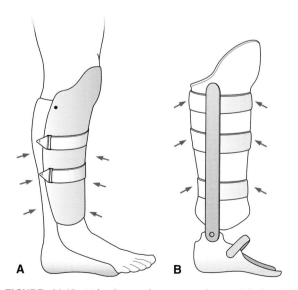

FIGURE 14.19. Unloading orthoses to reduce weight-bearing through the distal tibia. A molded proximal brim mimics the shape of a patellar tendon–bearing prosthetic socket. Solid **(A)** and articulated **(B)** ankle designs are used.

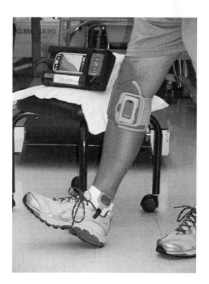

FIGURE 14.20. A functional electrical stimulation orthosis (neuroprosthesis) provides dorsiflexion and eversion assist by stimulating the common peroneal nerve. A calf band includes stimulating electrodes, stimulator, and batteries. Pressure sensors are located on a shoe insert. (Bioness Inc., Valencia, CA)

A GUIDE FOR PRESCRIPTION OF SHOE MODIFICATIONS AND FOOT ORTHOSES

The process of developing an orthotic prescription is described in Chapter 12. Specific prescriptions for AOs and AFOs are developed through the process of identifying the impairments, establishing specific goals related to the impairments, and designing a biomechanical device to apply the forces required to achieve the goals. Practitioners who contribute to developing orthotic prescriptions must also consider client performance while using trial or temporary AFOs as well as evidence for appliance effectiveness as reported in current research literature. Keywords and search terms to help clinicians identify relevant research studies that report on the efficacy of AOs and AFOs are provided at the end of this chapter. **Figure 14.21** provides a guide for

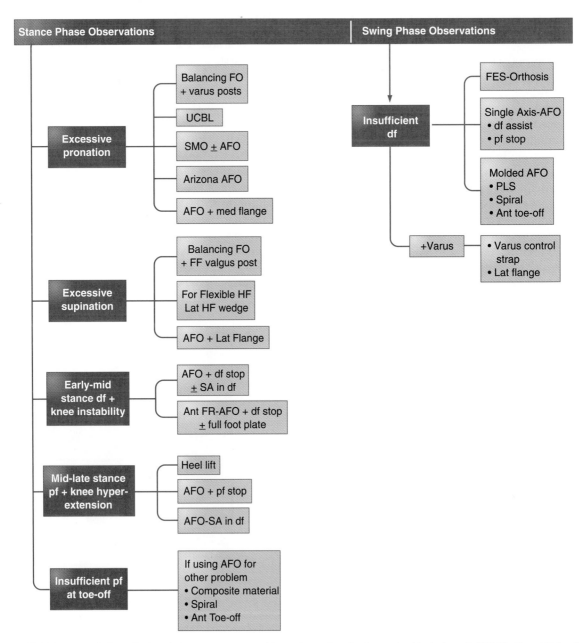

FIGURE 14.21. A guide for orthotic solutions to common problems observed at the foot and ankle during gait (HF, hindfoot; FF, forefoot; df, dorsiflexion; pf, plantarflexion; Lat, lateral; Ant, anterior; Med, medial).

prescription of FOs and AFOs that links commonly observed gait abnormalities with the types of orthoses that are likely to improve function. Because shoes function integrally with an orthosis, clients should be given a shoe prescription or instructions in the characteristics of shoes that are necessary to ensure that the orthosis functions optimally. The characteristics of shoes, shoe modifications, and their applications are discussed in Chapter 13.

ORTHOTIC CHECKOUT EXAMINATION AND TRAINING

When a new orthosis is received, a therapist must conduct an orthotic checkout examination of the client, the device, and the client wearing the device. This procedure is discussed in Chapter 11. Some specific features that should be examined in an AFO are listed in **Box 14.1**. The purpose of the checkout examination is to ensure that the device has been manufactured as prescribed and that its fit, function, comfort, and cosmesis are acceptable. The orthotist, therapist, and patient must work together to resolve any problems in any of these areas. When it is determined that the device is satisfactory, the therapist must review the orthotic goals to ensure that they have been achieved or implement a training program to accomplish them. Particularly for new orthosis

wearers, this requires patient instruction in proper methods of donning, doffing, and caring for the orthosis, as well as guidelines for appropriate footwear for use with the device. Some patients who use a plastic molded orthosis may need to wear a thin sock or stockinette between the orthosis and the skin because the plastic causes some patients to sweat excessively. A thin sock can wick perspiration away from the skin and keep it dry.

Functional training is usually necessary for new orthosis wearers, including gait training, as well as instruction in other types of functional activities such as steps, negotiating all types of indoor and outdoor surfaces, ramps, and getting up and down from the floor. If running and other higher-level functions are appropriate for the client, these should be included as well. Asking patients to identify functional activities that are important to or difficult for them helps clinicians individualize training and focus on relevant functional skills. To achieve optimal function, in addition to using the prescribed orthosis, patients may need to use ambulatory aids (canes, walkers) as well as continue with other interventions such as exercises to maintain or improve joint ROM, strength, cardiovascular fitness, and balance. Therapists must ensure that patients understand the roles of each of these interventions in optimizing and maintaining function.

BOX 14.1 | Specific Items to Include in the Checkout Examination of Ankle–Foot Orthoses

- For total contact molded orthosis
  - No excessive pressure at trimlines or over bony prominences
  - Molded relief areas properly match pressure-sensitive structures
  - No gapping occurs between the orthosis and limb during movement
  - The heel is secure and stable in the orthosis without pistoning or unwanted movements
  - Orthosis fits properly in shoe and is stable
  - Shoe has the required characteristics and holds the foot onto the orthosis without unwanted gapping or movement
  - After sustained wear, sweating of the skin covered by the orthosis is minimal and skin is reasonably dry and not irritated

- For conventional orthosis
  - Uprights conform to but do not contact the leg (~1 cm space)
- For articulated (hinged) orthosis
  - Proper alignment between anatomical and mechanical ankle axes
- No irritation of calf or fibular head
- Shoe with orthosis fits properly and does not exert excessive pressure on foot
- Closures/fasteners are secure and easy for the client to access and operate

SUMMARY

Many different types of AOs and AFOs are available to improve function in clients with impairments of the ankle. AOs are typically used with individuals with musculoskeletal disorders of the ankle, such as acute or chronic ankle sprains or instability. AFOs are prescribed for a wide range of musculoskeletal and neuromuscular disorders and are classified into three major groups by construction materials and methods: conventional (metal and leather), molded (plastics and composites), and hybrid (hinged or articulated) devices. AFOs are devices that function mechanically by applying forces to stabilize the ankle, control unwanted motions, or assist insufficient ones. An alternative type of orthosis for swing phase dropped foot uses functional electrical nerve stimulation to substitute for inadequate muscle function. AFOs should be prescribed individually based on preorthotic prescription clinical examinations, including biomechanical, gait, and functional analyses. Prescriptions should be based on these clinical assessments as well as patient performance with trial or temporary devices and information from the research literature concerning orthotic effectiveness and best practices for prescription. Appropriate shoes should be recommended with all orthotic prescriptions. An orthotic checkout examination to ensure proper orthotic fit, function, comfort, and cosmesis must be performed prior to providing functional training as well as other interventions that will allow the patient to maximize function.

KEYWORDS FOR LITERATURE SEARCH

For each search topic, select relevant terms from each domain of interest and execute a search using the Boolean term "AND".

Search Topic: What are the effects and effectiveness of ankle orthoses in management of acute and chronic ankle injuries?

Intervention
  Orthotic devices
  Bracing

Conditions
  Sprains or strains
  Ankle injuries
  Lateral ligament, ankle
  Ankle sprains
  Joint instability + ankle

Effects
  Efficacy
  Effectiveness

Search Topic: What are the effects and effectiveness of AFOs for patients with particular conditions?

Intervention
  Orthotic devices
  Ankle-foot orthosis
  Electrical stimulation therapy; functional electrical stimulation

Conditions (Examples):
  Cerebral palsy
  Hemiplegia
  Osteoarthritis; arthritis
  Equinovarus
  Cerebrovascular accident; stroke
  Meningomyelocele
  Neurological disorder
  Spinal cord injury
  Multiple sclerosis

Effects
  Efficacy
  Effectiveness
  Energy expenditure
  Gait analysis
  Stair locomotion; stair climbing
  Clinical guidelines
  Electromyography (EMG)

REFERENCES

1. Ubell ML, Boylan JP, Ashton-Miller JA: The effect of ankle braces on the prevention of dynamic forced ankle inversion. Am J Sport Med 31:933–940, 2003.
2. Gravlee JR, van Durme DJ: Braces and splints for musculoskeletal conditions. Am Fam Physician 75:342–348, 2007.
3. Sumiya T, Suzuki Y, Kasahara T: Stiffness control in posterior-type plastic ankle-foot orthoses: effect of ankle trimline. Part 2: Orthosis characteristics and orthosis/patient matching. Prosthet Orthot Int 20:132–137, 1996.
4. Thomas SS, Buckon CE, Jakobson-Huston S, et al: Stair locomotion in children with spastic hemiplegia: the impact of three different ankle foot orthosis (AFOs) configurations. Gait Posture 16:180–187, 2002.
5. Radka SA, Oliveira GB, Lindstrom KE, et al: The kinematic and kinetic effects of solid, hinged, and no ankle-foot orthoses on stair locomotion in healthy adults. Gait Posture 24:211–218, 2006.
6. Burtner PA, Woolacott MH, Qualls C: Stance balance control with orthoses in a group of children with spastic cerebral palsy. Devel Med Child Neurol 41:748–757, 1999.

7. Huang Y-C, Harbst K, Kotajarvi B, et al: Effects of ankle-foot orthoses on ankle and foot kinematics in patients with ankle osteoarthritis. Arch Phys Med Rehabil 87:710–716, 2006.

8. Huang Y-C, Harbst K, Kotajarvi B, et al: Effects of ankle-foot orthoses on ankle and foot kinematics in patients with subtalar osteoarthritis. Arch Phys Med Rehabil 87:1131–1136, 2006.

9. Lehneis H-R: Plastic spiral ankle-foot orthoses. Orthot Prosthet 28:3–13, 1974.

10. Madden M: Fabricating the spiral and hemi-spiral orthosis using a composite lay-up technique. J Prosthet Orthot 3:94, 1991.

11. Danielsson A, Sunnerhagen KS: Energy expenditure in stroke subjects walking with a carbon composite ankle foot orthosis. J Rehabil Med 36:165–168, 2004.

12. Davids JR, Rowan F, Davis RB: Indications for orthoses to improve gait in children with cerebral palsy. J Am Acad Orthop Surg 15:178–188, 2007.

13. Lima D: Overview of the causes, treatment, and orthotic management of lower limb spasticity. J Pediatr Orthop 2:33–40, 1990.

14. Radtka SA, Skinner SR, Dixon DM, et al: A comparison of gait with solid, dynamic, and no ankle-foot orthoses in children with spastic cerebral palsy. Phys Ther 77:395–409, 1997.

15. Crenshaw S, Herzog R, Castagno P, et al: The efficacy of tone-reducing features in orthotics on the gait of children with spastic diplegic cerebral palsy. J Ped Orthop 20:210–216, 2000.

16. Lohman M, Goldstein H: Alternative strategies in tone-reducing AFO design. J Prosthet Orthot 5:21–24, 1993.

17. Lam WK, Leong JCY, Li YH, et al: Biomechanical and electromyographic evaluation of ankle foot orthoses in spastic cerebral palsy. Gait Posture 22:189–197, 2005.

18. Nahorniak MT, Gorton GE, Gannotti ME, et al: Kinematic compensations as children reciprocally ascend and descend stairs with unilateral and bilateral solid AFOs. Gait Posture 9:199–206, 1999.

19. Park ES, Park CI, Chang HJ, et al: The effect of hinged ankle-foot orthoses on sit-to-stand transfer in children with spastic cerebral palsy. Arch Phys Med Rehabil 85:2053–2057, 2004.

20. Radtka SA, Skinner SR, Johanson ME: A comparison of gait with solid and hinged ankle-foot orthoses in children with spastic diplegic cerebral palsy. Gait Posture 21:303–310, 2005.

21. Romkes J, Hell AK, Brunner R: Changes in muscle activity in children with hemiplegic cerebral palsy while walking with and without ankle-foot orthoses. Gait Posture 24:467–474, 2006.

22. Balaban B, Yasar E, Dal U, et al: The effect of hinged ankle-foot orthoses on gait and energy expenditure in spastic hemiplegic cerebral palsy. Disabil Rehabil 29:139–144, 2007.

23. Sarmiento A: A functional below-the-knee cast for tibial fractures. J Bone Joint Surg 49A:855–875, 1967.

24. Lehmann JF, DeLateur BJ, Price R: Weight-bearing and other orthoses for skeletal and joint insufficiency. Phys Med Rehabil Clin North Am 3:185–192, 1992.

25. Liberson WT, Holmquest ME, Scot D, et al: Functional electrotherapy: stimulation of the peroneal nerve synchronized with the swing phase of the gait of hemiplegic patients. Arch Phys Med Rehabil 42:101–105, 1961.

26. Kottink AIR, Oostendorp LJM, Buurke JH, et al: The orthotic effect of functional electrical stimulation on the improvement of walking in stroke patients with a dropped foot: a systematic review. Artif Organs 28:577–586, 2004.

27. Hausdorff JM, Ring H: Effects of a new radio frequency-controlled neuroprosthesis on gait symmetry and rhythmicity in patients with chronic hemiparesis. Am J Phys Med Rehabil 87:4–13, 2008.

28. Yan T, Hui-Chan C, Li L: Functional electrical stimulation improves motor recovery of the lower extremity and walking ability of subjects with first acute stroke: a randomized placebo-controlled trial. Stroke 36:80–85, 2005.

15

Orthoses for Knee Impairments

OBJECTIVES

At the end of this chapter, all students are expected to:

1. Describe the types (categories) and functions of knee orthoses (KOs) and knee–ankle–foot orthoses (KAFOs).
2. Identify and describe the parts of KOs and KAFOs, including the materials and componentry used.
3. Discuss applications for KOs and KAFOs to improve function.

Physical Therapy students are expected to:

1. Determine the need for a KO or a KAFO for a client based on examination findings.
   a. Evaluate client examination findings, including preorthotic prescription clinical examinations, lower quarter biomechanical assessment, and functional and gait analyses, to diagnose impairments that may be improved by a KO or KAFO.
2. Develop goals for a KO or KAFO based on a client's impairments and functional requirements.
3. Describe the biomechanical methods employed in KOs and KAFOs to achieve the orthotic goals.
4. Prescribe a KO or KAFO to meet the orthotic goals and improve function.
5. Develop and execute a search strategy to identify research evidence for the effects and effectiveness of KOs and KAFOs and to identify best practices for orthotic prescription.
6. Recommend a KO or KAFO as a part of a plan of care to optimize function for an individual with impairments at the knee.
7. Recommend shoes with appropriate characteristics for use with specific KOs or KAFOs.
8. Examine and evaluate KOs and KAFOs for acceptable fit, function, comfort, and cosmesis.

CASE STUDIES

Ann O'Callahan is a 55-year-old elementary schoolteacher who reports right knee pain and has been given a diagnosis of medial compartment tibiofemoral osteoarthritis by her doctor. Her history and chief complaints are described in Chapter 11. In addition to the examination findings reported previously, today she is tender at the medial joint line and has a general complaint of pain throughout the anterior knee. The pain is accompanied by minimum swelling around the joint, but there are no signs of effusion. Knee strength is graded as 3+/5 by manual resistance, but her ability to produce force is limited by pain. Varus and valgus stress tests at the knee reveal mild laxity with some pain. Because she discontinued her walking exercise, she does daily straight-leg raise exercises instead and can perform 25 consecutively without difficulty or pain. Her hip, knee, and contralateral leg show no impairments. She is motivated to get started, as she is anxious to resume her walking exercise program.

Luis Sanchez is a 12-year-old sixth grader who has cerebral palsy and spastic diplegia. Luis' history and functional problems are described in Chapter 11. When you examine him today, you note that he has some limited joint range of motion (ROM): hamstrings contractures (popliteal angle of 145° on the 90-90 straight-leg raise test) and heel cord contractures (5° plantarflexion with the knee extended). Muscle strength assessment using manual resistance tests (in the available ROM) showed selective muscle weakness, including hip extension and abduction and ankle dorsi- and plantarflexion, 3/5; knee flexion and extension, 3+/5 and hip flexion, 4-/5. Poor muscle endurance is evidenced by reduced muscle strength grades when resistance tests are repeated after Luis walks and runs for about 15 minutes during various gait and functional assessments.

Walt Kawalski is a 61-year-old man who contracted poliomyelitis at age 6. The polio affected his right leg, and he was fit with a locked-knee KAFO. He became a community ambulator with the brace and has walked daily for 55 years, limited only by general endurance. He went to college and has been a small business owner for 30 years. He has had no history of falls, and other than various orthopedic surgeries on both legs, he has no significant medical history. He has no problems with his upper extremities and left leg, but he has developed worsening hip and back pain with walking. His orthopedic surgeon feels these symptoms may be related to gait abnormalities associated with his "stiff-knee," braced walking pattern and recommends an orthotic reevaluation. For many years, he has gotten new braces, as needed, but all have been of the same orthotic prescription. Walt is evaluated today by the orthotic team at a local rehabilitation hospital to determine if a new orthotic prescription is needed. The preorthotic examination findings include

- Both right knee and ankle are flaccid, with muscle atrophy and no voluntary movement
- Manual muscle tests of his right hip strength: extension 4/5, abduction 3/5, flexion 2/5, and adduction 2/5
- Right knee shows a 10° valgus deformity with no significant ligamentous laxity
- Right leg is 1 in. shorter than the left
- Left foot is shortened with rigid cavus and hammertoe deformities suggestive of intrinsic muscle weakness; left ankle ROM is 5° each of dorsi- and plantarflexion; plantarflexion strength is 3/5. He has never worn special shoes or bracing on the left leg, and he does not have any left leg problems or complaints.

Linda Schmidt, a 50-year-old pharmaceutical sales representative, sustained a grade 2 anterior cruciate ligament sprain during a skiing accident 8 weeks ago. She did not require surgery and has been attending physical therapy. She no longer has any signs or symptoms of acute inflammation and has returned to usual work and home activities. Although her knee does not "give way," she has an "unstable feeling" if she changes direction or moves quickly. She has decided not to return to skiing but would like to be able to play recreational tennis without sustaining more injuries.

Case Study Activities

All Students:

1. For each client, identify and discuss the functional problems and participation restrictions that may be improved with an orthosis.
2. Which joint or joints may benefit from an orthotic intervention? How do you expect an orthosis will affect each client's gait?
3. Identify advantages and disadvantages of using an orthosis for each client.
4. Describe biomechanically how an orthosis will affect each client's impairments and improve function.

Physical Therapy Students:

1. Identify and describe the impairments that contribute to each client's functional limitations.
2. Discuss the need for an orthosis for each client. If an orthosis is indicated, develop specific orthotic goals for each appliance.
3. Develop an orthotic prescription to achieve the best outcome and functional improvement for each client.
   a. Describe the type of orthosis and the orthotic componentry that will achieve the orthotic goals.
   b. Using biomechanical terminology, name the orthosis that you recommend for each client.
   c. Recommend the type of shoes that the client should wear with the prescribed orthosis. Explain why the characteristics of the recommended shoes are necessary.
   d. Is there evidence in the research literature to support your orthotic recommendations for each client? Describe the evidence and how it impacted your recommendation.
4. Develop a physical therapy plan of care for each client, which includes an orthosis, if appropriate, as well as other physical therapy interventions. How will you determine and measure the effectiveness and outcome of the interventions?

ORTHOSES FOR IMPAIRMENTS AT THE KNEE

Two major categories of orthoses have components that cross the knee joint. They are KOs, which enclose only the knee, and KAFOs, which extend across the knee and attach to and include orthotic ankle–foot components (see Chapter 14). KOs and KAFOs exert forces to limit or assist movements at the knee. To restrain unwanted motions they employ three- or four-point counterforce systems (**Fig. 15.1**). These counterforce systems can be applied to control unwanted movements in both the sagittal (flexion and extension) and the frontal planes. Deleterious frontal plane movements that KOs can restrain include tibial abduction or adduction, which result in positions of genu valgus or varus, respectively. Excessive knee motions in the transverse plane (tibial medial or lateral rotation) are difficult to restrain with orthotic components, and orthoses designed to control these rotations have little effectiveness unless they block all motion and lock the joint in a fixed position.

KOs and KAFOs, however, are not the only orthoses used to address impairments at the knee. Ground reaction ankle–foot orthoses (GR-AFOs), designed to manipulate the ground reaction force vector (GRFV) with respect to the knee axis, apply forces to the knee without physically extending across the knee joint. These GR-AFOs are described in Chapter 14 but are also discussed in this chapter as alternative orthotic solutions for knee impairments.

KNEE–ANKLE–FOOT ORTHOSES (KAFOs)

KAFOs are indicated for individuals who have significant weakness or deformity in the lower extremity, including the knee, as well as the hip in some cases.

At one time, most KAFOs were constructed from metal uprights, usually steel, with metal thigh and calf bands that were covered with leather and attached to the steel shank of rigid oxford-style shoes. The energy cost of walking with these heavy, bulky appliances was quite high, which limited their wearers' functional ambulation and caused many to reject them and choose other methods of mobility.[1,2] Although lightweight aluminum alloy metal uprights and bands are also available, they may not be strong enough for large, heavy, or very active individuals. As a result, most KAFOs in use today are manufactured using metal only for the joints (hinges) that connect the molded plastic thigh and shank (calf) shells. The foot plate and ankle component of this type of KAFO may be a single molded plastic piece that is contiguous with the calf shell or may include metal or plastic ankle articulating joints as described in Chapter 14. These modular metal–plastic KAFOs weigh less and reduce the energy cost of ambulation compared to metal and leather styles (**Fig. 15.2**).[3] Carbon fiber–reinforced composite plastics are also used to construct KAFO components. Because composite materials are very strong and lightweight, components made from composites can be quite thin and produce orthoses that are less bulky and more cosmetic in appearance.[4] However, because composite materials cannot be adjusted or significantly modified after

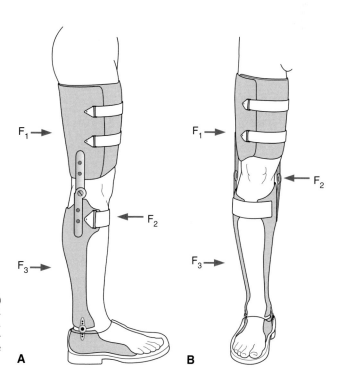

FIGURE 15.1. Knee-ankle-foot orthoses (KAFOs) use three-point counterforces to control movement. **(A)** Sagittal plane counterforces restrain knee flexion. **(B)** Frontal plane counterforces restrain tibial abduction and prevent an unwanted valgus position at the knee.

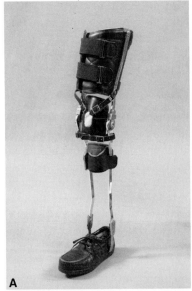

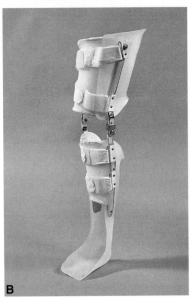

FIGURE 15.2. Knee–ankle–foot orthoses (KAFOs): **(A)** conventional double upright KAFO constructed from metal and leather, and **(B)** KAFO constructed from molded thermoplastic thigh and calf shells with metal knee joints.

molding, careful client selection and orthotic prescription and fitting are required.

Although plastic or composite orthoses are more commonly used today, there are indications for both types of KAFOs. Conventional, double upright devices are indicated when heavy-duty strength, adjustability, and the need to accommodate fluctuating edema or varying limb girth is important. The primary advantages

of KAFOs with molded plastic components are that they are lightweight, which reduces energy expenditure during function, they are easier to clean and maintain, and most clients feel they are more cosmetic and thus are less likely to abandon using them.

Orthotic Knee Joints

Although anatomical knee flexion and extension is a complex three-dimensional movement, orthotic knee joints are either single axis or polycentric (**Fig. 15.3**). Single-axis mechanical knee joints provide a simple hinge articulation that allows knee flexion and extension about a single fixed axis of rotation. Orthotic knee extension is needed to support the body during stance phase, while flexion is needed for sitting and, for those able to walk with an unlocked knee, during swing. However, because a single-axis mechanical

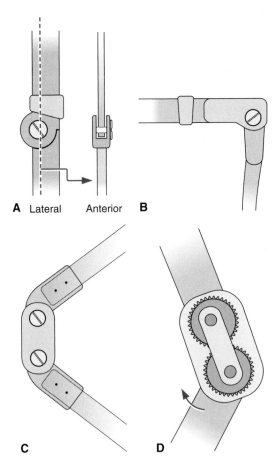

FIGURE 15.3. Orthotic knee joint axes. **(A)** Single-axis knee joints viewed laterally and anteriorly in extension, and **(B)** laterally in flexion. **(C,D)** Polycentric knee axes.

joint cannot continuously align with the anatomical knee joint as it moves through its range of motion, a KAFO with a single-axis joint moves and pistons to some extent on the limb. In an attempt to provide better coalignment between the orthotic knee joint and the instantaneous center of rotation of the anatomical joint, **polycentric orthotic knee joints** were developed. Polycentric joints have various designs that allow the axis to translate during joint rotation.

Components to Stop, Lock, and Control Knee Movement

The most common reason to prescribe a KAFO is to stop or limit an unwanted movement that interferes with function. At the knee, this is often unwanted knee flexion, or buckling, that occurs during stance phase. This stance phase knee instability (buckling) is usually caused by quadriceps weakness and is a common cause of falling. Various types of orthotic knee joint stops, locks, and control mechanisms are available to stabilize the knee and prevent knee flexion. These include a posterior offset knee joint, a drop ring lock, a cam (or pawl) lock with bail release, adjustable locks, stance control orthoses, and floor reaction AFOs.

Posterior Offset Knee Joint

The posterior offset orthotic knee joint, also called the eccentric free knee, is a single-axis mechanical joint that is displaced posteriorly (**Fig. 15.4**). This design enhances knee extension during stance phase by keeping the GRFV anterior to the mechanical axis, producing an extension moment at the knee. For individuals with good control of their hips and trunk, this may be an effective solution, because it enhances stance phase knee extension without interfering with swing phase flexion. However, individuals with poor control at the hip or trunk may find this type of orthotic knee joint ineffective. Lack of sufficient control of the proximal joint of the lower limb may allow the GRFV to move posterior to the orthotic joint axis, causing sudden knee buckling and possibly falling. To flex the knee for sitting, the wearer must shift weight off of the braced limb and slightly flex the hip to allow the GRFV to move posterior to the orthotic axis. This mechanism works best for individuals with good muscular control at the hip and who require only unilateral bracing.

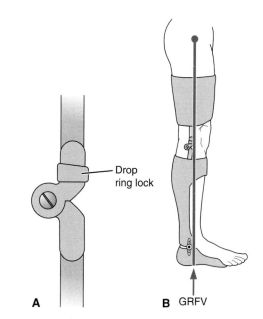

FIGURE 15.4. The posterior offset knee joint **(A)** provides knee extension assistance during stance phase **(B)** when the ground reaction force vector remains anterior to the mechanical axis and produces an extension moment at the knee.

Knee Locks and Stops

Knee locks are devices that when engaged hold the joint in a fixed position. The joint remains in the locked position until the device is released or disengaged. These locks are usually very reliable and can be used with clients who have difficulty controlling proximal or distal joints as well as the knee. A disadvantage is that when engaged, they remain locked in both stance and swing phases. When the knee is locked in extension during swing phase, gait alterations are required to advance the limb. Typical deviations that occur during locked-knee gait include lateral trunk lean to the nonswing side, hip hiking, and circumduction or vaulting. These gait deviations produce an uncosmetic gait pattern that is slow and inefficient and has a high energy cost.

There are various types of orthotic knee locks that are used to lock and unlock orthotic knee joints. Commonly used manual fixed locks that always lock the knee in the same extended position include drop-ring locks and cam (pawl) locks. An electromagnetic knee lock that is electronically controlled by a microprocessor is also available. This electronic knee lock is locked and unlocked by the patient using a wireless remote control unit that is hand-held or integrated into the handle of an ambulatory aid.[5] Adjustable locks allow practitioners to change the location of flexion, and extensions stops, thus restricting the ROM of the patient's knee. These locks are useful in postsurgical rehabilitation when limiting joint ROM is required to protect healing structures. A KAFO with a free knee is an orthosis in which the mechanical knee joints are unencumbered and free to move at any time through their full ROM. This type of knee is used with an orthosis designed to limit frontal plane movements without affecting sagittal plane movements.

Drop-Ring Lock

A drop-ring lock is a very simple manually operated lock that is mounted on the medial or both medial and lateral thigh uprights. The lock is a metal ring that slides down over the orthotic knee joint in extension. It is moved up off of the joint to release the knee and allow free movement (Fig. 15.5). This is the simplest type of knee lock. Usually there is a spring-loaded retention button above the knee to prevent the ring from dropping and locking the knee inadvertently. An

extended pull release is also available for those unable to bend forward to release the drop-ring lock.

Cam (Pawl) Lock With Bail Release

An alternative to the drop-ring lock is the cam or pawl lock with bail release (Fig. 15.5B). This type of lock is used for clients who would have difficulty operating a drop ring due to hand dysfunction, use of forearm crutches, or poor balance. These locks are present at both the medial and lateral orthotic knee joints and are connected by a bail release, which is a curved piece of metal that extends around the back of the knee. Raising the bail disengages the lock and allows knee flexion. The bail can be raised to disengage the lock without using hands, when it contacts the seat of a chair when sitting down.

Adjustable Knee Locks

Adjustable locks are particularly useful when a patient's condition is expected to change. For example, during the early postsurgical period, some patients who have had knee surgery may have ROM limitations to protect repaired tissues that are gradually decreased as tissue healing progresses. Adjustable locks permit practitioners to gradually reduce joint ROM restrictions as rehabilitation progresses without requiring multiple orthoses. Adjustable orthotic locks are also useful when progressive static stretching is utilized to reduce joint contractures. Two commonly used adjustable knee locks are the fan lock and the dial lock (Fig. 15.6). A *fan lock* allows a practitioner to preset the desired knee flexion angle of the brace by moving a screw into one of several positions on the fan-shaped joint mechanism. A drop-ring lock is used to hold the preset flexed knee position during standing and is released to allow flexion for sitting. As the patient's condition changes, the fixed knee flexion angle is changed by moving the adjustment screw. The *dial lock* is also adjustable and has the additional advantage of offering various types of ROM controls to the clinician. For example, the dial lock can be set and locked in a fixed position, permitting no movement in either direction. It can be set to limit motion in flexion, without limiting extension, or vice versa. It can also be set to offer specific flexion and extension stops, with unimpeded motion between the stops. A *ratchet lock* is another option. It is an orthotic joint that incorporates a one-way clutch that allows rotation in one direction but blocks all rotation in the opposite direction until it is released. This type of

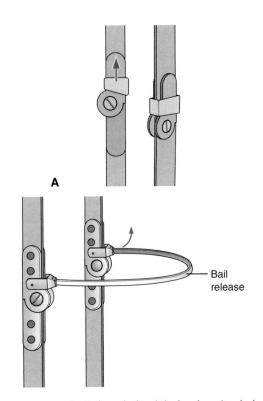

A

B

Bail release

FIGURE 15.5. Orthotic knee locks: **(A)** the drop-ring lock is released manually by sliding the metal ring up and is locked by sliding it down over the joint; **(B)** the cam (pawl) lock with bail release is disengaged, allowing the knee to flex, when the bail is lifted.

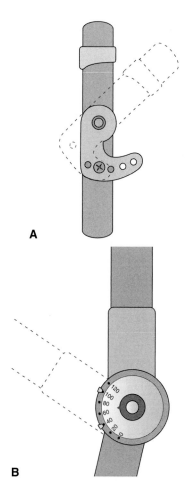

FIGURE 15.6. Adjustable knee locks: **(A)** a fan lock and **(B)** a dial lock.

joint and lock is used effectively in a KAFO for clients with a static or dynamic (spastic) knee flexion contracture to allow active knee extension but block all knee flexion, until it is released.

Stance Control That Permits Swing Phase Knee Flexion

Although the knee locks discussed above effectively prevent knee flexion during stance phase, most of them also prevent the flexion that is needed to shorten the leg and clear the foot from the floor during swing. The resulting slow, stiff-legged gait pattern makes it difficult to advance the braced leg without catching the foot on the floor, requires pelvic compensation that often leads to back and hip pain, and requires a high level of energy expenditure. As a result, as many as 60% to 80% of individuals with this type of locked-knee long leg brace

discontinue use in favor of other methods of mobility.[6] Further, about 40% of the individuals who continue to use their locked-knee KAFOs express dissatisfaction with their appliances.[7] Orthotic alternatives that provide enhanced stance phase stability without blocking swing phase knee flexion include anterior floor (ground) reaction AFOs (FR-AFOs) and **stance control orthoses** (**SCOs** or **SC-KAFOs**). A stance control orthosis is a KAFO that engages a knee control mechanism during stance phase only and disengages it for swing phase. Although FR-AFOs are not KAFOs, they are included in this section because they offer an alternative solution for the same knee impairment addressed by stance control KAFOs.

Anterior Floor Reaction Ankle–Foot Orthoses

Floor reaction AFOs are discussed in Chapter 14 because they are devices that address impairments at both the ankle and foot, as well as at the knee. They exert knee control by using specific ankle positioning to manipulate the location of the GRFV at the knee. The biomechanical explanation of how this type of appliance affects knee movements without extending orthotic componentry across the knee is presented in Chapter 2 on biomechanics and Chapter 14 on ankle–foot orthoses. Readers are encouraged to review the relevant sections of these chapters and the associated figures (see Figs. 2.6, 14.9C, 14.16, and related text). To summarize, anterior floor reaction AFOs provide enhanced stance phase knee extension by using a dorsiflexion stop set in neutral or a small amount of plantarflexion to keep the GRFV anterior to the knee joint axis throughout stance. A full- or sulcus-length foot plate, along with the dorsiflexion stop, also contributes to keeping the GRFV anterior to the knee joint axis. When this orthotic design is used with children or smaller adults, the orthosis does not extend above the knee. However, in larger or heavier individuals who require greater forces to produce the desired knee control, a **supracondylar GR-AFO**, which encases the anterior knee but does not extend above the knee, may be necessary. The higher supracondylar design increases the lever arm length and provides a larger surface area over which to distribute the force and reduce pressure (**Fig. 15.7**). The proximal shape and trimlines of the supracondylar floor reaction orthosis mimic those of the supracondylar suprapatellar transtibial prosthetic socket. To benefit from this orthosis, individuals must have some quadriceps and hip muscle strength (at least 3/5), as well as the ability to advance the leg in a

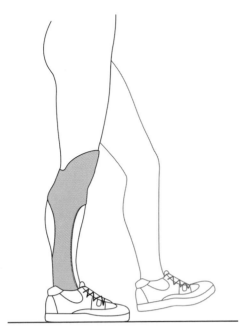

FIGURE 15.7. A floor reaction ankle–foot orthosis is used to enhance stance phase knee extension without preventing flexion during swing phase. (See Figure 14.9C for a photograph of the orthoses.)

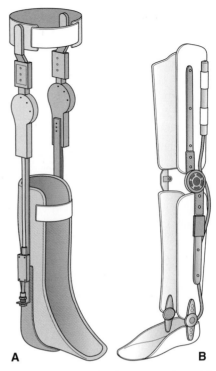

A   **B**

FIGURE 15.8. Stance control orthoses (SCOs) provide a stance phase lock or resistance but permit free knee flexion for swing phase. **(A)** The stance phase flexion control mechanism can be mechanical or **(B)** electronic with an on-board microprocessor.

reciprocal gait pattern. The presence of hip or knee flexion contractures interferes with the functioning of floor reaction orthoses and may be a contraindication for prescription. To effectively use floor reaction orthoses to enhance knee stability, any existing flexion contractures at the hip or knee must be less than 30° or 20°, respectively.[8]

Stance Control Knee–Ankle–Foot Orthoses

SCOs are KAFOs (SC-KAFO) that include a knee mechanism to stop flexion during stance but allow free knee motion during swing (**Fig. 15.8**). There are two parts to these systems: the knee lock and a controller that engages and releases the locking mechanism at the appropriate times during gait.[9,10] The locks are mechanical or electromechanical, and the controllers are mechanical or electronic using an onboard microprocessor that is operated by the patient using a remote control that is either hand-held or attached to an ambulatory aid. Mechanical stance control systems are gait activated, meaning that some physical component of the gait process locks and unlocks the knee mechanism, such as ankle ROM or inclination of the limb. For example, a knee lock may be automatically engaged when the knee reaches

extension at the end of swing and automatically released to swing freely when a knee extension moment and dorsiflexion occur simultaneously in terminal stance. Electronic- and microprocessor-controlled knee mechanisms use foot plate or tilt sensors to determine if the stance controls should be on or off. Some microprocessor-controlled orthotic knee joints provide stance phase flexion resistance in addition to a lock.[10] This mechanism is similar to the microprocessor-controlled transfemoral prosthetic knee mechanisms. It allows wearers to safely negotiate uneven and ascending or descending surfaces such as ramps or hills and provides for stumble recovery.

Clients with quadriceps paralysis or weakness due to polio, incomplete spinal cord injury, femoral neuropathy, or other disorders benefit from these orthoses, because they provide greater knee stability than other options such as FR-AFOs or KAFOs with posterior offset knee joints. A variety of stance control KAFO components are available, each with different advantages and disadvantages. Optimal patient outcome depends on a good match between the specific abilities and needs of the client and component selection. In addition to stance controls, some SC-KAFOs include a "pneumatic spring" to assist swing phase knee extension for those with significant muscle weakness at the hip.

Different stance control orthoses have specific patient requirements. However, in general, most require that clients have full knee extension ROM (or flexion contractures less than 10°), corrected knee varus or valgus less than 10°, and the ability to advance the leg for reciprocal stepping. Although studies with large numbers of subjects are not reported, preliminary investigations show that stance control orthoses improve some kinematic and spaciotemporal characteristics of gait when compared to locked-knee gait.[11] Experienced wearers who change from using orthoses with traditional orthotic knee locks to a stance control system require gait training to unlearn old gait compensations and to acquire an optimal gait pattern.[12]

Deweighting or Weight-Relieving Knee–Ankle–Foot Orthoses

At one time, fracture bracing was used as an effective method of treatment for distal femoral and proximal tibial fractures. However, since the development of better internal fixation hardware and surgical procedures, fracture bracing is only used as part of the care for distal femoral or proximal tibial fractures in people who are poor operative candidates or have complications that make surgery a high risk. The long leg femoral fracture brace was designed based on the principles of the ischial weight-bearing transfemoral prosthetic socket brim and was called an ischial weight-bearing orthosis. The femoral component of this fracture brace was shaped like the ischial weight-bearing socket in an attempt to partially unload the femur during weight-bearing. However, subsequent studies determined that this brace did not effectively unload the femur or the tibia.[13] KAFO fracture braces available today are prefabricated from polyethylene components and may include a femoral shell with an ischial weight-bearing or ischial containment (narrow ML) proximal component attached to hinged knee joints (with or without locks), a molded tibial shell, and a solid or hinged ankle–foot component (**Fig. 15.9**). More often, however, the thigh component of a contemporary long leg fracture brace is simply a snug-fitting cylinder designed to assist in immobilizing fracture fragments by increasing the hydrodynamic compressive effect of the thigh muscles on the enclosed femur.

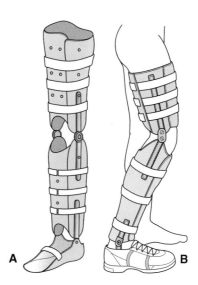

FIGURE 15.9. (A) Knee–ankle–foot orthosis fracture braces may have molded ischial weight-bearing or containment thigh components **(B)** or snug-fitting cylindrical thigh pieces.

KNEE ORTHOSES

Knee orthoses (KOs) are appliances that enclose the knee joint, usually extending as far as mid-thigh and mid-calf, but do not attach to ankle or hip componentry. There are two basic types of knee orthoses: soft and rigid. Soft appliances are usually made of some type of elastic fabric or neoprene (a synthetic rubber compound) and are typically constructed as "over-the-counter" prefabricated "pull-on" sleeves (Fig. 2.7) that apply compression forces to the limb. Many soft over-the-counter appliances are available that have little biomechanical control, other than to provide compression to control edema.

Rigid KOs have a rigid framework composed of either double (medial and lateral) or single (medial or lateral) uprights made of lightweight metal, plastic, or composite materials. The uprights have articulations at the knee joint that allow free flexion and extension movements around a single or a polycentric axis while restricting frontal plane movements (see **Fig. 15.3**). Appliances with two uprights are connected, either anteriorly or posteriorly, by thigh and calf bands, and the device is attached to the limb with various configurations of straps. Many KOs also include special strap and condylar adaptations designed to prevent migration of the orthosis on the limb, because freely suspended knee orthoses often migrate inferiorly or rotate on the limb during use. Although there are literally a myriad of different "styles" of KOs that are manufactured and sold, four groups of devices commonly seen in clinical practice are presented here. These include

■ Postoperative or rehabilitative orthoses
■ Functional orthoses
■ Orthoses for patellofemoral pain conditions
■ Off-loading or unloading KOs for knee osteoarthritis

Postoperative or Rehabilitative Knee Orthoses

Postoperative or **rehabilitative knee orthoses** are typically used after orthopedic surgery to protect structurally incompetent tissues from deleterious forces during healing (**Fig. 15.10**). Although a cast or knee immobilizer can also be used to protect these tissues, these alternatives totally immobilize the knee and prevent all joint motion, which has been shown to result in weaker tissues when healing is completed. For most surgeries, only some joint motions are deleterious, while "safe" joint movement actually protects the joint structures from atrophy and contractures caused by total stress deprivation. Rehabilitative orthoses have dial locks at the knee, which allow practitioners to adjust the motion stops so that safe knee flexion and extension is permitted (see Fig. 15.6). As healing progresses and the joint tissues are able to tolerate increased loads through larger ranges of motion, the stops can be adjusted accordingly. These devices are prefabricated and purchased by sizes based on simple linear measurement. Clinicians who instruct patients to exercise while wearing these devices must ensure that they fit properly and that the mechanical joints are properly aligned with the anatomical joints. Because after surgery these appliances are typically worn full time, except when exercising, they may slip inferiorly or rotate on the leg. Attempts to move the knee with improperly aligned orthotic joints can be painful and injurious to the knee joint structures. Rehabilitative KOs may be worn during walking. However, because they are bulky and usually extend as close to the ankle and groin as is comfortable, an ambulatory aid such as crutches or a walker should be used for safety.

Functional Knee Orthoses

Functional knee orthoses are also rigid appliances; however, they are shorter than rehabilitative devices, usually extending no farther than mid-thigh and

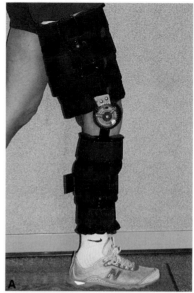

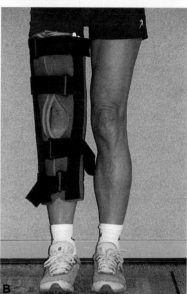

FIGURE 15.10. (A) Postsurgical or rehabilitative orthoses are used to protect healing tissues from movements that cause deleterious loads with adjustable ROM stops. **(B)** A knee immobilizer totally immobilizes the knee in full extension at all times.

mid-calf, and are less bulky. Designed to be worn during usual functional activities, they are constructed from lightweight, strong materials using configurations that minimize interference with movement. They have single-axis or polycentric knee joints without locks and, except for a 0° extension stop, most allow full movement in the sagittal plane. The most common application for functional braces is for individuals with ligamentous instability at the knee. Most are designed to employ three- or four-point counterforce systems to limit excessive movements, including varus and valgus stress and knee hyperextension (**Fig. 15.11**). Although many of these orthoses were developed to address the knee instability caused by anterior cruciate ligament (ACL) injury, most research has found that they are ineffective in restraining anterior translation of the tibia during functional activities.[14–16] As a result, they are no longer used as a routine part of post-ACL reconstruction surgery rehabilitation.[15] Some clients with ACL insufficiency without surgical reconstruction, however, report that they experience less sense of instability when wearing a functional brace.[16] Researchers are exploring other nonbiomechanical explanations for this improved sense of stability in selected populations of patients.[14]

Another type of functional knee brace is designed to restrain pathological knee hyperextension by using a three-point counterforce system. The original appliance, called a Swedish knee cage, employs a posterior to anterior (PA) force applied in the popliteal fossa countered by anterior to posterior (AP) forces at the distal thigh and proximal tibia (**Fig. 15.11B**). Although this prefabricated device is simple and does not limit knee flexion and extension, it is difficult to suspend in place, often migrates on the limb during use, and is reported by most as generally uncomfortable. When knee hyperextension co-occurs with impairments at the ankle which require an orthosis, a better solution is to restrain the knee hyperextension with an ankle plantarflexion stop or a solid ankle AFO in a small amount of dorsiflexion (Fig. 14.12). Another alternative for a mild knee hyperextension thrust when an AFO is not required is a small (less than ½-inch), wedge-shaped lift placed under the calcaneus of the involved limb. This small heel wedge causes the individual to flex the knee slightly to accommodate the small increased leg length. Clients who use this heel wedge must have sufficient quadriceps strength to prevent knee buckling.

Patellofemoral Knee Orthoses

Patellofemoral knee orthoses reduce anterior knee pain in some patients with patellofemoral pain syndromes.[17] Although the specific etiology of patellofemoral pain syndromes is still debated, abnormal tracking of the patella on the femur is believed to be a primary cause. There are many styles, but most patellofemoral orthoses are soft appliances made from an elastic material as a

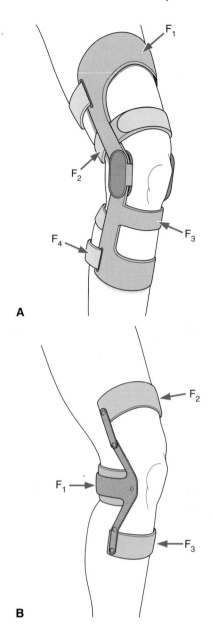

FIGURE 15.11. Functional knee orthoses (KOs): **(A)** functional KO with a four-point counterforce system in the sagittal plane and **(B)** Swedish knee cage with a three-point counterforce system to restrain knee hyperextension.

"pull-on" sleeve. Because many clinicians hypothesize that patellofemoral pain is associated with excessive lateral tracking of the patella, some patellar orthoses also have buttressing (C- or O-shaped built-up areas) around the patellar window or pull-straps that wrap around the lateral side of the patellar window to apply a medially directed force. These additions are attempts to stabilize the patella during functional activities (**Fig. 15.12**). Although this type of soft orthosis reduces knee pain in some patients with patellofemoral pain, other styles are not effective.[18] Studies that report the effects of orthoses that were successful in reducing pain show that in addition to achieving a small reduction in lateral patellar displacement, they increased patellofemoral joint contact area, which may reduce patellofemoral joint stress.[17,19] These findings led the investigators to propose that a mechanism by which these appliances relieve symptoms may be reducing joint stresses by increasing patellofemoral joint contact area.[17,19,20] Because our understanding of the use of orthoses to reduce pain in individuals with patellofemoral syndromes is not yet clearly determined, clinicians are encouraged to review current research evidence for effectiveness prior to prescribing any appliance. The Keywords for Literature Search section at the end of this chapter provides keywords and search terms to assist practitioners in finding relevant literature.

Off-Loading (Unloading) Knee Orthoses

Some patients with arthritis of the knee that affects only one compartment of the tibiofemoral joint may benefit from a knee orthosis. Off-loading knee orthoses are designed to reduce loads on the involved joint surfaces and may decrease pain and improve function.[21,22] The most common unicompartment arthritis is osteoarthritis (OA) of the medial compartment of the tibiofemoral joint with a varus deformity.

The goal of an unloading or off-loading brace for this type of osteoarthritic deformity is to produce an abduction moment to shift the joint contact force away from the overstressed medial joint surfaces.[23] A variety of different medial compartment unloader braces are available. They employ a mechanical method to reduce the adduction moment at the knee by applying a three-point counterforce system that produces a valgus force. To achieve this goal, different companies offer different brace styles for clients of various sizes, shapes, and levels of activity. Unloading braces may be custom-made from measurements at a central manufacturing site or prefabricated. Unloading braces may have a single upright or bilateral uprights, and they may provide mechanisms for the wearer to self-adjust the valgus correction or it may be predetermined. Some of the orthotic methods used to produce this valgus force include building the valgus correction into the frame of a custom-made brace, using a special polyaxial valgus-producing joint, attaching an adjustable ratcheting force strap to provide dynamic counterforces, or using other methods that increase either the middle or the counterforces of the valgus three-point force system (**Fig. 15.13**). Although less common, unloading braces are also available for individuals with lateral compartment tibiofemoral osteoarthritis with valgus deformity. For these individuals, unloading the lateral compartment is accomplished by using an orthosis that provides a varus force to produce an adduction moment at the knee.

GUIDES FOR PRESCRIPTION AND CHECKOUT OF KNEE–ANKLE–FOOT ORTHOSES AND KNEE ORTHOSES

As for all orthoses, a specific prescription is developed through the process of identifying impairments, establishing goals, and biomechanically designing an orthosis to apply the forces required to achieve the goals. This process is described in Chapters 11 and 12. A guide for prescription of knee–ankle–foot orthoses (KAFOs) is presented in **Figure 15.14**. Foot and ankle components that can be used with KAFOs are described in Chapter 14, and a guide for their selection is provided in Figure 14.21. Practitioners who contribute to developing orthotic prescriptions must also consider client performance with trial devices as well as reports of orthotic efficacy published in current research literature (see

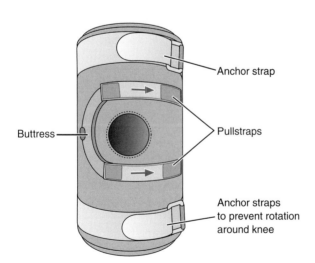

FIGURE 15.12. A typical patellofemoral orthosis is a soft, "pull-on" elastic sleeve, usually with some type of buttressing or pull-straps to stabilize the patella.

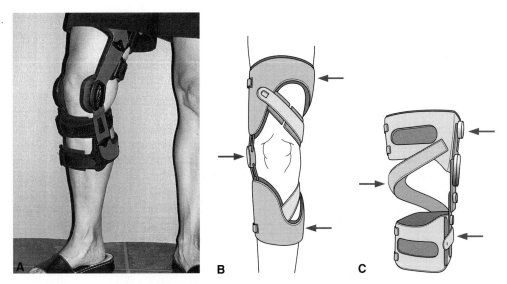

FIGURE 15.13. Unloading knee orthoses for medial compartment osteoarthritis apply a valgus force using three-point counterforces. Appliances are constructed with double uprights **(A)** or a single lateral **(B)** or medial **(C)** upright.

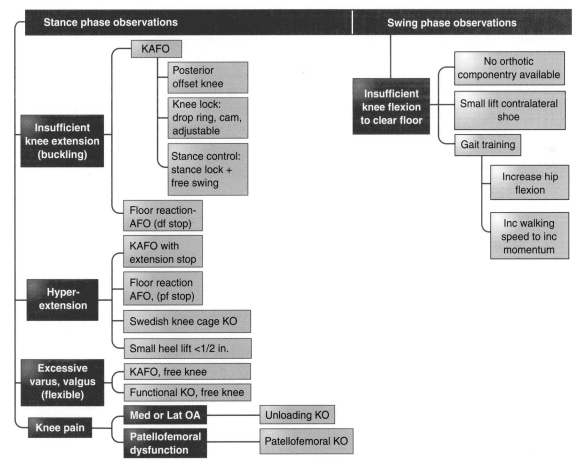

FIGURE 15.14. A guide for orthotic solutions for common problems observed at the knee during gait (pf, plantarflexion; df, dorsiflexion; med, medial; lat, lateral; inc, increase).

Keywords for Literature Search at the end of this chapter).

When a new orthosis is received, a therapist must conduct an orthotic checkout examination of the client, the device, and the client wearing the device. This procedure is also discussed in Chapter 11, and specific items relevant to the checkout examination of KAFOs and KOs are listed in **Box 15.1**. The purpose of the checkout examination is to ensure that the device has been manufactured as prescribed and that its fit, function, comfort, and cosmesis are acceptable. The orthotist, therapist, and patient must work together to resolve any problems in any of these areas. When it is determined that the device is satisfactory, the therapist must review the orthotic goals and ensure that they are achieved or implement a program to accomplish them. Particularly for new orthosis wearers, this requires patient instruction in proper methods of donning, doffing, and caring for the orthosis, as well as guidelines for appropriate footwear (Chapter 13) for use with the device. In addition, new wearers must be provided with a "wearing schedule" that guides the users to gradually progress wearing time with their new appliance over several days to a week, depending on the individual needs of each client. Increasing orthotic wearing time by an hour or two at an interval appropriate for the specific individual can avoid problems or make them easier to resolve if they do occur.

Functional training may also be necessary, including gait training as well as training for other types of functional activities such as steps, negotiating all types of indoor and outdoor surfaces, ramps, and getting up and down from the floor. If running and other higher-level functions are appropriate for the client, these should be included as well. Asking patients to identify functional activities that are important to them or difficult for them helps clinicians individualize training and focus on relevant functional skills.

SUMMARY

Two categories of orthoses are used to address impairments that originate at the knee. They include KAFOs that enclose the knee and attach to orthotic ankle and foot components and KOs that only cross the knee joint, leaving the hip and ankle free. In addition, FR-AFOs, discussed in Chapter 14, are used to address some knee impairments when the individual also requires an AFO.

KAFOs apply forces to the knee using three- or four-point counterforce systems to control movement in the sagittal and frontal planes. Orthotic knee joints are either single-axis or polycentric and may have various controls, including no controls (free), a posterior offset axis, extension or flexion stops, various types of locks, or several mechanisms that offer stance phase control without restricting swing phase flexion. Although KAFOs that prevent knee buckling improve walking safety and prevent falls in individuals with knee weakness, locking the knee in extension also produces gait deviations that significantly increase the energy cost of walking. To improve daily functioning, KAFOs must be selected which enhance the individual's ability to walk safely while minimizing the increased energy costs.

Knee orthoses are most commonly used by individuals with musculoskeletal disorders of the knee that produce pain, dysfunction, or both. Knee orthoses are either rigid or soft, depending on the materials from which they are constructed, and are grouped into four functional categories: rehabilitative or postoperative orthoses, functional orthoses, patellofemoral orthoses, and unloading orthoses for unicompartment arthritis. There are many additional

---

BOX 15.1	Specific Items to Include in the Checkout Examination for Knee–Ankle–Foot Orthoses and Knee Orthoses

■ Height of medial and lateral thigh uprights or thigh shell: They should be below and not impinging on the perineum and greater trochanter, respectively, in weight-bearing and non-weight-bearing positions.

■ Alignment between orthotic and anatomical knee axes: Check and recheck this before and after movement to determine if the orthosis is migrating on the limb.

■ If shank (leg) and thigh uprights are present, check the space between the limb and the uprights: There should be adequate clearance but not too much space that will make the appliance unnecessarily bulky.

■ If plastic calf and thigh shells: Check for total contact throughout, appropriate fit of relief depressions, and any areas of excessive pressure.

■ Strapping: Straps should be secure, easy to open and close, and have room for adjustment.

■ Knee locks: Locks should work properly and be easy for the client to engage and release.

soft, over-the-counter appliances, usually some sort of pull-on elastic sleeve, which have no significant biomechanical control mechanisms to affect impairments other than to provide compression to control edema.

When a new orthosis is received by a client, the therapist must perform an orthotic checkout examination to ensure proper fit, function, comfort, and cosmesis. In addition, therapists must provide functional training in donning and doffing the device as well as required care or maintenance of the device. Patient training and instruction are required to ensure that the functional goals established when the prescription was made are achieved.

KEYWORDS FOR LITERATURE SEARCH

Knee or Knee–Ankle–Foot Orthoses

Select appropriate terms (keywords, words in subject headings, MeSH terms) from each domain and search by combining the selected terms with the Boolean term "AND."

Intervention
  Orthotic devices + knee
  Knee–ankle–foot orthosis
  Bracing; braces + knee
  Knee brace
  Postoperative bracing
  Functional bracing

Conditions:
  Cerebral palsy
  Polio; postpolio syndrome
  Osteoarthritis; arthritis
  Multiple sclerosis
  Muscular dystrophy
  Meningomyelocele
  Spinal cord injury
  Patellofemoral; patellofemoral pain
  Anterior cruciate ligament
  Knee instability
  Knee reconstruction

Effects
  Efficacy
  Effectiveness
  Energy expenditure
  Activities of daily living
  Gait analysis
  Clinical guidelines
  Electromyography (EMG)
  Biomechanics
  Stress

REFERENCES

1. Barnett S, Bagley A, Skinner H: Ankle weight effect on gait: orthotic implications. Orthopedics 16:1127–1131, 1993.
2. Phillips B, Zhao H: Predictors of assistive technology abandonment. Assist Technol 5:36–45, 1993.
3. Taktak DM, Bowker P: Lightweight modular knee-ankle-foot orthoses for Duchenne muscular dystrophy: design, development and evaluation. Arch Phys Med Rehabil 76:1156–1162, 1995.
4. Hachisuka K, Makino K, Wada F, et al: Clinical application of carbon fiber reinforced plastic leg orthosis for polio survivors and its advantages and disadvantages. Prosthet Orthot Int 30:129–135, 2006.
5. E-MAG Control Joint 17B200; www.ottobockus.com, Select "Doctors-Therapists-Dealers", Select Custom Orthotics, Select KAFOs, accessed 5/10/2010.
6. Phillips B, Zhao H: Predictors of assistive technology abandonment. Assist Technol 5:36–45, 1993.
7. Fisher LR, McLellan DL: Questionnaire assessment of patient satisfaction with lower limb orthoses from a district hospital. Prosthet Orthot Int 13:29–35, 1989.
8. Davids JR, Rowan R, Davis RB: Indications for orthoses to improve gait in children with cerebral palsy. J Am Acad Orthop Surg 15:178–188, 2007.
9. Kaufman KR, Irby SE: Ambulatory KAFOs: a biomechanical engineering perspective. J Prosthet Orthot 18:175–182, 2006.
10. Kaufman KR, Irby SE, Mathewson JW, et al: Energy-efficient knee-ankle-foot orthosis: a case study. J Prosthet Orthot 8:79–85, 1996.
11. Irby SE, Bernhardt KA, Kaufman KR: Gait of stance control orthosis users: the dynamic knee brace system. Prosthet Orthot Int 29:269–282, 2005.
12. Irby SE, Bernhardt KA, Kaufman KR: Gait changes over time in stance control orthosis users. Prosthet Orthot Int 31:353–361, 2007.
13. Sarmiento A, Latta L: The evolution of functional bracing of fractures. J Bone Joint Surg 88-B:144–148, 2006.
14. Ramsey DK, Wretenberg PF, Lamontagne M, et al: Electromyographic and biomechanic analysis of anterior cruciate ligament deficiency and functional knee bracing. Clin Biomech 18:28–34, 2003.
15. McDevitt ER, Taylor DC, Miller MD, et al: Functional bracing after anterior cruciate ligament reconstruction: a prospective, randomized multicenter study. Am J Sports Med 32:1887–1892, 2004.
16. Swirtun LR, Jansson A, Renstrom P: The effects of a functional knee brace during early treatment of patients with a nonoperated acute anterior cruciate ligament tear: a prospective randomized study. Clin J Sport Med 15:299–304, 2005.
17. Powers CM, Ward SR, Chan L-D, et al: The effect of bracing on patella alignment and patellofemoral joint contact area. Med Sci Sport Ex 36:1226–1232, 2004.
18. Powers CM, Doubleday KL, Escudero C: Influence of patellofemoral bracing on pain, knee extensor torque and gait function in females with patellofemoral pain. Physiother Theory Pract 24:143–150, 2008.
19. Powers CM, Ward SR, Chen Y-J, et al: The effect of bracing on patellofemoral joint stress during free and fast walking. Am J Sports Med 32:224–231, 2004.

20. Powers CM, Ward SR, Chen Y-J, et al: Effect of bracing on patellofemoral joint stress while ascending and descending stairs. Clin J Sport Med 14:206–214, 2004.

21. Matsumo H, Kadowaki KM, Tsuji H: Generation II knee bracing for severe medial compartment osteoarthritis of the knee. Arch Phys Med Rehabil 78:745–749, 1997.

22. Kirkley A, Webster-Bogaert S, Litchfield R, et al: The effect of bracing on varus gonarthrosis. J Bone Joint Surg 81-A:539–548, 1999.

23. Sharma L: Nonpharmacologic management of osteoarthritis. Curr Opin Rheumatol 14:603–607, 2002.

16

Orthoses for Paraplegia or Hip Impairments

OBJECTIVES

At the end of this chapter, all students are expected to:

1. Describe the types (categories) and functions of hip orthoses and orthoses used with individuals with paraplegia.
2. Identify and describe the parts of hip orthoses and orthoses prescribed for individuals with paraplegia, including the materials and componentry used.
3. Describe impairments that may be improved by hip orthoses (HOs) or hip–knee–ankle–foot orthoses (HKAFOs).
4. Discuss applications for HOs and orthoses to improve function for individuals with paraplegia.

Physical Therapy students are expected to:

1. Determine the need for a HO or an HKAFO based on examination findings.
   a. Evaluate client examination findings, including preorthotic prescription examination, lower quarter biomechanical assessment, and gait and functional analyses, to diagnose impairments that may be improved with a HO or HKAFO.
2. Develop appropriate goals for a HO or HKAFO based on a client's impairments and functional requirements.
3. Describe the biomechanical methods employed in HOs and HKAFOs to achieve the orthotic goals.
4. Develop and execute a search strategy to locate research evidence for the effects and effectiveness of HOs or HKAFOs and to identify best practices for orthotic prescription.
5. Recommend an appropriate orthosis to optimize function as a part of a plan of care for individuals with paraplegia or impairments of the hip.
6. Recommend shoes with appropriate characteristics for use with specific HKAFOs.
7. Examine and evaluate HOs and HKAFOs for acceptable fit, function, comfort, and cosmesis.

CASE STUDIES

Tyrone O'Neal is a 17-year-old high school football player who sustained a T8 fracture in an auto accident in which he was thrown from the car. The accident occurred 3 months ago, and he received immediate decompression and spine stabilization surgery at a trauma center. Despite prompt treatment, he has a complete spinal cord injury (ASIA level A: complete lesion with no motor or sensory function preserved in the sacral segments S4 through S5) with neural motor and sensory levels at T12 bilaterally. Initially, he required a postoperative spinal orthosis; however, he no longer needs additional external spine stabilization and does not have surgical restrictions. His upper extremity strength is 5/5, and his range of motion in both upper and lower extremities is full and pain free. Abdominal muscle strength is 3+/5. He is independent in a wheelchair and requires only minimal assistance to close supervision for transfers. He is otherwise healthy. Muscle tone in his paralyzed limbs using the modified Ashworth Scale is 2 to 2+ (marked increase in muscle tone through most of the range of motion (ROM), but affected parts are easily moved). He very much wants to walk and is highly motivated to achieve that goal.

Sasha Bogdonova is a 3-year-old child with cerebral palsy, spastic diplegic type. She is able to walk but displays scissoring gait characterized by both significant adduction and internal rotation at both hips. Using the modified Ashworth scale, her spasticity is rated 4, but she does not demonstrate fixed contractures, and passive range of motion (PROM) at both hips includes the following: abduction, 30°; external rotation, 20°; hip extension, 5°; knee extension, 0°; ankle dorsiflexion, 3°. Standing x-rays reveal hip displacement with a Migration Percentage of 30%. Sasha is not using any orthoses at the present time. She walks independently indoors but uses a posterior walker outdoors or in the community where her scissoring causes her to fall. Sasha has supportive parents who are very involved in her therapy.

Case Study Activities

All students:

1. Discuss whether each client may benefit from an orthosis and justify your decision.
   a. Discuss the functional problems that may be improved with an orthosis.
   b. Identify and discuss functional activities and possible participation restrictions that may be affected by use of an orthosis.
   c. What joint or joints may benefit from an orthosis? What would an orthosis need to do at the joint(s) to improve function?
2. How do you expect an orthosis to affect each client's ability to walk, gait pattern, and ability to perform other functional activities?
3. Identify and discuss advantages and disadvantages of using an orthosis with each client.

Physical Therapy students:

1. Describe the impairments that contribute to each client's functional limitations.
2. If an orthosis is indicated, develop specific orthotic goals for each client.
3. Develop a specific orthotic prescription to achieve the best outcome and functional improvement.
   a. Describe the type of orthosis, the orthotic componentry, and the biomechanical methods of force application that will achieve the specific orthotic goals.
   b. Using biomechanical terminology, name the orthosis that you recommend for each client.
   c. If specific shoes are required, describe the shoes you recommend for use with the orthosis and why specific shoe characteristics are required.
   d. Is there evidence in the research literature to support your orthotic recommendations for each client? Describe the evidence you found and how it impacted your orthotic recommendation.
4. Develop a physical therapy plan of care for each client, which includes an orthoses, if appropriate, as well as other physical therapy interventions.
5. How will you determine and measure the effectiveness and functional outcome of your interventions?

ORTHOSES FOR IMPAIRMENTS AT THE HIP

Two major categories of orthoses have components that cross the hip joint. They are HKAFOs and HOs. HKAFOs include orthotic components that cross the hip joint and are attached to various knee and ankle and foot components that are discussed in Chapters 15 and 14, respectively. HKAFOs are usually prescribed for patients with paraplegia or significant paraparesis due to spinal cord injury, including those with acquired injuries due to accidents, congenital deficiencies such as spina bifida with meningomyelocele, or paralyses that develop gradually due to progressive neuromuscular diseases. HOs are most often used as part of the management of childhood skeletal disorders, such as congenital hip dysplasia, or to restrict hip movement during the postoperative period following hip surgery in children and adults.

In an HKAFO or HO, the orthotic hip joint is an articulation that connects the thigh upright and its attached cuff or molded shell to the pelvic component. It is oriented to align with the anatomical hip joint and is located externally at a point slightly anterior and superior to the greater trochanter (see Table 2.1). The pelvic component, called a **pelvic band**, is made of a rigid material that spans the distance between the greater trochanter and the iliac crest (**Fig. 16.1**). Compared to the length of the leg lever, the orthotic pelvic lever arm is quite short and requires that the orthosis apply a large force over a relatively small area of contact with the body. Thus, for some individuals, particularly those with weak hip extensor and trunk muscles, a pelvic band may be inadequate to provide effective hip and pelvic control (**Fig. 16.2**). For these individuals, effective orthotic control of the pelvis requires supporting the trunk as well. Thus, rather than a pelvic band, some HKAFOs have an extended structure to provide stabilization to the pelvis and trunk together (**Fig. 16.3**). Those HKAFOs that include componentry over the lumbar or lumbar and thoracic regions of the spine are called LS-HKAFOs and TLS-HKAFOs, respectively. Regardless of the level of the superior extent of the pelvic or trunk portion of the orthosis, biomechanically they function similarly to achieve hip and trunk stabilization for walking in paraplegic individuals and are thus discussed collectively with HKAFOs

HKAFOs and HOs restrain unwanted motion in the hip joint via three- or four-point counterforce systems or force couples applied in the sagittal (flexion)

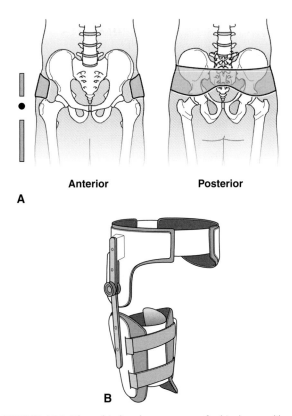

FIGURE 16.1. The pelvic band component of a hip–knee–ankle–foot orthosis extends between the iliac crest and greater trochanter. **(A)** Pelvic bands are constructed from rigid materials, such as padded metal or molded plastic. **(B)** All pelvic bands offer a short lever arm to control the trunk and pelvis.

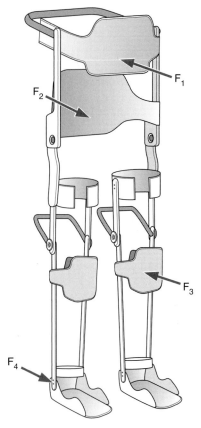

FIGURE 16.3. A hip guidance orthosis (HGO) or ParaWalker extends superiorly to stabilize the trunk as well as the pelvis. Orthotic forces are applied using a four-point counterforce system.

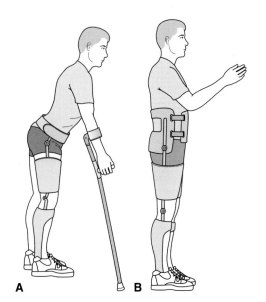

FIGURE 16.2. Clients with poor trunk and pelvic control are inadequately stabilized with a pelvic band alone **(A)**. An orthosis that extends to the thoracic spine provides trunk and pelvic control **(B)**.

or frontal (adduction) planes (see Fig. 16.3). Transverse plane motion, however, is poorly controlled with hip orthoses. Straps that spiral around the leg and attach to a pelvic strap have been used to restrain excessive internal or external rotation of the limb when the deformity is flexible. However, their effectiveness is limited, and they are more often used as a therapy aid rather than a definitive orthotic device (Fig. 16.4).

HOs and HKAFOs, however, are not the only orthoses used to address impairments at the hip. Ground reaction knee–ankle–foot orthoses (GR-KAFOs), designed to manipulate the ground reaction force vector (GRFV) with respect to the hip axis, apply forces to the hip without physically extending across the hip by holding the ankle in a dorsiflexed position while the knee is locked in extension. The biomechanical explanation of how these GR-KAFOs stabilize the hip is described in this chapter as an orthotic option for individuals with paraplegia.

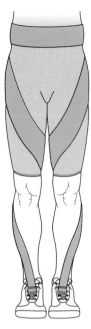

FIGURE 16.4. Straps attached to a waist or pelvic belt are designed to limit hip internal rotation in individuals with flexible deformities. However, effectiveness is limited.

HIP CONTROL USING ORTHOTIC HIP JOINTS

Orthotic hip joints are mechanical articulations that extend across and encase the hip joint and use various components to control unwanted hip motions. Although the anatomical hip joint allows movement in all three planes, most orthotic hip joints are uniaxial and permit only sagittal plane flexion and extension movements. Various orthotic components are available to control or limit movements at the hip in the sagittal plane. Categories of orthotic hip joints and components include free motion joints, limited motion joints, orthotic locks, and reciprocal motion joints.

Orthotic Components to Stop or Lock Sagittal Plane Hip Movement

A **free motion joint** is a single-axis orthotic hip joint that does not limit movement in the sagittal plane but blocks both frontal and transverse plane motions and holds the hip in a neutral position in these planes. A **limited motion joint** is an orthotic joint that has either a flexion or extension stop or both extension and flexion stops. Orthotic stops are components that are added to the single-axis joint to stop motion at a predetermined point in a particular direction. Thus, a 0° extension stop limits or stops hip extension at 0°. An orthotic hip joint with both flexion and extension stops limits motion to that available between the two stops (**Fig. 16.5**). An **orthotic lock** is a mechanism that, when engaged, locks or holds the joint in a predetermined position and prevents all movement. When the lock is disengaged, free joint movement is permitted. The most common type of hip joint lock is the *drop-ring lock*, which is also used to lock the knee in extension (see Fig. 15.5). This lock is composed of a simple metal ring that fits over and slides on the pelvic upright (**Fig. 16.6**). When it slides down over the hip joint, it prevents both flexion and extension.

Reciprocating Orthotic Hip Joints

Although the joints described above may be used in unilateral or bilateral orthoses, **reciprocal orthotic hip joints** are used only on bilateral KAFOs or HKAFOs with a pelvic band or a trunk stabilizing component. Reciprocal orthotic hip joints are interconnected by cables or other mechanisms that limit step length.[1] When the wearer advances one leg by rotating the trunk or flexing the hip for swing phase, the coupled hip mechanism results in concurrent extension of the other hip (in stance phase). Additionally, when the reciprocal hip mechanism is engaged, both hips cannot flex simultaneously during stance, thus restraining

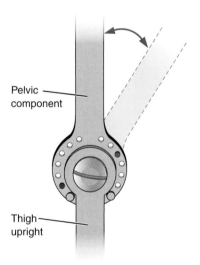

Pelvic component

Thigh upright

FIGURE 16.5. A limited motion hip joint has orthotic components called stops that restrict joint movement between preset, but usually adjustable, limits.

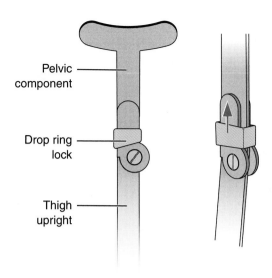

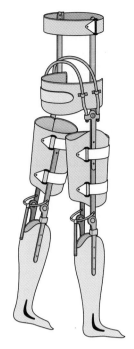

FIGURE 16.6. A drop-ring lock slides down over the hip joint to lock or hold the joint at 0°. When it is disengaged, free hip flexion and extension occur.

FIGURE 16.7. The Louisiana State University reciprocating gait orthosis has two cables that link the hip joints, one connecting anterior and the other posterior to the hip joints. The cables transmit the force that couples flexion of one hip with concurrent extension of the other hip.

"jackknifing" or unwanted trunk flexion. The reciprocal mechanism, however, can be disengaged to allow the wearer to sit down or get up from a chair. This reciprocal mechanism was developed at the Ontario Crippled Children's Center and revised by researchers at Louisiana State University (LSU), New Orleans, Louisiana (**Fig. 16.7**). Orthoses with reciprocating hip mechanisms are called *reciprocating gait HKAFO* (RG-HKAFOs) or most commonly, simply *reciprocating gait orthoses* (RGOs). The *LSU-RGO* has two Bowden cables, one attaching anterior and the other posterior to the hip joints. These cables couple the hip joints so that flexion of one hip in swing results in concurrent stance phase extension of the other hip. A modification of this system, called the *advanced RGO* (ARGO), has a single push–pull cable that links the mechanical hip joints to produce the reciprocal hip joint movement.[2] It also has a cable link between the orthotic hip and knee joints and a pneumatic assist to aid knee extension. These features make it easier to rise from the sitting position by eliminating the need to manually straighten and lock the knees before standing.[3] A third variation of the RGO-type appliance is called the *isocentric RGO* (IRGO). This type of RGO produces reciprocal hip motion by replacing the cables used in other RGO designs with a specially designed pelvic band with a centrally located pivoting bar and tie rod arrangement, which is simple and durable (**Fig. 16.8**).

Another type of reciprocating system developed in Australia in the early 1990s for individuals with

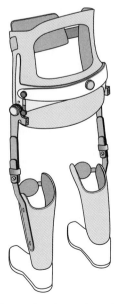

FIGURE 16.8. An isocentric reciprocating gait orthosis uses a centrally pivoting bar and tie rod arrangement, which eliminates the cables used by other reciprocating gait orthosis designs to produce reciprocal hip motion.

paraplegia is called the *WalkAbout system*.[4] This device provides an alternative to HKAFOs with laterally placed external hip joints and is composed of a pair of KAFOs connected with a removable single medial hip joint. This medial connecter, which includes two center balls linked together with a spacer, attaches to the proximal ends of the medial uprights of both KAFOs and allows reciprocal movement of the legs (**Fig. 16.9**). This system is lightweight, easy to don and doff, and easy to use with a wheelchair. Some individuals with spinal cord injuries also report improved standing balance with this device when compared to using unlinked KAFOs.[5] However, because of the misalignment of the orthotic and anatomical hip joints, individuals walking with this device demonstrate very short step length (37% of normal) and excessive horizontal rotation of the pelvis, resulting in a slow, energy-expensive gait.[6] Several other medially linked KAFO systems for individuals with lower-level thoracolumbar paraplegia were developed to minimize these problems, including the Primewalk and a hip and ankle linked orthosis. The Primewalk uses a sliding mechanism to bring the orthotic and physiological hip centers closer together. The hip and ankle linking orthosis connects both ankles to the single medial hip joint, which enables the user to keep both feet parallel to the floor throughout gait and provides assistance for leg swing.[7]

Orthotic Components for Frontal and Transverse Plane Positioning of the Hip

Adjustable positioning orthotic joints are composed of a moveable single-axis hip joint with additional componentry that allows the orthotist to position the thigh upright in positions other than frontal and transverse plane neutral. Thus, the orthosis can be used to place the thigh in positions such as abduction or medial or lateral rotation, while allowing sagittal plane flexion and extension movements. This adjustable feature is used therapeutically to position the hip in abduction, or it may also be used to accommodate a hip deformity. Various mechanisms are employed to achieve this joint positioning, including adjustable serrated plates in the frontal plane to control abduction positioning or in the transverse plane to position the thigh in a selected position of rotation (**Fig. 16.10**). An alternative orthotic mechanism consists of a free moving ball surrounded by a ring with two set screws. Tightening the screws allows the orthotist to lock the joint in a desired three-dimensional position (**Fig. 16.11**).

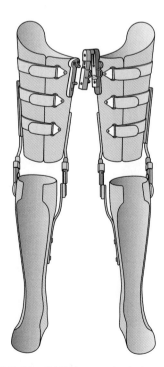

FIGURE 16.9. The WalkAbout orthosis is made up of two knee–ankle–foot orthoses connected at the proximal ends of their medial uprights with a mechanism that enables reciprocal gait.

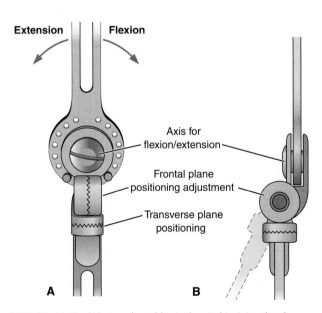

FIGURE 16.10. **(A)** An adjustable single-axis hip joint that has opposed serrated plates to adjust the positioning of the thigh upright in the frontal and transverse planes. **(B)** The adjustable single-axis hip joint is adjusted from a neutral (gray) to an abducted position (pink).

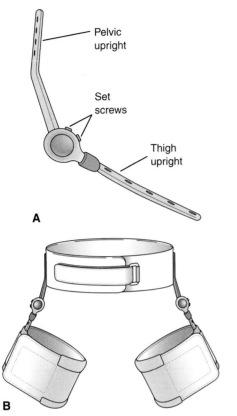

FIGURE 16.11. (A) An adjustable spherical joint is adjusted to a desired position and locked with set screws. (B) The joint is used in an abduction positioning hip orthosis.

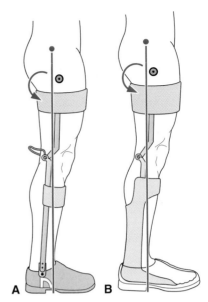

FIGURE 16.12. Scott-Craig knee–ankle–foot orthoses provide a stance phase hip extension moment by manipulating the ground reaction force vector posterior to the hip joint axis. Both conventional (A) and a hybrid of metal and molded plastic components (B) are used (●, center of mass; ◉ joint axis).

HIP CONTROL USING GROUND REACTION FORCES

An alternative to an orthotic hip joint to provide sagittal plane stance phase control is use of the ground reaction force vector (GRFV). When the GRFV passes posterior to the hip joint, it produces a hip extension moment (Figs. 2.2 and 16.12). Hip extension is limited by the large iliofemoral ligament (Y-ligament or Ligament of Bigelow), which is a strong connective tissue thickening that reinforces the anterior hip joint capsule and prevents excessive hip hyperextension. Thus, when the posteriorly positioned GRFV produces a hip and trunk extension moment, hyperextension is anatomically limited by the iliofemoral ligament. *Scott-Craig KAFOs* are designed to use the GRFV to provide hip stability in the sagittal plane during stance phase for individuals with hip extensor weakness and paraplegia.[8] These braces direct the GRFV to a position posterior to the hip joint axis by using orthotic componentry to hold

the ankle in a small amount of dorsiflexion while locking the knee in full extension (see Fig. 16.12). The plantarflexion stop of this slightly dorsiflexed solid ankle joint forces the leg to rotate anteriorly as the foot moves from heel strike to foot flat (weight acceptance). As a result, during midstance, the GRFV passes anterior to the knee and posterior to the hip, facilitating knee and hip extension, respectively (Fig. 16.13). This biomechanical design can be constructed using either conventional metal and leather long leg brace components, as originally designed, or a combination of metal and molded plastic materials.[9] Regardless of the materials used, clients who ambulate with Scott-Craig KAFOs use a swing-to or swing-through tripod gait pattern with bilateral crutches. Although these appliances were specifically developed for clients with paraplegia due to spinal cord injury, many paraplegic individuals are unable to successfully use them for function due to frontal and transverse plane instabilities. For example, patients with spinal cord injuries who experience involuntary muscle spasms may have difficulty if their spasms cause their legs to swing forward unevenly, scissor (adduct), or slide apart uncontrollably, producing loss of balance and falls. Several devices were developed to address these issues. One device is a spreader-bar that attaches to the medial uprights, keeping the legs

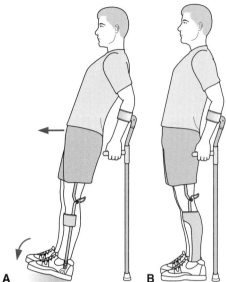

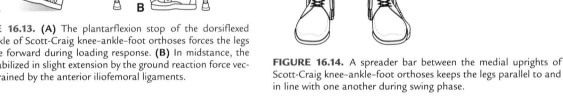

FIGURE 16.13. (A) The plantarflexion stop of the dorsiflexed solid ankle of Scott-Craig knee–ankle–foot orthoses forces the legs to rotate forward during loading response. **(B)** In midstance, the hip is stabilized in slight extension by the ground reaction force vector, restrained by the anterior iliofemoral ligaments.

FIGURE 16.14. A spreader bar between the medial uprights of Scott-Craig knee–ankle–foot orthoses keeps the legs parallel to and in line with one another during swing phase.

parallel and in-line with one another throughout stance and swing (**Fig. 16.14**). The medially linked KAFOs (see Fig. 16.9) discussed with the reciprocating orthotic components also help to control the legs in the frontal and transverse planes and may be an effective solution for individuals who do not require the more extensive bracing of HKAFOs.

ORTHOTIC APPLIANCES FOR INDIVIDUALS WITH PARAPLEGIA

A major challenge for individuals with paraplegia is to find a practical and relatively energy-efficient method for functional mobility inside, outside, and in the community. Using a wheelchair on level surfaces is a highly efficient means of locomotion, with an average speed, rate of oxygen uptake, and oxygen cost that approximate that of normal walking.[10] Although the Americans with Disabilities Act (www.ada.gov) requires architectural accessibility in all public places and reasonable accommodations in schools and work environments, depending totally on a wheelchair for all mobility can be difficult. Additionally, remaining seated in a wheelchair has negative effects on health, including the possible development of muscle atrophy, joint contractures, and pressure ulcers, as well as osteoporosis, urinary and

intestinal stasis, and cardiovascular deconditioning.[11] Children with congenital spinal cord deficiencies also require weight-bearing through their lower limbs to stimulate normal skeletal development and maturation. Because of these negative psychosocial and physiological effects of remaining totally in a wheelchair, two types of appliances have been developed to help individuals with spinal cord injuries achieve upright postures. The first group of devices includes standing devices or frames that are used primarily to achieve and maintain a static upright posture to facilitate weight-bearing through the legs. The second group includes various orthotic systems used for therapeutic or functional ambulation. **Therapeutic ambulation** includes part-time walking for the purpose of exercise and to reduce the health risks of wheelchair sitting. Functional ambulation refers to the use of ambulation as the primary method of mobility during daily functional activity. Appliances used by individuals with paraplegia or paraparesis for functional ambulation include various combinations of KAFOs and AFOs, bilateral KAFOs, HKAFOs, RGOs, and functional electrical stimulation, used either alone or in conjunction with orthoses. Although the orthotic components used in these orthoses are described earlier in this chapter, commonly prescribed appliances used by paraplegic individuals to achieve standing and walking are described here.

Standing Frames

Orthotic devices to support static standing are commercially available in sizes for both children and adults. However, most **standing frames** are used with young children with paraplegia to enable weight-bearing through the lower limbs to facilitate development and to provide hands-free (no crutches required) standing so the child can play and experience various environments. Most of these devices have a series of alternating anterior and posterior straps or pads that create a four-point counterforce system to stabilize the trunk, hips, and knees, while securing the feet to a large, stable base (**Fig. 16.15**). These devices are applied over clothing and shoes. *Prone standers* provide similar experiences for children who are unable to stand independently, but the support framework contacts the anterior surface of the body and can be adjusted from fully prone to fully upright and a variety of intermediate positions (**Fig. 16.16**). The *Rochester Parapodium* is a modified standing frame that has articulations at the hips and knees that allow the child to sit down and stand again (**Fig. 16.17**). To sit down, the child rotates the levers located at hip level on the lateral uprights. To rise from a chair, the child pulls on the central rod that extends from the footplate. The hips can also be bent while keeping the knees extended, which permits the child to bend over to retrieve a toy from the floor.

Another version of the standing frame, called a **Swivel Walker**, was developed at the Orthotic Research and Locomotion Assessment Unit (ORLAU)

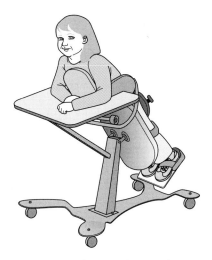

FIGURE 16.16. Prone standers are adjustable from a prone to a fully upright position, as well as intermediate postures.

in England. It is similar in design to other standing frames in that it has a frame to which are attached a series of pads or straps to provide four-point counterforces that stabilize the trunk, hips, and knees for upright standing. Its footplate, however, is different from other standing frames, because it is designed to

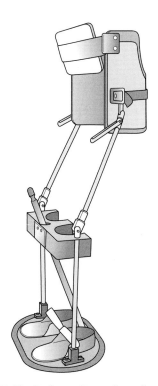

FIGURE 16.17. The Rochester Parapodium allows a paraplegic child to stand, sit, and bend over to retrieve an object from the floor.

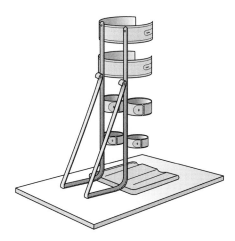

FIGURE 16.15. Standing frames are primarily used with young children with paraplegia to provide hands-free weight-bearing experiences.

permit swivel walking by tilting or shifting weight from side to side (**Fig. 16.18**). The lower surface of the footplate has two swiveling plates that slope upward and laterally to allow the user to rock from side to side. The sideways inertial forces produced during this side-to-side rocking create a forward turning moment resulting in forward movement or ambulation over smooth, flat surfaces.[12,13] Certain Parapodiums, although they do not have this specially designed footplate, also offer the opportunity for self-actuated ambulation using side-to-side alternate rocking and pivoting.

Orthoses for Ambulation

At the present time, there are many orthotic options for individuals with spinal cord injury and paraplegia who are motivated to ambulate. Thus, it can be difficult to select the most appropriate appliance for a particular individual. Because there is so much variation among individuals with spinal cord injury, it is important to complete a carefully performed and thorough preorthotic prescription client examination and to thoroughly discuss the client's goals and expectations prior to considering orthotic options.

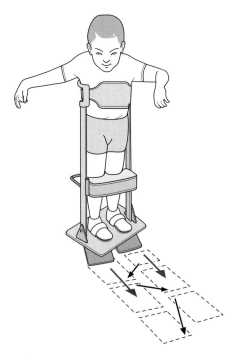

FIGURE 16.18. The Swivel Walker consists of a standing frame with a specialized footplate. The child ambulates by rocking from side to side and pivoting forward.

Table 16.1 presents important client factors and their implications for making orthotic prescriptions with paraplegic individuals.

A major factor to consider when selecting orthoses for individuals with spinal cord injuries is the high energy cost of ambulation. Although some research has been conducted to identify and compare the energy costs of ambulation with various orthotic devices, components, and combinations of appliances, the numbers of subjects in these studies is small, which limits the generalizability of the findings. Additionally, it is difficult to directly apply these research findings to a specific client because so many individual factors affect the actual energy cost of ambulation for a particular individual. For example, at the neurological level, whether the injury is complete or incomplete and the presence or degree of spasticity or spasms represents a few factors that vary among individuals with spinal cord injury and affect energy expenditure during ambulation. Despite these limitations, clinicians who prescribe orthoses for individuals with spinal cord injuries with paraplegia need current information regarding the energy costs of ambulation with various orthoses or other devices and must factor this information into their orthotic recommendations. Using the Keywords for Literature Search terms at the end of this chapter can help clinicians to find and access up-to-date research concerning the energy costs of new orthotic devices as they develop.

There are six major categories of orthoses used by individuals with spinal cord injuries who want to ambulate functionally or for exercise. They are listed in **Table 16.2**. The components used in these orthoses are described in this chapter under the headings of "Hip Control Using Orthotic Hip Joints" and "Hip Control Using Ground Reaction Forces."

Bilateral Hip–Knee–Ankle–Foot Orthoses With Pelvic Band or Thoracolumbar Orthosis

Bilateral HKAFOs with a pelvic band (with or without thoracolumbar orthosis) were the traditional appliances prescribed for paraplegic individuals, particularly children with spina bifida with thoracic-level spinal lesions requiring external hip and pelvic control. Originally, these orthoses were constructed from metal and leather, but more modern versions use molded plastic thigh and calf components with metal uprights and pelvic band (**Fig. 16.19**). When these

TABLE 16.1	Client Factors and Implications for Orthotic Prescription for Individuals With Paraplegia Due to Acquired or Congenital Spinal Cord Injury	
Client Factors	**Implications for Orthotic Prescription**	
Upper extremity dexterity and strength	■ Ability to use crutches ■ Ability to don/doff appliances	
Active muscle control of the trunk and pelvis	■ Need for orthotic components to control trunk/pelvis	
Ability to stabilize the hips in extension (active hip extensor muscles)	■ Need for orthotic control of unwanted hip flexion in stance (hip joints/stops, GR-KAFOs, etc)	
Ability to actively advance each leg by hip flexion or trunk rotation	■ Selecting orthoses to use with reciprocal versus swing-through gait patterns	
Ability to control the hip in the frontal plane (unwanted abduction or adduction?)	■ Separate KAFOs versus connected KAFOs or HKAFOs	
Ability to control the hip in the transverse plane (unwanted medial or lateral rotation?)	■ Separate KAFOs versus connected KAFOs or HKAFOs	
Presence of involuntary muscle spasms during upright posture that produce jackknifing, scissoring, or unwanted hip or knee flexion	■ Significant spasms may require more restrictive HKAFOs or pharmacological management of spasms before orthotic prescription	
Ability to actively stabilize the knees in extension (quadriceps control)	■ KAFO versus AFO	
Ability to actively control the foot and ankle (active dorsiflexion, eversion, plantarflexion)	■ Foot/ankle orthotic componentry	
Presence of muscle imbalance deformity (eg, equinovarus, calcaneous)	■ Surgical/pharmacological correction of deformity to make the foot plantigrade	
Presence of joint contractures, particularly hip or knee flexion	■ Stretching prior to orthotic prescription	
Presence of sensation, including joint proprioception	■ Protection ■ Impaired sensation may require more orthotic controls	
Cardiovascular fitness	■ Ability to tolerate the high level of energy expenditure of ambulation	

AFO, ankle–foot orthosis; GR-KAFO, ground reaction knee–ankle–foot orthosis; HKAFO, hip–knee–ankle–foot orthosis; KAFO, knee–ankle–foot orthosis.

appliances are used, the hip and knee joints are locked in extension, the ankle joints have plantarflexion stops, and the child ambulates using crutches and a swing-through gait pattern. These devices may be heavy, bulky, and unsightly, but most importantly, the required gait pattern results in a high energy cost.[14,15] As a result, few individuals are able to use these devices for functional mobility. In addition, negotiating stairs or walking on any surface other than smooth, flat surfaces is very difficult.[16]

TABLE 16.2 Types of Orthoses Used for Ambulation by Individuals With Congenital or Acquired Spinal Cord Lesion

Types of Orthoses	Considerations
Bilateral HKAFOs + pelvic band	■ Bulky, heavy ■ Locked hips and knees require swing-through gait ■ High energy expenditure
Bilateral KAFOs ■ Unattached (Scott-Craig) ■ Medially attached (WalkAbout)	■ Scott-Craig requires swing-through gait; high energy expenditure ■ WalkAbout—very slow gait; high energy expenditure ■ Both require active trunk and hip frontal plane control
Reciprocal orthoses ■ HGO or ParaWalker ■ LSU-RGO ■ ARGO ■ IRGO ■ IRGO + stance control knee joint ■ WalkAbout, Primewalk KAFOs	■ All require ability to advance each leg individually by hip or trunk flexion ■ HGO very stable, wear over clothing ■ WalkAbout KAFOs very short step, slow gait, very high energy cost ■ Locked knee requires lateral trunk lean to clear opposite foot for swing ■ RGO + stance control knee allows knee flexion during swing, leading to increased step length and reduced energy cost compared to locked-knee RGO
FES (Parastep®)	■ Very slow gait; very high energy expenditure ■ Fatigue of stimulated muscles ■ Easy to don/doff ■ Easier to get out of chair; do not have to lock knees before arising
FES-orthosis hybrids ■ FES + AFOs ■ FES + RGOs	■ Easier to get out of chair with FES-assisted knee extension ■ In FES-RGOs, improved hemodynamics in legs but no improvement in energy cost of ambulation
AFOs	■ For low lumbar or sacral SCI levels ■ Improved sagittal plane ankle motion in gait, but increased transverse plane knee motion, which may produce knee instability and early DJD

AFO, ankle–foot orthosis; ARGO, advanced reciprocating gait orthosis; DJD, degenerative joint disease; FES, functional electrical stimulation; HGO, hip guidance orthosis; HKAFO, hip–knee–ankle–foot orthosis; IRGO, isocentric reciprocating gait orthosis; KAFO, knee–ankle–foot orthosis; LSU-RGO, Louisiana State University reciprocating gait orthosis; SCI, spinal cord injury.

Bilateral Knee–Ankle–Foot Orthoses

Bilateral unattached KAFOs, such as the *Scott-Craig orthoses* (see Fig. 16.12), provide hip control by using the GRFV rather than an orthotic hip joint. These orthoses may be used by individuals who have sufficient trunk control and do not require trunk or pelvic orthotic support. Individuals typically walk using crutches and a swing-through gait pattern, which has a very high energy cost, although some individuals are able to use a reciprocal four-point gait, which is much slower.[16] Individuals who have difficulty with spasticity and involuntary spasms in the trunk and hip flexor muscles may be unsafe as the spasms may cause jackknifing,

uneven leg swing, scissoring, or unwanted leg rotation, which disrupt balance and cause falls. Scott-Craig KAFOs also feature cam locks with bail releases at the knee (see Fig. 15.5B). This feature may make sitting down in a chair easier, because the bail is meant to release or unlock the knee locks when they contact the chair seat during descent, thus eliminating the need to manually release the locks. Although this eliminates the need to manually release the locks, this sitting-down maneuver requires a high level of skill and precise positioning, which are not achievable by all users.

The *WalkAbout* component (and modifications of this design) attaches to and links the proximal medial

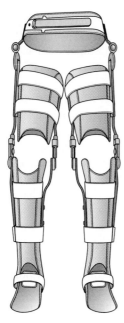

FIGURE 16.19. Bilateral hip-knee-ankle-foot orthoses with molded plastic and conventional components. The molded footplate is worn inside oxford-style shoes with a cushion heel.

uprights of bilateral KAFOs (see Fig. 16.9). This device allows a reciprocal gait pattern but also severely restricts step length and thus walking speed. When compared to other reciprocal orthoses, walking with the WalkAbout medially attached KAFO appliance is slower and has significantly greater energy demands.[17] An advantage of this device, however, is that because it attaches to the KAFOs medially, it does not add width to the wearer and thus makes it easy to get into and out of a wheelchair. This feature may be advantageous for the individual who uses a wheelchair for functional mobility but requires the ability to stand and walk short distances from the wheelchair for certain activities.

Reciprocal Gait Orthoses

Reciprocal gait orthoses (RGOs) are bilateral HKAFOs that have lateral orthotic hip joints aligned with the anatomical joints and a pelvic band or thoracolumbar orthosis (see Figs. 16.7 and 16.8). The primary characteristic of these appliances is that they have componentry that couples the orthotic hip joints so that they cannot flex simultaneously, thus preventing jackknifing. They also facilitate a reciprocal gait pattern because hip flexion on one side facilitates concurrent hip extension on the contralateral side. There are three major types of RGOs: the LSU-RGO, the ARGO, and the IRGO. The different characteristics and

componentry used in each type are described in this chapter under the topic heading "Hip Control Using Orthotic Hip Joints." Although these appliances were first developed for children as an alternative to bilateral long leg braces with pelvic band, versions for adults were soon developed, and today all types are available for both children and adults. Although all three types of RGOs can be constructed using various configurations, the ARGO typically has only lateral uprights and hip–knee links and pneumatic-assisted knee extension that facilitates sitting down and rising from a chair. Another reciprocating orthosis is the *hip guidance orthosis* (HGO), designed for children, and its adult counterpart, the *ParaWalker*, that was developed in England (see Fig. 16.3). These devices are TLS-HKAFOs (thoracolumbosacral-hip-knee-ankle orthoses), but instead of having a linking mechanism connecting the hip joints, the ParaWalker hip joints are very sturdy and have adjustments to restrict the arc of hip motion. This appliance is worn over clothing and has shoe plates to which the wearer's shoes are strapped. Although these reciprocating devices improved paraplegic gait efficiency, it is still very low when compared to normal gait and even to wheelchair ambulation.[18–20]

Most RGOs include orthotic knee locks that fix the knees in extension and require users to lean posterolaterally to advance the contralateral leg and clear the advancing foot over the floor. Ambulation with this stiff-knee gait pattern causes an increase in oxygen uptake by as much as 23% per limb.[21] The stance control orthotic knee joint (discussed in Chapter 15) provides knee stability in stance phase while allowing free knee flexion during swing. When it is used in a unilateral KAFO, it decreases oxygen consumption and energy cost compared to a similar appliance with a locked knee.[22] Building on this experience, the locked-knee joints of an IRGO were replaced with stance control joints for a single client with a T10 complete spinal cord injury.[23] The addition of the stance control knee joints to the IRGO used by this subject doubled his walking speed and stride length and improved the consistency of his gait pattern. Although oxygen consumption was not measured, the client reported that he preferred the stance control knee joints to the locked joints.

Functional Electrical Stimulation

Functional neuromuscular **electrical stimulation** (FES) is also used as an orthotic option with paraplegic individuals. It can be used as an orthosis to provide trains of electrical stimulation to selected paralyzed muscles and peripheral nerves to produce muscle contractions in a pattern that allows ambulation. A FES device to provide unbraced ambulation for short distances by paraplegic individuals was developed by Daniel Graupe and colleagues at the University of Illinois at Chicago in the 1980s.[24] This device, called the *Parastep*® (Sigmedics Inc, Northfield, Illinois), received approval from the United States Food and Drug Administration (FDA) in 1994 and is commercially available by prescription. It can be used with paraplegic individuals whose lesions are at T12 or higher, with intact lumbar peripheral nerves. It consists of a belt or pocket-held microcomputer and electrical stimulation unit, push-button switches located on the handles of a walker to input commands to the computer, and four or six pairs of adhesive surface electrodes with lead wires from the stimulator (**Fig. 16.20**). Pairs of stimulating electrodes are placed on both legs over the quadriceps to stimulate knee extension, over the common peroneal nerve to stimulate flexion and stepping, and over the paraspinal or gluteal muscles to stimulate trunk/hip extension and pelvic stability.[25] Others have developed FES orthoses for paraplegia that use implanted electrodes rather than surface electrodes.[26] Generally,

the microprocessor generates trains of impulses that grossly imitate the neural triggers that would have traveled through the spinal cord to the appropriate peripheral nerves below the injury level. These trains of stimuli trigger action potentials in the peripheral nerves and cause muscle contraction. The push buttons on the handles of the specially equipped walker allow the user to select from the computer's program menu: stand up, sit down, step left, step right, increase stimulation, or decrease stimulation.[25] Although the walking abilities of different users are quite variable, one study reports that on average subjects were able to walk 115 meters (about 377 feet) at an average speed of 5 meters/minute (about 0.2 mph).[27] However, the physical effort involved in standing and walking with a FES system alone is estimated as at least six times that of normal walking by an unimpaired individual, as indicated by oxygen uptake tests.[25] Although the energy cost of FES-assisted ambulation is quite high, even higher than the energy costs of walking with mechanical orthotic systems, electrical stimulation of the leg muscles during walking improves venous return and stroke volume, which are reduced in paraplegic individuals due to pooling of blood in the legs as a result of loss of the muscle pump. In addition, FES-stimulation builds some

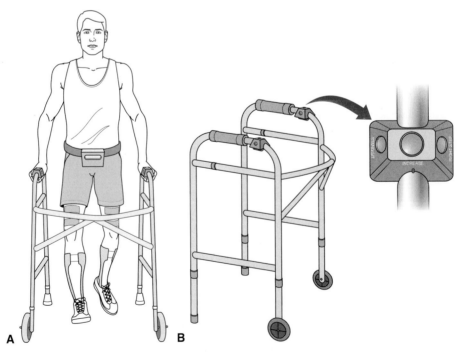

FIGURE 16.20. The Parastep® is a functional electrical stimulation device that provides standing and walking opportunities for individuals with paraplegia, shown here in use with bilateral ankle-foot orthoses. The microprocessor/electrical stimulator unit is worn on the body (**A**) with a push-button controller on the walker handle (**B**).

muscle mass in paralyzed atrophied muscles.[20] Despite these benefits, the high energy expenditure and fatiguing of the stimulated muscles limits the application of this FES-assisted ambulation system primarily to therapeutic walking rather than functional ambulation.

Functional Electrical Stimulation–Orthosis Hybrid Appliances

To overcome the limitations of using FES alone for ambulation, hybrid devices that combine a FES device with mechanical orthoses have been developed. These include using FES stimulation with AFOs, various types of RGOs, as well as stance control KAFOs. Various combinations of mechanical orthotic components and FES configurations have been tried, but basically, the mechanical orthoses provide joint stabilization and the FES provides propulsion. A major advantage of the FES in these hybrid orthoses is that the quadriceps contraction provides controlled knee flexion during rising from and returning to a sitting position, which uses less energy and effort than performing that task with braced knees that are locked in extension. Another advantage of FES-hybrid orthoses that have orthotic knee locks or controls is that during static stance, the quadriceps stimulation (and contraction) can be turned off. This reduces the energy cost of sustained muscle contraction and reduces the energy expenditure and muscle fatigue that limits ambulation using FES alone.[20] The FES configurations used in various hybrid orthoses also differ considerably. For example, one study of hybrid orthoses used AFOs or SMOs coupled with implanted FES electrodes to muscles in both legs, including the quadriceps, gluteus maximus and medius, and posterior fibers of the adductor magnus.[28] Some studies report the effects of hybrid orthoses that combine various types of RGOs with FES using surface electrodes to the quadriceps and hamstring only, while others used implanted electrodes in the quadriceps, gluteus maximus and medius, tensor fascia lata, iliopsoas, sartorius, and gracilis.[20,29] Bilateral KAFOs with stance control knee joint mechanisms have also been combined with surface electrode FES to the quadriceps and common peroneal nerve.[30] Because this technology is still evolving, definitive generalizable conclusions for orthotic prescription cannot be made. Clinicians working with children and adults with spinal cord injury should follow prescription recommendations as they emerge from ongoing research (see Keywords for Literature Search at the end of this chapter).

Ankle–Foot Orthoses

Individuals with spinal cord injuries with low lumbar lesions are often very difficult to manage with available orthoses. Individuals with lesions that spare the quadriceps (innervation from L2 L3 L4) but produce significant weakness in the gluteus maximus (innervation from L5 S1 S2) and gluteus medius/minimus (innervation from L4 L5 S1) are often fit with AFOs because they have sufficient quadriceps strength to prevent stance phase knee buckling. However, the lack of abductor power produces gait deviations, including a contralateral posterior-lateral lurch at the hip during stance as well as abnormal valgus and rotatory stress at the knee.[31] These muscular deficiencies, particularly when they occur in children with spina bifida, can produce rotatory instabilities at the knee that may eventually lead to degenerative joint changes.[32,33] Individuals prescribing orthoses for these patients must consider possible deleterious effects of long-term orthotic use and provide ongoing reevaluation to prevent joint degeneration due to repetitive abnormal loading.

HIP ORTHOSES FOR INDIVIDUALS WITH SELECTED MUSCULOSKELETAL HIP CONDITIONS OR THOSE RECOVERING FROM HIP SURGERY

HOs are appliances that include components that cross and enclose the hip joint but leave the distal portions of the lower limb free. HOs may be unilateral (applied to only one hip) or bilateral, but are typically composed of thigh and pelvic components with some type of articulation for the hip joint. These devices are used in the conservative management of certain musculoskeletal disorders, particularly in children where orthoses can provide effective corrective forces. HOs are also used with both children and adults to provide postoperative protection or stabilization for patients who have had hip surgery.

Orthoses Used With Developmental Dysplasia of the Hip

Developmental dysplasia of the hip (DDH) covers a spectrum of congenital conditions including hip dislocation, subluxation, and hip instability (a located hip that is dislocatable). These abnormalities result from an abnormal relationship between the developing femoral head and acetabulum. Without adequate contact between these two skeletal components of the hip, neither develops properly. When hip instability is discovered in children younger than 6 months of age, treatment usually includes bracing that holds the hip in flexion and abduction, because this position maximizes and normalizes contact between the acetabulum and femoral head. The *Pavlik harness* is the device most often used to achieve this positioning (**Fig. 16.21**).[34] It is a device made of canvas or another washable fabric with straps that run from the chest to the feet to produce the desired hip positioning. It is effective, does not interfere with the child's kicking movements, and is easy for parents to manage during dressing and diaper changes. The chest strap should be located at the child's nipple level with about two finger's width of space between the strap and the body. The anterior straps located at the mid-axillary line set the hips at 100° to 110° hip flexion. Too much flexion can produce femoral nerve compression or inferior dislocations.[35] The posterior straps are located at the level of the child's scapulae and allow for comfortable hip abduction. This strap prevents adduction and dislocation, but excessive abduction should be avoided to prevent the development of avascular necrosis. With the Pavlik harness correctly applied, ultrasound is used to image the hip and confirm proper hip positioning.[36] Bracing with this device is continued until the hip is stable on clinical exam. If the Pavlik harness is not successful, manual reduction is performed following skin traction, and the corrected position is maintained with a hip spica cast. Ambulatory children between the ages of approximately 9 to 24 months who require fixed abduction positioning of their hips may be fit with a "Rhino Cruiser," a rigid plastic orthosis that holds the hips in the desired abduction position without limiting movements of the active toddler (**Fig. 16.22**).

Orthoses Used With Legg-Calvé-Perthes Disease

Legg-Calvé-Perthes disease consists of a sequence of stages that starts with the temporary loss of blood supply to the femoral head in a growing child (usually between the ages of 4 to 10 years), resulting in avascular necrosis of the femoral head. The etiology of this loss of blood supply is usually unknown. However, the condition is usually self-limiting and is followed by revascularization and new bone formation. During the period of avascular necrosis, the femoral head may collapse and flatten. If the head ossifies with a flattened shape that is incongruent with the acetabulum, it may lead to early degenerative joint disease of the hip as the child grows into adulthood. At one time, children were treated with non-weight-bearing to prevent collapse of the femoral head; however, this treatment approach is no longer valid. The current treatment is to maintain hip range of motion, particularly abduction, as well as containment of the femoral head within the acetabulum so that as the femoral head reforms, it will develop a spherical shape matching that of the acetabulum. Various approaches are used to achieve containment, including no intervention, casting or weight-bearing bracing to position the hip in

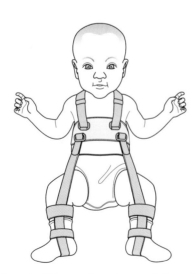

FIGURE 16.21. A Pavlik harness is used to treat infants with developmental dysplasia of the hip.

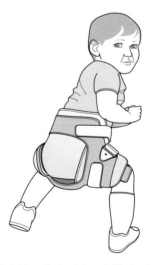

FIGURE 16.22. A "Rhino Cruiser" is a rigid plastic hip orthosis designed to maintain abduction hip positioning in the ambulatory toddler.

abduction, or surgical osteotomies to maximize bony containment. Many different types of orthoses have been used over the years. Current orthotic approaches include the *Atlanta (Scottish Rite) abduction orthosis* and the Petrie cast or brace (**Fig. 16.23**). The Atlanta hip orthosis consists of a pelvic band and movable hip joints that are connected to abducted thigh cuffs.[37] For larger children, the orthosis is constructed with a bar between the thigh cuffs to reinforce the abducted position. This abduction bar is attached to the thigh cuffs with a special joint that does not prevent reciprocal flexion and extension movements of the legs. Thus, children wearing these appliances are allowed full weight-bearing using a reciprocal gait pattern, albeit abducted from the usual leg positions. *Petrie casts*, or orthoses, are long leg devices with abduction bars between the legs to hold the femurs in a position of abduction and internal rotation to maximize femoral head containment in the acetabulum.[38,39] Children are permitted full weight-bearing and ambulation using these appliances. The efficacy of bracing or casting compared to surgical interventions is still controversial.[39]

Hip Control Hip Orthoses

Hip control HOs are used with individuals who have poor muscular control at the hip, such as children with cerebral palsy, or with individuals following hip surgery. Post-operative HOs are used to protect healing joint structures from deleterious positions or motions without immobilizing the joint. These devices may be unilateral or bilateral and are made up of a pelvic band (see Fig. 16.1) connected to a thigh cuff or cuffs by orthotic hip joints. Various types of orthotic hip joints may be selected, depending on the particular needs of the patient. Options for orthotic hip joints are discussed earlier in this chapter under the heading "Hip Control Using Orthotic Hip Joints." The simplest hip control HO employs a simple single-axis joint that allows hip flexion and extension but blocks movements in the frontal and transverse planes. Orthotic stops can be used with these single-axis joints to limit flexion and extension to a particular range of motion (see Fig. 16.5).

Many conditions, however, require positioning in abduction. For example, some children with cerebral palsy have excessive adductor muscle tone and abductor weakness that impair balance and restrict functional activities. These children may benefit from bilateral HOs that restrict excessive adduction and internal rotation and provide some abduction positioning to improve balance. Adjustable orthotic hip joints (see Figs. 16.10 and 16.11) permit abduction positioning; however, this fixed abducted position may make walking difficult for children with muscle weakness. An alternative is the *SWASH (standing, walking, and sitting hip) orthosis* (**Fig. 16.24**). This orthosis has unique articulations that connect the posterior aspect of a pelvic shell and padded waistband to the lateral sides of bilateral thigh cuffs. These unique joints provide wide abduction during hip flexion when the wearer is sitting and narrower abduction when standing erect and walking, but they do not interfere with reciprocal

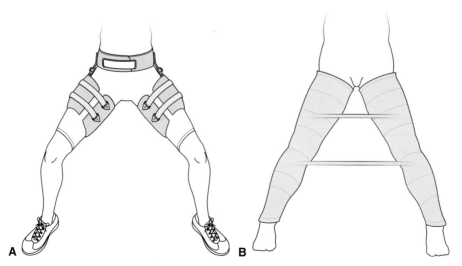

FIGURE 16.23. Abduction orthoses or casts are used to treat some children with Legg-Calvé-Perthes disease to enhance femoral head containment: **(A)** Atlanta (Scottish Rite) hip orthosis and **(B)** Petrie cast or orthosis.

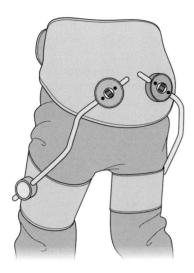

FIGURE 16.24. The standing, walking, and sitting hip (SWASH) orthosis provides variable hip abduction to restrict scissoring and improve balance.

the child's condition changes. Postoperative HOs, typically constructed from molded plastic pelvic and thigh shells linked by adjustable hip joints, provide an alternative to casting that allows adjustment of joint positioning as healing and rehabilitation progresses as well as the ability to remove the appliance easily for hygiene and wound care (**Fig. 16.25**).

Hip control HOs are most commonly used in adults who have sustained a dislocation of their total hip arthroplasty or who required revision of their total joint replacement. These revision procedures necessitate extended periods of joint immobilization to facilitate joint stability and healing. These postoperative appliances are usually unilateral, restricting movement only of the involved hip, and are purchased from central manufacturers based on patient measurements. An important advantage of contemporary postoperative appliances is that a range of orthotic hip joints are available that offer multiple adjustments to accommodate specific positioning and movement requirements in all three planes (**Fig. 16.26**). For example, some postoperative HOs

leg movements. During ambulation, the wearer's legs are almost parallel, thus preventing the scissoring gait pattern that disrupts balance. Studies of the effectiveness of SWASH orthoses in various applications are limited. However, some have used these appliances along with Botox-A injections as part of treatment for children with spastic cerebral palsy with progressive hip migration (lateral displacement of the femoral head on the acetabulum, which may lead to hip subluxation or dislocation).[40]

Many surgical procedures performed at the hip require either positioning in abduction or restriction of adduction during the postoperative period to promote hip stability and enhance healing. Hip stabilization HOs are used in both children and adults. A common application for these orthoses in children is to immobilize and stabilize the hip and surrounding soft tissues following surgery for management of spasticity, contractures, or subluxation and dislocation. In the past, immobilization was accomplished with **hip spica casts**, which are difficult to maintain, cumbersome, and require changes and recasting as

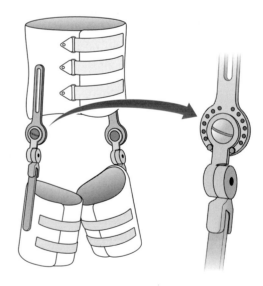

FIGURE 16.25. Postoperative hip control hip orthoses have adjustable hip joints to maintain required hip positioning without limiting allowed motions.

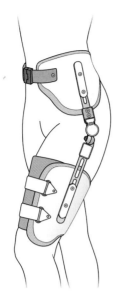

FIGURE 16.26. A postoperative hip orthosis may be used by individuals who have dislocated or required revision of a total hip arthroplasty.

provide orthotic joints that increase abduction positioning during sitting and reduce it in standing and walking when less abduction is required. Other options include variations in the size of the pelvic component, which can be increased or decreased, depending on the amount of orthotic control required. The real clinical advantage of these alternative orthotic joints is that they permit effective positioning and movement controls to protect the joint without interfering with allowable joint motions. This balance between protection and movement facilitates optimal progression in rehabilitation.

GUIDES FOR PRESCRIPTION AND CHECKOUT OF HIP–KNEE–ANKLE–FOOT ORTHOSES AND HIP ORTHOSES

As for all orthoses, the specific prescription is developed through the process of identifying patient impairments, establishing goals, and biomechanically designing an orthosis to apply the forces required to achieve the goals. This process is described in Chapter 11. A guide for prescription of HKAFOs based on gait analysis is presented in **Figure 16.27**. Foot, ankle, and knee components used in HKAFOs are described in Chapters 14 and 15, respectively. When developing orthotic prescriptions, practitioners must also consider client performance with trial devices and evidence of orthotic efficacy published in the current research literature (at the end of this chapter).

When a new orthosis is received, a therapist must conduct an orthotic checkout examination of the client, the device, and the client wearing the device. The general checkout procedure is discussed in Chapter 11, and specific items relevant to the checkout of HKAFOs and HOs are listed in **Box 16.1**. The purpose of the checkout examination is to ensure that the device has been manufactured as prescribed and that its fit, function, comfort, and cosmesis are acceptable. The orthotist, therapist, and patient must work together to resolve problems in any of these areas. When it is determined that the device is satisfactory, the therapist must review the orthotic goals and ensure that they have been achieved or implement a program to accomplish them. Particularly for new orthosis wearers, this requires patient instruction in proper methods of donning, doffing, and caring for the orthosis, as well as guidelines for appropriate footwear (Chapter 13) for use with the device. In addition, therapists must provide new wearers with a "wearing schedule" that guides the user to gradually increase the time the user wears his or her new appliance over several days to a week, depending on the individual needs of the client. Increasing orthotic wearing time by an hour or two at an interval appropriate for the specific individual can avoid problems or make them easier to resolve if they do occur.

Functional training may also be necessary, which includes gait training, as well as training in how to perform other types of functional activities such as steps, negotiating all types of indoor and outdoor surfaces, ramps, and getting up and down from the floor. Asking patients to identify functional activities that are important to or difficult for them helps clinicians individualize training and focus on relevant functional skills.

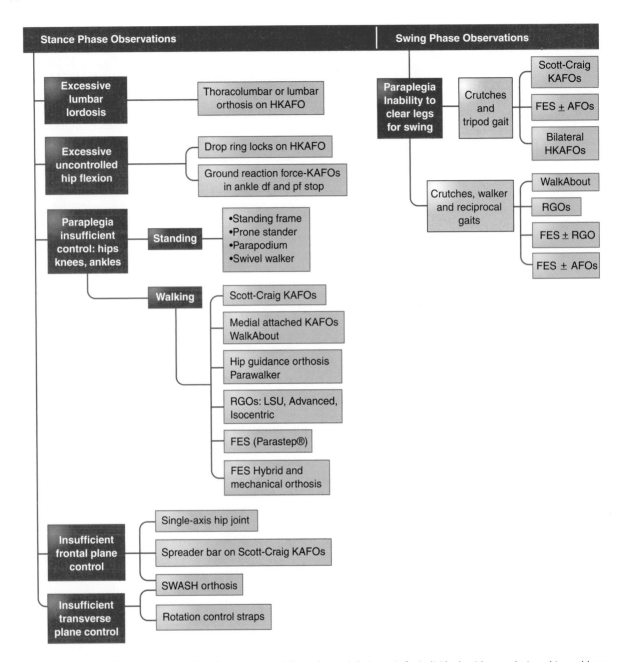

FIGURE 16.27. A guide to orthotic solutions for common problems observed during gait for individuals with paraplegia or hip problems.

BOX 16.1	Specific Items to Include in the Checkout Examination for Hip–Knee–Ankle–Foot Orthoses (HKAFOs) and Hip Orthoses (HOs)

- If examining an HKAFO with knee and foot and ankle components, see Chapters 14 and 15 for checkout items specific to these components.
- Height of medial thigh uprights or shells. They should be below and not impinging on the perineum in weight-bearing and non-weight-bearing positions.
- Alignment between orthotic and anatomical hip axes (slightly anterior and superior to the greater trochanter). Check and recheck before and after movement to determine if the orthosis is migrating on the limb.
- If thigh and pelvic uprights are present, check the space between the limb and the uprights. There should be adequate clearance but not too much space that will make the appliance unnecessarily bulky.
- If plastic pelvic and thigh shells are present, check for total contact throughout, for appropriate fit of relief depressions, and for any areas of excessive pressure and the effectiveness of padding.
- Strapping. Straps should be secure, easy to open and close, and have room for adjustment.
- Hip locks. Locks should work properly and be easy for the client to engage and release.
- Limited motion joints. If orthotic joints are prescribed to limit joint range of motion or position, the anatomical motion or position in the orthosis should match the prescription requirement.

types of bilateral KAFOs and HKAFOs are available to provide the necessary support for the legs and trunk so that the individual can walk using crutches or walkers with either a tripod (swing-to or swing-through) or a reciprocal gait pattern. Various mechanisms that link the hip joints and facilitate reciprocal gait are used in HKAFOs called RGOs. However, walking with these appliances is still very slow and energy expensive. The use of FES with an orthosis may improve the walking ability of individuals with paraplegia, as the FES can provide some active propulsion while the orthosis provides stability.

HOs are primarily used to control hip position. People who need hip control or positioning orthoses include individuals who lack adequate muscular control at the hip, children who require abduction positioning to facilitate proper development or healing of the hip joint, and those who have had hip surgeries that require positioning to protect healing tissues from deleterious stresses. Most hip control HOs have adjustable hip joints that provide position and motion regulation in all three planes. In most cases, these lightweight adjustable HOs have replaced the need for heavy, cumbersome hip spica casts, which are difficult to keep clean and manage functionally.

When a new orthosis is received by a client, the therapist must perform an orthotic checkout examination to ensure proper fit, function, comfort, and cosmesis. In addition, therapists must provide functional training in donning and doffing the device as well as required care or maintenance of the device. Patient training and instruction are required to ensure that the functional goals established when the prescription was made are achieved.

SUMMARY

This chapter presents the orthotic components used to apply forces to the hip or control hip positioning and range of motion to improve function. Two major categories of appliances are used in the management of hip problems: HKAFOs—appliances that combine componentry at the hip and pelvis as well as the knee and foot and ankle, and HOs—appliances that have componentry only at the hip and pelvis.

The primary application for HKAFOs is with paraplegic individuals who have thoracic spinal lesions, including children with spina bifida and meningomyelocele, as well as children and adults with acquired or traumatic spinal cord injuries. Various

KEYWORDS FOR LITERATURE SEARCH

For each topic, select appropriate keyword, subject heading words, or MeSH terms from each domain and search using the Boolean term "AND".

Search Topic: What are the Energy Costs of Ambulation for Individuals With Paraplegia?

Intervention
Orthotic devices
Hip–knee–ankle–foot orthosis
Reciprocating gait orthosis
Functional electrical stimulation

Application
  Paraplegia
  Meningomyelocele
  Spinal cord injury

Effect
  Walking
  Oxygen consumption
  Oxygen cost
  Energy expenditure
  Energy metabolism

Search Topic: What is the Effectiveness of Hip–Knee–Ankle–Foot Orthoses or Hip Orthoses in the Management of Particular Conditions at the Hip?

Intervention
  Orthotic devices
  Hip orthosis
  Post-operative bracing
  Functional electrical stimulation

Conditions
  Cerebral palsy
  Hip dislocation, congenital
  Developmental dysplasia of the hip
  Hip dislocation, adult
  Arthroplasty, replacement, hip
  Osteogenesis imperfecta
  Legg-Calvé-Perthes disease; Legg-Perthes disease
  Hip migration
  Spasticity

Effects
  Efficacy
  Effectiveness
  Energy expenditure
  Activities of daily living
  Gait analysis
  Clinical guidelines
  Walking
  Biomechanics

REFERENCES

1. Douglas R, Larson PF, D'Ambrosia R, et al: The LSU reciprocation-gait orthosis. Orthopedics 6:834–839, 1983.
2. Lissens MA, Peeraer L, Tirez B, et al: Advanced receiprocating gait orthosis (ARGO) in paraplegic patients. Eur J Phys Med Rehabil 3:147, 1993.
3. Campbell JH: Linked hip-knee-ankle-foot orthoses designed for reciprocal gait. J Prosthet Orthot 18:204–208, 2006.
4. Middleton JW, Yeo JD, Blanch L, et al: Clinical evaluation of a new orthosis, the "Walkabout," for restoration of functional standing and short distance mobility in spinal paralyzed individuals. Spinal Cord 35:574–579, 1997.
5. Middleton JW, Sinclair PJ, Smith RM, et al: Postural control during stance in paraplegia: effects of medially linked versus unlinked knee-ankle-foot-orthoses. Arch Phys Med Rehabil 80:1558–1565, 1999.
6. Genda E, Oota K, Suzuki K, et al: A new walking orthosis for paraplegics: hip and ankle linkage system. Prosthet Orthot Int 28:69–74, 2004.
7. Suzuki T, Sonoda S, Saitoh E, et al: Prediction of gait outcome with the knee-ankle-foot orthosis with medial hip joint in patients with spinal cord injuries: a study using recursive partitioning analysis. Spinal Cord 45:57–63, 2007.
8. Scott BA: Engineering principles and fabrication techniques for the Scott-Craig long leg brace for paraplegics. Orthot Prosthet 25:14–17, 1971.
9. Lobley S: Orthotic design from the New England regional spinal cord injury center. Phys Ther 65:492–493, 1985.
10. Waters RL, Lunsford BR: Energy cost of paraplegic locomotion. J Bone Joint Surg 67-A:1245–1250, 1985.
11. Brissot R, Gallien P, Le Bot M-P, et al: Clinical experience with functional electrical stimulation-assisted gait with Parastep in spinal cord–injured patients. Spine 25:501–508, 2000.
12. Stallard J, Farmer IR, Pointer R, et al: Engineering design considerations of the ORLAU swivel walker. Eng Med 15:3–7, 1986.
13. Stallard J, Lomas B, Woollam P, et al: New technical advances in swivel walkers. Prosthet Orthot Int 27:132–138, 2003.
14. Cerny K, Waters R, Hislop H, et al: Walking and wheelchair energetics in persons with paraplegia. Phys Ther 60:1133–1139, 1980.
15. Merkel KD, Miller NE, Westbrook PR, et al: Energy expenditure of paraplegic patients standing and walking with two knee-ankle-foot-orthoses. Arch Phys Med Rehabil 65:121–124, 1984.
16. Miller NE, Merritt JD, Merkel KD, et al: Paraplegic energy expenditure during negotiation of architectural barriers. Arch Phys Med Rehabil 65:778–779, 1984.
17. Harvey LA, Davis GM, Smith MB, et al: Energy expenditure during gait using the Walkabout and isocentric reciprocal gait orthoses in persons with paraplegia. Arch Phys Med Rehabil 79:945–949, 1998.
18. Beillot J, Carre F, Le Claire G, et al: Energy consumption of paraplegic locomotion using reciprocating gait orthosis. Eur J Appl Physiol 73:376–381, 1996.
19. Lotta S, Fiocchi A, Giovannini R, et al: Restoration of gait with orthoses in thoracic paraplegia: a multicentric investigation. Paraplegia 32:608–615, 1994.
20. Merati G, Sarchi P, Ferrarin M, et al: Paraplegic adaptation to assisted-walking: energy expenditure during wheelchair versus orthosis use. Spinal Cord 38:37–44, 2000.
21. Mattsson E, Brostrom L-A: The increase in energy cost of walking with an immobilized knee or an unstable ankle. Scand J Rehab Med 22:51–53, 1990.
22. Kaufman KR, Irby SE, Mathewson JW, et al: Energy-efficient knee-ankle-foot orthosis: a case study. J Prosthet Orthot 8:79–85, 1996.
23. Rasmussen AA, Smith KM, Damiano DL: Biomechanical evaluation of the combination of bilateral stance-control knee-ankle-foot orthoses and a reciprocating gait orthosis in an adult with a spinal cord injury. J Prosthet Orthot 19:42–47, 2007.

24. Graupe D, Kohn KH, Basseas S, et al: Electromyographic control of FES in paraplegics. Orthopedics 7:1134–1138, 1984.

25. Graupe D, Kohn KH: Functional neuromuscular stimulator or short-distance ambulation by certain thoracic-level spinal-cord-injured paraplegics. Surg Neurol 50:202–207, 1998.

26. Marsolais EB, Kobetic R: Functional electrical stimulation for walking in paraplegia. J Bone Joint Surg 69-A:728–733, 1987.

27. Klose KJ, Jacobs PL, Broton JG, et al: Evaluation of a training program with SCI paraplegia using the Parastep-I ambulation system: part I. Ambulation performance and anthropometric measures. Arch Phys Med Rehab 78:789–793, 1997.

28. Bonaroti D, Akers JM, Smith BT, et al: Comparison of functional electrical stimulation to long leg braces for upright mobility for children with complete thoracic level spinal injuries. Arch Phys Med Rehabil 80:1047–1053, 1999.

29. Ferguson FA, Polando G, Kobetic R, et al: Walking with a hybrid orthosis system. Spinal Cord 37:800–804, 1999.

30. Stein RB, Hayday F, Chong SL, et al: Speed and efficiency in walking and wheeling with novel stimulation and bracing systems after spinal cord injury: a case study. Neuromodulation 8:264–271, 2005.

31. Katz DE: The use of ambulatory knee-ankle-foot-orthoses in pediatric patients. J Prosthet Orthot 18:192–198, 2006.

32. Williams JJ, Graham BP, Dunne KB, et al: Late knee problems in myelomeningocele. J Pediatr Orthop 13:701–703, 1993.

33. Thomson JD, Ounpuu S, Davis RB, et al: The effects of ankle-foot orthoses on the ankle and knee in persons with myelomeningocele: an evaluation using three-dimensional gait analysis. J Pediatr Orthop 19:27–33, 1999.

34. Pavlik A: The functional method of treatment using a harness with stirrups as the primary method of conservative therapy for infants with congenital dislocation of the hip, 1957. Clin Orthop Relat Res 281:238–244, 1992.

35. Viere RC, Birch JG, Herring JA, et al: Use of the Pavlik harness in congenital dislocation of the hip. An analysis of failures of treatment. J Bone Joint Surg 72-A:238–244, 1990.

36. Suzuki S: Ultrasound and the Pavlik harness in CDH. J Bone Joint Surg 75-B:483–487, 1993.

37. Meehan PL, Angel D, Nelson JM: The Scottish Rite abduction orthosis for the treatment of Legg-Perthes disease. J Bone Joint Surg 74-A:2–12, 1992.

38. Petrie JG, Bilenc I: The abduction weight-bearing treatment in Legg Perthes' disease. J Bone Joint Surg 53-B:54–62, 1971.

39. Grezgorzewski A, Bowen RJ, Guille JT, et al: Treatment of collapsed femoral head by containment in Legg-Calvé-Perthes disease. J Pediatr Orthoped 23:15–19, 2003.

40. Boyd RN, Dobson F, Parrott J, et al: The effect of botulinum toxin type A and variable hip abduction orthosis on gross motor function: a randomized controlled trial. Eu J Neurol 8(Suppl 5):109–119, 2001.

17

Orthoses for Trunk, Cervical, or Cranial Impairments

OBJECTIVES

At the end of this chapter, all students are expected to:

1. Describe the types (categories) and functions of trunk, spinal, and cranial orthoses.
2. Identify and describe the parts of trunk, spinal, and cranial orthoses, including the materials, componentry, and designs that are used in contemporary appliances.
3. Describe the impairments that may be improved by trunk, spinal, or cranial orthoses.
4. Discuss applications for trunk, spinal, and cranial orthoses and their impact on patients' functional abilities.

Physical Therapy students are expected to:

1. Determine the need for a trunk, spinal, or cranial orthosis based on examination findings.
   a. Evaluate client examination findings, including preorthotic prescription examinations, lower quarter biomechanical assessment, and gait and functional analyses, to diagnose impairments that may be improved with a trunk, spinal, or cranial orthosis.
2. Develop appropriate goals for a trunk, spinal, or cranial orthosis based on a client's impairments and functional requirements.
3. Describe the biomechanical methods employed in trunk, spinal, and cranial orthoses to achieve the orthotic goals.
4. Develop and execute a search strategy to locate research evidence for the effects and effectiveness of trunk, spinal, and cranial orthoses and to identify best practices for orthotic prescription.
5. Recommend an appropriate orthosis as part of a plan of care for individuals with specific impairments of the trunk, spine, or cranium.
6. Examine and evaluate trunk, spinal, or cranial orthoses for acceptable fit, function, comfort, and cosmesis.

CASE STUDIES

Tyrone O'Neal is a 17-year-old high school football player who sustained a T8 fracture in an auto accident in which he was thrown from the car. Tyrone is also presented as a case study in Chapter 16. His accident occurred 2 weeks ago, and he received immediate decompression and spine stabilization surgery at a trauma center. Despite prompt treatment, he still has a complete spinal cord injury (ASIA level A) with neural motor and sensory levels at T12 bilaterally. His medical condition is stabilizing, and he will be discharged to a rehabilitation hospital shortly to begin more intense rehabilitation. Although hardware to stabilize his spine and support the segmental fusion was put in place during his surgery, Tyrone's surgeon wants him to use a spinal orthosis during his active rehabilitation for protection of the fusion.

Janice DiSimone is a 12-year-old child who was just diagnosed with adolescent idiopathic scoliosis (AIS). She has a double thoracolumbar curve. The thoracic curve, which is the primary curve, is a right 30° curve with the apex at T9, and the secondary lumbar curve is a left 26° curve at L3. She is premenarche, and her iliac apophyses are rated as Risser 1. Janice is very athletic and participates in many very active sports, including soccer, gymnastics, as well as other sports.

Sarah Schultz is a 72-year-old retired secretary and widow who has just recently been diagnosed with osteoporosis. Unfortunately, this diagnosis was not made until she went to the doctor with complaints of unrelenting back pain and spinal radiographs revealed evidence of compression fractures of T5 through T6. She was referred to and has attended physical therapy for 3 weeks and is experiencing some improvement in her symptoms. However, she continues to have significant pain that makes her unable to do the cooking and gardening that she enjoys and does not wish to give up.

Father Mahoney is a 60-year-old priest who was involved in a multivehicle auto accident in which his car was "rear-ended." Immediately after the accident, he experienced "numbness" and moderate weakness in both arms and minimal weakness in both legs. He was moved by helicopter to the closest trauma center for treatment. The doctors determined that he had suffered a nondisplaced fracture at C5 and C6 during the accident but also had preexisting cervical arthritis and foraminal stenosis. It was determined that surgery and other invasive interventions were not indicated. Over the course of 5 to 7 days, he spontaneously recovered from the numbness and leg weakness. He continued to experience mild weakness in his hands. After 3 weeks of strict bedrest and cervical immobilization, he is permitted to get up and begin physical therapy. Father Mahoney is 6' 2" tall, weighs 300 lbs, and his BMI (body mass index) is 30.

Case Study Activities

All students:

1. Discuss whether each client may benefit from an orthosis and justify your decision.
   a. What regions of the body may benefit from an orthotic intervention? Identify and discuss the general purpose of an orthosis.
   b. Discuss how an orthosis might affect functional activities and community participation.
2. Discuss how you expect an orthosis to affect each client's ability to walk, gait pattern, and ability to perform activities of daily living?
3. Identify and discuss the advantages and disadvantages of using an orthosis with each client, as well as other treatment options that may be available to address the client's problems.

Physical Therapy students:

1. Identify and describe the impairments that contribute to each client's problem and functional limitations.
2. If an orthosis is indicated, develop specific orthotic goals for each client.
3. Develop an orthotic prescription to meet the orthotic goals and achieve the best functional outcome.

   a. Describe the type of orthosis, the orthotic componentry and design, as well as the biomechanical methods of force application that will achieve the orthotic goals.
   b. Using biomechanical terminology as well as terminology currently used in clinical settings, name the orthosis that you recommend for each client.
   c. Identify evidence in the research literature to support your orthotic recommendations for each client. Describe the evidence that you found and how it impacts your orthotic recommendation.
4. Develop a physical therapy plan of care for each client, which includes an orthosis, if appropriate, as well as other physical therapy interventions.
5. Describe how you will determine and measure the effectiveness and functional outcome of your interventions.

ORTHOSES FOR IMPAIRMENTS OF THE TRUNK AND CERVICAL REGION

Although orthoses worn on the trunk or neck are typically named according to the spinal segments enclosed (cervical, thoracic, lumbar), the spinal vertebrae are surrounded and affected by many other anatomical structures. These include soft tissue structures, such as muscles, ligaments, and in the case of the lumbar region, the abdominal viscera, as well as other bony structures such as the ribs and the pelvic and pectoral girdles. Spinal orthoses prescribed to affect the sacral and lumbar regions must work through and accommodate the hard and soft tissues of the pelvis and abdomen. Orthoses prescribed to affect the thoracic spine must be designed to accommodate the ribs and their movements during ventilation as well as the effects of pectoral girdle movements. Prescriptions for cervical orthoses must take into account the effect of movements of the head and thoracic spine on the neck. As a result, orthoses for the sacral, lumbar, and thoracic regions are collectively termed **trunk orthoses**, although they are individually named, respectively, as follows:

■ Sacroiliac orthoses or belts (SIOs)
■ Lumbosacral orthoses (LSOs)
■ Thoracolumbosacral orthoses (TLSOs)

■ Orthoses designed for the cervical spine are called cervical orthoses (COs) or collars when they encase only the neck, occipital, mandibular, and clavicular regions

■ Cervicothoracic orthoses (CTOs) when they include anterior and posterior thoracic extensions that connect under the axillae

In addition to the acronym indicating the joints enclosed in the orthosis, complete biomechanical terminology requires that the type of control exerted by the orthosis is also described. Thus, an orthosis designed to limit lumbar flexion and extension is termed *LSO-FE control*. Although most practitioners use biomechanical terminology to name orthoses, many eponyms continue to be used to name trunk and cervical appliances. Thus, in this chapter, both biomechanical and commonly used eponyms are used to name the appliances discussed.

Orthoses used to address impairments and conditions affecting the trunk and cervical region are usually prescribed to achieve one or more of the following goals:

■ Limit motion, either regionally or segmentally, to reduce pain, protect unstable segments, or facilitate healing following injury or surgery

■ Support the trunk or neck to reduce the loads applied to various trunk, cervical, or spinal structures during functional activities

■ Correct or limit the progression of deformity

■ Provide a reminder to wearers to maintain or initiate active postural corrections

Current trunk and cervical appliances do not apply forces to impart or assist movement. Thus, dynamic orthoses that apply forces to assist or substitute for missing muscle function which are used in both the upper and lower extremities are not available for the trunk. One type of dynamic spinal orthosis is discussed in this chapter. However, this appliance uses a dynamic (elastic) force to correct deformity, not substitute for missing function.

In addition to categorizing spinal orthoses based on the regions to which they are applied, trunk and cervical orthoses are grouped according to the materials from which they are constructed as soft or rigid devices. **Soft orthoses** for the trunk are often referred to as corsets or belts and are made from materials such as fabrics (eg, canvas), elastic, or neoprene. Soft trunk appliances may have rigid elements added to particular regions, such as metal or rigid plastic paraspinal "stays" (rod-like

reinforcements) or a molded plastic lumbar lordosis support that is slipped into a posterior pocket. In general, these corset-type devices are designed to compress the abdomen and increase lumbar stiffness and passive stability.[1] Soft cervical orthoses or collars are constructed from polyurethane foam covered with stockinette. **Rigid orthoses** are most commonly made from molded polyethylene or another type of plastic, either as one piece or as several pieces attached together by straps.

However, whether made from soft or rigid materials, most spinal appliances are prefabricated as "over-the-counter" or "off-the-shelf" devices that are selected for a client based on sizes derived from client measurements. Some prefabricated appliances are custom-fit by orthotists, and others are constructed with multiple straps that allow a health-care practitioner to adjust the fit to an individual client. A few trunk orthoses are custom-made for a particular individual from a custom-mold; however, this is usually reserved for those with structural deformities that make successful fitting with prefabricated devices difficult.

TRUNK ORTHOSES

Trunk orthoses, composed of soft or rigid materials, are referred to by the region of the spine to which they are applied. Thus, soft spinal orthoses include thoracolumbosacral corsets, lumbosacral corsets or belts, and sacroiliac belts. Rigid trunk orthoses for the thoracic or lumbar regions are typically called TLSOs or LSOs, respectively. A third category of trunk orthoses is used in the management of some individuals with scoliosis. Although most scoliosis orthoses are rigid, a few are constructed from soft materials.

Soft Trunk Orthoses: Corsets and Belts

Corsets and belts have been used for a very long time, particularly to help in symptom management for individuals with back pain. These appliances lack rigid horizontal components, although they may have vertical "stays" to prevent the fabric from rolling or metal or molded plastic inserts to provide additional support in particular areas. *Lumbosacral corsets*, the most common soft trunk orthoses, cover the lumbar and sacral regions as well as the abdomen with fabric or elastic materials. Many designs are available: older versions consist of canvas with elastic inserts and lacings for adjustments; newer versions are composed of elastic or neoprene and various adjustable Velcro straps (**Fig. 17.1**). The height of the appliances also varies. Traditionally, lumbosacral corsets extend from the xiphoid to the pubic symphysis anteriorly, and posteriorly they extend from just inferior to the scapulae to as low on the buttocks as possible without interfering with sitting. The material over the abdomen, often called an apron, usually provides an opening and closure method for donning and doffing the appliance. Some have proposed that corsets improve back pain symptoms by compressing the abdominal contents, altering the contraction of trunk and abdominal muscles, and increasing intra-abdominal pressure (IAP), thus unloading, to some degree, the lumbar intervertebral discs. Although some corsets can increase IAP, it does not appear to produce the putative unloading effect.[2] Other researchers have demonstrated that lumbosacral belts or corsets can contribute to passive lumbar stiffness or stability and slightly reduce erector spinae activity but have no effect on abdominal muscle activity or lumbar joint stability.[1,3] Additionally, pelvic motion in the sagittal and transverse planes is only minimally affected by wearing a corset, although moderate frontal plane movement restriction can occur.[4] Others suggest that in addition to minimal benefits, continued use of a corset may actually have a negative effect on its wearer by reducing back and abdominal muscle strength. However, in a study in which normal subjects wore lumbosacral corsets for 21 days, no loss of muscle strength was identified.[5]

Thoracolumbosacral (TLS) soft orthoses include all the components of lumbosacral soft appliances, but they extend further into the thoracic region, between or over the scapulae, and typically have axillary straps that wrap around the axillae (from posterior to anterior) to limit thoracic flexion (**Fig. 17.2**). Individuals with increased thoracic kyphotic curves often find these axillary straps uncomfortable, which may contribute to poor adherence to a prescribed orthotic wearing schedule or discontinuance of orthotic use. Although some TLS corsets only have posterior contact with the ribs, others are circumferential in the thoracic region. Wearing these circumferential corsets for at least one hour has been shown to alter the breathing patterns of normal individuals by reducing the tidal volume and increasing the breathing rate.[6] These findings may have prescription implications for individuals with medical conditions that cause respiratory or ventilatory difficulties and also require a thoracolumbosacral orthosis to stabilize the thoracic spine. Examples of clients with compromised pulmonary ventilation who may also need a thoracolumbar orthosis include individuals with a thoracic spinal cord injury and those with muscular dystrophy.

Another type of soft thoracic orthosis, called a *postural training orthosis* (PTO) or a *weighted kyphoorthosis* (WKO), was developed for individuals with

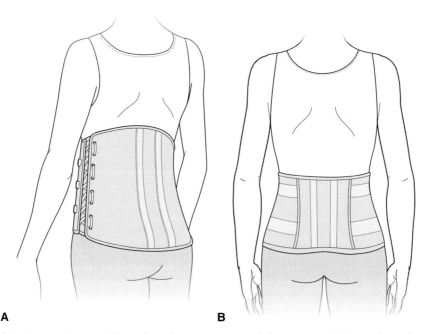

A   **B**

FIGURE 17.1. Soft lumbosacral corsets: **(A)** traditional corset constructed from canvas, elastic, and metal paraspinal inserts and **(B)** contemporary corset constructed from elastic or neoprene with reinforcements.

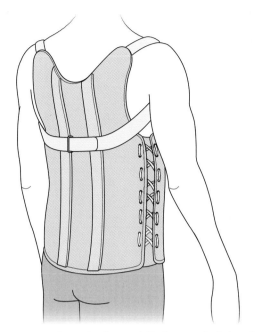

FIGURE 17.2. Thoracolumbosacral (TLS) corset includes all the components of a lumbosacral corset with the addition of a thoracic extension and axillary straps.

osteoporosis, excessive thoracic kyphosis, and balance issues that could lead to falls and fractures.[7] This device, designed to be worn like a backpack, increases its wearer's perception of spinal joint position or proprioception, improves balance and some gait parameters, increases back extensor muscle strength, and reduces back pain (**Fig. 17.3**).[8] Unlike some spinal orthoses, this appliance is not intended to passively correct the kyphotic deformity through full-time wear. This appliance has a pocket located posteriorly at about T10 into which is placed a 1- to 2-lb weight. The orthosis is worn from 30 minutes to 2 hours per day during exercise sessions that focus on trunk extension, balance, and posture. Some individuals who wear the appliance also report improvements in the amount and level of their daily physical activities.[7]

Sacroiliac orthoses are usually constructed as belts that are worn around the pelvis between the iliac crests and the greater trochanters, although some are a bit wider and extend to the inguinal region or pubic symphysis (**Fig. 17.4**). Sacroiliac belts are used by patients with back pain that is attributed to sacroiliac joint (SIJ) hypo- or hypermobility. Proponents suggest that these appliances, when used in conjunction with manipulation or spinal stabilization exercises, relieve pain by contributing to SIJ compression, which assists in stabilizing the joints. Pregnancy-related pelvic girdle pain and low back pain are commonly associated with SIJ hypermobility. Use of a sacroiliac belt with these patients may decrease SIJ mobility and reduce pain symptoms during functional activities as well as during a provocative maneuver, which is highly correlated with SIJ instability.[9]

Rigid Trunk Orthoses: Lumbosacral and Thoracolumbosacral Orthoses

For many years, rigid trunk orthoses were constructed from a metal framework of vertical uprights and horizontal bands covered in leather with a canvas and

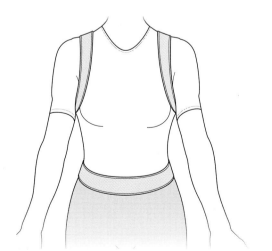
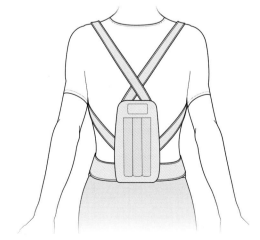

FIGURE 17.3. A weighted kyphosis orthosis or postural training orthosis. Weight (1 to 2 lbs) is placed in a posterior pocket as kinesthetic feedback.

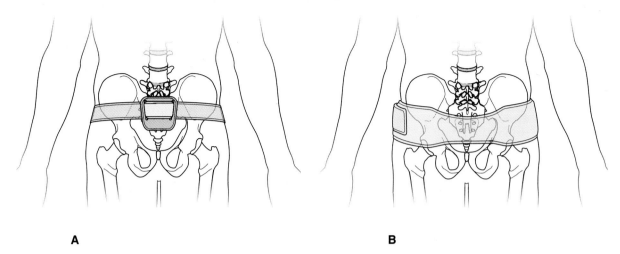

A   **B**

FIGURE 17.4. Sacroiliac belts are designed to compress the sacroiliac joints to improve joint stability. (A) A sacroiliac belt with an optional stabilization pad. (B) Sacroiliac belts are located between the iliac crests and the greater trochanter.

elastic abdominal apron. Although metal orthoses are still available, most rigid trunk orthoses used today are made from molded plastic (usually polyethylene) as one piece or multiple pieces connected by straps. Regardless of the materials from which they are made, most rigid appliances are prescribed to limit spinal motion, either regionally or segmentally, to protect the spine or facilitate healing. Rigid orthoses employ three-point counterforce systems to restrict spinal motion and can be applied in more than one plane in

one orthosis. For example, the appliance depicted in **Figure 17.5** restricts sagittal plane (flexion, extension) and frontal plane (lateral bend) movements by placing rigid components where force applications are required to form the three-point counterforce systems. In order to control the lumbar spine effectively with these counterforce systems, an appliance must have sufficient lever arm length to produce effective forces. Thus, rigid LSOs, whether made from molded plastic or metal uprights and bands, typically extend from

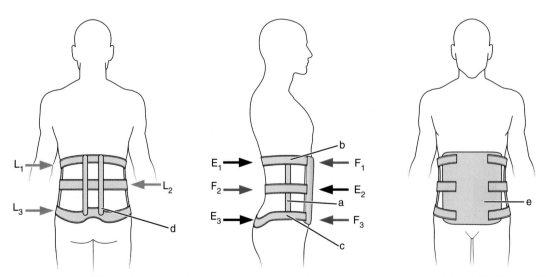

FIGURE 17.5. A rigid LSO employs three-point counterforces to control flexion, extension, and lateral bend. F1, F2, and F3 control lumbar flexion; E1, E2, and E3 control extension; L1, L2, and L3 control left lateral bend. [**a,** lateral upright; **b,** thoracic band; **c,** pelvic band; **d,** paraspinal upright; **e,** abdominal apron].

slightly below the inferior angle of the scapulae to as caudal on the buttocks as is possible without interfering with sitting, including firm contact over the sacrum. Appliances that are shorter have reduced ability to apply forces and control spinal motions. LSOs are less effective in controlling trunk rotation because little anatomical trunk rotation occurs in the lumbar region. TLSOs are more effective when rotary control of the trunk is important. However, whether a LSO or a TLSO is selected, rigid plastic **body jackets** are more effective in controlling rotation because their "total contact" design has more contacts to provide three-point counterforces in the transverse plane (**Fig. 17.6**). Pelvic rotation is also difficult to control in a spinal orthosis. In order to affect the pelvis, the orthotic pelvic band or inferior aspect of the body jacket must extend inferiorly as far as possible without interfering with sitting and maintain solid contact with the sacrum and buttocks.

Most spinal orthoses are worn under clothing. Some wearers may experience rubbing or skin irritation if the orthosis migrates or moves on the trunk during daily activities. To protect the skin and minimize slippage of the orthosis, clients are instructed to wear a T-shirt or "body sock" between their skin and the appliance (see Fig. 17.6). When a large surface area of skin is covered by a solid piece of molded plastic as with a molded body jacket, sweating may also become a problem, since evaporation of perspiration from the skin surface is impaired. A T-shirt or **body sock** interface between

the orthosis and the skin can serve to wick away perspiration and protect the skin. Additionally, perforations or holes may be drilled into solid plastic orthoses to facilitate evaporation and prevent excessive sweating that can lead to skin irritation or maceration. Some molded orthoses are also lined with a foamed polyethylene plastic material to provide cushioning for a softer interface with the trunk. Although this may increase comfort, particularly over bony prominences, these linings often increase sweating in the appliance. Clinicians who prescribe spinal orthoses must carefully consider these options and select those that meet the individual needs of specific clients.

Rigid Lumbosacral Orthoses

Figures 17.5, 17.6, and **17.7** feature four rigid LSOs which employ three-point counterforce systems to limit motion in the lumbar spine. Each spans the lumbar region as described above and applies three-point counterforces to achieve motion control. **Table 17.1** presents their specific names and summarizes the features that characterize these devices. Because most are prefabricated in a wide variety of designs, health-care providers who select devices for clients must evaluate these commercially available orthoses to determine if a particular appliance meets the biomechanical needs of a particular patient.

Rigid Thoracolumbosacral Orthoses

There are also many different designs used in the manufacture of TLSOs (see Fig. 17.8 through Fig. 17.13). Selection of the most appropriate orthotic design for a particular individual depends on the specific purpose or goal of the appliance. Common goals for use of TLSOs include:

- Restricting spinal motion following thoracic spinal surgery
- Limiting thoracic flexion or supporting an excessive thoracic kyphosis to minimize thoracic back pain
- Preventing the progression of scoliotic curves in certain individuals with adolescent idiopathic scoliosis
- **Table 17.2** summarizes commonly used TLSOs and the primary features that characterize them, excluding the TLSOs used with scoliosis.

Most TLSOs, although intending to affect a thoracic spinal segment, also include the lumbar and sacral regions within the orthosis (**Figs. 17.8** and **17.11**). This is required to provide sufficient lever arm length

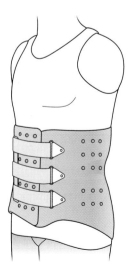

FIGURE 17.6. An anterior overlap total contact body jacket LSO is worn with a body sock to protect the skin. Perforations (holes) in the plastic facilitate evaporation and prevent excessive sweating.

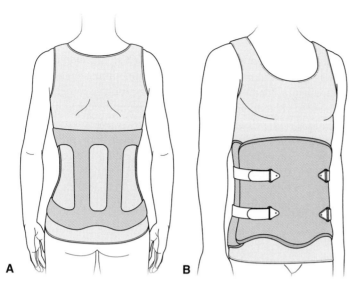

A   B

FIGURE 17.7. Rigid LSOs: **(A)** posterior view of LSO, FE control (chairback); **(B)** anterior view of body jacket LSO, FELR (flexion, extension, lateral bend, and rotation) control (clamshell).

to effectively control the thoracic spine, as well as to minimize migration of the orthosis on the wearer's trunk. Typically, the effective range of stabilization in a TLSO is from T5 through L4. Orthoses that are expected to affect spinal segments above T5 require an additional rigid extension to the subclavicular or cervical regions which accommodates the arms but allows application of orthotic counterforces at higher levels (see Fig. 17.13). The addition of a hip joint and thigh cuff extends effective orthotic control inferiorly.

Because TLSOs that are used following thoracic spinal surgery must control motion in all directions, most postoperative appliances are a type of molded body jacket. Postoperative body jackets must facilitate donning and doffing in the supine position,

because some patients may not be permitted to sit up without orthotic support. For these individuals, **bivalved** or clamshell devices (those with separate front and back components) are advantageous as the posterior half can be slid under a supine patient and the anterior shell placed and secured on top prior to sitting up (**Fig. 17.12**). One-piece anterior- or posterior-opening devices may have a gap with or without a tongue to protect the skin from pinching or may simply overlap (see Fig. 17.11). Individuals with excessive adipose tissue or pendulous abdomens may find it easier to don their appliances correctly in supine where gravity will assist in distributing tissues more evenly. Health-care providers who select appliances for clients must consider the method and

TABLE 17.1 **Types of Rigid Lumbosacral Orthoses (LSOs)**		
Biomechanical Terminology (see Figure for Picture)	**Eponymous Terminology**	**Features**
LSO, FE control (see Fig. 17.7A)	Chairback orthosis	Thoracic, pelvic bands; paraspinal uprights; no lateral uprights
LSO, FEL control (see Fig. 17.5)	Knight spinal orthosis	Thoracic, pelvic bands; paraspinal, lateral uprights
LSO, FELR control (see Fig. 17.6) (see Fig. 17.7B)	• Anterior overlap body jacket • Clamshell body jacket	• Anterior opening, total contact molded plastic • Bivalved, total contact molded plastic

E, extension; F, flexion; L, lateral bend; R, rotation.

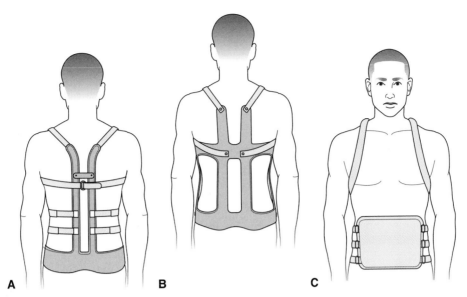

FIGURE 17.8. Conventional TLSO. **(A)** TLSO, FE control (Taylor spinal); **(B)** TLSO, FEL control (Taylor Knight spinal); **(C)** both have axillary loops as part of three-point counterforces to limit flexion and an abdominal apron.

ease of donning and doffing the appliances as well as the biomechanics of force application when selecting spinal supports for specific patients.

A common complication of spinal osteoporosis is compression fractures of the vertebral bodies, particu-larly in the thoracic region where the physiological curve is kyphosis. Although compression fractures do not present instability or neural compromise, they often cause back pain and the deformity of excessive and progressive thoracic kyphosis. This increased

TABLE 17.2	**Type of Rigid Thoracolumbosacral Orthoses (TLSOs)**	
Biomechanical Terminology	**Eponymous Terminology**	**Features**
TLSO, F control • (see Fig. 17.9A,B) • (see Fig. 17.9C)	• Jewett • CASH	Anterior sternal and suprapubic PA forces to limit flexion + posterior pad for PA force • Lateral uprights • Cruciform
TLSO, F control • (see Fig. 17.10)	Spinomed®	Backpack design; facilitates active postural extension
TLSO, FE control • (see Fig. 17.8A)	Taylor spinal	Axillary loops for AP forces to limit flexion; posterior spinal upright(s); abdominal apron
TLSO, FEL control • (see Fig. 17.8B)	Taylor Knight spinal	Knight spinal LSO + Taylor paraspinal uprights with axillary loops
TLSO, FELR control • (see Fig. 17.11) • (see Fig. 17.20) • (see Fig. 17.12) • (see Fig. 17.13)	Body jackets: • Anterior opening • Posterior opening • Clamshell • Sternal, subclavicular extensions	Total contact molded plastic; custom-made or custom-fitted prefabricated

AP, anterior to posterior; CASH, cruciform anterior sternal hyperextension; E, extension; F, flexion; L, lateral bend; PA, posterior to anterior; R, rotation.

kyphosis can result in poor balance, falls, and more fractures. Through medical and public health attention that focuses on preventing and minimizing the negative effects of osteoporosis, more aging individuals take advantage of treatment options to minimize bone loss or improve spinal stability. Treatment options include medications as well as surgical procedures, such as vertebroplasty and kyphoplasty, to stabilize or correct deformity when it occurs. Despite these options, some individuals with thoracic back pain and kyphotic deformity continue to experience functional limitations and a higher risk of falling. For these individuals, an orthosis that limits thoracic flexion and supports the thoracic spine may improve function. A variety of thoracic orthoses have been developed and used over the years. Traditional thoracic orthoses that limit flexion include the Taylor spinal and Taylor Knight spinal orthoses (see Fig. 17.8), which are similar in design, and the Jewett and CASH (Cruciform Anterior Sternal Hyperextension) orthoses (see Fig. 17.9), which are also based on similar design principles. A newer orthosis, the Spinomed® device, uses active rather than passive controls (see Fig. 17.10).

The *Taylor orthosis* consists of a pelvic band, bilateral posterior paraspinal uprights with axillary loops that attach posteriorly, and an anterior abdominal apron. This design provides for three-point counterforces to limit thoracic flexion and extension only (TLSO, FE control). To limit lateral bend in addition to flexion and extension, the Taylor thoracic paraspinal uprights and axillary loops are added to the top of a Knight spinal LSO. This composite orthosis is called a TLS, FEL control orthosis or a *Taylor Knight spinal orthosis* (see Fig. 17.8B). These appliances, constructed from rigid metal or plastic materials to apply passive counterforces, are often poorly tolerated as they are bulky and uncomfortable. Additionally, the axillary loops may exert excessive pressure that is painful and restricts arm movement. As a result, some clients loosen the axillary strap, which reduces the effectiveness of the orthosis.

The Jewett and CASH orthoses, often referred to as hyperextension appliances, use a three-point counterforce system to restrict flexion, without limiting other spinal movements. These appliances are prefabricated and purchased in sizes according to client measurements. Both are similar in that they apply anterior to posterior forces through sternal and suprapubic pads, which are opposed by a central posterior to anterior force (Fig. 17.9). These devices are intended to provide a hyperextension force to unload healing vertebral compression fractures. However, in individuals who have a thoracic kyphotic deformity, the pressure applied by the sternal and suprapubic pads is usually intolerable. The CASH orthosis has also been used by some therapists to stimulate active correction as part of a postural training program to increase thoracic extension. However, because of their design, these appliances typically migrate and rotate on the trunk during functional activities, which makes them uncomfortable to wear, causing poor compliance and early abandonment.

For individuals with back pain and compression fractures due to osteoporosis, a newer thoracic orthosis was developed called the *Spinomed®* spinal orthosis (Medi-USA, Whitsett, North Carolina). This device is worn like a backpack and consists of a back pad, which is hand-moldable as a cold material, and a system of belts with Velcro straps and closures (see Fig. 17.10). When used in conjunction with other appropriate interventions, individuals with osteoporotic compression fractures can improve back extensor and abdominal muscle strength and reduce back pain, body sway, and thoracic kyphotic deformity.[10] Unlike the Taylor-type and hyperextension orthoses, this appliance is not designed to passively hold the wearer erect but is used to provide feedback to stimulate the active correction of posture during exercise as well as functional activities. The hand-bendable, lightweight frame is also adjustable, if the deformity improves.

Similarly to rigid LSO body jackets, rigid *TLSO body jackets* provide the greatest amount of motion control in all planes. Using biomechanical terminology, they are termed rigid TLSO with FELR (flexion, extension, lateral bend, and rotary) control. These devices may be custom-made for a particular individual but are more frequently custom-fitted from centrally manufactured modules. A wide range of designs are manufactured by orthotic and orthopedic companies; however, most are equivalent in terms of restriction of motion and added passive trunk stiffness.[11] Thus, practitioners must select devices that are biomechanically appropriate for the needs of a specific client as well as acceptable in terms of other factors that affect the practical side of orthotic wear and compliance. Additional factors to consider when prescribing a body jacket orthosis include the location of the openings and the method for donning and doffing the device, its effects on breathing and arm movement, as well as the skin and general comfort. **Figures 17.11, 17.12,** and **17.13** show several

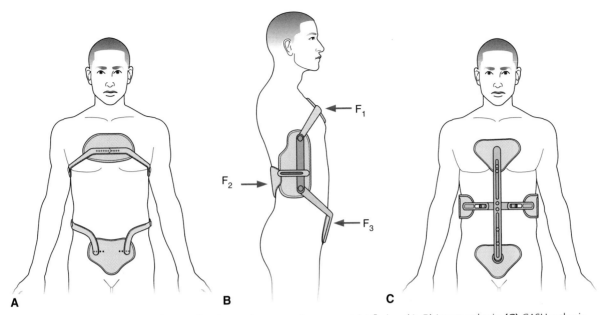

FIGURE 17.9. TLSO, F control orthoses using three-point counterforces to restrict flexion. **(A, B)** Jewett orthosis; **(C)** CASH orthosis.

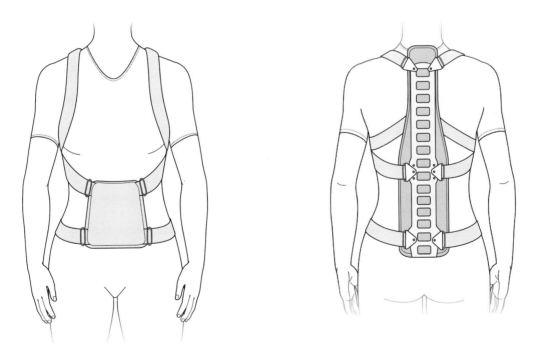

FIGURE 17.10. The Spinomed® backpack-type thoracolumbosacral orthosis is used with clients with excessive kyphosis due to osteoporotic compression fractures.

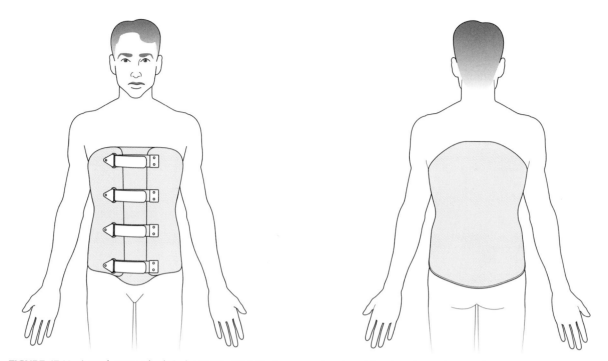

FIGURE 17.11. A total contact body jacket TLSO, FELR (flexion, extension, lateral bend, and rotary) control, with anterior opening and tongue to protect the skin.

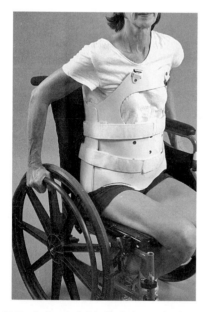

FIGURE 17.12. A clamshell (bivalved) thoracolumbosacral orthosis, FELR control. This type of opening is easier for clients who must don and doff in a supine position.

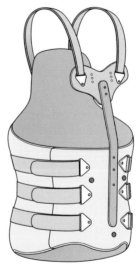

FIGURE 17.13. TLSO body jacket with sternal extension outrigger to provide counterforce for flexion control in subclavicular region.

biomechanically effective TLSO body jacket designs that are commonly used for postsurgical immobilization. Some clients who need trunk support are unable to tolerate an appliance that is made totally from rigid materials. These individuals may benefit from a **soft body jacket**. This device is molded for total contact, just like a rigid body jacket, but it is constructed from dense foamed polyethylene, rather than hard plastic, and is attached to a rigid framework (**Fig. 17.14**). These soft body jackets may be helpful for individuals with poor muscular control of the trunk, such as individuals with muscular dystrophy. Rigid TLSO body jackets are also used in the management of some individuals with scoliosis; however, this application and the devices involved are discussed in a separate section.

Thoracolumbar Orthoses for Management of Scoliosis

Scoliosis is a spinal deformity in which the spine curves laterally in the frontal plane, producing C- or S-shaped curves. Because spinal lateral bending and rotation are biomechanically coupled, scoliosis also includes abnormal spine rotation in the transverse plane. As a result, when a scoliotic curve involves thoracic vertebrae, in addition to the lateral curvature, the deformity includes a "*rib hump*," reflecting the rotation of the vertebrae to which ribs are attached (**Fig. 17.15**). Some scoliosis deformities

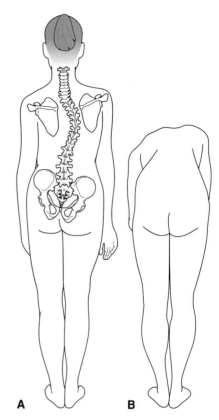

FIGURE 17.15. Scoliosis is a three-dimensional spinal deformity that includes abnormal lateral curves (**A**) and a "rib hump" (**B**) when the structural curve involves the thoracic spine.

also include a sagittal plane component, which is usually abnormal *kyphosis*. Thus, although scoliosis is typically characterized by its lateral curvatures in the frontal plane, it is actually a three-dimensional spinal deformity. Like all deformities, scoliosis can be structural or functional (flexible). It is termed *structural* when the abnormal curve is fixed and cannot be corrected by active or passive means. Various other terms are used to describe scoliotic curves, including terms to describe the location of the curve, its configuration, the side of the convexity, as well as the amount of the curve. A good understanding of this descriptive terminology is necessary for the clinician working with clients with scoliosis, because different types of curves require different types of treatment. The largest structural curve is called the *major (primary) curve.* A single C-type major curve is termed thoracic or lumbar when it occurs only in the thoracic or lumbar region, respectively. It is called thoracolumbar when it spans both regions. *Compensatory curves* may develop above or

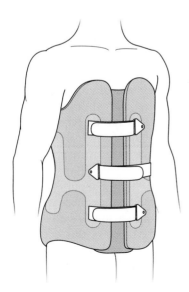

FIGURE 17.14. A soft TLSO is composed of a rigid framework to support a total contact molded foamed thermoplastic body jacket.

below the major curve to maintain normal alignment. A double major curve is an S-type curve in which both curves are primary and structural. The *apex of the curve* designates the most rotated vertebra in a curve and the one that is most deviated from the vertical axis. A curve that is convex to the right is called a right-sided scoliosis. *Trunk decompensation* or loss of trunk balance describes the relative position of the head with respect to the sacrum. When the trunk is balanced, a plumb line dropped from the spinous process of C7 should pass through the first spinous processes of the sacrum (or the gluteal cleft). A decompensated scoliosis is a curve in which the trunk is also displaced laterally with respect to the pelvis (**Fig. 17.16**). Notation of this feature is important, as it is often a predictor of curve progression (worsening). The *amount of the curve* is designated in degrees as measured on a standing radiograph. The most common method of measurement is called the *Cobb method*, which is illustrated in **Figure 17.17**.

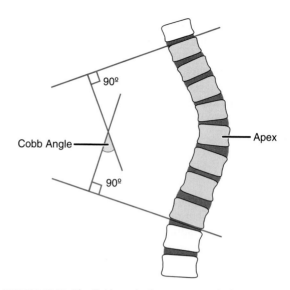

FIGURE 17.17. The Cobb method to measure spinal curves. Lines are drawn parallel to the upper and lower vertebral endplates of the uppermost and lowermost vertebrae that tilt toward the concavity. The Cobb angle is made by the intersection between perpendiculars to these two lines.

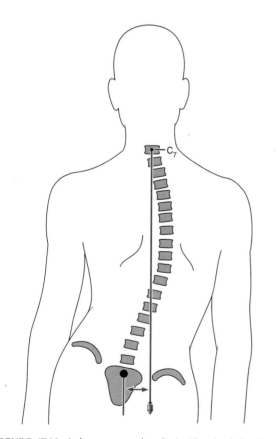

FIGURE 17.16. A decompensated scoliosis. The plumb line from C7 falls to the right of S1. The distance between these lines is the amount of decompensation or lateral displacement of the trunk.

Scoliosis is classified as congenital, neuromuscular, or idiopathic. *Congenital scoliotic curves* are present at birth. *Neuromuscular scoliosis* develops in individuals with neuromuscular disorders characterized by abnormalities of nerve or muscle function that produce muscle imbalances. Neuromuscular disorders that may cause scoliosis include cerebral palsy, muscular dystrophy, and spinal cord injury. However, in 80% to 90% of individuals diagnosed with scoliosis, the cause is classified as idiopathic, or unknown. Idiopathic scoliosis is further described by the age of the individual at the time that the curve is detected: infantile scoliosis is identified after birth but before age 3 years; juvenile scoliosis is detected between ages 3 and 10 years; adolescent scoliosis is noted around the time of puberty; and adult scoliosis is identified after the age of 18 years. By far, the most common type is adolescent idiopathic scoliosis (AIS), and it is the most common type managed with orthoses. Although the cause of idiopathic scoliosis is unknown, much is known about the condition. That information is important for those who participate in the management of individuals with scoliosis; however, it is beyond the scope of this book. This chapter focuses on the orthotic options for this particular subset of individuals with scoliosis. Practitioners must consider this information on orthotic management of scoliosis as just one piece in the context of management of all types of scoliosis.

The goal of using a spinal brace in the management of scoliosis in an individual who does not have a neuromuscular disorder is to support the trunk and hold the curve to prevent progression, or worsening, of the curve.[12,13] The type of scoliosis most amenable to brace treatment is AIS that is progressing. Curve progression is greatest during times of rapid growth; thus, individuals with AIS are the most frequent recipients of scoliosis braces. Because the presence of a significant progressive curve in an adolescent is seven times more likely to occur in a girl than a boy, most scoliosis brace wearers are girls. Individuals with idiopathic scoliosis for whom brace treatment is recommended are those with curves that measure between 25° and 45° that have progressed by at least 5° since detection and who have significant growth potential remaining as indicated by largely open growth plates, and in girls, lack of menses.[13] At least one-third of curves in this range do not progress. Nonprogressing curves and those less than 25° are observed but not treated. Progressive curves that are greater than 45° to 50° are treated with surgery to correct and fuse the spine.[12] Although research to identify the specific parameters to predict the most effective treatment for individuals with scoliosis is not totally definitive, the factors that most influence treatment choices include the amount of the curve, evidence of curve progression, and potential for continued growth.[13] The goal of brace treatment for individuals with AIS is to hold a progressing curve (one that is worsening) until growth stops and the individual is skeletally mature. The curves of some individuals may decrease during bracing; however, they typically regress to the prebrace amount after brace treatment is complete.

Braces currently used to treat adolescent idiopathic scoliosis can be grouped into several categories. The first grouping is according to the time and amount of daily brace wear. Most AIS braces are prescribed to be worn during the day and night, from a minimum of 16 to 18 hours per day to the preferred 23 hours per day. A second group of orthoses, called nocturnal (nighttime) braces, are worn only at night during sleep (8 to 10 hours per day) on at least 5 of 7 nights per week. Nighttime braces are passive appliances that apply forces as three-point counterforce systems to passively overcorrect the scoliotic curves. Daytime orthoses are subclassified according to how forces are applied: passive, both passive and active, and dynamic. Like nighttime braces, braces that apply forces passively employ some mechanism to provide three-point

counterforces to support and correct as many aspects of the curve as possible, including curve components in all three planes, as well as trunk decompensation if it is present (**Fig. 17.18**). Braces that employ active correction with passive correction have voids or reliefs opposite to the passive correction pads. Wearers are encouraged to actively pull away from the pads into the voids, thus exerting active forces to their curves. Most scoliosis braces use passive or a combination of passive and active methods to apply corrective forces and are made from rigid materials, usually molded thermoplastics. However, one category of orthoses employes dynamic forces exerted by elastic bands that apply corrective tensile forces that move with the wearer during activities.[14]

One last brace characteristic also used to categorize scoliosis appliances is the height of the device. Most scoliosis orthoses are thoracolumbosacral appliances that do not extend above the axilla and are thus termed TLSOs. However, one appliance, the Milwaukee brace, has a superstructure, or one anterior and two posterior uprights that extend from the pelvic mold and are connected at the cervical spine with a neck ring (**Fig. 17.19**). This is the original scoliosis brace that was developed in the 1940s as a

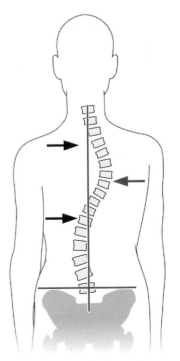

FIGURE 17.18. Scoliosis braces apply three-point counterforces to apply passive corrective forces to the curves.

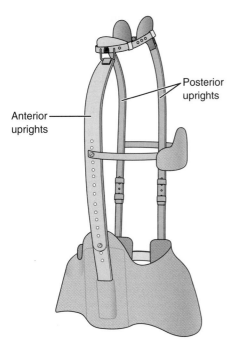

Anterior—uprights

Posterior uprights

FIGURE 17.19. The Milwaukee CTLSO applies three-point counterforces to the scoliosis curves through the lateral thoracic and lumbar pads attached to the anterior and posterior uprights.

conservative method of treating scoliosis. The Milwaukee brace, termed a cervicothoracic lumbosacral orthosis (CTLSO), is used when the apex of the thoracic curve is superior to T6. Lower or under-arm orthoses (TLSOs) do not have sufficient leverage to provide effective three-point counterforces to correct high thoracic curves. The Milwaukee brace is also used to correct excessive kyphosis, because this abnormal curve usually has a high thoracic apex. The original Milwaukee brace was heavy, bulky, and unsightly under clothing. Today's version, however, does not make contact with the mandible or the occiput, because earlier versions that did contact these cranial structures produced temporomandibular problems. **Table 17.3** summarizes the categories of scoliosis braces and provides examples of commonly used appliances in each group.

Day and Night Wear Braces: The Boston Thoracolumbosacral Orthosis and the Wilmington Thoracolumbosacral Orthosis

The *Boston TLSO* (Boston Brace, Avon, Massachusetts) was the first low-profile (without a superstructure) scoliosis brace that was developed from the Milwaukee brace. It was developed at the Children's Hospital of Boston in the 1970s. In addition to lacking the anterior and posterior uprights and neck ring, the Boston TLSO has other features that differ from the Milwaukee brace. Although a Boston brace may be custom fabricated for a specific client from an individual cast or by using CAD-CAM (computer-assisted design/computer-assisted manufacture) methods, most are made from prefabricated copolymer modules selected for a particular client based on measurements (**Fig. 17.20**). Trimlines are cut on the selected module, based on the child's x-ray, to provide contact points to apply three-point counterforces for curve correction. Additional pads are added to the inside of the module to focus the counterforces. Voids or reliefs are located opposite to the curve to provide space for active curve correction as the child moves away from the pads. For individuals with a curve apex above T6, a superstructure can be added to the Boston module to provide a point for higher force application (**Fig. 17.21**).

TABLE 17.3	Types of Braces Used in Nonoperative Management of Adolescent Idiopathic Scoliosis		
Time of Wear	**Type of Orthotic Force Application**		
	Passive	**Passive + Active**	**Dynamic**
Day and Night (16/18–23 hr/day; daily)	• Wilmington TLSO	• Milwaukee CTLSO • Boston TLSO	• Spine Cor TLSO (soft)
Night Only (8–10 hr/day; at least 5 days/wk)	• Charleston Bending TLSO • Providence TLSO		

CTLSO, cervicothoracic lumbosacral orthosis; TLSO, thoracolumbosacral orthosis.

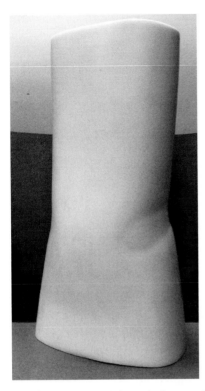

FIGURE 17.20. The Boston TLSO is made from prefabricated copolymer modules, available in 30 sizes. The opening is posterior, and iliac crest rolls secure the appliance to the pelvis.

The Wilmington TLSO, a passive appliance fabricated from a thermoplastic material such as orthoplast, is custom-made for each client from an individual cast. This device was developed at the DuPont Hospital for Children in Wilmington, Delaware. The negative cast of the child is made while traction and transverse forces are applied to achieve as much curve correction as possible. The positive cast made from this mold is modified, and the thermoplastic material is formed over the mold. No additional correction pads are added to the inside of the appliance. The orthosis is fit to the patient with inferior trimlines to the level of the greater trochanters and pubic symphysis, and the superior aspect of the brace is trimmed to fit as high in the axillae as possible. There is an anterior overlapping opening to facilitate easy donning and doffing (**Fig. 17.22**).

For best results, clients are encouraged to wear their braces (Boston or Wilmington) for 23 hours per day, removing the brace only for bathing and exercise. Although some report successful outcomes with brace wear as little as 16 to 18 hours per day, there is a direct correlation between the amount of time spent in the brace and the effectiveness of the brace in preventing curve progression.[15] Brace efficacy is also significantly

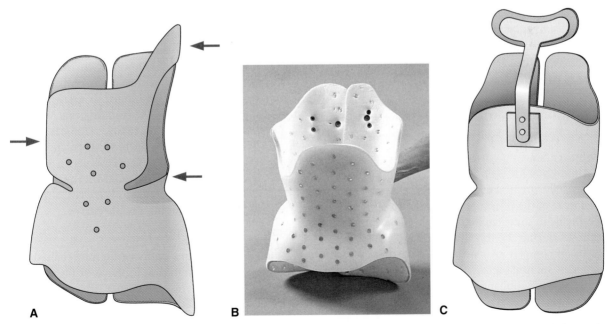

A   **B**   **C**

FIGURE 17.21. The Boston thoracolumbosacral orthosis: **(A)** cut to provide three-point counterforces to a thoracic scoliosis; **(B)** posterior opening with Velcro closures; **(C)** a superstructure can be added to apply forces to a curve with apex above T6.

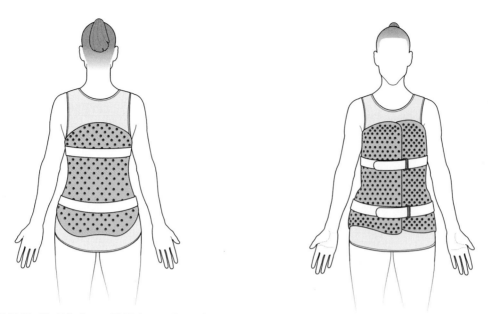

FIGURE 17.22. The Wilmington TLSO is a passive scoliosis orthosis made from a cast taken with maximum curve correction.

influenced by the location of pressure pads (Boston) and how tightly the closures are fastened.[16] Because patients usually wear their orthoses for years while awaiting skeletal maturity, adherence to a prescribed wearing schedule is extremely important to achieve the best outcome. To maximize treatment compliance, therapists must help clients solve problems and address concerns that might otherwise reduce wearing time. When skeletal maturity is reached and bracing is discontinued, a gradual weaning process is followed to ensure that curve stability is maintained as brace wear is reduced. The weaning process may take a year or more to complete.

Nocturnal Orthoses: The Charleston Bending Brace and the Providence Scoliosis System

Nighttime braces are used with the same population of children with AIS as the day and night wear braces. The treatment goal is also the same. The advantage of the nocturnal braces is that they may be acceptable to some children who do not want to wear orthoses during the day due to cosmesis, self-image issues, or complaints that the orthosis interferes with activities such as sports. Nighttime orthoses differ from day wear appliances in that they place the trunk in an overcorrected side-bent position that is not compatible with walking and performing daily activities. Two nighttime braces are available: the Charleston bending brace and the Providence scoliosis system. Like other scoliosis braces, the *Charleston*

bending brace is a molded plastic TLSO that is formed over a cast of the child's trunk. However, the mold for this brace is taken while the child is standing and side-bending toward the convexity of the curve. With a stabilizing force at the trochanter and a laterally directed force at the apex of the curve, side-bending toward the convexity unbends and overcorrects the scoliosis (**Fig. 17.23**). This orthosis is most effective with single curves with their apices below T7.

The *Providence scoliosis system*, a second-generation nocturnal brace, also employs overcorrection in a molded plastic appliance. However, in this system, casting occurs in a recumbent position with a series of corrective pads precisely positioned to apply forces to produce hypercorrection. The resulting brace applies controlled direct lateral and rotational forces on the trunk, resulting in greater in-brace correction than other braces (**Fig. 17.24**). The Providence brace is fabricated with the aid of CAD-CAM technology and is used with a wider range of curves than the Charleston brace, including double curves.

Dynamic Scoliosis Braces

Although their designs and wearing protocols differ, both day wear and nighttime scoliosis orthoses, made from rigid plastics, restrict normal movements and may cause skin irritation. An alternative conservative treatment method for the same skeletally immature children with mild to moderate progressive idiopathic scoliosis was developed by two pediatric orthopedic surgeons in Montreal, Quebec, Canada.[14] This

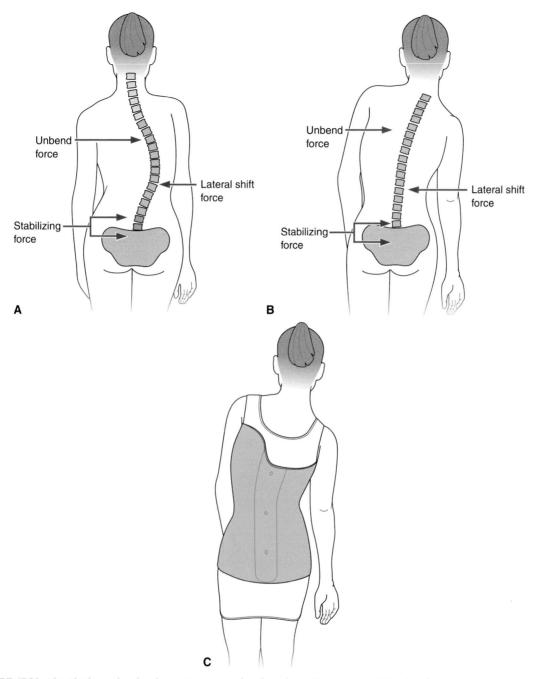

FIGURE 17.23. The Charleston bending brace is a nocturnal scoliosis brace that applies side-bending forces toward the convexity of the curve (**A**) to overcorrect the curve (**B, C**).

device, called *SpineCor*, is constructed from flexible materials and applies dynamic forces to maintain or improve the spinal deformity while reeducating the body to return to a more normal posture. The SpineCor appliance consists of a free-moving configuration of belts, straps, and pads fixed at one end to a plastic pelvic base and at the other end to a fabric vest. Four adjustable elastic bands work together dynamically to maintain and improve spinal deformity while allowing movement and posture reeducation (**Fig. 17.25**). The configuration and lengths of the bands are determined with the aid of software that

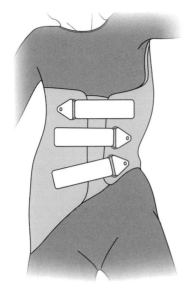

FIGURE 17.24. The Providence nocturnal brace applies carefully controlled direct lateral and rotational forces to the trunk to overcorrect the scoliotic curves.

monitors clinical, radiological, and postural variables; classifies the curve pattern; and describes the specific corrective movement strategy for the particular curve type identified. Similarly to rigid orthoses, clients must wear this dynamic device 20 hours per day (under clothing) for at least 18 months or until skeletal maturity. The device is not successful with obese children or girls who have already reached menarche. Although long-term studies are not yet available, one comparison between the flexible SpineCor and a rigid scoliosis orthosis showed that client acceptance of both devices was comparable, but a greater proportion of those wearing the dynamic orthosis experienced unacceptable curve progression.[17]

Efficacy of Orthotic Treatment for Idiopathic Scoliosis

A considerable amount of research has been conducted to test and validate the effectiveness of various orthotic devices to stop the progression of mild to moderate scoliosis curves while awaiting skeletal maturity as well as to compare effectiveness among devices. However, making comparisons among studies has been difficult because different research groups used different parameters. In 2005, the Scoliosis Research Society established parameters for all future AIS bracing studies so that meaningful comparisons can be made.[18] As more studies are conducted using these designated parameters, more meaningful comparisons among orthoses can be made that may assist clinicians in selecting the most appropriate appliance for each client. The Keywords for Literature Search section that appears at the end of this chapter lists terms that clinicians can use to find relevant literature to guide clinical decision making concerning orthotic management of clients with idiopathic scoliosis.

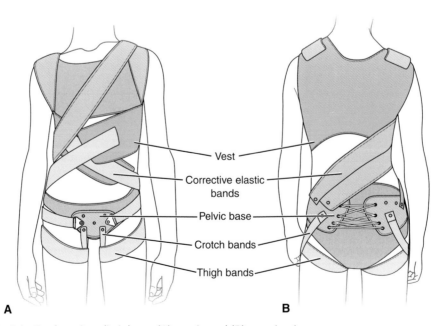

Vest

Corrective elastic bands

Pelvic base

Crotch bands

Thigh bands

A   **B**

FIGURE 17.25. The SpineCor dynamic scoliosis brace: **(A)** anterior and **(B)** posterior views.

CERVICAL ORTHOSES

Cervical orthoses, like trunk orthoses, are used primarily to

- Stabilize unstable cervical spine joints or fractures
- Limit cervical spine motion to protect healing tissues following injury or surgery
- Protect the cervical spine during extrication and transportation to definitive medical care following trauma in which a spinal cord injury is possible

Cervical orthoses are classified as COs or collars and CTOs. **Table 17.4** summarizes the categories and commonly used types of cervical orthoses.

Cervical Collars

Cervical collars encase the neck and may also make contact with the occiput and mandible as well as the clavicular or sternal areas and the upper back superior to the scapular spines. Collars are further

TABLE 17.4 Types of Cervical Orthoses		
Biomechanical Terminology (see Figures for Pictures)	**Subtype**	**Applications**
Cervical orthosis (CO); head cervical orthosis (HCO), collar	Soft collars Semirigid collars • Philadelphia (Fig. 17.26A) • Miami J (Fig. 17.26B) • Aspen (Fig. 17.26C) • NeckLoc®	Extrication collars; general cervical support and FE control Moderate midcervical motion restriction
Cervicothoracic orthosis (CTO)	Semirigid collar with thoracic extension • Philadelphia CTO (Fig. 17.27) • Miami J CTO • Aspen CTO (Fig. 17.28) • Etc	Mid and low C-spine control; FEL control
	Poster-CTOs • Two-poster (Fig. 17.29A) • Four-poster (Fig. 17.29B) • Three-poster (SOMI) (Fig. 17.30)	• FE control • FEL control • C1 through C3 F control
	Vest-CTO • Minerva (Fig. 17.33) • Halo (noninvasive halo) (Fig. 17.32) • Halo (invasive) (Fig. 17.31)	FELR control; maximum available motion restriction

E, extension; F, flexion; L, lateral bend.

designated by the nature of the materials from which they are constructed as soft or semirigid.

Soft Collars

Soft collars, constructed from foamed polyurethane covered in stockinette, are applied by wrapping them around the neck and are secured with a Velcro closure, which is usually posterior. These "over-the-counter" devices are slightly wider posteriorly with an anterior "cut-out" to accommodate the chin and are sold in varying lengths and widths. Soft collars, however, do not significantly limit cervical spine motion and thus are ineffective when motion limitation is important for protection or stabilization.[19] At one time, soft collars were used to rest soft tissues injured by whiplash trauma or other mechanical disorders. Research, however, does not validate the effectiveness of cervical collars in the management of acute or chronic whiplash or other mechanical disorders.[20,21]

Semirigid Collars

Semirigid cervical collars are made from a variety of materials including foamed polyethylene thermoplastic (Plastizote), sheet thermoplastics, and injection-molded plastics (**Fig. 17.26**). In addition to encasing the neck, they cover the occipital and mandibular regions of the head and the clavicular, sternal, and upper back (above the spines of the scapulae) regions and are sometimes termed head cervical orthoses (HCOs) or collars. These devices are prefabricated and sold as "over-the-counter" appliances based on client measurements. Most are bivalved, with front and back components connected by adjustable Velcro

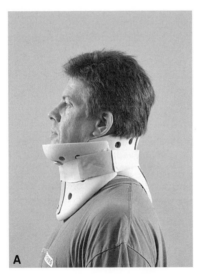
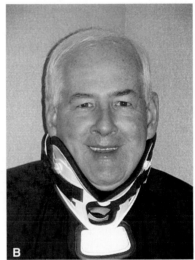
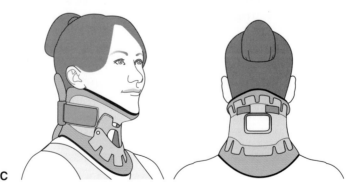

FIGURE 17.26. Semirigid cervical collars: **(A)** the Philadelphia collar, **(B)** the Miami J collar, and **(C)** the Aspen collar.

closures, which makes donning and doffing easier for clients who are not permitted to sit up without orthotic support. Catalogs and Web sites for companies that manufacture or sell these appliances offer many versions of each device with various options to accommodate sizing and specific applications. Most are available in sizing to fit children as well as adults. Because they are used as extrication orthoses to stabilize the cervical spine following trauma, most have an anterior hole to accommodate tracheotomy care and palpation of the carotid pulse without having to remove the anterior stabilizing section of the orthosis. Some also provide an opening in the posterior portion of the collar to allow for airflow, fluid drainage, and palpation of the cervical spine. Most of these semirigid collars provide adequate general restriction of cervical motion, although they control flexion better than extension and are least effective in limiting lateral bend and rotation. The best segmental motion control occurs in the midcervical spine, but they are only moderately effective in the lower cervical regions.[22] Motion control in the lower cervical spine requires a cervicothoracic orthosis (CTO), which is discussed later in this chapter ("Cervicothoracic Orthoses").[22,23] One study showed that the NecLoc collar (Jerome Medical, Moorestown, New Jersey) was most effective in limiting motion, followed by the Aspen (International Healthcare Devices, Long Beach, California) and Miami J (Jerome Medical, Moorestown, New Jersey).[24] The Philadelphia collar (Philadelphia Collar Company, Philadelphia, Pennsylvania) was least restrictive of motion. For conditions that require general support but not rigid immobilization, any of the semirigid cervical collars are reasonably effective and adequate.[21] Another application for the lightweight, Plastizote Philadelphia collar is as a static splint to maintain neck alignment and range of motion in individuals with significant burns over the neck and trunk regions.

For all collars, proper sizing, fit, and application of the appliance with the spine in a neutral position are important and greatly influence the efficacy of the orthosis as well as patient comfort. Although the mandibular piece of the collar is needed to help the orthosis provide support and motion control, it also restricts mouth opening.[25] This can hinder definitive airway placement in an emergency situation as well as simple daily activities like eating. When use of an orthosis makes daily activities difficult, many patients abandon their appliances. A therapist working with a client wearing an orthosis is responsible to ensure that the client can perform his or her daily activities safely, comfortably, and efficiently while wearing the appliance.

Cervicothoracic Orthoses

CTOs enclose the same regions as the semirigid cervical collars but also extend onto the trunk with anterior and posterior thoracic components that attach to one another by rigid or flexible connectors under the arms. The sizes of the thoracic components vary from narrow anterior and posterior chest pieces to a full rigid vest. However, in general, CTOs provide greater segmental and regional motion restriction, particularly in the lower cervical region. Additionally, they provide more effective motion control of cervical lateral bending and rotation.[22]

Three types of CTOs are available: semirigid cervical collars with thoracic extensions, posttype CTOs, and maximum immobilizing appliances. Most of the semirigid cervical collars discussed above are available with thoracic extension kits that, when added to the collar, convert the HCO to a CTO (**Fig. 17.27** and **Fig. 17.28**). Many of these devices are modular so that the thoracic extension can be added when greater stabilization or immobilization is required and removed when it is no longer needed. This feature makes them attractive for use as a postsurgical orthosis, because the thoracic extension can be removed as healing progresses and less restriction is required.

Post cervical braces are composed of separate mandibular, occipital, and anterior and posterior thoracic components with rigid vertical posts that extend from the thoracic components to the chin or occiput. The anterior and posterior thoracic components are connected by flexible straps over the shoulders and around the chest under the arms. In general, post-type orthoses are more restrictive and cooler than collars, but they are also more difficult to don and doff correctly. There are three types of post-CTOs: two-post, three-post, and four-post appliances. Two-post orthoses have anterior and posterior midline posts that restrict flexion and extension but provide little control of cervical lateral bend and rotation (**Fig. 17.29**). Four-post orthoses are similar to two-post CTOs, but they

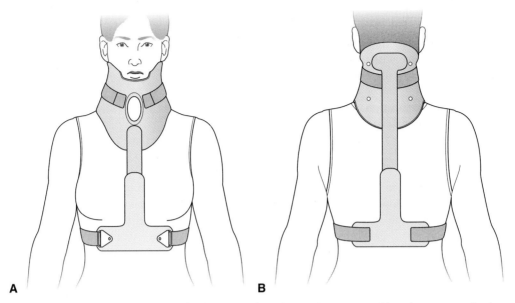

FIGURE 17.27. Philadelphia CTO. **(A)** Anterior and **(B)** posterior thoracic extensions connected by Velcro straps under the arms convert the Philadelphia cervical orthosis to a CTO.

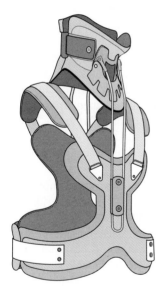

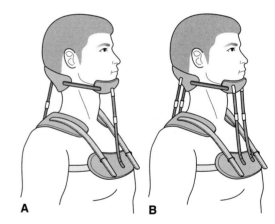

FIGURE 17.29. Post-type CTOs: **(A)** two-post CTO; **(B)** four-post CTO.

FIGURE 17.28. Aspen CTO. A two- or four-post apparatus connects anterior and posterior thoracic plates to the Aspen CO.

provide two anterior and two posterior posts that attach on either side of the mandibular and occipital supports, respectively. Thus, four-post orthoses are able to provide greater restriction of cervical side-bend and rotation. The *SOMI (sternal occipital mandibular immobilizer) orthosis* has three posts, all of which extend

from the anterior thoracic component. The center post terminates at the mandibular plate, and the two lateral posts bend backward and attach to the occipital plate **(Fig. 17.30)**. This orthosis was designed to be applied to a supine patient who is not permitted upright posture without orthotic support. Because it does not have a posterior thoracic plate, it may be more comfortable for patients who must remain supine. It is able to restrict movement in all three planes, but it is most effective in limiting flexion at C1 through C3 and is

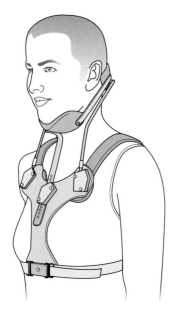

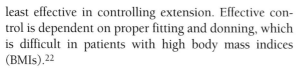

FIGURE 17.30. The SOMI orthosis is a three-post CTO.

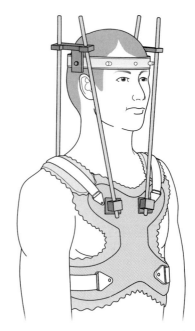

FIGURE 17.31. A skeletal (invasive) halo-vest CTO.

least effective in controlling extension. Effective control is dependent on proper fitting and donning, which is difficult in patients with high body mass indices (BMIs).[22]

CTOs with the greatest ability to restrict cervical motion include the halo-vest or body jacket orthosis and the Minerva orthosis. These appliances are used following cervical fractures with or without spinal cord injury or with other conditions that require the maximum possible immobilization. The halo-vest orthosis, however, has become the "gold standard" when immobilization in the upper cervical spine and restriction of rotation and side bend are critical.[26] The halo-vest orthosis also allows precise three-dimensional positioning and has been used to obtain cervical realignment with ligamentous reconstruction.

The halo-vest orthosis includes a cranial ring that is attached to the skull by four or six pins that are inserted by a surgeon through the scalp into the outer layer of the compact bone of the cranium. The ring or halo is then attached to the vest by rods (Fig. 17.31). Originally, the halo, pins, and rods were metal, but now they are made of ceramics, carbon fiber composites, or other materials that are compatible with magnetic resonance imaging. Although these invasive orthoses are attached to the cranium, a small amount of cervical motion still occurs, particularly in the lower cervical spine.[27]

Patients who wear these devices are permitted to participate in normal daily activities, including walking if the individual is able. However, because of its size and effect on redistribution of the patient's center of mass, it may increase the risk of falling.[28] Complications that may occur while wearing the halo-vest orthosis include skin breakdown or irritation under the vest, pin track infections, and pin loosening.[29] Diligent daily pin site cleaning and conscientious follow-up with the surgeon are essential with this treatment. Children are more likely to experience halo-related complications, probably because of their thinner scalps and calvariae.[30] As a result, early surgical internal fixation and external fixation with pinless appliances are used when possible.

A pinless *noninvasive halo orthosis* has been used following pediatric surgery for congenital muscular torticollis release, C1 to C2 rotary subluxation reduction, postoperative cervical immobilization, tumor removal, and odontoid fracture, and in some adults with neurologically intact non- or minimally displaced cervical fractures.[31] The device consists of a padded carbon composite anterior-only chest plate with connector posts that attach to an open ring frontal bone band (halo) that is lined with a silicone material that adheres to the skin and prevents migration. A posterior occiput support holds the head against the frontal band, and a mandibular sling supports the chin (**Fig. 17.32**). This device is particularly effective in controlling cervical lateral bending and rotation.[22]

The *Minerva orthosis*, another pinless cervical immobilizer, was originally developed as a custom-made cast to immobilize the cervical spine after cervical fracture. Currently, it is available as a prefabricated custom-fit appliance for both children and adults (**Fig. 17.33**). The cervical stabilization component can be attached to either a TLSO body jacket or anterior and posterior chest plates that are less restrictive of the trunk. The cervical unit connects to the thoracic component by anterior and posterior posts. The cervical unit includes a molded shell that covers the posterior neck as well as the occiput. A forehead band extends from this shell to stabilize the head against the posterior component. The mandibular piece that is supported by the anterior post is also attached to the posterior occipital shell. The Minerva CTO has shown adequate immobilization in children and adults and is considered a reasonable alternative to a halo device.[22,32]

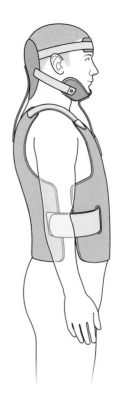

FIGURE 17.33. A Minerva orthosis with a body jacket TLSO. The Minerva cervical attachment includes a large posterior neck and occipital shell, a forehead band, and a mandibular support.

CRANIAL REMODELING ORTHOSES

Deformational plagiocephaly is a condition in which an infant's head is asymmetrically shaped, usually with

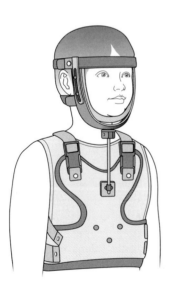

FIGURE 17.32. A pinless noninvasive halo-vest CTO employs a nonslip silicone lining on the halo ring to attach the frontal band to the head without pins.

a flattened surface, which is easiest to identify when viewed from the top. There are many possible causes of plagiocephaly, some of which may occur before birth and some after. Causes of plagiocephaly that occur in utero include multiple fetuses that limit space and the ability to move, as well as uterine fibroids that create an abnormally shaped uterine space. Premature children, developmentally delayed children, and children with congenital muscular torticolis may also show plagiocephaly caused by a limited ability to move and change position. However, there has been an increase in plagiocephaly since the early 1990s when the American Academy of Pediatrics began to recommend a supine sleeping position for infants to reduce the incidence of sudden infant death syndrome. When congenital muscular torticolis, craniosynostosis (premature closing of the cranial sutures), and other conditions have been ruled out as possible causes, treatment options for mechanical deformational plagiocephaly include teaching the parents to reposition the child frequently and a cranial remodeling orthosis, which is also called a molding helmet or headband (**Fig. 17.34**). The process of fitting a cranial orthosis starts with making a negative mold of the child's head, usually by using a digital scanning device. A positive cast is made and modified to a symmetrical shape, and then the helmet or head band is formed around this corrected mold. When fit to the infant, the device applies a mild holding pressure to the prominences while leaving room for growth in the adjacent flattened regions.[33] During treatment, infants and their helmets are checked and modified as needed on a weekly or biweekly schedule to ensure that appropriate contacts and reliefs are present in the orthosis.

Cranial orthoses are approved by the FDA (United States Food and Drug Administration) for use with infants from ages 3 to 18 months with moderate to severe deformational plagiocephaly who have not shown improvement after 6 to 8 weeks of repositioning therapy.[34] The average length of treatment is 3 to 5 months; however, when treatment is initiated in children older than 12 months, treatment time may be longer. Some researchers report that earlier intervention significantly improves outcomes, independent of the severity of the presenting asymmetries.[35] Other studies demonstrate that treated infants exhibit normal growth trajectories and plot appropriately for all parameters on pediatric growth charts.[36] Finally, a study that evaluated children 5 years after completion of treatment showed that cranial orthoses are safe and effective in correcting cranial asymmetries caused by mechanical deformation.[37]

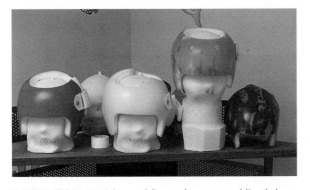

FIGURE 17.34. Cranial remodeling orthoses or molding helmets are used to treat deformational plagiocephaly.

GUIDES FOR PRESCRIPTION AND CHECKOUT OF TRUNK AND CERVICAL ORTHOSES

Prescriptions for trunk or cervical orthoses are developed to meet specific goals developed for each client which are based on a sound understanding of the client's pathology, impairments, and functional needs, as well as on his or her lifestyle requirements. A guide for prescription of trunk and cervical orthoses to meet specific goals is presented in **Figure 17.35**. When developing orthotic prescriptions, practitioners must also consider best practice guidelines and reports of orthotic efficacy published in current research literature (see Keywords for Literature Search section at the end of this chapter).

When a new orthosis is received, a therapist must conduct an orthotic checkout examination of the client, the device, and the client wearing the device. The general checkout procedure is discussed in Chapter 11, and specific items relevant to the checkout of trunk and cervical orthoses are listed in **Boxes 17.1, 17.2,** and **17.3.** Because many spinal orthoses are prefabricated and ordered from catalogs by selecting a size according to client measurements, therapists must ensure that the appliance received is actually the correct size and that any adjustments that may be needed are made by the appropriate practitioner.

Spinal orthoses are not always easy to apply correctly and are often applied incorrectly, which makes their use at best uncomfortable and at worst harmful to the client's condition. The therapist must ensure that the appliance is applied properly and that the client or a caregiver can also apply the device correctly. If the appliance is custom-made by an orthotist, the therapist, patient, and orthotist must work together to make sure that the appliance fits properly, is as comfortable as possible, and does not unnecessarily restrict daily activities and exercise. Most new appliance wearers adapt to their orthoses more comfortably when they gradually increase wearing time over several days to a week, depending on the individual needs of the client. Increasing orthotic wearing time by an hour or two at an interval appropriate for the specific individual can avoid problems or make them easier to resolve if they occur. Obviously, when an orthosis is prescribed to restrict deleterious motions

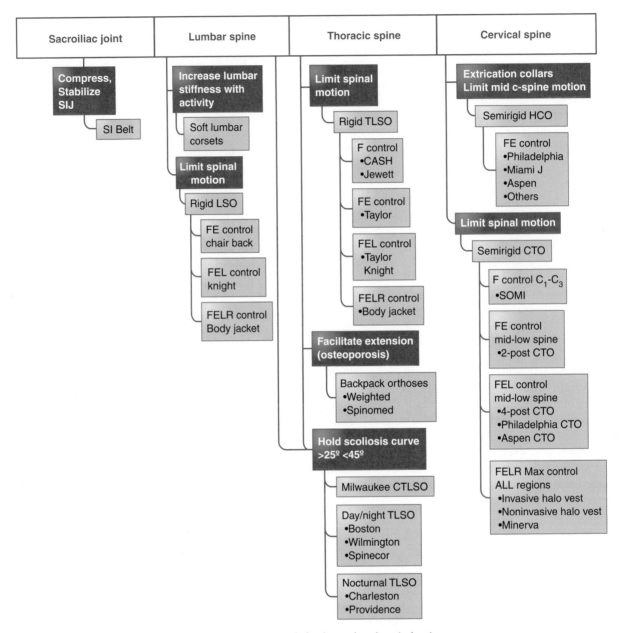

FIGURE 17.35. A guide to orthotic solutions for treatment goals for the trunk and cervical regions.

after trauma, gradually increasing wearing schedules is inappropriate. In these cases, orthoses are usually worn full time until evidence of healing indicates that it is safe to wean from the appliance. During full-time brace wear, clients may lose some muscle strength and become dependent on the appliance. In these cases, the client must gradually increase his or her time out of the orthosis, while gradually discontinuing brace use. Functional training with a new appliance may also be necessary, because wearing a trunk or cervical orthosis that limits motion may require developing alternative methods of doing usual daily activities. Asking patients to identify functional activities that are important or difficult for them helps clinicians individualize training and focus on relevant functional skills.

BOX 17.1	Specific Items for the Checkout Examination of Rigid Trunk Orthoses (LSOs)

- Orthosis is comfortable
- Pelvic band or inferior trimline lies between iliac crest and greater trochanter
- Thoracic band or superior trimline lies below inferior angle of scapulae
- Any uprights or horizontal bands follow the contour of the body, are not too far away from the body, but do not contact the body or exert pressure
- Total contact jackets exert even pressure without high-pressure areas over bony prominences such as spinous processes, trochanters
- If there is an abdominal apron, it extends from xiphoid to pubic symphysis and does not roll at edges
- Client can sit with hips flexed to 90° without impingement of brace on thighs and without orthosis "riding-up" due to posterior contact on chair
- T-shirt or body sock between orthosis and skin lies flat without wrinkles
- Fasteners for closure have adjustability and can be tightened to appropriate tension
- Orthosis does not migrate on body during movement or appropriate functional activities

BOX 17.2	Specific Items for the Checkout Examination of Rigid Thoraco-lumbosacral Orthoses (TLSOs) or Scoliosis TLSO or CTLSO

For Milwaukee CTLSO
- For neck ring: Occipital pads lie below occiput, and nothing contacts mandible
- For uprights: conform to body without contact; do not interfere with chest expansion during respiration

For All Total Contact Rigid TLSOs
- Pelvic girdle is total contact without excessive pressure on bony prominences (eg, iliac crests, trochanters, ribs)
- If appliance is for daytime wear, client can sit with 90° hip flexion without excessive pressure on thighs and without superior migration of orthosis
- Appropriate abdominal compression
- Closures provide appropriate adjustability and can be fastened with appropriate tension
- Interior pressure pads (scoliosis brace) apply firm pressure to apices of curves
- T-shirt or body sock between skin and orthosis is smooth, without wrinkles
- Appliance does not migrate on trunk during appropriate movement

BOX 17.3	Specific Items for the Checkout Examination of Cervical and Cervicothoracic Orthoses (COs and CTOs)

- Orthosis is comfortable
- If a prefabricated orthosis, size delivered was appropriate
- Orthosis can be and is applied properly
- Neck is maintained in appropriate position
- Occipital support is located appropriately under the occiput
- No excessive pressure on mandible
- Thoracic components are comfortable, located appropriately for the orthotic function, and do not exert excessive pressure
- Closures or fasteners have appropriate adjustability and are fastened with appropriate tension

SUMMARY

This chapter discusses trunk and cervical orthoses that are used to apply forces to the axial skeleton and related nonosseous structures. These appliances are typically prescribed to provide support for unstable structures, protect healing structures, or limit regional or segmental range of motion. Scoliosis and cranial remodeling orthoses present special applications in which braces are used during rapid skeletal growth to influence skeletal remodeling to improve deformity.

Trunk and cervical orthoses are broadly classified according to the materials from which they are constructed as soft (flexible), semirigid, or rigid appliances. Soft appliances are able to apply compressive forces; however, their clinical effectiveness during function is largely regarded as minimal. Rigid appliances are primarily used to protect unstable fractures or other types of injuries or to support the spines of individuals with neuromuscular diseases that produce trunk weakness or muscle imbalance deformity. Although still used for postoperative stabilization following spine surgeries, more effective internal fixation hardware and surgical procedures have minimized the importance of orthoses in this role.

The use of lightweight plastics and composites in rigid orthoses, rather than metal and leather, has improved the appearance of spinal orthoses. However, in general, they are still restrictive, uncomfortable, and visible under clothing. As a result, patient compliance with spinal brace treatment requirements and adherence to wearing schedules is difficult for some clients. Therapists must monitor the possible negative aspects of brace wear and minimize their effects on function and daily life activities in order to optimize treatment outcome. Long-term brace wear can have negative effects on spinal and girdle joint range of motion, trunk or cervical muscle strength, pulmonary function (for orthoses that encase the thorax), exercise tolerance and fitness, as well as self-esteem and psychological affect. In order for an orthosis to be effective, it must be worn as prescribed; thus, therapists must monitor and address quality of life issues.

Most trunk and cervical orthoses are prefabricated and mass produced and ordered for patients by size selection based on client measurement. Orthoses that do not fit properly or are applied improperly and thus hold the spine in improper positions are uncomfortable and ineffective and may actually be harmful. Thus, therapists must be able to evaluate orthotic fit, application, and joint position in the orthosis and assume responsibility to initiate necessary corrections by the appropriate practitioner.

KEYWORDS FOR LITERATURE SEARCH

For each topic, choose relevant keywords, subject heading words, or MeSH terms from each domain and search using the Boolean term "AND".

Search Topic: What are the Effects of Orthoses in the Management of Clients With Adolescent Idiopathic Scoliosis?

Conditions
  Scoliosis; classification, prevention and control, therapy, rehabilitation
  Adolescent idiopathic scoliosis

Intervention
  Orthotic device
  Braces

Effect
  Effectiveness
  Treatment outcome
  Lung volume measurement
  Respiratory function test
  Disease progression
  Patient compliance
  Patient satisfaction

Search Topic: What are the Effects of Using Trunk, Cervical, and Cranial Orthoses in the Management of Individuals with Selected Conditions?

Conditions
  Plagiocephaly, nonsynostotic
  Cervical vertebrae
  Thoracic vertebrae
  Lumbar vertebrae
  Joint instability
  Spinal fractures
  Fractures, compression
  Osteoporosis
  Kyphosis
  Neck injuries
  Sacroiliac joint
  Pregnancy

Intervention
  Orthotic device
  Braces
  Lumbar corsets
  Cervical collar

Effects
  Effectiveness
  Treatment outcome
  Lung volume measurement
  Respiratory function test
  Range of motion
  Trunk muscle strength
  Posture
  Balance
  Lifting
  Low back pain
  Biomechanics, spine kinematics
  Patient compliance
  Patient satisfaction
  Quality of life

REFERENCES

1. Ivancic PC, Cholevicki J, Rabebold A: Effects of the abdominal belt on muscle-generated spinal stability and L4/L5 joint compression force. Ergonomics 45:501–513, 2002.

2. Arjmand N, Shirazi-Adl A: Role of intra-abdominal pressure in the unloading and stabilization of the human spine during static lifting tasks. Eur Spine J 15:1265–1275, 2006.

3. Cholewicki J, Reeves NP, Everding VQ, et al: Lumbosacral orthoses reduce trunk muscle activity in a postural control task. J Biomech 40:1731–1736, 2007.

4. Vogt L, Pfeifer K, Portscher M, et al: Lumbar corsets: their effect on three-dimensional kinematics of the pelvis. J Rehabil Res Dev 37:495–499, 2000.

5. Fayolle-Minon I, Calmels P: Effect of wearing a lumbar orthosis on trunk muscles: study of the muscle strength after 21 days of use on healthy subjects. Joint Bone Spine 75:58–63, 2008.

6. Puckree T, Lauten VA, Moodley S, et al: Thoracolumbar corsets alter breathing pattern in normal individuals. Int J Rehabil Res 28:81–85, 2005.

7. Sinaki M, Lynn SG: Reducing the risk of falls through proprioceptive dynamic posture training in osteoporotic women with kyphotic posturing: a randomized pilot study. Am J Phys Med Rehabil 81:241–246, 2002.

8. Sinaki M, Brey RH, Hughes CA, et al: Significant reduction in risk of falls and back pain in osteoporotic-kyphotic women through a spinal proprioceptive extension exercise dynamic (SPEED) program. Mayo Clin Proc 80:849–855, 2005.

9. Mens JMA, Damen L, Snijder CJ, et al: The mechanical effect of a pelvic belt in patients with pregnancy-related pelvic pain. Clin Biomech 21:122–127, 2006.

10. Pfeifer M, Begerow B, Minne MW: Effects of new spinal orthosis on posture, trunk strength, and quality of life in women with postmenopausal osteoporosis: a randomized trial. Am J Phys Med Rehabil 83:177–186, 2004.

11. Cholewicki J, Alvi K, Silfies S, et al: Comparison of motion restriction and trunk stiffness provided by three thoracolumbosacral orthoses (TLSOs). J Spinal Disord Tech 16:461–468, 2003.

12. Peelle MW, Luhmann SJ: Management of adolescent idiopathic scoliosis. Neurosurg Clin N Am 18:575–583, 2007.

13. Shaughnessy WJ: Advances in scoliosis brace treatment for adolescent idiopathic scoliosis. Orthop Clin N Am 38:469–475, 2007.

14. Coillard C, Vachon V, Circo AB, et al: Effectiveness of the SpineCor brace based on the new standardized criteria proposed by the scoliosis research society for adolescent idiopathic scoliosis. J Pediatr Orthop 27:375–379, 2007.

15. Rowe DE, Berstein SM, Riddick MF, et al: A meta-analysis of the efficacy of non-operative treatments for idiopathic scoliosis. J Bone Joint Surg 79-A:664–674, 1997.

16. Wong MS, Mak AFT, Luk KDK, et al: Effectiveness and biomechanics of spinal orthoses in the treatment of adolescent idiopathic scoliosis. Prosthet Orthot Int 24:148–162, 2000.

17. Wong MS, Cheng JCY, Lam TP, et al: The effect of rigid versus flexible spinal orthosis on the clinical efficacy and acceptance of the patients with adolescent idiopathic scoliosis. Spine 33:1360–1365, 2008.

18. Richards BS, Bernstein RM, D'Amato CR, et al: Standardization of criteria for adolescent idiopathic scoliosis brace studies: SRS committee on bracing and nonoperative management. Spine 30:2068–2075, 2005.

19. Carter VM, Fasen JA, Roman JM, et al: The effect of a soft collar, used as normally recommended or reversed on three planes of cervical range of motion. J Orthop Sport Phys 23:209–215, 1996.

20. Vassiliou T, Schnabel M, Ferrarc R, et al: Randomized, controlled outcome study of active mobilization compared with collar therapy for whiplash injury. Emerg Med J 21:306–310, 2004.

21. Kongsted A, Qerama E, Dasch H, et al: Neck collar, "act-as-usual" or active mobilization for whiplash injury?: a randomized parallel-group trial. Spine 32:618–626, 2007.

22. Schneider AM, Hipp JA, Nguyen L, et al: Reduction in head and intervertebral motion provided by 7 contemporary cervical orthoses in 45 individuals. Spine 32:E1–E6, 2007.

23. Sandler AJ, Dvorak J, Humke T, et al: The effectiveness of various cervical orthoses: an in vivo comparison of the mechanical stability provided by several widely used models. Spine 21:1624–1629, 1996.

24. Askins V, Eismont FJ: Efficacy of five cervical orthoses in restricting cervical motion: a comparison study. Spine 22:1193–1198, 1997.

25. Goutcher CM, Lochhead V: Reduction in mouth opening with semi-rigid cervical collars. Br J Anesthes 95:344–348, 2005.

26. Johnson RM, Hart DL, Simmons EF, et al: Cervical orthoses: a study comparing their effectiveness in restricting cervical motion in normal subjects. J Bone Joint Surg 59-A:332–339, 1977.

27. Botte MJ, Byrne TP, Abrams RA, et al: Halo skeletal fixation: techniques of application and prevention of complications. J Am Acad Orthop Surg 4:44–53, 1996.

28. Richardson JK, Ross ADM, Riley B, et al: Halo vest effect on balance. Arch Phys Med Rehabil 81:255–257, 2000.

29. Dormans JP, Crisciliello AA, Drummond DS, et al: Complications in children managed with immobilization in a halo vest. J Bone Joint Surg 77-A:1370–1373, 1995.

30. Baum JA, Hanley EN, Pullekines J: Comparison of halo complications in adults and children. Spine 14:251–252, 1989.

31. Mueller DG, Mueller K: Three case studies involving the use of a noninvasive halo for cervical stabilization. J Prosthet Orthot 17:40–47, 2005.

32. Gaskill SJ, Marlin AE: Custom fitted thermoplastic Minerva jackets in the treatment of cervical spine instability in pre-school age children. Pedriatr Neurosurg 16:35–39, 1990.

33. Littlefield TR: Cranial remodeling devices: treatment of deformational plagiocephaly and postsurgical applications. Semin Pediatr Neurol 11:268–277, 2004.

34. Larsen J: Orthotic treatment protocols for plagiocephaly. J Prosthet Orthot 16(4S):31–34, 2004.

35. Kelly KM, Littlefield TR, Romatto IK, et al: Importance of early recognition and treatment of deformational plagiocephaly with orthotic cranioplasty. Cleft Palate Craniofac J 36:127–130, 1999.

36. Kelly KM, Littlefield TR, Pomatto IK, et al: Cranial growth unrestricted during treatment of deformational plagiocephaly. Pediatr Neurosurg 30:193–199, 1999.

37. Lee RP, Teichgraeber JF, Baumgartner JE, et al: Long-term treatment effectiveness of molding helmet therapy in the correction of posterior deformational plagiocephaly: a five year follow-up. Cleft Palate Craniofac J 45:240–245, 2008.

Orthoses for Upper Extremity Impairments

OBJECTIVES

At the end of this chapter, all students are expected to:

1. Describe the types and functions of upper extremity orthoses.
2. Identify and describe the parts of upper extremity orthoses, including the materials, componentry, and orthotic designs used in these appliances.
3. Describe the impairments and functional activities that may be improved by the use of an upper extremity orthosis.
4. Discuss the ways in which an upper extremity orthosis may affect the wearer's ability to perform his or her activities of daily living.
5. Discuss applications for upper extremity orthoses to improve function.

Physical Therapy students are expected to:

1. Determine the need for an upper extremity orthosis for a client based on examination findings.
   a. Evaluate examination findings, including those from preorthotic prescription examinations, upper quarter biomechanical assessment, and functional analysis, to diagnose impairments that may be improved by use of an upper extremity orthosis.
2. Develop appropriate goals for an upper extremity orthosis based on a client's impairments and functional limitations.
3. Describe the biomechanical methods employed in upper extremity orthoses to achieve the orthotic goals.
4. Develop and execute a search strategy to identify research evidence for the effects and effectiveness of upper limb orthoses and to identify best practices for upper extremity orthotic prescription.
5. Name an upper extremity orthosis using both biomechanical terminology and the Splint Classification System (SCS) developed by the American Society for Hand Therapists.

6. Recommend an orthosis to improve and optimize function as part of a plan of care for an individual with impairments in the upper extremity.
7. Examine and evaluate upper extremity orthoses for acceptable fit, function, comfort, and cosmesis.

CASE STUDIES

Harry Green is a 67-year-old African American widower who suffered a thrombotic cerebral vascular accident (stroke) with right hemiparesis. His history and chief complaints are described in Chapter 2. Mr. Green's acute care hospitalization progressed without complication, and he was discharged to a rehabilitation facility for intensive therapies. From that facility he was discharged to home, where he received some continued home care therapy for several weeks. It is now 6 months after his stroke, and Mr. Green is living alone in his own home with community services. He walks safely with a lower extremity orthosis and an ambulatory aid, but his upper extremity function has not improved very much, and he uses his hand only to hold things down. He has also developed shoulder pain that is not incapacitating but definitely impedes functional activities. He realizes that to continue to be independent at home, he needs to have more use of his upper extremity.

Marjorie Harris is a 40-year-old owner of a music school and violinist in the community symphony orchestra. Marjorie is an active mother of three sons. She teaches violin to children in her music school, plays violin in various community orchestra and theater performances, and also fills in as needed as a musician at her synagogue. Marjorie has experienced lateral elbow pain in her "bowing" arm on and off, but it has always been nagging, and never limiting. Recently, the pain worsened and is not responding to several days of rest as it always has in the past. She went to an orthopedist who diagnosed lateral epicondylitis.

Anthony DiSalvo is a 24-year-old young man who sustained a traumatic brain injury in an auto accident when he was 19 years old, which resulted in spastic quadriparesis as well as speech and cognitive impairments. After extensive rehabilitation, he was discharged and is living with his parents where he requires minimal assistance for most activities. He uses a wheelchair for community mobility but had been able to use a walker and lower extremity orthoses to stand and walk independently for short distances at work and at home. These abilities are necessary for him to continue with his job at the sheltered workshop. Several months ago, he had a heterotopic ossification removed from his right biceps brachii muscle, and subsequent to that he developed a urinary tract infection. These medical issues prevented him from walking for a month. He is now healthy and ready to resume walking and work; however, he has developed a right elbow flexion contracture that makes him unable to use the walker, which is necessary because his balance is not sufficient to walk without it.

Dong Wen is a 27-year-old laid-off loading dock worker who sustained a laceration of his right forearm 3 months ago when he returned home and interrupted a burglary in his apartment. When the burglar pulled a knife on him, he punched out a window to escape and lacerated his arm in the process. He was taken to the emergency room, and his wound was evaluated, cleaned, and sutured. The emergency department doctor told him that he was lucky that he had not injured any tendons. He did not receive follow-up care, other than suture removal, as he is uninsured. He is currently seeking care at a pro bono clinic, because he is now having difficulty using his right hand. The clinic doctor diagnosed a combined median and ulnar nerve injury.

Case Study Activities

All students:

1. Discuss whether each client may benefit from an orthosis, and justify your decision.

a. Identify and discuss the functional problems that may be improved with an orthosis.
b. Identify and discuss functional activities and possible participation restrictions that may be affected by use of an orthosis.
c. List the joint(s) and impairments contributing to each client's functional limitations. How could an orthosis address the impairments?

2. How do you expect an orthosis to affect each client's ability to perform their activities of daily living?

3. Identify and discuss advantages and disadvantages of using an orthosis with each client.

Physical Therapy students:

1. If an orthosis is indicated, develop specific goals for the orthosis for each client.

2. Develop a specific orthotic prescription to achieve the best outcome and functional improvement.

a. Describe the type of orthosis, the orthotic componentry, and the biomechanical methods of force application that will achieve the specific orthotic goals.
b. Using biomechanical and Splint Classification System (American Society of Hand Therapists) terminology, name the orthosis you recommend for each client.
c. Is there evidence in the research literature to support your orthotic recommendations for each client? Describe the evidence you found and how it impacted your orthotic recommendation.

3. Develop a physical therapy plan of care for each client, which includes an orthosis, if appropriate, as well as other physical therapy interventions.

4. If an orthosis is prescribed and provided to a client, how will you determine or measure its effectiveness or impact on function?

UPPER EXTREMITY FUNCTION AND ORTHOTIC INTERVENTIONS

Functional activities carried out by the upper extremity are more complex and variable, compared to lower extremity functional activities. Although the joints of the lower extremity are also capable of complex movement patterns, in most functional activities, the legs are used for support and propulsion of the body and for mobility in the environment. To accomplish these tasks, the joints of the lower extremity are used in repetitive movement patterns, such as the strides and steps that make up walking or running and are described in gait analyses. The upper extremity joints' functions, however, are broad in scope and variable. For example, the shoulder complex, the most mobile joint in the body, allows an individual to place the hand in a large range of positions all around the body without having to move the trunk; the elbow allows the individual to reach away from and bring objects toward the body as well as transmit forces from the trunk to the environment through pushes and pulls; the wrist is a stable link between the arm and hand; and the hand provides an interface with the environment that can produce a powerful grip or delicate fine manipulations. Thus, to function well, the upper extremity joints must be stable to transmit forces but also very mobile to make possible its wide range of functional uses. This need for the joints of the upper extremity to be both stable and mobile during optimal function makes designing an effective orthosis that is acceptable to its user difficult. In fact, few orthoses that are currently available are able to substitute for insufficient joint stability as well as mobility and be acceptable in appearance, size, and bulk. Thus, most upper limb orthoses are prescribed to provide stability, although some are able to impart mobility by using elastic bands, springs, or functional electrical stimulation.

Because the upper limb functions in such a wide range of tasks, many appliances are task specific, and individuals choose devices that facilitate tasks that are specifically important to them. As a result, there is a huge range of devices available, limited only by the creativity of the orthotist or therapist attempting to meet a client's need. The purpose of this chapter is not to present an exhaustive array of every device available, but to provide readers with examples of typically used appliances that demonstrate the major categories of upper limb orthoses and the terminology used to identify and describe them. Readers who require a more comprehensive presentation of orthoses must consult atlases of upper limb orthoses and hand splints.[1,2]

Upper Limb Orthotic Terminology

Orthotic devices for the upper extremity, particularly those used for impairments of the forearm, wrist, and hand, are often referred to as splints, implying that there is a difference between an orthosis and a splint. To lessen confusion among physicians, therapists, orthotists, and insurers, the American Society of Hand Therapists appointed a task force to examine and standardize this terminology.[3] The task force concluded that the terms **splint**, brace, support, and orthosis all refer to devices that apply external forces to the body to improve function and that these terms can be used interchangeably.

However, the use of the term *splint* versus *orthosis* was not the only confusing terminology issue. In the 1970s, orthotists developed a system of orthotic terminology based on the joints enclosed in the appliance and the type of biomechanical control applied (see Chapter 12). Using this system of biomechanical terminology, upper limb orthoses are described as follows:

- SEWHO—Shoulder, elbow, wrist, hand orthosis
- EO—Elbow orthosis
- WHO—Wrist, hand orthosis
- HdO—Hand orthosis

These terms are then followed by a term to describe the orthotic control exerted by the appliance (stop, resist, hold, assist). Although this terminology works well for lower limb appliances, it is not precise enough to accurately describe and distinguish among the wide range of upper limb appliances used. Traditionally, the name of a hand splint included a string of terms that described their form and location on the limb.[4] However, this form-based nomenclature led to misunderstandings and miscommunication among practitioners. Thus, the American Society of Hand Therapists task force also developed a new method to name upper extremity orthoses in a clear and complete way that effectively distinguishes among similar appliances.[3] This system of terminology, called the **Splint Classification System** (SCS), is used today to name upper limb orthoses, rather than the biomechanical system used to name lower limb appliances. SCS terminology, which provides a function-based description of a device, includes a term to describe each of the following characteristics of an orthosis:

- *Articular or nonarticular:* articular splints cross a joint and nonarticular splints do not. For example, an articular splint that crosses the wrist joint is called a wrist splint; a nonarticular humeral splint is applied only to the humerus and does not cross any joints.
- *Location:* identifies the part of the client's anatomy to which the appliance is applied. An articular orthosis names the primary joint affected, and a nonarticular orthosis names the body region to which the orthosis is applied.

- *Direction:* describes the direction of the applied forces or the joint position supported and is referred to as flexion, extension, radial or ulnar deviation, supination or pronation, and abduction.
- *Purpose of the orthosis:* names the purpose of the splint: to (1) *immobilize* a joint or structure, (2) *mobilize* tissue or assist movement, or (3) *restrict* an aspect of joint motion.

An example of the effectiveness of SCS terminology in distinguishing among similar orthoses is presented in **Figure 18.1**. The three splints shown all affect the fourth and fifth metacarpophalangeal (MP) joints of the hand. The SCS name for each splint distinguishes it from the others by identifying the specific purpose of each device as the root of its name: immobilization (Fig. 18.1A), flexion mobilization (Fig. 18.1B), and extension restriction (Fig. 18.1C). This SCS terminology is used throughout the remainder of this chapter. Practitioners, however, must also be familiar with some additional descriptor terms that continue to be used, particularly by those who fabricate complex hand splints, to designate particular splint designs and parts. These terms are listed and defined in **Box 18.1**. Hand–wrist splint parts are labeled in **Figure 18.2**.

Purposes for Upper Limb Orthoses

The general purposes for using any type of orthoses are discussed in Chapter 12. **Table 18.1** lists the general orthotic purposes that can be achieved with each type of SCS functionally named appliance with examples of specific goals for commonly prescribed upper extremity orthoses.

In addition to the goals listed in Table 18.1, upper extremity orthoses may be prescribed for two other specialized purposes. The first specialized purpose is to substitute for hand grip in individuals who are unable to grasp utensils due to paralysis, but have sufficient strength at the shoulder and elbow to move the hand toward the body. For example, splints designed to hold utensils may be useful for individuals with a C5–C6 complete spinal cord injury who can elevate the shoulder but lack hand function (**Fig. 18.3**).

The second group of specialized splints are constructed to be used as an exercise or therapy tool rather than to assist function. These exercise splints transmit forces longitudinally or transversely from unimpaired joints to assist movement in an adjacent impaired joint. For example, a "buddy taping" splint (**Fig. 18.4A**) attaches an impaired digit to an unimpaired digit. When the stronger digit moves, it transmits force transversely and assists joint movement in the attached impaired digit. A "blocking splint" (**Fig. 18.4B**) is an exercise tool used to assist active range of motion (ROM) exercise. By blocking or restricting movement of the more mobile joints in a ray (in this example, the metacarpophalangeal joints), the mobilizing force is transmitted longitudinally to the more restricted joint (the proximal interphalangeal joints). A functional electrical stimulation wrist splint is also available and can be used by individuals with upper motor neuron injuries with active exercises to restore grasp and release (**Fig. 18.5**).[5]

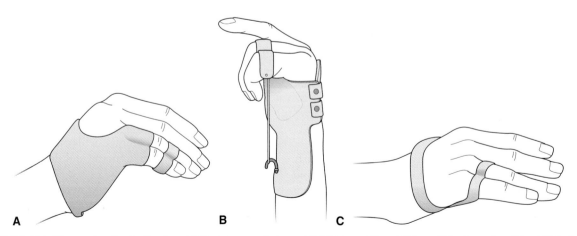

FIGURE 18.1. Three splints for the fourth and fifth metacarpophalangeal (MP) joints: **(A)** an MP immobilization splint, **(B)** a MP flexion mobilization splint, and **(C)** a MP extension restriction splint.

BOX 18.1 | Descriptor Terms for Hand Splints

Location of the splint base on the limb:

Circumferential	Splint base that wraps around the entire circumference of a body part
Gutter	Splint base that wraps around only one side of a limb; usually refers to a radial gutter or ulnar gutter splint that encompasses only the radial or ulnar side of the forearm, respectively
Volar	Splint-base located on the anterior surface of the limb
Dorsal	Splint-base located on the posterior surface of the limb

Origin or base of the splint:

Digit-based	Originates on the digit; free metacarpophalangeal joint motion
Hand-based	Originates on the hand; free wrist motion
Forearm-based	Originates on the forearm; free elbow motion

Names of parts of a splint:

Opponens bar	Supports the thumb in an opposed position opposite to the index and long fingers
C-bar	Abducts the thumb and maintains the web space between the thumb and palm
Outrigger	Structure added to a splint base from which finger cuffs are suspended on a dynamic or static progressive splint
Finger cuffs	Slings or loops that fit around digits that transmit forces from the splint outrigger to the body in a dynamic or static progressive splint
Thumb post	Splint part that wraps around the thumb
Forearm trough	Supports the forearm
Metacarpal bar	Distal end of wrist orthosis that supports metacarpal heads; ends proximal to distal palmar crease
Hypothenar bar	Splint return that supports the ulnar side of the hand

Categories of Upper Limb Orthoses

There are two major categories of upper limb orthoses: static and dynamic. **Static splints** are passive supports that hold a joint or body part in a particular predetermined position. Two additional subcategories or specialized types of static splints include serial static and static progressive splints. These splints are used as part of a treatment program to increase ROM by increasing tissue length. **Dynamic splints** impart forces to the target joint to substitute for missing muscle contraction or to apply low load prolonged stresses to increase tissue length.

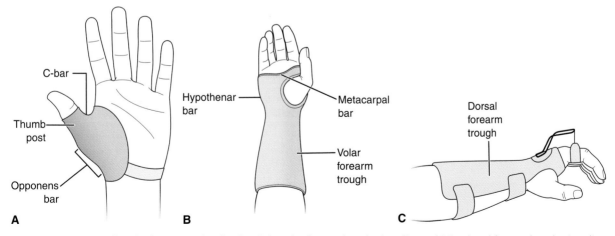

FIGURE 18.2. Parts of hand splints: **(A)** a thumb splint, **(B)** a volar forearm-based wrist splint, and **(C)** a dorsal forearm-based wrist splint.

TABLE 18.1   Purposes for Upper Extremity Orthoses

Function-Based Upper Extremity Splint Type	General Purposes for Any Orthosis	Examples: Specific Upper Extremity Orthotic Goals
Immobilization	*Stabilize* joints, tissues by stopping excessive, abnormal movements	Stabilize unstable, painful joints • Rest joints to reduce inflammation, pain • Prevent muscle imbalance deformities • Facilitate fracture healing
	Manage deformity by *preventing* formation of contractures	• Prevent loss of range of motion or contracture formation
	Protect structures from deleterious loads, forces	• Facilitate healing of injured or repaired tissue (tendons, ligaments)
Mobilization	*Assist* weak or missing joint movements	• Substitute for lost movement due to nerve injury
	Manage deformity by applying *corrective* forces	• Mobilize and elongate shortened tissues to increase passive range of motion
Restriction	*Protect* structures from deleterious loads	• Prevent joint movements in unsafe ranges of motion

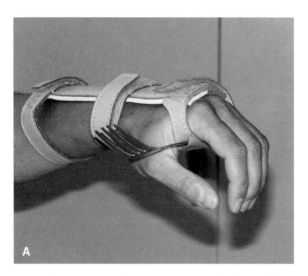 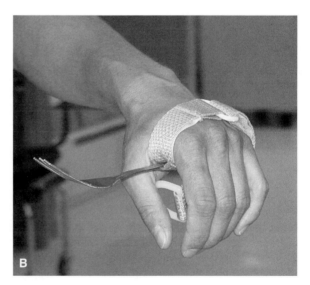

FIGURE 18.3. (A) A wrist extension immobilization splint is modified to hold a utensil for a client who does not have active grip. **(B)** A hand-based utensil holder is sufficient for an individual who does not need external wrist support.

Static Splints

Static splints are the most common type of appliances. They are either articular (cross a joint) or nonarticular. In both cases, they are devices that immobilize and support the body part, usually in a stable position

of rest or a functional position. A rest position for a joint is a position in which the tendons, ligaments, and other joint structures are neither maximally shortened nor maximally lengthened. Resting positions are usually used to protect inflamed or healing

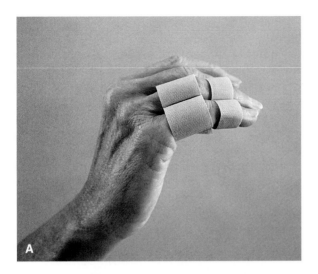

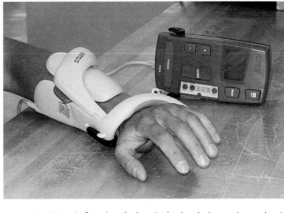

FIGURE 18.5. A functional electrical stimulation wrist orthosis has a portable microprocessor-controlled stimulation unit to help patients practice grasp and release.

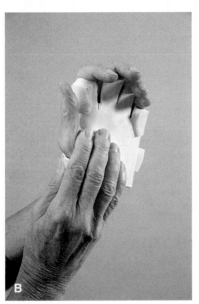

FIGURE 18.4. Exercise splints are used to transmit forces from unimpaired joints to an adjacent impaired joint during exercise: (A) "buddy taping" and (B) "blocking splint."

joint structures. Thus, positioning in **resting splints** must also prevent the formation of joint contractures. If a joint is rested in a static splint with the joint tissues in a shortened position, contractures will develop, resulting in loss of ROM. Thus, static resting splints typically hold joint tissues in elongated positions, but not at the absolute end point. For example, the collateral ligaments of the MP joints in the hand are shortened or "on slack" when the joints are extended. If the hand is placed in a static splint with

the MP joints immobilized at 0°, the ligaments will shorten and form contractures that limit finger flexion and grasping (**Fig. 18.6A**). Clinicians who prescribe and fit upper limb orthoses must have a good understanding of the anatomy and biomechanics of the joints in order to avoid these disastrous potential pitfalls. The functional position of the hand and wrist is a position that includes 20° to 30° of wrist extension, 40° to 45° MP flexion, 45° of proximal interphalangeal (PIP) joint flexion, and relaxed flexion of the distal interphalangeals (DIPs), with the thumb abducted and opposite to the index and long fingers. Immobilization in this position places ligaments in a midposition that is compatible with usage of the hand in most functional activities (Fig. 18.6B). Another simple but important static functional splint immobilizes the thumb and maintains the web space between the thumb and the hand (Fig. 18.6C). An example of a nonarticular static upper extremity splint is a humeral fracture brace. These are used to stabilize closed oblique or spiral fractures of the mid- and proximal diaphysis of the humerus. They achieve fracture stabilization through soft tissue compression within a circumferential bivalved molded plastic brace (**Fig. 18.7**).[6,7]

Serial Static and Static Progressive Splints

Serial static and *static progressive splints* are specialized static splints that are used as part of a program to increase joint ROM by increasing connective tissue length. Thus, they are classified by function as mobilization orthoses. These splints mobilize shortened tissues and increase their length by applying low load, but prolonged tensile stresses at the end point of the available passive joint ROM. This low load prolonged tensile stress (LL-PS) produces stress relaxation and stimulates the connective tissue cells to increase tissue turnover and remodeling. When this occurs while the tissues are maintained in an elongated position, the remodeled tissues are longer than before treatment and allow greater joint ROM.[8,9] Maintaining the joint at its end range position can be achieved either with a series of static splints or casts that are replaced weekly or at another appropriate interval (**serial static**) or with a single splint that is adjustable (**static progressive**). Serial casts, which are worn full time (24 hours per day) until they are replaced, are commonly used to reduce flexion contractures at the PIP joints (**Fig. 18.8**).

Static progressive splints can be custom-made for an individual or purchased or rented as a prefabricated device. Patients use these devices at home and must wear them for at least 30 minutes, three times per day.

The static progressive device, whether custom made or prefabricated, must have a method to adjust the position of the treatment joint so that whenever the appliance is worn, the joint is held at its current end range. As tissue elongation occurs, the joint position is adjusted to take up any slack in the joint caused by the increased tissue length and joint ROM. Different splint components are available to provide various methods to adjust the joint position. For example, in custom-made splints that use finger cuffs and string to hold the end range joint position, a component that resembles and functions like a tuning peg for a guitar string can be used to tighten the string that holds the treatment joint (**Fig. 18.9**). A turnbuckle is another component that allows adjustment of joint position in a static progressive splint (**Fig. 18.10**).[10] Although they are available in different sizes and can be used at many joints, they are frequently used at the elbow. Because the elbow is particularly prone to stiffness following trauma, and aggressive or forceful stretching promotes

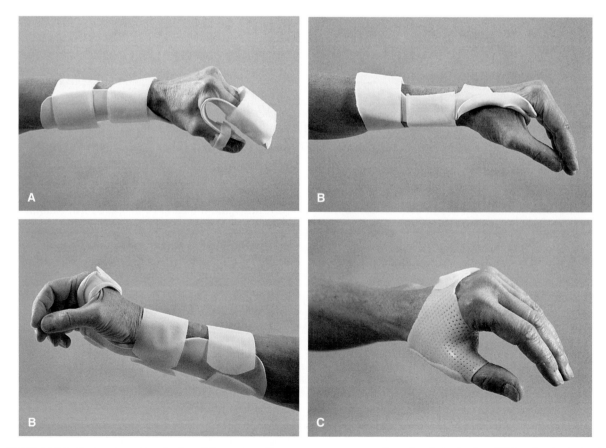

FIGURE 18.6. Static wrist and hand splints: **(A)** a resting splint to prevent contracture formation during healing, **(B)** functional wrist hand splints, and **(C)** a thumb abduction immobilization splint to maintain thumb web space.

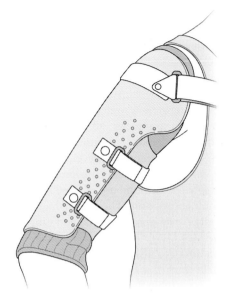

FIGURE 18.7. A humeral fracture brace is a nonarticular static splint used to stabilize selected closed humeral diaphyseal fractures by soft tissue compression.

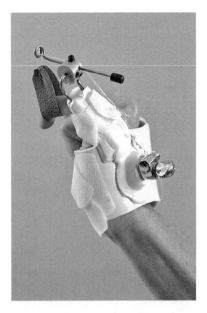

FIGURE 18.9. A static progressive splint to increase proximal interphalangeal joint extension uses a nonelastic cord to hold the joint at the end range extended position. The knob (Merit static progressive component) is adjusted to tighten the cord as range of motion improves.

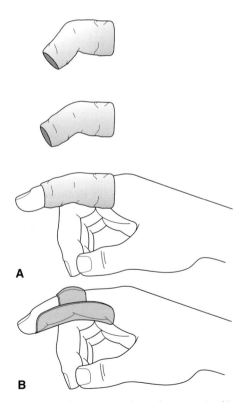

A

B

FIGURE 18.8. Serial casts are used to reduce a proximal interphalangeal joint flexion contracture by holding the joint at maximum end range extension with a series of progressively more extended casts **(A)** or splints **(B)**.

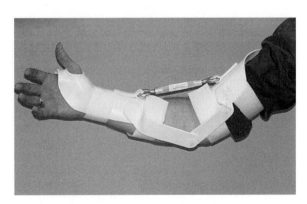

FIGURE 18.10. A static progressive splint with a turnbuckle component to incrementally increase elbow extension.

the formation of heterotopic ossification, static progressive elbow splinting provides a safe and effective method to increase elbow flexion or extension passive ROM.[11] End range positions can be maintained in many different "low-tech" ways, including simple inelastic strings secured with Velcro tape (**Fig. 18.11**). Commercially available static progressive devices are also available for purchase or rental for almost any joint in the body, such as the JAS line of appliances (Joint Active System, Bonutti Healthcare, Effingham, Illinois).

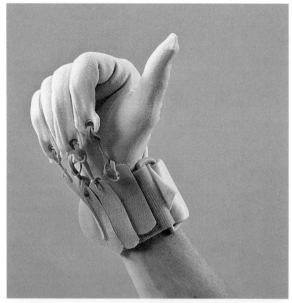

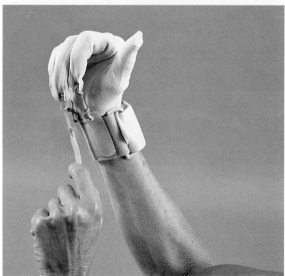

FIGURE 18.11. A simple "low-tech" device to increase finger flexion uses a glove and adjustable Velcro fasteners for each digit. The cord on each digit may be nonelastic (static progressive loading) or elastic (dynamic loading).

Dynamic Splints

Dynamic splints are mobilization devices that apply dynamic forces to the body, usually by using elastic bands, springs, or other materials with elastic memory that store and release energy. Like static progressive splints, dynamic splints are also used to provide low load prolonged stress to increase joint ROM. However, the end range force is dynamic and is usually produced by a spring or elastic material. Dynamic splints that

increase joint ROM may look exactly like static progressive splints, except that the material holding the end range position is elastic (**Figs. 18.11 and 18.12**). Although static progressive and dynamic splints are both used to mobilize contractures, when the joint's end feel is hard, as with mature, long-standing contracture, static tension is preferred.[12] Additionally, static tension usually produces ROM increases more quickly than dynamic loading, regardless of the nature of the end feel.[12] Both splints, however, produce best results when end range time is maximized. Thus, splints must apply only the amount of force required to hold the end range position. The use of high tensile loads that produce pain and limit total end range time is less effective.[13]

Dynamic splints are also used to substitute for a missing muscle function and may be helpful for individuals with peripheral nerve injuries. For example, a radial nerve injury, which causes weakness of the wrist extensor muscles and the extensor digitorum communis muscle (MP extension), may benefit from a wrist immobilization and MP extension mobilization splint (**Fig. 18.13**). This splint assists function by stabilizing the wrist to facilitate grasp and by providing grasp release via elastic band–driven MP extension. Additionally, the brace prevents the

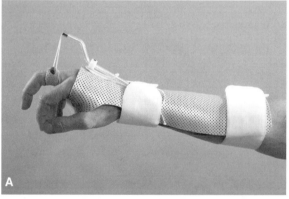

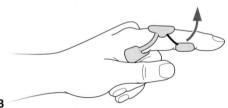

FIGURE 18.12. Dynamic mobilizing splints to increase joint range of motion: **(A)** a splint with an elastic band to increase metacarpophalangeal joint extension and **(B)** a digit-based spring PIP extension splint.

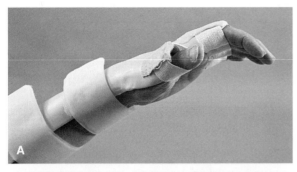

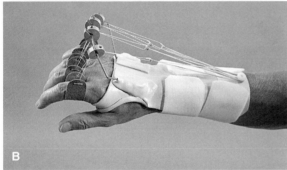

FIGURE 18.13. (A) A dynamic splint substitutes for lost muscle function from a radial nerve injury. (B) Elastic bands from the outrigger to the finger cuffs produce metacarpophalangeal extension.

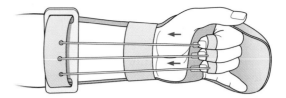

FIGURE 18.14. A postoperative dynamic splint. The elastic bands substitute for and protect the repaired flexor tendon.

The device consists of an orthosis that supports the wrist in a position of about 20° wrist extension with a portable microprocessor–controlled electrical stimulator (see Fig. 18.5). The muscle groups that receive stimulation include the extensor digitorum communis, extensor pollicis brevis, flexor digitorum superficialis, flexor pollicis longus, and the thenar muscle group. The wearer can choose one of the preprogrammed stimulation patterns, which includes three for therapeutic exercise and muscle conditioning and three for functional activities, such as grasp, release, and key grip.

Types of Orthoses: Classification by How They Are Made

Orthotic devices for the upper limb can be *custom made* for an individual patient or prefabricated and purchased by matching sizes to patient measurements. **Prefabricated orthoses** can be obtained from manufacturers or suppliers that require that orders be placed by professional health-care providers, such as physicians, therapists, or orthotists, or they can be obtained directly by the consumer from drugstores and durable medical equipment stores. Prefabricated appliances ordered by health-care professionals for patients are usually delivered to the practitioner, who then fits the device to the patient and ensures that it functions properly. **Custom-made orthoses** are made by practitioners, usually therapists or orthotists for a specific individual. Because they do not need to be as strong as lower limb devices, upper extremity orthoses are usually constructed from low-temperature plastics that are molded directly on the client. Material properties and the types of thermoplastics materials are discussed in Chapter 12. Hand and wrist splints are often custom made because splinting components and materials in sheets and precut splint forms can be purchased, which makes it relatively easy for a trained and skilled clinician to fabricate a device in a clinical setting with the patient

development of contractures and deformity that result from muscle imbalances at a joint.

Dynamic splints are also used to protect repaired tendons while they are healing. After a lacerated tendon has been surgically repaired, it must be protected from tensile forces that could disrupt the repair site. The contraindicated, potentially disruptive forces are produced by joint motions that would elongate the tendon and by contraction of the tendon's muscle. For example, the flexor tendons in the hand are often lacerated and surgically repaired. Following the surgical repair, patients use a protective dynamic splint with a dorsal restriction (block) to limit MP extension and elastic bands from their fingertips to the volar aspect of the wrist. The elastic bands substitute for and protect the flexor tendons during healing (**Fig. 18.14**).

Another type of dynamic wrist hand splint does not use either elastic bands or springs to produce the dynamic force. This device (Bioness, Valencia, California) provides functional electrical stimulations (FES) to the finger flexors and extensors to assist in grasp and release. This appliance is appropriate for individuals with hand weakness due to upper motor neuron disorders, such as stroke, traumatic brain injuries, and spinal cord injuries (C5–C6 complete).[5]

present. Appliances for the elbow and shoulder are less often custom made by clinicians and may be purchased from a supplier and fit by the clinician. Custom-made and fitted hand and wrist splints are preferred for postoperative patients as well as other situations when frequent changes are expected as the patient progresses or when complicated and individualized splint designs are necessary. Custom devices are also preferable for clients with significant hand and wrist deformities, such as arthritic deformities. Other factors that influence whether an appliance is custom made or prefabricated include the type of orthotic componentry required to achieve the orthotic goal, the experience and splint-making skill of the clinician, the availability of the equipment required to construct custom-made splints, as well as the clinician's time requirement. The process of custom splint fabrication is beyond the scope of this book, but many excellent texts are available that provide this information.[1,14] Clinicians who wish to become proficient in splint fabrication should enroll in courses that provide hands-on instruction as well as gain experience working with experienced hand therapists.

SHOULDER ORTHOSES

Shoulder orthoses are most often prescribed to support or immobilize the shoulder after surgery or to provide stabilization following traumatic injuries such as joint dislocation and fracture. In these cases, the purpose of the orthoses is to protect the injured structures and facilitate healing. Devices to achieve these goals are grouped generally as sling-type immobilizers, articulated abduction stabilizers, and nonarticular splints, such as the humeral fracture brace (see Fig. 18.7).

There are many different designs or styles of *shoulder slings*. However, all of them attempt to support the shoulder in a nonstressful rest position and reduce the inferior pull that the weight of the arm places on the glenohumeral joint and capsule. The traditional orthopedic sling, which places the glenohumeral joint in a position of adduction and internal rotation, is used for general posttraumatic or postsurgical immobilization as well as to immobilize the shoulder following nondisplaced proximal humeral fracture or glenohumeral dislocation (**Fig. 18.15**). Although these devices usually provide adequate immobilization for short-term use, usage for long durations may produce glenohumeral as well as elbow flexion contractures that impair function and are difficult to

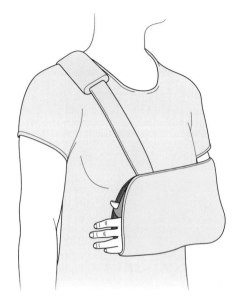

FIGURE 18.15. An orthopedic shoulder immobilization sling.

reduce. Additionally, the strap over the back and at the neck can be irritating, and the decreased hand usage imposed by the sling may cause stiffness and loss of grip strength. An alternative for those who require long-term shoulder support is the humeral cuff and shoulder saddle sling. This device has a cuff lined with a nonslip material that grips the skin as it encircles the upper arm. The humeral cuff is suspended from a shoulder saddle and chest harness that shares the support of the upper limb and reduces loading of the glenohumeral joint (**Fig. 18.16A**). Another humeral cuff-type sling is called the Wilmer carrying orthosis (**Fig. 18.16B**). Constructed of a shoulder–chest harness and a lightweight tubular metal forearm frame, this appliance uses the weight of the forearm as a counterbalance to force the humerus into the shoulder complex. Unlike other slings, it does not prevent humeral internal and external rotation but still provides some support and protection of the forearm. These appliances are used to reduce shoulder subluxation or pain in individuals with significant upper limb weakness, such as those with hemiplegia or brachial plexus injury. However, the nature of shoulder pain in these conditions is complex, and the effectiveness of the various types of slings in reducing shoulder subluxation has not been clearly determined.[15–17] Because studies that report the effects and effectiveness of these devices are sparse, clinical decision-making regarding the use of slings and supports for clients with upper limb

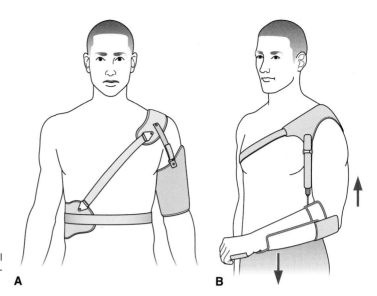

FIGURE 18.16. Humeral suspension slings: **(A)** humeral cuff and shoulder saddle sling to minimize humeral subluxation and **(B)** Wilmer carrying orthosis.

A   **B**

paralysis should be guided by the clinical responses of individual clients and current research evidence as it emerges. Please see Keywords for Literature Search at the end of this chapter.

Other soft shoulder appliances are used to restrict specific shoulder motions following surgery or trauma. The purpose of these appliances is to restrict joint motions or positions that may disrupt repaired or healing tissues. For example, an abduction sling (**Fig. 18.17A**) may be used following rotator cuff repair surgery to minimize tension on the repaired tendons and prevent shoulder movements that might disrupt the repair. Another device restricts the amount of shoulder abduction and external rotation that can occur and may be helpful during rehabilitation following a glenohumeral dislocation (Fig. 18.17B). Figure-eight clavicle straps have been used to immobilize closed clavicular fractures in the middle one-third; however, standard orthopedic slings are also used (Fig. 18.17C).

Rigid orthoses with adjustable positioning rods and articulations are also used when more precise positioning or immobilization is required. These are most often used following shoulder surgeries, but they are also used to provide low load prolonged stress for individuals with axillary contractures. Most are prefabricated and have adjustments to accommodate patients of various sizes and different joint positioning requirements. Practitioners who work with clients wearing these devices must closely monitor the three-dimensional position of the shoulder in the brace, as improper positioning can apply deleterious

forces to the joint. Using the SCS terminology, these orthoses are called rigid shoulder abduction immobilization appliances. However, older terms remain in clinical usage. For example, an orthosis that holds the shoulder in maximum abduction is called an "airplane splint," and similar devices that place the shoulder in less than full abduction are called "gunslinger" or "holster" orthoses (**Fig. 18.18**).

Orthoses to assist or substitute for lost muscle function at the shoulder are available but are not particularly practical. Clients who require this type of assistance include patients with spinal cord injuries and those with brachial plexus injuries. Some individuals with brachial plexus injuries have used an orthosis that employs the cable and harness system of an upper extremity prosthesis to produce elbow flexion and even to operate a terminal device, if the hand is paralyzed. This allows the arm to be used as an assist to the other dominant unimpaired arm. A device called a balanced forearm orthosis (BFO) or mobile arm support (MAS) has been used by some patients with spinal cord injuries (usually C5–C6 complete). This mechanical device attaches to the upright of the wheelchair and assists with simple hand-to-mouth and reaching activities that might be helpful for activities such as self-feeding (**Fig. 18.19**). It has a series of pivoting ball bearing joints and a forearm platform. The person using the device uses available muscles to position the forearm support so that gravity will produce the missing motion, usually elbow extension, which is needed for reaching. A utensil holder attached to a hand splint is also required. Although simple mechanically, precise

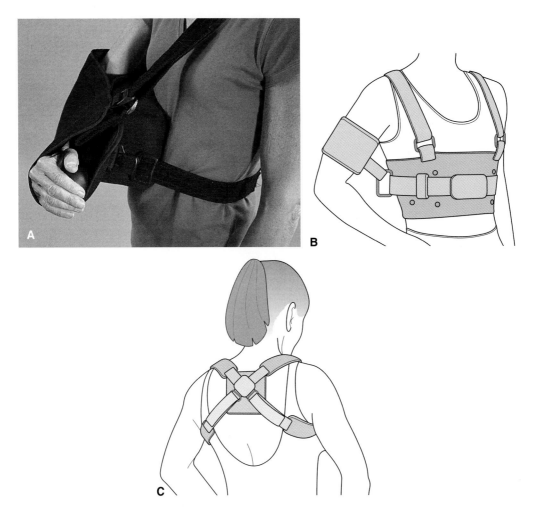

FIGURE 18.17. Soft shoulder orthoses to restrict motions or positions that are deleterious to healing following surgery or trauma: **(A)** abduction positioning sling, **(B)** abduction restriction harness, and **(C)** clavicle strap.

positioning and balancing are required for this device to function properly, which limits the practicality of using this device for daily function.

ELBOW ORTHOSES

Elbow orthoses are most commonly used to either restrict motion to protect healing of repaired structures or mobilize contractures that are limiting joint ROM. Orthoses with adjustable limited motion hinges can be used for both purposes (**Fig. 18.20**). Like the limited motion hinges used in knee orthoses, this orthotic articulation allows the clinician to set ROM stops that allow free active motion between the stops in a safe range. Because the stops are easily adjusted in the clinic, changes in the amount of allowable ROM can be made as the patient progresses.

These stops can also be used to position an elbow with joint contracture at its ROM end point to provide low load prolonged stress. Static progressive stretching to increase elbow joint passive ROM may also employ an articulated elbow orthosis with an adjustable turnbuckle device (see Fig. 18.10).

Nonarticulated elbow orthoses molded from low-temperature thermoplastics are custom made and applied to the anterior or posterior surfaces or circumferentially on the arm to immobilize the elbow (**Fig. 18.21**). These appliances extend from the shoulder to the wrist to maximize force application through long levers while minimizing contact pressure by distributing the forces over a large surface area. Like the articulated elbow orthoses, they are used to immobilize the elbow joint as part of a static progressive stretching program to increase joint ROM

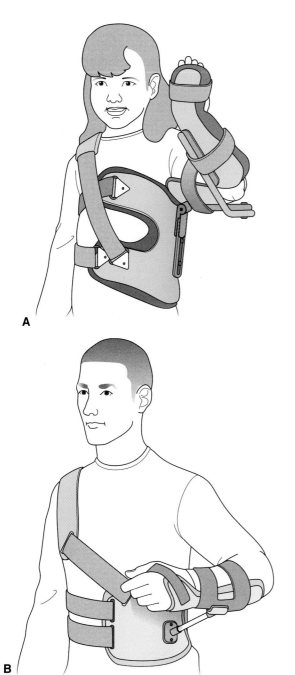

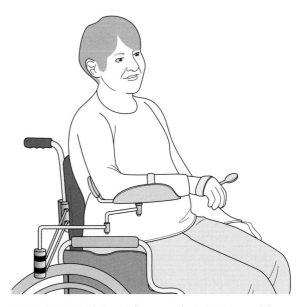

FIGURE 18.19. A balanced forearm orthosis (BFO) or mobile arm support (MAS).

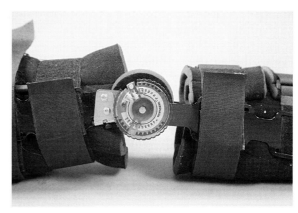

FIGURE 18.20. An articulated adjustable elbow orthosis. The range of motion stops can be set to restrict flexion, extension, or both motions.

FIGURE 18.18. Rigid shoulder abduction orthoses are used to immobilize a healing joint or mobilize contracture: (A) abduction rotation orthosis with adjustable articulations and (B) "gunslinger" abduction orthosis.

or to prevent contracture formation. For example, individuals with upper motor neuron pathologies and elbow flexor spasticity may use this simple, nonbulky device at night to maintain elbow extension ROM and prevent flexion contractures.

FOREARM ORTHOSES

ROM of the forearm joints can become restricted not only due to primary injury to the forearm, but also secondary to immobilization or treatments for injuries of the elbow or wrist. Supination is necessary to perform most daily activities performed on the body, like feeding and personal hygiene, while pronation is required for most reaching activities. As a result, restoration of supination and pronation ROM is an important upper extremity rehabilitation goal. Increasing forearm ROM with therapeutic exercises alone may not be successful. However, the addition of

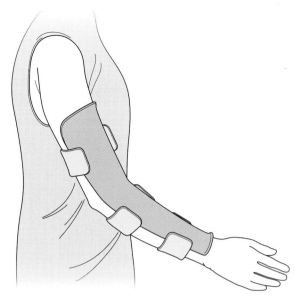

FIGURE 18.21. A nonarticulated elbow immobilization orthosis.

a low load prolonged stress technique using splinting usually adds significantly to functional success. Many custom and prefabricated devices can be used to achieve this goal; however, clinicians should choose devices that are readily available and easy for them to use safely and effectively (Fig. 18.22).

As in other regions of the body, surgeries to repair or reconstruct structures in the forearm or wrist may require restriction of forearm motion during the healing period. To effectively control forearm rotation, a splint must incorporate both the humeral epicondyles and the wrist. To achieve this goal, an orthosis is usually constructed to hold the forearm in a neutral

position (neither supinated nor pronated) that allows elbow flexion and extension between 30° and 120°. This orthosis is called a forearm neutral rotation immobilization orthosis or may be referred to as a sugartong splint (Fig. 18.23).

Tendinopathy is a common cause of pain around the elbow. It may be caused by inflammation or degeneration of the tendons of the wrist extensor muscles where they attach to the humeral lateral epicondyles. This condition is called lateral epicondylitis or epicondylosis, respectively. A similar, but less common, condition involving the common tendon attachments of the wrist flexors to the medial epicondyle produces medial elbow pain called medial epicondylitis or epicondylosis. These conditions, caused by microtrauma, are usually attributed to repetitive motion during daily activities. A variety of noninvasive interventions have been used to treat these conditions, including rest, ice, analgesics, eccentric exercise, and compression band orthoses. To treat lateral epicondylosis, compression bands are placed around the forearm with a compression pad located on the lateral side of the elbow just distal to the humeral epicondyle and radial head (Fig. 18.24). It is proposed that these appliances work by compressing the tendons and reducing some of the load on them during muscle contraction. Although research evidence for the effectiveness of these devices is weak, some studies report improvement when used in conjunction with physical therapy and when worn during functional activity.[18,19]

WRIST AND HAND ORTHOSES

A huge number of wrist and hand orthoses are available from a variety of sources, including off-the-shelf and over-the-counter prefabricated appliances as well

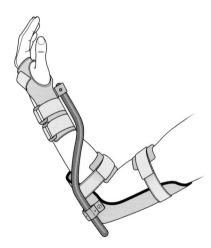

FIGURE 18.22. A dynamic forearm splint applies sustained gentle force to increase forearm motion.

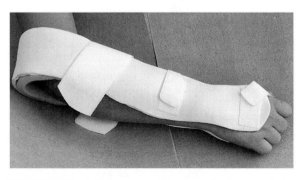

FIGURE 18.23. A forearm immobilization splint is also called a sugartong splint.

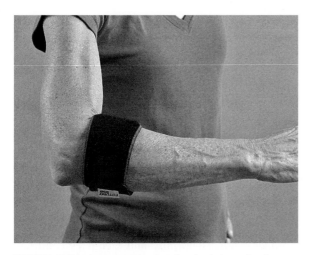

FIGURE 18.24. A compression band orthosis is used to improve symptoms of lateral epicondylitis.

as custom-made and individually designed splints. As with the other upper extremity joints, orthoses are used to immobilize joints, mobilize tissues to increase ROM, and restrict unwanted or harmful joint motions. Additionally, orthoses are used in conjunction with other interventions to reduce impairments and improve function. Thus, hand and wrist splints, like all interventions, are selected to improve or prevent impairments that detract from function. Impairments commonly encountered by therapists when treating patients with hand and wrist pathologies are presented below with examples of splints that may help to reduce the impairments and improve function. Readers are encouraged to use their knowledge of joint anatomy and biomechanics to apply the principles of splint selection presented here to develop applications at other joints.

Splints for Reduced Range of Motion

The small joints of the hand and wrist are susceptible to trauma when aggressive or excessively forceful stretching is used to increase ROM. Static progressive and dynamic splints that apply sustained low mobilizing loads are usually more effective. Examples of static progressive and dynamic splints that employ the principles of low load, prolonged stress to increase joint ROM are presented in Figures 18.1B and 18.8 to 18.12. Some of the splints shown apply mobilizing forces to a part of the hand or a digit through cuffs or slings that are attached by string (fish line) or elastic bands to the splint base (see Figs. 18.1B and 18.9). The string or elastic band represents the line of pull of the mobilizing force and must be oriented perpendicularly to the body part to which the force is applied so that the cuff provides even contact and pressure and does not migrate (**Fig. 18.25**).

Static splints are also used to prevent loss of ROM when a patient has a condition in which it is likely that contractures may develop, such as inflammation and healing. Static resting splints (see Fig. 18.6) must support the immobilized joints in positions that are compatible with proper joint biomechanics and alignment. Splints must also support and maintain the transverse and longitudinal arches of the hand (**Fig. 18.26**). These mobile arches are necessary for complete ROM during full opening and closing of the fist. Improper joint positioning and flattening of the arches of the hand within splints designed to prevent contractures can lead to improper joint function, impairment, and additional contracture.

Splints for Pain

Splints can help to reduce pain caused by acute inflammation by providing rest, protection, and immobilization of the injured or inflamed joint structures. The splint allows its wearer to rest the painful hand or wrist while maintaining movement in the other noninvolved joints of the upper extremity. When splinting is coupled with elevation and compression dressings, the edema associated with acute inflammation or injury may also be reduced. Resting splints must maintain the soft tissue structures of the immobilized joints in elongated positions to prevent development of contractures during the resolution of the inflammation (see Fig. 18.6 and related text). Clients should use resting splints only when necessary, as they limit functional use of the hand and may lead to dysfunction if used too long. Patients should

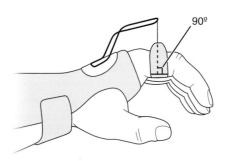

FIGURE 18.25. The line of tension of a mobilizing force must be maintained at 90° to the long axis of the bone to which the force is applied.

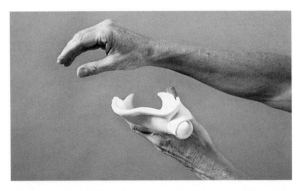

FIGURE 18.26. The longitudinal and transverse arches of the hand must be incorporated into hand splints to maintain full range of motion and function.

reduce their use of resting splints as soon as possible, although they may continue to use the splints part time to protect the injured area at night or when out or in crowds where reinjury may occur.

Immobilization splints are also used to manage pain in chronic disorders, such as osteoarthritis, carpal tunnel syndrome, and other chronic joint disorders. The goal of splinting in management of chronic symptoms is to position the involved joints to minimize the stresses that produce pain during function. For example, osteoarthritis of the basal joint of the thumb produces pain with activities that require pinch grips. A thumb neutral position immobilization splint can reduce this pain and protect the joint (see Fig. 18.6C). The symptoms of carpal tunnel syndrome increase with activities and positions that increase pressure in the carpal tunnel, such as wrist flexion. A wrist neutral position (0°) immobilization splint maintains the carpal tunnel in its position of lowest pressure, which may reduce pain and other symptoms in some individuals.

Splints for Impaired Muscle Function

Injury to the peripheral nerves that innervate the muscles of the hand can produce muscle weakness and muscle imbalance deformities. Dynamic hand splints can be used to substitute for the lost muscle function. For example, a radial nerve injury produces weakness in wrist and MP joint extensor muscles. The elastic bands from the dorsal outrigger of the dynamic splint shown in Figure 18.13 produce MP joint extension and substitute for lost muscle function caused by the nerve injury.

Peripheral nerve injuries also lead to the development of muscle imbalance deformities that interfere

with hand function. For example, an ulnar nerve injury produces paralysis of the ulnarly innervated intrinsics, which leads to muscle imbalance at the MP and interphalangeal (IP) joints. If preventative measures are not taken, the result can be a hand deformity in which the MP joints of the fourth and fifth digits are hyperextended, and the IP joints are flexed. This deformity interferes with use of the ulnar side of the hand in grasp and release. A splint to prevent the progression of the muscle imbalance to a fixed deformity can preserve function. In this case, a MP extension restriction splint that blocks MP extension facilitates IP extension by stabilizing the proximal phalanx in flexion (**Fig. 18.27**). This splint prevents the development of a fixed deformity and facilitates continued functional usage of the hand. A median nerve injury results in paralysis of the muscles of the thenar eminence. A thumb extension restriction splint that positions the thumb in abduction and maintains the web space between the thumb and index finger is required to maintain functional opposition for pinch and activities that require manipulation.

Splints for Joint Instability

Joint instability develops when the ligaments and other structures that stabilize the joint become lax and incompetent. Functional usage of unstable joints produces pain and abnormal joint movements and mechanics, which further degrades joint stability and may cause destruction of the articular surfaces. Individuals with connective tissue disorders, such as Ehlers Danlos syndrome (hypermobility type) and inflammatory arthritis, are at risk for developing joint instability and related joint deformities. Individuals with inflammatory arthritis, such

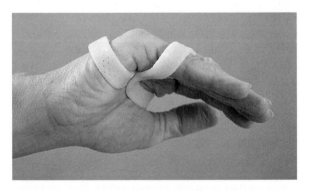

FIGURE 18.27. A metacarpophalangeal extension restriction splint prevents muscle imbalance deformity and maintains function with an ulnar nerve injury.

as rheumatoid arthritis, experience episodes of joint inflammation during periods of disease exacerbation. These episodes of joint inflammation weaken the joints' connective tissue stabilizers and produce joint instability. To prevent joint destruction, individuals with arthritis should employ joint protection techniques during their daily activities and use restrictive splints to prevent unstable joints from abnormal positions and movements. Examples of preventable hand deformities that may occur in individuals with joint instability are swan neck (hyperextension at the PIP joints) and ulnar drift (ulnar deviation at the MP joints) deformities. Both deformities are predictable and thus preventable by using restriction splints before deformity develops. **Figure 18.28** shows commonly used restriction splints that prevent the unstable joint positions. Because restriction splints for individuals with

chronic diseases and joint instability must be worn long-term to be effective, the poor cosmesis of the plastic splints that are used to manage short-term trauma is unacceptable for many patients. Therapists must consider splint appearance and include the client in decision-making concerning selection of hand splints. Attractive-looking splints may increase clients' adherence to splint wearing schedules on a long-term basis. Restrictive splints that look like jewelry are available for most of the usual hand deformities and may increase adherence for long-term splint wear (The Silver Ring Company, Charlottesville, Virginia; www.silverringsplint.com).

GUIDES FOR PRESCRIPTION AND CHECKOUT OF UPPER EXTREMITY ORTHOSES

As for all orthoses, the specific prescription is developed through the process of identifying impairments, establishing goals, and designing an orthosis to apply the forces required to achieve the goals. This process is described in Chapter 12. When developing orthotic prescriptions, practitioners must also consider reports of orthotic efficacy published in current research literature. Although research reports on the effectiveness of orthotic devices commonly used in the management of many upper extremity conditions are not plentiful, clinicians must monitor research findings as they emerge and modify their practices accordingly. Keywords and search terms to help clinicians track relevant research are listed at the end of this chapter.

When a new orthosis is received, whether prefabricated or custom made, a therapist must conduct an orthotic checkout examination of the client, the device, and the client wearing the device. The general checkout procedure is discussed in Chapter 11, and specific items relevant to the checkout of upper extremity orthoses are listed in **Box 18.2**. The purpose of the checkout examination is to ensure that the device is acceptable in terms of fit, function, comfort, and cosmesis. Clients require instruction in proper methods of donning, doffing, and caring for the orthosis. For example, an appliance made from low-temperature thermoplastics can be deformed if left in a sunny window or car on a hot day or if washed in hot water. Since most upper limb splints are constructed from plastic, some clients have difficulty with sweating under the splint that may cause skin maceration. A thin stockinette worn between the skin and splint

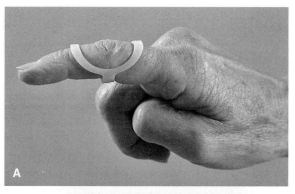

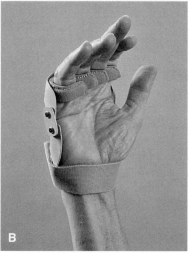

FIGURE 18.28. Restriction splints used to prevent joint instability deformities: **(A)** proximal interphalangeal hyperextension restriction splint for swan neck deformity and **(B)** metacarpophalangeal ulnar deviation restriction splint for ulnar drift deformity.

■ Orthosis is comfortable

■ Orthosis has an acceptable appearance

■ No excessive pressure on bony prominences; padding or relief areas appropriately located

■ Palmar splint base supports the arches of the hand

■ Splint base is properly contoured to provide total contact with the body

■ Splinted joints are positioned as prescribed

■ Restriction and immobilization splints adequately control movement as prescribed

■ Splint does not impede movement at joints that should be free to move normally

■ All mechanical joints are properly aligned with the anatomical joint

■ Trimlines are smooth and rounded, and there are no sharp edges

■ Orthosis does not gap away from or migrate on the limb during movement

■ Straps have appropriate adjustability and fit snugly, without pinching or "digging into" the client

■ Splint does not impede circulation

■ Straps are properly located to maintain total contact between orthosis and limb

■ Outriggers and splint components are securely and safely fastened to the splint base

■ For a functional orthosis that is worn during activity:

  ■ Distal trimline does not interfere with metacarpophalangeal flexion

  ■ Palmar splint permits thumb opposition to index and long fingers

  ■ Thumb palmar abduction is maintained

■ If a stockinette is worn under the orthosis, it fits properly

  ■ There are no wrinkles when worn under the splint

  ■ The patient has extra so that the stockinette can be laundered

may assist with managing excessive moisture and protecting the skin. New wearers must be given a "wearing schedule" that guides the user to gradually increase wearing time with his or her new appliance over several days to a week, depending on the individual needs of the client. Increasing orthotic wearing-time by an hour or two at an interval appropriate for the specific individual can avoid problems or make them easier to resolve if they do occur. Appliances that are applied for postsurgical stabilization are typically worn full time immediately; however, a gradual weaning schedule may be required when it is time to discontinue splint use. Protective splints may be used for extended periods of time at night, even after splint wear has been discontinued during the day. Although this may seem counterintuitive, sleeping individuals have no control of limb and joint positioning. Thus, newly healed structures may inadvertently be placed in sustained stressful positions.

If the device is worn during functional activities, a therapist must observe the client performing usual functional activities with the device in place to ensure that the appliance is functioning properly. Asking patients to identify functional activities that are important to or difficult for them helps clinicians individualize training and focus on relevant functional skills.

SUMMARY

This chapter presents selected orthotic devices that are commonly used in the upper extremity. Upper extremity appliances are named using the SCS terminology developed by a task force of the American Society of Hand Therapists rather than the biomechanical terminology used to name lower extremity and spinal orthoses. SCS terminology distinguishes upper extremity orthoses by their location on the limb, type of force applied, and primary function (immobilization, mobilization, or restriction). Generally, immobilization orthoses are used to rest or protect joints to reduce pain and facilitate healing; mobilization splints are used to increase ROM; and restriction splints are used to prevent deleterious or unwanted joint movements. Upper extremity appliances are either prefabricated or custom made from low-temperature materials that can be molded directly on the patient. Selected examples of shoulder, elbow, wrist, hand, and digit orthoses that are used to improve impairments are presented. Readers are encouraged to combine their knowledge of joint anatomy and biomechanics with the splinting principles presented to develop orthotic solutions for upper extremity conditions and impairments that are not discussed.

KEYWORDS FOR LITERATURE SEARCH

For the research topics listed below, choose relevant keywords, subject headings, and MeSH terms from each domain and search using the Boolean term "AND".

Search topic: What Are the Effects and Effectiveness of Slings and Supports for the Shoulder?

Conditions

Hemiplegia
Brachial plexus injury
Stroke
Shoulder subluxation
Shoulder dislocation/pc – prevention and control;
  rh – rehabilitation; th – therapy
Shoulder pain
Shoulder fracture

Intervention
Orthotic devices
Orthotic devices + shoulder

Effect
Biomechanics, kinematics
Arthropometry
Treatment outcome

Search topic: What Is the Evidence for Best Practice When Using an Orthosis in the Management of Patients with Upper Extremity Disorders?

Conditions (add terms relevant to specific clients and clinical questions)

Upper extremity: pathology, pathophysiology,
  physiology, injuries
Carpal tunnel syndrome
Tennis elbow
Tendinitis
Tenosynovitis; de Quervain's tenosynovitis
Wrist injuries
Cumulative trauma disorders

Intervention
Intervention
Orthotic device
Splints

Effects
Treatment outcome

REFERENCES

1. Fess EE, Gettle KS, Philips CA, et al: Hand and upper extremity splinting: principles and methods, 3rd ed. St. Louis, MO, Elsevier Mosby, 2005.
2. Raphael J, Skirven T (eds): Atlas of the hand clinics: contractures and splinting. Philadelphia, PA, WB Saunders, 2001 March.
3. American Society of Hand Therapists: Splint Classification System. The American Society of Hand Therapists, Garner, North Carolina, 1992.
4. Tenney CG, Lisak JM: Atlas of hand splinting. Boston, Little Brown, 1986.
5. Ring H, Rosenthal N: Controlled study of neuroprosthetic functional electrical stimulation in sub-acute post-stroke rehabilitation. J Rehabil Med 37:32–36, 2005.
6. Sarmiento A, Zagorski JB, Zjch GA, et al: Functional bracing for the treatment of fractures of the humeral diaphysis. J Bone Joint Surg 82-A:478–486, 2000.
7. Sarmiento A, Waddell JP, Latta LL: Diaphyseal humeral fractures: treatment options. Instr Course Lect 51:247–269, 2002.
8. McClure PW, Blackburn LG, Dusold C: The use of splints in the treatment of joint stiffness: biological rationale and an algorithm for making clinical decisions. Phys Ther 74:1101–1107, 1994.
9. Bonutti P, Windau J, Ables B, et al: Static progressive stretch to reestablish elbow range of motion. Clin Orthop Rel Res 303:128–134, 1994.
10. Gelinas JJ, Faber KJ, Patterson SD, et al: The effectiveness of turnbuckle splinting for elbow contractures. J Bone Joint Surg 82-B:74–78, 2000.
11. Doornberg JN, Ring D, Jupiter JB: Static progressive splinting for posttraumatic elbow stiffness. J Orthop Trauma 20:400–404, 2006.
12. Schultz-Johnson K: Splinting the wrist: mobilization and protection. J Hand Therapy 9:165–176, 1996.
13. Flowers K, LaStayo P: Effect of total end range time on improving passive range of motion. J Hand Therapy 7:150–157, 1994.
14. Coppard BM, Lohman H: Introduction to splinting, 2nd ed. St. Louis, MO, Mosby, 2001.
15. Spaulding SJ: Biomechanical analysis of four supports for the subluxed hemiparetic shoulder. Can J Occup Ther 66:169–175, 1999.
16. Lo SF, Chen SY, Lin HC, et al: Arthrographic and clinical findings in patients with hemiplegic shoulder pain. Arch Phys Med Rehabil 84:1786–1791, 2003.
17. Paci M, Nannetti L, Taiti P, et al: Shoulder subluxation after stroke: relationships with pain and motor recovery. Physiother Res Int 12:95–104, 2007.
18. Callaghan M, Holloway J: Tennis elbow and the epicondyle clasp. Emerg Med J 24:296–297, 2007.
19. Wilson JJ, Best TM: Common overuse tendon problems: a review and recommendations for treatment. Am Fam Physician 72:811–818, 2005.

Living with a Prosthesis/Orthosis

Training for Sports and Leisure

By Robert S. Gailey, PT, PhD

19

OBJECTIVES

At the end of this chapter, all students are expected to:

1. Describe appropriate prosthetic components for sports and leisure activities for any patient with an amputation.
2. Refer patients to appropriate sports organizations and websites for the disabled.

Physical Therapy students are expected to:

1. Outline a training program to improve strength, balance, and endurance without increasing the risk of injury for any amputee interested in returning to sports activities.
2. Identify accessory equipment that might assist in sports participation.

CASE STUDIES

Richard Canto, the 20-year-old soldier who lost his left leg as a result of a roadside bomb in Iraq, is now 8 months postamputation. He is doing well with his prosthesis and is currently going through reclassification as he wants to stay in the Army. He has learned from his fellow service members that many of them participate in the Challenged Athletes Foundation San Diego Triathlon Challenge, where for more than 20 years, over 100 other amputee athletes have swum, cycled, and run with hundreds of able-bodied athletes. They compete in teams of three athletes, each athlete competing in one event. In high school, Richard played football and baseball, and now he wants to train for all three events so he can compete with some fellow service members. He has 9 months to train for the triathlon event. The spirit of the event is not to win but to participate with people who share similar life experiences.

Angie Thompson is a 56-year-old, right-handed female with a left transfemoral amputation performed 14 months ago secondary to peripheral vascular disease without diabetes. She has a history of hypertension; however, she has lost weight through diet and exercise over the past year and is ready to return to sports. She has lived in New Hampshire all her life; she was an avid golfer and alpine skier prior to limb loss and would like to return to both sports. Her doctor has cleared her to participate but suggests that she progress slowly.

Case Study Activities

All Students:

1. Describe why training for an event like the Challenged Athletes Foundation San Diego Triathlon Challenge is more appropriate for Richard than the Paralympics.
2. Describe the special prosthetic components each person would need for the selected activities.
3. Describe skiing techniques that would best be used by Angie.

Physical Therapy Students:

1. Develop a training program for each patient.

Innovation in surgical techniques, assistive technology, and physical rehabilitation has afforded people with disabilities great opportunities to participate in leisure activities and sports than any prior generation. Unfortunately, in the United States, the gap between people with disabilities who participate in regular exercise and those who do not appears to continue to widen. Obesity is ranked among the top ten leading health indicators by Healthy People 2010.[1] Obesity increases the risk for type 2 diabetes, hypertension, **dyslipidemia**, cardiovascular disease, respiratory problems, osteoarthritis, and lowers life expectancy.[2,3] The obesity rates for people with and without disabilities have increased over the past two decades; however, the prevalence in people with disabilities is significantly higher, ranging between 8% and 14% depending on gender, race, and state.[4] To improve overall health, the President's Council on Physical Fitness and Sports recommends a healthier diet and 2 hours and 30 minutes of moderate-intensity exercise per week.[5] Evidence suggests that regular participation in exercise can lead to better functional health, reduce obesity, and reduce symptoms of anxiety and depression.[6]

The goal of the rehabilitative team should be to assist the person with a disability in the transition to a comfortable regimented exercise program to maintain the physical conditioning achieved during rehabilitation and then introduce the concept of leisure exercise or, in some cases, to competitive sports. This does not mean that the rehabilitation team is involved every step of the way. The team's responsibility is to educate and motivate the person. Education includes prescribing a personalized regimented exercise program including precautions to prevent further injury as well as providing contacts for outside support groups and suitable special interest organizations. Equally important is providing the motivation to start the person on the road to meet his or her long-term goals by impressing upon the person the benefits that come with a lifelong commitment to sports or recreational activities.

SPORTS ORGANIZATIONS FOR THE DISABLED AND PARALYMPICS

After World War II, in the United States and Europe, returning soldiers with disabilities such as spinal cord injuries and amputations were eager to return to sports and competition. Sports such as skiing, basketball, swimming, and athletics were very popular forms of motivation for rehabilitation. The military hospitals, Veterans Administration (VA) (currently Veterans Affairs), and veteran service organizations (VSO) such as the Paralyzed Veterans of America (PVA) and the Disabled American Veterans (DAV) strongly supported adaptive sports as a means to keep veterans physically fit and involved in organized activities. After the Viet Nam war, veterans became even more proactive in sports and recreational therapy as a means to provide peer support and maintain physical fitness. Programs such as National Handicapped Sports (currently Disabled Sports USA) provided venues for training, competition, and peer socialization for veterans after discharge from the military. These programs today are very popular for both veterans and civilians with disabilities.

At present, wounded soldiers in military hospitals and veterans within the VA are exposed to a variety of sports programs for the disabled, often while still in rehabilitation. Likewise, many civilian rehabilitation centers offer the same experience. The philosophy is simple—introduce the person to a recreational environment that may lead to a lifetime of physical fitness, healthy activities, and friendships. Throughout the United States, there are now local and regional chapters of disability and sport-specific organizations eager to recruit new members who share the same interest in sport and recreation. The Resources section at the end of this chapter provides a partial list of sports organizations for people with disabilities in the United States.

In the United States, there are disabled sports organizations (DSOs) sanctioned as governing bodies to the International Paralympic Committee (IPC) (**Table 19.1**). They are disability specific or organizations that are founded on the athlete's disability rather than sport. The DSOs sponsor national competitions,

TABLE 19.1 Disability-Specific International Sports Federations		
Name	**Abbreviation**	**Website**
Cerebral Palsy International Sports and Recreation Association	CPISRA	www.cpisra.org
International Blind Sports Federation	IBSA	www.ibsa.es
International Sports Federation for Persons with Intellectual Disability	INAS-FID	www.inas-fid.org
International Wheelchair and Amputee Sports Federation	IWAS	www.iwasf.com

assist athletes who qualify for the Paralympics with travel and outfitting, and maintain the integrity of the sports for their disability groups. Although the Paralympics often receives the attention of the media and aspiring athletes, the DSOs are involved in developmental programs for athletes of all ages and abilities. The Paralympics, like the Olympics, is the pinnacle of competition within many sports for athletes, requiring that an athlete qualify within specific "standards" of performance. The standards are usually set within 5% or 10% of the world record performance regardless of how an athlete may have placed in a national Paralympic trials competition. In short, the Paralympics are reserved for the most elite of athletes, regardless of the sport or disability.

The majority of people, with or without disability, enjoy participating in sports on a recreational level for the pure pleasure of the sport, without aspirations of participating at the elite level. All too often a young person who was an amateur athlete prior to acquiring a disability is told by well-meaning supporters that they can "go to Paralympics," which is rarely the case. As clinicians, it is important to realize that returning an individual to recreational sports is first and foremost. The truly gifted athlete will aspire to the Paralympics.

Providing the contact information of local or national DSOs is one way to begin the process of returning someone to recreational sport. There is a variety of information on each organization's website to provide an adequate introduction to the athlete. Attending a competition or training workshop is a wonderful way to meet other athletes and become comfortable with the difference that may be encountered in a sport by the athlete with disability.

The International Paralympic Committee (IPC) is the international organizer for the Summer and Winter Paralympic games. The IPC is a nonprofit organization run by 162 National Paralympic Committees (NPCs) that supervise and coordinate the World Championships and other competitions worldwide. The most notable event is the Paralympic games that occur every 4 years, at the same site, shortly after the Summer or Winter Olympic games.

The IPC serves as the International Federation for the nine multidisability sports, and the four disability-specific international sports federations (IOSDs) govern the sports specific to their respective disability groups. There are 27 sports (20 Paralympic Summer sports, 5 Paralympic Winter Sports, 2 Non-Paralympic sports) that fall under the responsibility of different governing bodies, as outlined in **Box 19.1.**

To create an equal playing field between athletes with similar or different disabilities, a functional classification system was implemented. The broad disability groups are amputee, cerebral palsy, visual impairment, spinal cord injury, intellectual disability, and *les autres,* which is a French term, literally translated as "the others," or athletes with a disability that is not appropriately represented by the aforementioned disability groups. The classification process is conducted by trained professionals, known as classifiers, who perform physical and technical assessments and observe the athletes in and out of competition. Classifiers are composed of physicians, physical therapists, and sports specialists who are certified within a particular disability group or sport. The specific classification groups for each sport are beyond the scope of this chapter but can be found on the IPC website.

In addition to organizing the competitions, the IPC services the disabled athletes in many other capacities. Currently, the IPC coordinates with the World-Anti-Doping Agency (WADA) to ensure that drug-free participation occurs at every sanctioned event. The Sports Science Committee is committed to the advancement of knowledge of Paralympic sports. The Development and Education program creates programs and initiatives aimed at supporting member countries in the promotion and education of sport for people with disabilities and the Paralympic movement throughout the world. To learn more about all the programs and functions of the IPC, their website is the best resource for up-to-date information.[7]

ROLE OF PHYSICAL THERAPY IN PREPARING PEOPLE WITH DISABILITY FOR A LIFETIME OF SPORT AND RECREATIONAL ACTIVITIES

Preparing the Amputee for Recreation Sports

Clinicians such as physical therapists and prosthetists are often placed in the role of coaching early in the rehabilitation process as the amputee or any athlete with a disability is preparing to return to athletics. One of the most common obstacles for the athletes, coaches, therapists, prosthetists, and parents is how to encourage a disabled potential athlete to improve his or her performance, or to initiate participation in a particular event. Often the easiest and most

---

BOX 19.1 | International Paralympic Committee Sports and the Governing Bodies[7]

International Paralympic Committee Sports

- Alpine skiing
- Athletics
- Biathlon
- Cross-country skiing
- Ice sledge hockey
- Power lifting
- Shooting
- Swimming
- Wheelchair dance sport (currently a non-Paralympic sport)

Governed by the Cerebral Palsy International Sports and Recreation Association (CPISRA)

- Boccia
- Football seven-a-side

Governed by the International Blind Sports Federation (IBSA)

- Football five-a-side
- Goalball
- Judo

Governed by the International Wheelchair and Amputee Sports Federation (IWAS)

- Wheelchair fencing
- Wheelchair rugby

International Federation Sports

- Governed by international federations (IFs)
- Archery (International Archery Federation)
- Cycling (International Cycling Federation)
- Equestrian (International Equestrian Federation)
- Rowing (International Rowing Federation)
- Sailing (International Foundation for Disabled Sailing)
- Table tennis (International Table Tennis Federation)
- Volleyball (sitting) (World Organization for Volleyball for Disabled)
- Wheelchair basketball (International Wheelchair Basketball Federation)
- Wheelchair curling (World Curling Federation)
- Wheelchair tennis (International Tennis Federation)

---

frequently used approach is "just get out there and try it!" However, under ideal situations, a qualified coach would instruct the athlete in the proper skills necessary for a given event, and with time and training, the athlete would comfortably return to his or her sport. Unfortunately, rarely is this the case in disabled athletics. Because of the scarce number of amputee athletes in any one region and even fewer coaches, the opportunity to work with enough athletes to develop any real expertise is difficult. Although there are several excellent coaches around the country, many current and former athletes themselves, only a small number of developing athletes are afforded the opportunity to work with them, usually because of geographic location. As a result, most amputee athletes must rely on themselves, other athletes, parents, interested able-bodied coaches, and clinicians.

Most coaches of athletes with disabilities have learned to become resourceful when working toward enhancing the performance of their athlete. Because there are few formal resources pertaining specifically to disabled sports performance, therapists and coaches must seek out several sources of knowledge, synthesizing the information to determine what is applicable

to their athlete's specific training program. A problem-solving approach to training can be a challenging and rewarding aspect of coaching with disabled athletics. Box 19.2 outlines some guidelines.

SPORT PROSTHETIC COMPONENTS

Sports and Prosthetic Ankle/Foot Options

The choice of prosthetic feet for sports is limited because there are very few sport-specific prosthetic feet. The most popular sports feet are primarily designed for running. Fortunately, most sports do not require extensive running, so an everyday prosthesis with the appropriate components and suspension may allow recreational athletes to participate. Some people who are comfortable with their socket will elect to change just their prosthetic foot. A small adapter called a Ferrier Coupler (Ferrier Coupler Inc., North Branch, Michigan) provides athletes with a quick-changing self-aligning device to quickly swap over prosthetic feet or knee–shin systems. Those athletes who have the resources may choose to have a

BOX 19.2 | Training and Coaching Tips for the Athlete With a Disability

Listen to the athlete. Training with disabled athletes must be a cooperative effort. No absolute system of training has been developed, so novice coaches should listen to the athlete and discuss technique variances together.

Seek other disabled athletes competing in the same sport. Most of the developments in equipment and performance techniques have been achieved through the experiential knowledge and efforts of the athletes. Many of the top coaches are disabled athletes, either retired or still competing. In addition, a training partner can help to make the practices easier.

Recruit able-bodied coaches. Disabled coaches are often difficult to find. Many elite disabled athletes train with able-bodied sport teams and athletes, under the direction of able-bodied coaches. Often the coordinated efforts of a coach and a therapist who is aware of the abilities and constraints of the athlete's physical capabilities work well when the athlete is working on improving technique or performance.

Read texts and publications pertaining to both able-bodied and disabled athletics. In recent years, there have been a number of significant contributions to the body of literature concerning disabled sport. Unfortunately, there is still a tremendous void in many particular sports and for many specific disability groups. However, reading and learning about able-bodied training methods and techniques is still an excellent way to gain insight into a particular sport.

Contact the appropriate disabled sports organizations for information and names of people to assist with training. Disabled sports organizations try to maintain information on a variety of topics, including athletes and coaches. Disabled sports organizations are generally underutilized as resources and should be contacted to assist with providing direction in the training process.

Video record practices and competitions. Video recording practice sessions and competitions for immediate visual feedback or for more detailed critique later is an excellent method of instruction. Moreover, prior recordings of elite competitors with similar disabilities can be reviewed for a comparative analysis and to allow the athlete to visualize the technique. Caution must be taken not to imitate another athlete, as each athlete should experiment to learn what works best for him or her.

Consult with technical experts about adaptive equipment. Many disabled athletes utilize adaptive equipment such as wheelchairs, prostheses, orthotics, and other assistive devices. Prosthetists, orthotists, biomedical engineers, and other adaptive technology specialists can assist in providing specially designed equipment that will meet the individual needs of the athlete and enhance performance. Only a few clinical professionals specialize in adaptive technology for sports because of the infrequent demand. Because poorly fitting equipment can be more harmful than helpful and in some cases even dangerous, the coach and athlete should seek out and collaborate with these clinical professionals.

Investigate motivational methods that will assist in maintaining the athlete's interest in training and the sport. Maintaining an athlete's level of intensity when training for a sport can sometimes be a real challenge. A wide variety of literature, motivational recordings, and other resources are available to coaches interested in the inspirational aspects of coaching. As with any athlete, maintaining a balance between level of difficulty and level of frustration is important. Continuing to experience success with training and competition is positive reinforcement that will ensure that the athlete continues in the sport.

Become familiar with the rules or rule changes that may influence the performance techniques. As disabled sports evolve, classifications, rules, and competition formats will continue to change. Athletes and coaches alike must keep abreast of these changes to prevent any last-minute confusion and alterations in competition strategies.

Attend coach's conferences for both the able-bodied and disabled athlete. Conferences and seminars are excellent forums in which to exchange ideas and learn innovative approaches to sport techniques.

Experiment with new techniques. Experimenting with new and unique techniques may help overcome a particular obstacle or enhance performance. Be careful of new styles that emerge from a single athlete, as they may lack mechanical advantages and provide only a psychological edge. Keep an open mind.

Maintain written records. Keeping journals of training sessions and competitions provides a log that may be reviewed by the coach and athlete to determine trends that may enhance or hinder performance. There is also a tremendous need for the publication of positive and negative outcomes with regard to athletic performance to assist other athletes who are in similar situations.

*With permission from Advanced Rehabilitation Therapy, Inc., Miami, Florida.

sport leg because the cover does get damaged and will lose the cosmetic appeal with wear.

When selecting a prosthetic ankle–foot system, it is important to discuss recreational and sports interest thoroughly, because the amputee will likely try to participate in his or her favorite sport within the first year after amputation. If the prosthetic components do not respond to the demands of the sport, the probability of success will diminish, resulting in frustration and embarrassment that may keep the person from ever participating in that sport again. Many prosthetic feet are suitable for walking but are not dynamic enough for sport. Without sufficient energy release, the athletic performance becomes unacceptable to the amputee. Therefore, it is important to prescribe the correct prosthetic foot that not only permits a natural gait but also allows the amputee to participate in recreational sports.

During the initial evaluation, the clinician should explore the recreation interests of the amputee. Not all sports require ultradynamic prosthetic feet. In fact, many amputees participate in sports such as golf, bowling, shuffleboard, and boating which require more mobility than dynamics.

Multiaxial foot systems with dynamic keels provide the advantages of a movable ankle, and the carbon footplate offers the benefits of a dynamic response foot (see Chapter 6). Because of the mobility present at the ankle, it is believed that some of the "energy release" generated in dynamic response feet with movable ankles is not as great. But, a multiaxial foot system should be considered for people who walk on hills or uneven terrain, such as golfers, hikers, or those who need a certain degree of movement in all planes of motion, such as bowlers, shuffleboarders, or those who require ankle motion for standing balance, such as boaters.

The source and degree of mobility available in prosthetic feet have changed tremendously through the years. No longer does the motion come from only the ankle, the "split toe"—a divide running the length of the footplate—permitting motions that replicate inversion and eversion without absorbing as much elastic energy as rubber bumpers in ankle joints. The advantage is motion with limited loss of the dynamic properties. Another design that has become very popular is **elastomer** or another type of hard rubber sandwiched between a primary and a secondary footplate. Once again, the frontal and some transverse plane ankle motion can be mimicked while maintaining foot dynamics. Another foot design incorporates shock absorbers and rotators into the shin rising above the traditional ankle location, providing long axis rotation (see Chapter 6). These shock absorbers and rotators can be coupled with any number of foot designs. Many of these types of dynamic feet with secondary motion components use the "J"-shape footplate and pylon to create dorsiflexion and have a dynamic heel for plantarflexion.

The degree of motion required should be determined by the everyday environment that an amputee must negotiate and the recreational activities in which the amputee chooses to participate. A golfer who lives in a hilly part of the country will need a fairly large degree of motion in all planes to negotiate hills when walking, adopting a stance on uneven terrain, or permitting some rotation during the swing. In contrast, a bowler may require a significant degree of sagittal plane movement, with dorsiflexion and plantarflexion, but may not want as much frontal or transverse plane motion. Boaters, however, want to keep their prosthetic feet flat on the deck of the boat and would therefore prefer some motion at the ankle to absorb the rocking motion of the boat.

There are far too many variables to try and match a sport with a particular prosthetic foot. Suffice it to say that there are a wide variety of dynamic feet available today to meet everyone's activity level. What is important is that the amputee's recreational interests be explored at the time of prosthetic prescription and that an appropriate choice be made.

Prosthetic Running Foot Options

Össur Cheetah®

Designed primarily for unilateral and bilateral transtibial amputees, the Össur Cheetah® foot component has become the prosthetic foot of choice for transfemoral amputees as well. The Cheetah foot is plantarflexed to keep sprinters on their toes. The distal posterior pylon is bowed, lengthening the footplate to increase the moment arm for maximal deflection so that, as the material energy is returned, it will propel the athlete's limb into the acceleration phase of swing (**Fig. 19.1A,B**). Because of the forces applied to the foot during sprinting, the height of the prosthetic limb is typically 1 to 2 inches taller than the sound limb, allowing a decrease in body height when the foot is compressed. The goal is to have the pelvis level during stance and to eliminate any unnecessary trunk or head movement.

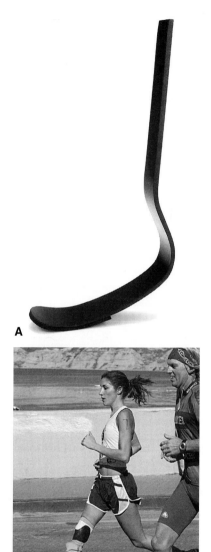

FIGURE 19.1. **(A)** An Össur Cheetah® carbon fiber running foot. **(B)** A transtibial distance runner with a Cheetah Flex-Foot competing in the Challenged Athletes Foundation Annual San Diego Triathlon Challenge. *(Courtesy of Össur America.)*

Össur Flex-Sprint™

The Össur Flex-Sprint™ is the sprinting foot popular with some transfemoral sprinters. There is no posterior bow which makes alignment with the knee a little more stable. Transfemoral sprinters tend to bounce off the prosthetics foot and have a marked reduction in hip flexion with both the prosthetic and sound limb (**Fig. 19.2A,B**).

Both the Cheetah and the Flex-Sprint are designed for running. Sprinting feet typically provide no medial–lateral mobility, so all motion occurs in the sagittal plane. Although novice runners will not need these specialized feet to start training, no elite track athletes have competed over the past decade without using these specialized feet.

Össur Flex-Run™

The Össur Flex-Run™ is designed for long-distance running or jogging. Because of the exaggerated posterior bow shape, the vertical compliance is much greater than any other running foot design (**Fig. 19.3A,B**). The Flex-Run can be fabricated for unilateral transtibial amputees, transfemoral amputees, and bilateral amputees who want to run longer distances. To take full advantage of this foot, the athlete lands on the prosthetic toe, extending the hip throughout the support phase, achieving maximal deflection of the foot. As the prosthetic limb is about to enter the acceleration or swing phase, the effort for jogging is minimized by allowing the foot to initiate the upward motion. Then, as the spring effect reaches a peak, upward acceleration is continued by flexing the hip as the limb moves into the float phase. Runners perceive less muscular effort after they gain a sense of the foot's compression and release, allowing the foot to initiate upward momentum while they use the hip flexors to continue the forward progression of the limb. There is no evidence to support reduced work of running with the Flex-Run. Nevertheless, the "bouncy" sensation that amputee runners experience with a little training results in a more rhythmic running pattern. This may increase the chance that they can reach a physiological steady state during training runs. The benefit of being able to establish a comfortable pace is that amputee runners can develop muscular and cardiopulmonary endurance with their prostheses while allowing the residual limb to gradually develop a tolerance to the high forces being applied within the socket. Although few amputees choose to run for long distances as a method for endurance training, this option is possible for many athletes with limb loss.

Prosthetic Running Knees

Transfemoral amputees have additional considerations when learning to run with a passive prosthetic knee. The basics for running can be learned on almost any

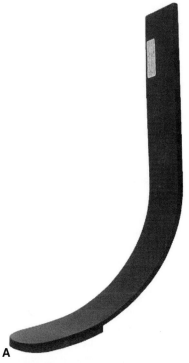

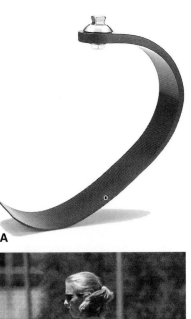

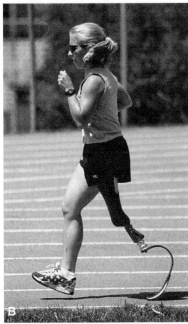

FIGURE 19.3. (A) Össur Flex-Run™ carbon graphite running foot. *(Courtesy of Össur America.)* (B) Transfemoral amputee trains for distance-running events with Flex-Run. *(Courtesy of Advanced Rehabilitation Therapy Inc.)*

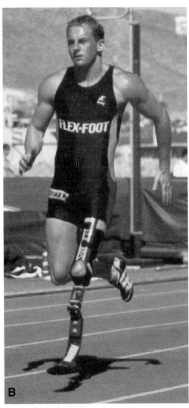

FIGURE 19.2. (A) An Össur Flex-Sprint™ carbon fiber running foot, (B) Transfemoral sprinter with Flex-Sprint foot and Otto Bock 3R55 polycentric hydraulic knee. *(Courtesy of Össur America.)*

knee system. However, friction-control knees are too slow to respond to any speed greater than a fast walk, and prosthetic knees without some type of stance control are not recommended to teach running as they are not designed for running and are not safe. Pneumatic systems are also not sufficiently cadence-responsive for the demands of running or agility sports. The two preferred knee systems for athletics are the Mauch Swing'n'Stance (SNS) (Össur) Type Hydraulic or S-Type Swing Only Hydraulic knee (Fig. 19.4A,B) or the Otto Bock Modular Polycentric

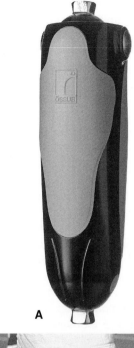

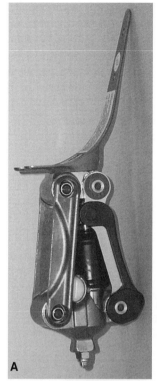

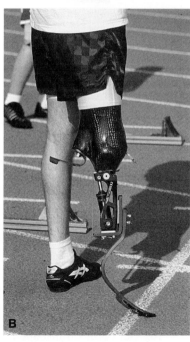

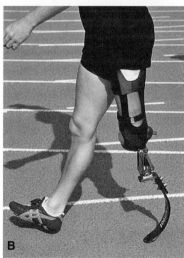

FIGURE 19.4. (A) Össur Mauch SNS hydraulic knee. **(B)** Mauch Hydraulic Knee and Cheetah Foot on a transfemoral amputee. *(Courtesy of Advanced Rehabilitation Therapy Inc.)*

FIGURE 19.5. (A) Otto Bock 3R55 polycentric hydraulic knee, **(B)** 3R55 hydraulic knee, and Össur Sprint-Flex on runner with knee disarticulation amputation. *(Courtesy of Otto Bock USA.)*

Axis Joint (3R55) with Hydraulic Swing Phase Control **(Fig. 19.5A,B)**. The Mauch hydraulic cylinder uses a single-axis frame, and the SNS type offers athletes a wide range of resistance adjustment and stance control. Most competitive athletes, however, use the S-Type Swing Only hydraulic unit, because stance control is no longer necessary with athletes who are successful runners. The Otto Bock 3R55 Polycentric Axis Joint is a favorite for athletes with knee disarticulation because of the instantaneous center of rotation capabilities of a four-bar design, providing increased toe clearance and greater stride symmetry.

Learning how to maximize knee performance during running requires transverse rotation of the pelvis to generate a full stride length and striking the ground with a backward force during the support phase as described in **Box 19.3**. For lateral movements, keeping the prosthetic limb slightly posterior to the sound limb will keep the weight line anterior to the knee joint, ensuring a knee extension moment to decrease the risk of the knee buckling.

ANCILLARY COMPONENTS

Shock absorbers are thought to reduce ground reaction forces during high-impact activities (Chapter 6). This can be a tremendous benefit for athletes who run long distances or participate in high-impact sports. Because shock absorbers also absorb an undetermined amount of energy, they do not return much stored energy, which reduces acceleration as the athlete moves into swing phase. As a result, many athletes who participate in high-speed sport do not incorporate a shock absorber into their sport prosthesis.

Torsion adapters are often chosen by athletes who participate in multidirection sports such as tennis or generate rotation about the long axis as with a golfer swinging a club (Chapter 6). Theoretically, torsion adapters reduce the shear forces within the socket and permit greater rotation for improved performance. Not all athletes who participate in tennis or golf find the added motion beneficial. Some find the additional motion difficult to control or conclude that the benefits are not worth the additional weight and maintenance.

Knee rotation adaptors allow the amputee to move the foot and shin components into a variety of positions that would otherwise be impossible. For example, to facilitate recreational activities that involve sitting, such as gardening, just being able to move the foot out of the way is very convenient. Knee rotators also facilitate greater ease with dressing, changing shoes, and similar routine tasks.

SPORTS AND LEISURE ACTIVITIES

The recreational activities most enjoyed by amputees are swimming, fishing, walking, dancing, boating, golf, bowling, and cycling.[8] These activities are very similar to the top ten activities in the general population ranked by participation: walking, camping, swimming, fishing, bowling, bicycling, billiards, hiking, and aerobic exercise. Not surprisingly, amputees and nonamputees enjoy exactly the same recreation sport activities, regardless of level of amputation. Running is not within the top ten activities with either group, yet it is the one skill most amputees want to have.

Across all age groups, the reasons for limiting participation in recreational activities were similar. Amputees have identified the inability to run and to jump as the two most common limitations to returning to sport.[8] Decreased endurance, increased fatigue, decreased balance, and reduced speed of mobility are also problems that impede participation in sports, or that allow the amputee to maintain the level of physical skill achieved prior to the loss of limb. Many amputees find learning the skills necessary to participate in recreational activities intimidating. Providing a comfortable environment is initially required. The environment can be as simple as the tone of instruction or creating a support group situation with other amputees. Support and motivation are key ingredients for getting people involved in leisure activities.

Running

Although running does not rank very high as a preferred sport or leisure activity, it is one of the most common reasons for lack of participation in recreational activities, primarily because of the misconception that it is a prerequisite skill for sports. Many amputees who do not have a strong desire to run for sport or leisure may have an interest in learning to run simply for the peace of mind that comes with the knowledge that they could move quickly to avoid a threatening situation. Running, as with all advanced skills, requires time and practice to become proficient. Amputees should be exposed to basic running skills during rehabilitation so that they can pursue sports if they wish. The basics of running can be performed by most amputees in the Five Basic Steps of Amputee Running[9] (**Box 19.3**).

Learning to run can occur on just about any type of prosthesis. Initially, the prosthetic foot or knee is not critical. However, if the amputee decides that running is going to be part of his or her active lifestyle, the amputee should discuss with his or her prosthetist the various available prosthetic options. The same principles of running apply regardless of the prosthetic foot and knee systems; however, prosthetic feet and knees designed for running can reduce the effort and improve performance.

BOX 19.3 | Five Basic Steps to Amputee Running

Step 1: Prosthetic Trust
The runner must first gain trust in the prosthesis and develop the confidence that the prosthetic limb is going to be there and will not collapse when striking the ground. This is accomplished by reaching out with the prosthetic limb and landing squarely on the foot. The runner should ignore everything else, knowing that the prosthetic limb will be reliable and comfortable.

Step 2: Backward Extension
The runner reaches out with the prosthetic foot during swing. Just as the prosthetic limb strikes the ground, the runner pulls the prosthetic leg back forcefully, creating a backward force, to accelerate the forward. This movement has two effects: First, it will accelerate the body forward causing increased speed. Second, this movement produces the power to shift the body's weight over the prosthesis and fully load the prosthetic foot, resulting in maximum prosthetic foot performance as the forefoot is loaded.

Step 3: Sound Limb Stride
The focus now shifts to the sound limb. The runner concentrates on taking a longer stride with the sound limb, which is accomplished by continuing to pull down and back through the prosthetic limb. Pulling back during the prosthetic foot's initial contact with the ground initiates the movement pattern. The runner should continue to extend the hip by pulling down and back into the socket. This generates more power and a stronger push-off with the prosthetic limb, which enable the sound limb to reach out to complete a full stride.

Step 4: Stride Symmetry
This phase is designed to decrease the enormous effort being exerted, and to simply relax and jog a little. The runner should choose a comfortable jogging pace that produces an equal stride length for both limbs. There is no concern for the arms. Attention is focused on maintaining stability over the prosthetic limb using the muscles of the hips to create equal and relaxed strides.

Step 5: Arm Carriage
The runner is focused on arm swing. The arms and legs move in opposition to each other during running, so as the right leg moves forward, so will the left arm. The elbows should flex to about 90°, and the hands should be loosely closed and rise to just below chin level when brought forward.

Putting It All Together
The runner should be ready to combine all the elements of running together. The runner should relax and think about only a couple of elements of running with each pass. Many long-distance runners augment their endurance training program by utilizing low-impact activities such as swimming or stationary biking or stair-climbing machines. In time, the runner will develop his or her own comfortable running style, depending on the sports or recreational activities chosen for participation.

*With permission from Advanced Rehabilitation Therapy, Inc., Miami, Florida.

Sport Wheelchairs

Since the 1980s, sport-specific wheelchair designs have grown into a highly scientific field of assistive technology sports performance, generating research and development in centers and universities throughout the United States. Manufacturers today offer a line of sports wheelchairs that are suitable for introduction to a sport for the novice and intermediate athlete. Once an athlete reaches the elite level of competition, custom-fitted and custom-designed equipment is mandatory to reach the athlete's full athletic potential. Within each sport, the seating, posture, propulsion techniques, and, in team sports, player position must be considered for the individual athlete. Rarely at a competition today could one athlete use another athlete's wheelchair because of fit and performance—each wheelchair is as individual as the athlete (Fig. 19.6).

The science of fitting a sports wheelchair is a specialty area that requires the expertise of the athlete, coach, assistive technologist, manufacturer, and engineer.[10] Clinicians should be aware of the components of a sports wheelchair and the performance characteristics. Because the materials and designs change so frequently, each component will be presented in general terms (Box 19.4).

Road Racing Wheelchairs, Hand Cycles, and Recumbent Bikes

For many people with mobility limitations, a traditional bicycle is not a viable option because of the balance requirements. As the popularity in road racing and aerobic training continues to attract new participants, special wheelchairs for road racing, hand

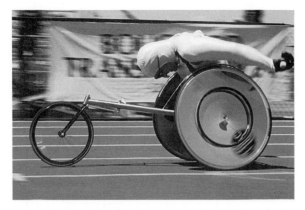

FIGURE 19.6. Aerodynamically designed track wheelchair. *(Courtesy of Advanced Rehabilitation Therapy Inc.)*

cycles, and recumbent bikes have emerged. Many athletes who compete consider the use of these three assistive devices for separate and unique sports, with a different skill set required to train for competition. As a result, road racing and track events will identify three separate categories for the competition.

For the individual athlete, these three assistive devices have offered multiple options for participation in sport that were not always available. Historically, wheelchair racing dates back to post–World War II when Sir Ludwig Guttman introduced the use of wheelchair sports as a means of rehabilitation. The evolution of wheelchair designs and technology has permitted numerous athletes with mobility limitations such as spinal cord injury, cerebral palsy, amputation, and other neuromuscular impairments to participate in sport (**Fig. 19.7**). Today, the excitement of wheelchair sports has developed a tremendous

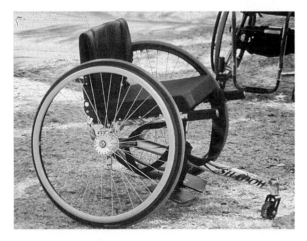

FIGURE 19.7. Tennis wheelchair with a single caster and handbars and a wide camber for stability. *(Courtesy of Advanced Rehabilitation Therapy Inc.)*

following of sports enthusiasts as participants and spectators.

Wheelchair competition is fast and exhilarating, requiring a high level of fitness. Wheelchair athletes who maintain rigorous training programs for extended durations or distance are more prone to a variety of overuse and acute injuries.[12] The most common injuries reported in athletes competing in wheelchairs are soft tissue injuries of the shoulder, elbow, and wrist; abrasions and contusions of the arms and hands; and blisters of the hands.[10,11] The loss of the ability to propel the wheelchair because of injury not only limits training time and the ability to compete, but in most cases reduces mobility with everyday life, in the home, at work, and in the community. Because of the associated injuries and the need to reduce the incidence of injuries associated with pushing, hand cycles were developed as a means of maintaining training time with a reduction in overuse injuries. Because of the reduction of injuries, increased speed, and greater ease of learning to maneuver hand cycles, participation rapidly grew.

Hand cycles and recumbent bikes offer people with mobility issues numerous options. Both are available premanufactured and are adequate for the majority of novice riders. However, most companies also have the ability to fabricate custom cycles and bikes designed to fit the individual athlete. A custom-fit cycle or bike helps create a comfortable riding posture, reduce strain to soft issues, improve performance, and can aid in the ease of mounting and dismounting. For these reasons, most competitive cyclists will take the time to obtain a custom-fit cycle or bike.

Cycling

Cycling for the amputee affords a chance to enjoy speed and cover great distance at both competitive and recreational levels. Many amputees choose cycling as a form of exercise that offers excellent aerobic conditioning without the high impact on the residual limb that occurs during running. Another advantage is that little is required in the way of adaptive equipment for any level of lower limb amputation.

Amputee cyclists of all levels may have difficulty in achieving maximum power when they push downward on the pedal. Biomechanically, the best way to achieve optimum power is to place the prosthetic shank directly over the pedal, unlike the intact side, where the metatarsal heads are centered over the

BOX 19-4 | Sports Wheelchair Components

- *Frame:* Sports wheelchairs typically have a rigid frame design to reduce unwanted motion that would reduce performance. The need to collapse the wheelchair for ease of transportation as in everyday wheelchairs is not a concern. Elite athletes will have a custom-made frame constructed to their height, weight, sports, and disability. For example, an athlete with SCI may not find it uncomfortable to tuck his or her legs under the bucket, whereas an athlete with full sensation might find the position very awkward and would prefer to extend his or her legs. A road racer will want to have minimal weight and maximum aerodynamics, whereas a wheelchair rugby player will fortify his or her chair frame with extra tubing and protective aluminum panels to decrease damage during competition.

- *Length*: Sports such as road racing use the longer three-wheel design, whereas sports such as tennis, basketball, and wheelchair rugby use short, more compact styles for great maneuverability.

- *Wheels*: Lightweight wheels are preferred in most sports. The wheel can have traditional spokes, carbon spokes, or the carbon discs that can improve aerodynamics and tire rotation. In team sports, where collisions are common, wheels will have spoke protectors to reduce damage to the spoke protectors.

- *Tires*: The technology of tires has evolved tremendously. Issues such as tire diameter, width, inflation pressure, and tread need to be considered. Road racers prefer high-pressure tubeless tires with a tread that varies depending on the weather and road conditions. Off-road wheelchairs, similar to mountain bikers, prefer low-pressure, wider tires with a heavy tread for more traction.

- *Camber*: To increase maneuverability and lateral stability, the wheels may be set in a negative camber where the bottom of the wheel is wider than the top. The wider bottom permits faster turns and allows the athlete to lean further over the chair laterally during competition, such as in tennis or basketball. The narrow top brings the hand rim closer to the athlete's arms for greater power generation and ease of hand contact.

- *Casters*: Track and road racers use three wheels, with a single smaller wheel for efficiency with moving in a straight line. Tennis, basketball, and rugby players use one or two small casters in the front of the chair depending on player position and preference. The caster is often placed under the feet for quicker turning and greater responsiveness (see **Fig. 19.7**).

- *Push-rim*: The diameter, shape, and surface of the push-rim vary between sports. Road racers prefer a smaller, sometimes slightly wider, and stickier push-rim because of the turning ratio and contact area. Tennis and basketball players prefer a push-rim close to the diameter of the tire so that hand contact will be immediate as their hand maneuvers their chair and they focus on the ball.

- *Seat*: A steep seat angle is referred to as bucketing, where the athlete with reduced sitting stability would prefer to have a greater backward angle or to sit down and back in the bucket with trunk flexing forward creating more trunk stability. Conversely, a basketball player with better trunk control looking for greater mobility and height would want a taller seat with fewer restrictions.

- *Steering*: Steering compensators are often incorporated into track and road racing wheelchairs to reduce the effort of steering with the hand rims and can make large turns more precise, especially when coasting downhill. For subtle steering adjustments, racers in tightly fitted buckets will swing the upper body or hips to turn or maintain direction; this action is known as "hipping" the chair.

- *Gloves*: Most wheelchair athletes use gloves to protect the skin, reduce repetitive stress injuries to the joints of the hand and wrist, and improve performance. The design of gloves has changed over time. For example, road racers once used a glove with a taped thumb so that the thumb and wrist action would contact the push-rim resulting in overuse injuries to the thumb and wrist. Today, gloves are designed so the back of the hand contacts the push-rim with a more fist-like position, reducing finger and wrist injuries.

With permission from Advanced Rehabilitation Therapy, Inc., Miami, Florida.

pedal. Recreational riders should simply place the midfoot directly over the pedal. Competitive cyclists may wish to use a toe-clip to hold the prosthetic foot in place. To fit the forefoot into the toe-clip and still position the shank over the pedal, amputee cyclists may cut the prosthetic forefoot off or use an adapted toe-clip or stirrup that provides extra depth (**Fig. 19.8**).

Transtibial amputees generally experience minimum difficulty in riding with prosthesis, but additional suspension may be needed for which there are many alternatives. For transfemoral amputees who ride with their prosthesis, seating and hip range of motion (ROM) present the greatest problems. The transfemoral amputee cyclist requires a saddle that is wide enough to balance upon, yet narrow enough so that the upper thigh is not pinched between the socket and the saddle. A racing saddle is generally used for this reason because of its narrow design. Some riders initially choose a wider saddle for the added balance obtained by a wider posterior portion. Soft-tissue pinching may be greatly reduced with the addition of a padded seat cover and a well-padded pair of cycling shorts. The thinner, more flexible polyethylene plastic sockets also aid in maintaining balance and reducing pinching.

Although most competitive cyclists prefer to ride with their prostheses for the added power from using both legs, many transfemoral amputees find it more

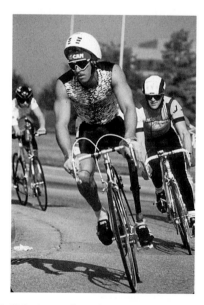

FIGURE 19.8. A transfemoral amputee cyclist competing in a road race. Most transfemoral amputees choose to compete without a prosthesis. *(Courtesy of Advanced Rehabilitation Therapy Inc.)*

comfortable to ride without it. They simply remove the pedal on the prosthetic side and use a toe-clip on the sound side to apply power.

Swimming

Swimming is both a competitive and a recreational sport enjoyed by amputees of all ages. The freedom of the water, cardiovascular benefit, and muscular endurance gained from swimming make it an ideal activity. Competitive swimmers are not permitted to wear prostheses while competing, and as a result, these athletes learn to swim extremely well unaided. When first learning to swim, lower limb amputees experience some difficulties such as drifting toward the amputated side when kicking with the sound limb. Others describe difficulty in maintaining their trunk and shoulder parallel to the water surface, thus reducing their speed, resulting in additional exertion to propel through the water. On the whole, most amputees, young and old, learn to swim easily.

Advantages to wearing a prosthesis during swimming include having two limbs to enter and exit the water and shower facilities and to facilitate poolside activities. In addition, the prosthesis can add propulsion during swimming and wading. Amputees who have problems with limb volume fluctuations may also have difficulty donning their prostheses after swimming and may therefore benefit from wearing one while in the water.

Wheelchair-mobile people may require assistance in and out of the pool if they are unable to perform floor-to-chair transfers independently. Many public and private pools are equipped with Hoyer lifts as a result of public awareness and public policy such as the Americans with Disabilities Act. Once in the pool, the water provides accommodating resistance to movement, which is an excellent method of strengthening.

Golf

Good balance and the ability to weight shift are probably the two key skills necessary to play golf well. Training for both of these skills can begin early during rehabilitation and continue at home until the amputee is ready to return to the driving range. Consistent practicing of trunk rotation and weight shifting will help develop balance and ambulation skills to prepare the amputee to return to the golf course.

The mechanics of the golf stroke are relatively individual to each golfer. The amputee will invariably lose distance on his or her swing; however, if the swing keeps the ball in play or on line, then the golfer's objective has been met. The key to teaching amputees to golf is that they play within their own individual limitations; this means that they need to learn to maintain balance and weight shift whether they are standing or swinging from a wheelchair.

Assistive devices in golf and the manner in which golfers choose to play are almost as varied as their golf strokes. Many amputees prefer not to wear a prosthesis; others use a wheelchair, tripods, or other devices to lean on as they swing. Some amputees who do wear their prostheses and stand independently prefer some type of rotator or swivel device, but others find the additional weight or additional rotational movement to be a disadvantage. Typically, the back limb (right-handed golfer's right leg) is stationary during the backswing, and very little motion should be permitted at the knee or ankle. As a result, no torsion or rotation device is used (**Figs. 19.9** and **19.10**). Conversely, the forward limb (right-handed golfer's left leg) requires rotation during the forward swing; therefore, a torsion or rotator device would be appropriate. A number of golfers will take the spikes out of their golf shoes so that the shoe will be able to rotate directly on the ground.

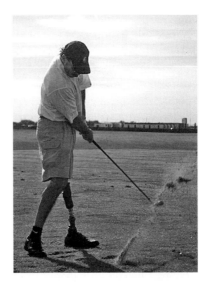

FIGURE 19.10. Prosthetic foot with torsion control on golfer with transfemoral amputation. *(Courtesy of Advanced Rehabilitation Therapy Inc.)*

Golfers who have limited standing ability, such as SCI individuals with spinal cord injuries, or bilateral lower limb amputees can play with adaptive golf carts that enable play from a variety of postures. Adaptive golf carts are lightweight, enabling the golfer to ride anywhere on the golf course, including the greens. The seat positions swivel so that the golfer can address the ball from a seated or leaning posture with both feet on the ground. Access to the golf bag is easy so that the golfer with a disability can play a round independently (**Fig. 19.11**).

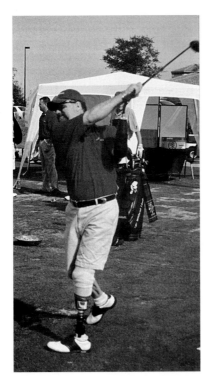

FIGURE 19.9. Golfer with transtibial and transradial amputation uses torsion control on prosthetic foot. *(Courtesy of Advanced Rehabilitation Therapy Inc.)*

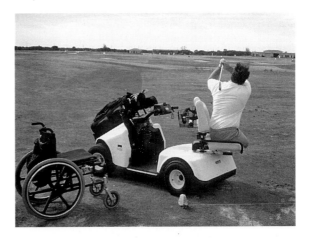

FIGURE 19.11. A bilateral transfemoral amputee golfer using the SoloRider golf cart as he begins a round of golf. Note the golf bag secured to the front of the cart for easy access. *(Courtesy of Advanced Rehabilitation Therapy Inc.)*

Golf is one of the most popular sports enjoyed by amputees and people with disabilities of all ages and functional abilities. Very few recreational activities encourage people to get outside, compete within their comfort level, and enjoy social exchange with friends the way golf does. Interestingly, golf is also one of the most beneficial activities that anyone can use as a means to improve balance, coordination, strength, ROM, and endurance. In many ways, golf is the perfect rehabilitation therapy.

Adaptive Winter Sports

Adaptive Snow Sports

Alpine skiing has become a disability-friendly environment over the past two decades thanks to many adaptive technology innovations. The majority of mountain resorts now offer some form of adaptive-ski program with instruction and equipment. Finding a certified Professional Ski Instructors of America (PSIA) instructor is recommended to ensure that the instructor has received formal training and has demonstrated the minimal level of competency. Certification programs are available for Alpine skiing (PSIA) and snowboarding (American Association of Snowboard Instructors [AASI]). Because there are a variety of disabilities and needs for adaptive equipment, there are numerous prefabricated and custom equipment designs available to skiers and snowboarders. Learning terminology related to adaptive equipment can assist the clinician in becoming familiar with the sport. Volunteering at winter adaptive sports events to spend time with athletes and professional instructors will assist in learning the sport and all the variations (**Box 19.5** and **Fig. 19.12**).

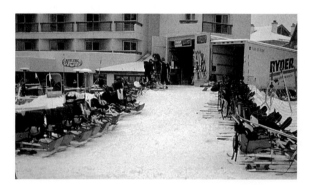

FIGURE 19.12. Adaptive ski equipment ready for use at the Disabled American Veterans Winter Ski Clinic. *(Courtesy of Advanced Rehabilitation Therapy Inc.)*

BOX 19.5 | Alpine Skiing Adaptive Equipment

■ *Snow Sliders*: Snow sliders are skies with a walker mounted to offer maximum stability with the ability to steer. They are usually introduced to novice skiers who prefer slower speeds but may progress to four-tracking in the future. Visually impaired skiers or those skiers requiring both upper and lower body stability use snow sliders.

■ *Outriggers*: Outriggers are typically adapted forearm crutches mounted on ski tips. They are used to provide balance when skiing with the ability to "flip" the ski tips up; the metal serrated brake on the tail prevents slipping and permits ease of crutch walking before and after skiing, sometimes referred to as "flip skis" (**Fig. 19.13**).

■ *Three-Tracking*: Three-tracking refers to a skier using two outriggers and a single full-length alpine ski. This is the most common method for unilateral amputees who cannot ski with a prosthesis; people with developmental or neuromuscular disease that affects a single limb may adopt the three-tracking method as well.

■ *Four-Tracking*: Four-tracking skiers use two skies and two outriggers. This population has either partial or complete use of their lower limbs but prefers to have the additional stability provided by the outriggers. People with cerebral palsy, spina bifida, incomplete spinal cord injuries, multiple sclerosis, muscular dystrophy, or lower limb amputations use this method of skiing.

■ *Ski-Bras*: Ski-bras are small adaptive accessories that attach to the tips of a four-tracker's ski, preventing separation of the skies because of muscular weakness or poor technique. There are numerous ski-bra designs available to skiers depending on their individual needs (**Fig. 19.14**).

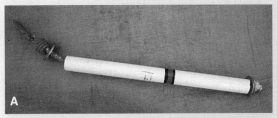

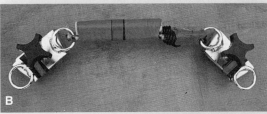

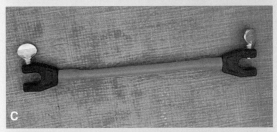

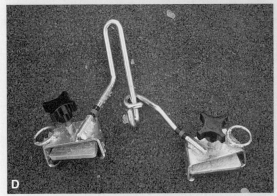

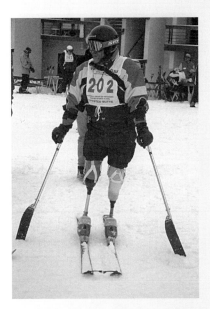

FIGURE 19.13. A bilateral transtibial amputee four-track skier, using an outrigger to transverse the level area at the base of the mountain. Note the ski-bra attached to the tips of the skis. *(Courtesy of Advanced Rehabilitation Therapy Inc.)*

FIGURE 19.14. (A) A semirigid ski-bra, **(B)** Ski-bra made with ski tip clamps and bungee cord. **(C)** A flexible rubber ski-bra. **(D)** A sliding rigid ski bra. *(Courtesy of Advanced Rehabilitation Therapy Inc.)*

Continued

BOX 19.5 | Alpine Skiing Adaptive Equipment—cont'd

■ *Mono-Ski*: A mono-ski has a molded seat or "cab" that is mounted over a suspension mechanism and a single ski. A shorter pair of outriggers is used for balance, turning, and mobility on flat snow. The cab can be either premanufactured or custom fabricated for the skier. Mono-skiers have the greatest skill level with regard to trunk control, balance, and upper limb strength; however, the mono-ski also offers the greatest mobility and speed on the mountain (**Fig. 19.15**).

■ *Bi-ski*: Bi-skis have a seat mounted on two shorter and often wider skis, used with a pair of outriggers. For those skiers who require greater balance, the design of the skis permits greater stability. Additionally, a fixed outrigger can be attached to the bi-ski for even greater stability, especially with turns, reducing the risk of rolling (**Fig. 19.16**). The bi-ski is frequently used as an introductory ski for people who will progress to a mono-ski (**Fig. 19.17**).

Both the mono-ski and bi-ski have a lever mechanism for the chair lift that raises the cab for great ease of boarding the bench when getting on the ski lift (**Fig. 19.18**). Dismounting from the chair lift requires a forward lean to initiate the momentum to drop off the bench and ski down the slope. People whose primary mode of mobility is a wheelchair, such as people with spinal cord injury, cerebral palsy, spina bifida, brain injury, multiple sclerosis, muscular dystrophy, and

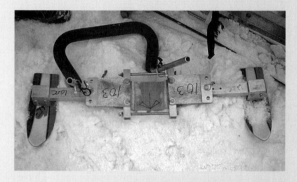

FIGURE 19.17. Bi-ski fixed outrigger or stabilizer used to prevent falls and rolling with a bi-ski. *(Courtesy of Advanced Rehabilitation Therapy Inc.)*

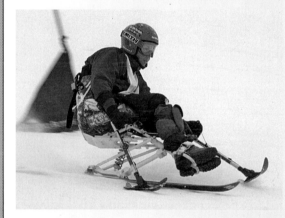

FIGURE 19.15. Mono-skier with outriggers. *(Courtesy of Advanced Rehabilitation Therapy Inc.)*

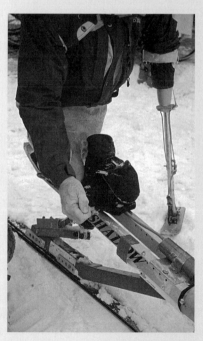

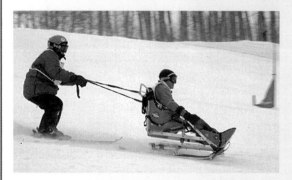

FIGURE 19.16. A student learning to ski on a bi-ski tethered to the instructor. *(Courtesy of Advanced Rehabilitation Therapy Inc.)*

FIGURE 19.18. Mono-ski lift mechanism for mounting chair lifts. *(Courtesy of Advanced Rehabilitation Therapy Inc.)*

BOX 19.5 | Alpine Skiing Adaptive Equipment—cont'd

bilateral lower limb amputations, are typically most comfortable with mono-skiing or bi-skiing.

■ *Ski Bikes*: A ski-based platform with two half skis and seat is ridden traditionally with ski boots that act as outriggers to provide better balance. Ski bikes are often used to introduce snow sports to skiers with weak or poor standing balance.

■ *Sighted Guides*: Visually impaired skiers can often ski well but because of sight limitations need assistance. Sighted guides ski in front of the visually impaired skier shouting directions with regard to turns or obstacles. Skiers may be completely blind or may have visual difficulties contrasting the snow terrain. Competitive visually impaired skiers and guides develop a tremendous amount of trust and teamwork to maneuver the course at high speeds (Fig. 19.19).

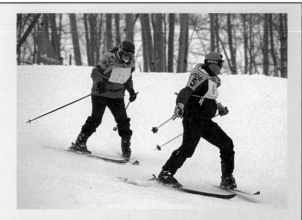

FIGURE 19.19. Sighted guide leads a visually impaired skier down the mountain. *(Courtesy of Advanced Rehabilitation Therapy Inc.)*

SUMMARY

Participation in sport and recreational activities is important for achieving life satisfaction and successful community integration. People with disabilities share the same interests and aspirations as people without disabilities. Clinicians should appreciate that the path to independence in sports and recreational activities has not been paved for athletes with disabilities, but rather by them. The demand for specialized programs, venues for competition, and the development of assistive technology has been created primarily by the athletes and people with disabilities, as a result of encountering obstacles and exploring ways to overcome the obstacles. Clinicians who recognize this truth learn to listen to those they serve. Consequently, they value the need to seek council from others, including successful disabled athletes and appropriate disabled organizations.

Understanding the biomechanics of a sport, the rules, and the assistive technology is a complex task. There are often too few athletes with similar disabilities within a given geographic region to develop expertise. As a result, athletes, coaches, and clinicians are all learning together, forming teams to exchange information with each other. This chapter summarized the current information regarding the disabled organizations, sports, and assistive technology available today. This will change. The level of competition will improve. The need to work together toward a common goal will always remain.

KEYWORDS FOR LITERATURE SEARCH

Handicapped sports

Paralympics

Sport orthoses

Sport prostheses

REFERENCES

1. Healthy People 2010. Services USDoHaH, 2nd ed. U.S. Department of Health and Human Services, 2000.
2. Rippe JM, Crossley S, Ringer R: Obesity as a chronic disease; modern medical and lifestyle management. J Am Diet Assoc 98:9–15, 1998.
3. Solomon C, Manson J: Obesity and mortality: a review of the epidemiologic data. Am J Clin Nutr 66:1044–1050, 1997.
4. Centers for Disease Control and Prevention (CDC): State-specific prevalence of disability among adults—11 States and the District of Columbia, 1998. MMWR 49:711–714, 2000.
5. The President's Council on Physical Fitness and Sports, Department of Health and Human Services, 2008.
6. 2008 Physical Activity Guidelines for Americans. Department of Health and Human Services. www.health.gov/paguidelines; http://www.health.gov/paguidelines/pdf/paguide.pdf
7. International Paralympic Committee website www.paralympics.org
8. Gailey R: Recreational pursuits of elderly amputees. Top Geriatr 8(1):39–58, 1992.
9. Gailey R: The essentials of lower limb amputee running and sports training. Miami, FL, Advanced Rehabilitation Therapy, 2004.
10. Copper RA, Ohnabe H, Hobson DA: An introduction to rehabilitation engineering. New York, Taylor & Francis, 2007.
11. Curtis KA, Dillon DA: Survey of wheelchair athletic injuries: common patterns and prevention. Paraplegia 23:170–175, 1985.
12. Ferrara MS, Davis RW: Injuries to elite wheelchair athletes. Paraplegia 28:335–341, 1990.

RESOURCES

Company List

Ferrier, Inc.
3461 Burnside Road
N. Branch, MI 48461
800.437.8597

Otto Bock Industries
3000 Xenium Lane N.
Minneapolis, MN 55441
800.328.4058

Össur
27412 Laguna Hills Drive
Alsio Viejo, CA 92656
800.233.6263

SoloRider
7315 South Revere Parkway
Suite 604
Centennial, CO 80112
800.898.3353

United States Disabled Sports Organizations

BlazeSports America/National Disability Sports Alliance
25 West Independence Way
Kingston, RI 02881
401.792.7130
www.blazesports.org

Disabled Sports Organizations
Disabled Sports, USA (DSUSA)
451 Hungerford Drive #100
Rockville, MD 20850
301.217.0960
www.dsusa.org

United States Association of Blind Athletes (USABA)
33 North Institute Street
Brown Hall, Suite #015
Colorado Springs, CO 80903
719.630.0422
www.usaba.org

Wheelchair Sports, USA (WSUSA)
1236 Jungermann Road, Suite A
St. Peters, MO 63376
636.614.6784
www.wsusa.org

Additional Resources

Amputee Coalition of America (ACA)
900 E. Hill Ave., Ste. 205
Knoxville, TN 37915-2566
888.267.5669
www.amputee-coalition.org

Challenged Athletes Foundation
PO Box 910769
San Diego, CA 92191
858.866.0959
www.challengedathletes.org

Disabled American Veterans (DAV)
National Headquarters
P.O. Box 14301
Cincinnati, OH 45250-0301
877.426.2838
www.dav.org

Eastern Amputee Golf Association
2015 Amherst Drive
Bethlehem, PA 18015
888.868.0992
www.eaga.org

National Amputee Golf Association (NAGA)
11 Walnut Hill Road
Amherst, NH 03031
800.633.6242
www.nagagolf.org

National Center on Physical Activity and Disability
University of Illinois at Chicago
1640 West Roosevelt Road
Chicago, IL 60608-6904
312.355.4058
www.ncpad.org

Paralyzed Veterans of America
National Headquarters
801 18th Street, NW
Washington, DC 20006-3517
800.424.8200
www.pva.org

Professional Ski Instructors of America
133 S. Van Gordon Street
Ste. 200
Lakewood, CO 80228
303.987.9390
www.thesnowpros.org

Shake-A-Leg Miami
2620 South Bayshore Drive
Miami, FL 33133
305.858.5550
www.shakealegmiami.org

The President's Council on Physical Fitness and Sports Department of Health and Human Services
www.fitness.gov

Physical Activity Guidelines for Americans Department of Health and Human Services
www.health.gov/paguidelines

20

Clinical Decision-Making for Prosthetics and Orthotics

OBJECTIVES

At the end of this chapter, Physical Therapy students are expected to:

1. Diagnose problems that may lead to patient complaints of pain or dysfunction when using a prosthetic or orthotic device.
2. Analyze the gait of individuals using a prosthesis or orthosis to determine possible biomechanical or neuromuscular abnormalities.
3. Differentiate between problems caused by
   a. The appliance
   b. Patient impairment
   c. Use of the appliance
4. Select appropriate interventions to reduce pain and improve function.
   a. Appropriately refer patients to the prosthetist or orthotist.
5. Implement a plan of care as needed for remediation.
   a. Determine the effect of wearing a prosthesis or orthosis on other parts of the body.

Physical Therapist Assistant students are expected to:

1. Evaluate patient responses or statements regarding prosthetic or orthotic wear to
   a. Appropriately inform the physical therapist regarding the patient's status and needs.
   b. Differentiate between critical and noncritical problems and respond appropriately.
   c. Implement a remediation program as developed by the physical therapist.

CASE STUDIES

Betty Lukas, a 50-year-old teacher for the deaf, has *Charcot-Marie-Tooth* disease. She developed equinovarus deformities at both ankles that caused pressure ulcers on the plantar surfaces of both fifth metatarsal heads. The ulcers were treated and are healed. To prevent reulceration, she underwent bilateral Achilles tendon lengthening and was fit with bilateral ankle–foot orthoses (AFO) to stabilize her ankles during gait and prevent the development of fixed equinovarus deformities. She has been wearing the orthoses for 3 months. She returns stating that she is having difficulty going up and down steps and getting up from a low chair. She also states that she has pain in her knees when she walks longer distances which she did not have before she received the orthoses. She states that her gait is stiff and awkward. She is basically unhappy with the appliances.

Harry Green, a 67-year-old man, suffered a cerebral vascular accident causing a right hemiplegia (see Chapter 2 for details). He was discharged from rehabilitation one year ago using a floor reaction AFO to facilitate knee extension and a single-point cane. He has been living independently in his home with support from members of his extended family, church, and community agencies. He is happy with his functional abilities and uses his orthosis to walk around his home, the local senior center, as well as for short distances within his community. He has not experienced any falls and is confident in his walking. However, over the last month he has developed right posterior knee pain that gets worse when he walks longer distances or is on his feet for longer periods of time and is relieved with rest. Harry is afraid this knee pain will cause him to fall or restrict his ability to maintain his independence. His doctor diagnosed mild tibiofemoral osteoarthritis and suggested that he take acetaminophen to relieve pain and that he work with his orthotist and therapist to determine if his orthosis or his gait pattern can be modified to improve his knee pain.

Janice Simmons (see Chapters 4 through 7 for previous case study information) was discharged from physical therapy 6 months ago wearing her patellar tendon–bearing (PTB) prosthesis. At the time of discharge, she was independent in all mobility and self-care activities with her PTB shuttlelock suspension prosthesis with gel liner and moderate response foot. At the time of discharge, she was wearing one ply of sock between the liner and the socket and everything checked out well. She does not use any ancillary devices inside the house but likes to use a cane outside. She has not returned to work as a waitress but has found a part-time job at the local senior center as a receptionist. She can sit most of the time in that job. She wears her prosthesis from 12 to 14 hours a day and has not been back to the prosthetist for any reason. She returns to the follow-up clinic today complaining of some discomfort in her back and in her left knee after walking a while. When she walks, her left hip seems to drops on prosthetic stance.

Jacob Kearn, a 32-year-old Air Force captain, lost his right leg above the knee and part of his left foot at the metatarsal level in a helicopter crash. He also sustained a simple fracture of the right radius. He was treated and rehabilitated at Brooks Army Medical Center in San Antonio, Texas. He has been fitted with a right ischial containment suction prosthesis with "C" leg and high return foot and a modified shoe for the left foot with a carbon fiber footplate and foam filler within the shoe. He completed all rehabilitation approximately 3 months ago and is independent in all mobility and self-care activities without any ancillary devices. As part of his rehabilitation program, he spent a month at the Center for the Intrepid learning advanced activities such as running, rock climbing, and working out with weights. He is currently assigned to a desk job with a helicopter squadron but is spending considerable time at the gym and on the track to try and regain flight status. He reports to the orthopedic screening clinic today complaining of pain in his right hip, the right groin area, and his left knee. He describes the right hip and groin pain as aching and sharp when he puts weight on the leg. The left knee feels stiff and generally sore after he works out.

Case Study Activities

Physical Therapy Students:

1. From the information given, hypothesize possible diagnoses or causes for each patient's complaint.

2. Select appropriate examination methods to gather the data needed to establish appropriate diagnoses for each patient's problem.
   a. Hypothesize potential results of your examination for each patient.
3. Differentiate between biomechanical, neuromuscular, or improper use issues that may contribute to the stated problems.
4. Develop a plan for intervention or referral for each patient.

Physical Therapist Assistant Students:

1. What data would you need to gather from each patient to help the physical therapist make a diagnosis?
2. Differentiate between problems with the appliance, problems with the patient's activities, and biomechanical problems.

THE CLINICAL DECISION-MAKING PROCESS: IMPLICATIONS FOR RESOLVING PROSTHETIC AND ORTHOTIC PROBLEMS

As indicated in Chapter 1, diagnosing is a process. It requires, among other things, finding relationships between elements of the problems and developing an algorithm that will lead to potential courses of action. Although many clinical decisions are routine and repetitive, others are complex and unique. Thus, therapists must diagnose individual problems and adapt treatment options to the unique characteristics presented by each patient. Each therapist brings an individual knowledge base, set of values, decision rules, and past experiences to the situation.[1] Research indicates that experienced clinicians use a **hypothetico-deductive system** of decision-making. Using this method, experts develop pictures of similar problems, if–then relationships, hypothesize one or more probable diagnosis, and then gather data to verify or eliminate the hypotheses. The novice, on the other hand, reasons forward, gathers relevant and irrelevant data, and then analyzes the data to form differential diagnoses.[2–4] Much of the research in this area has shown that expert decision-making is more effective and efficient, and educational programs teach students these models of clinical reasoning and diagnosing.[1,5]

This, however, is a simplified explanation of a complex process. Generally, problems that fall into familiar patterns are resolved quickly, based on past experiences and pattern recognition. Although making diagnoses by pattern recognition is quick and efficient, clinicians are at risk for cognitive dispositions to respond (biases) that may lead to diagnostic error.[6] A common cognitive error with this type of decision-making is **anchoring**, the tendency to lock onto salient features in the patient's initial presentation too early in the diagnostic process and failure to consider other alternatives properly.[6,7] Diagnostic errors due to anchoring are compounded by **confirmation bias**, the tendency to look for confirming evidence to support a diagnosis while minimizing disconfirming evidence.[6,7] Complex problems or those that do not fit familiar patterns require a more systematic process of analytical thinking and decision-making.

The diagnostic or clinical reasoning process is used to respond to many stimuli, including new patient referral, patient responses to interventions, as well as finding resolution to patient complaints. Although the general diagnostic process is similar for most situations, the necessary knowledge base varies. The specific process must be tailored to particular applications. In this chapter, the clinical decision-making process is presented as a systematic method that clinicians can use to diagnose the causes of complaints in clients who are using prosthetic or orthotic devices. Accurate diagnosis of the source(s) of patient complaints is required to effectively and efficiently find appropriate solutions to the problems and restore satisfaction with the appliance and optimal function.

PROSTHETIC OR ORTHOTIC PROBLEMS

Physical therapists who work with clients using prosthetic and orthotic devices must analyze patient complaints and make appropriate decisions regarding a plan of action to resolve the problem. Common complaints of clients who wear appliances include the following:

- Pain in the part of the body encased by the appliance
- Pain or weakness in other body areas
- Poor appliance fit
- Inefficient appliance functioning
- Damage to the appliance or broken components
- Dissatisfaction with their level of function with the appliance (unmet expectations)

Not all problems have simple solutions; not all problems have acceptable solutions. However, when multiple poorly thought-out attempts to improve a situation fail, patients often become frustrated, abandon the device, and may settle for functioning at a lower level than is necessary.

Types of Prosthetic or Orthotic Problems

An appliance problem may be identified by the patient as a complaint or concern or by a therapist as an observation of less than optimal functional performance. For example, a patient may complain: "My left knee hurts when I walk." Alternatively, a therapist may observe a gait deviation or an abnormal movement pattern during a functional activity, which may or may not be painful for the client. Regardless of the nature of the specific problem, an effective decision-making process must provide clinicians with a method to identify the source or sources of the problem so that an appropriate plan to resolve the problem can be developed. **Figure 20.1** depicts an algorithm that clinicians may use to approach the problem in a systematic way.

The cases presented at the beginning of this chapter provide examples of common patient complaints concerning prosthetic or orthotic devices. Mr. Green has pain in the back of his knee when he walks: Is he hyperextending the knee on stance? Ms. Simmons' hip drops when she walks, and she occasionally has back pain: Is she dropping down too far into the socket? These patients present familiar or typical complaints, which therapists who are experienced in working with prosthetic and orthotic problems will have seen many times before. The experienced therapist will quickly form several hypotheses about each problem and gather relevant data quickly and efficiently. Making probable hypotheses for the cause of the problem focuses the data-gathering process on the most relevant examination procedures. Effective data gathering includes some or all of the following:

- Careful and specific questioning to describe the symptom and the symptom behavior
- Observation of patient movements during functional activities
- Examining the appliance both on and off the patient
- Reexamination of the patient to identify any physical changes since appliance fitting

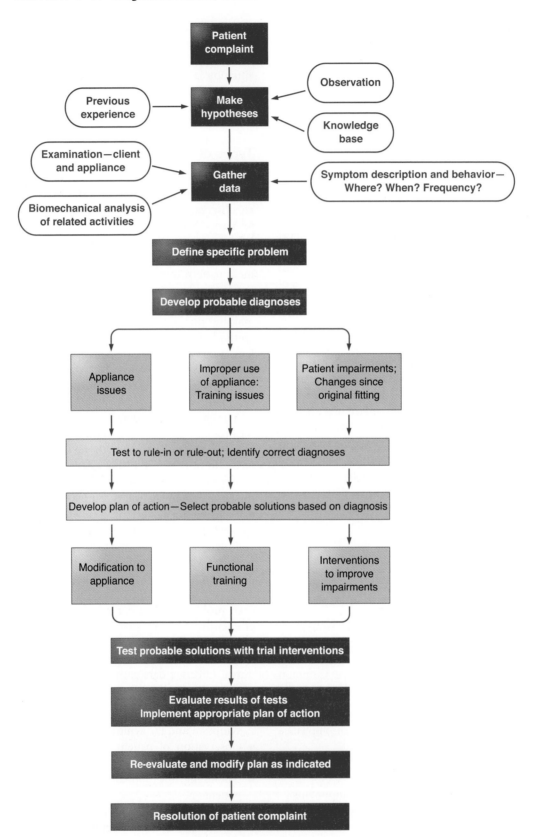

FIGURE 20.1. A clinical decision-making approach to resolve client problems.

Using a Clinical Decision-Making Algorithm for Prosthetic or Orthotic Problems

Figure 20.2 provides an example of the use of the decision-making algorithm depicted in Figure 20.1 to hypothesize probable causes, diagnose the specific cause, and find relevant solutions for Ms. Lukas, one of the case study clients described at the beginning of this chapter. Ms. Lukas's AFOs were prescribed to stabilize her ankles and prevent equinovarus deformities, which often develop in individuals with Charcot-Marie-Tooth neuropathy. Although she has been wearing and caring for her orthoses daily as prescribed, she comes to physical therapy at this time with the common complaint of, "my knees hurt when I walk." This patient complaint, as is often the case, is general and vague and provides little useful guidance to the clinician to perform an examination to gather relevant data. Direct questioning to determine the specific nature and behavior of the complaint symptoms is necessary to help the clinician develop probable hypotheses. For example, careful questioning helped the clinician (see **Fig. 20.2**) to clarify the general complaint to a more specific description of the symptoms. By asking specific questions, the clinician clarified the patient's complaint: "It hurts on the front of both knees when I walk, as soon as I put weight on my feet. It also hurts when I do the steps foot-over-foot, particularly when I go down steps." This specific description of the pain and its behavior directs the clinician to focus on problems aggravated by weight-bearing that occur early during the stance phase of gait and other functional activities. Biomechanical analysis to reveal the kinematics and kinetics affecting the involved limbs at this specific part of function helps the clinician to identify possible sources and solutions for the problem. The process of gait and functional analyses are described in Chapters 2 and 7.

Once the patient complaint is clearly described, the next step is to develop hypotheses for probable sources or causes of the problem. Prosthetic and orthotic problems can be grouped into three major areas:

- Problems with the appliance and its components
- Problems related to patient impairment, such as limited joint range of motion (ROM), muscle strength or endurance, or changes in residual limb volume
- Problems related to how the client is using the device

Clinicians can avoid anchoring biases (cognitive dispositions to respond) by considering possible problems in each of these three categories that are consistent with the specific symptoms presented by the patient. Because functional problems rarely fall into just one category, clinicians must be open to the possibility that a combination of issues contributes to the patient complaint. Clinicians may need to address a problem with interventions that include a modification to the device as well as therapeutic activities to reduce patient impairment or improve how the individual uses the device. Some problems may be resolved with a simple modification to the device or how it is used; however, often multiple or incremental adjustments are required to achieve the optimal functional outcome. Therapists must provide follow-up reassessments and maintain communication with the patient and prosthetist or orthotist until the best possible resolution is achieved and the client is satisfied and able to function at his or her highest level.

Clinicians work with clients using a wide range of prosthetic and orthotic devices that are fabricated from various designs, components, and materials. Thus, learning lengthy lists of possible problems for specific devices with particular componentry is not practical or effective. Clinicians must learn to recognize patterns of biomechanical and neuromuscular problems regardless of the specific appliances used by a particular client. Development of this generalizable skill allows practitioners to identify problems in many different clients, regardless of the specific devices used, including prostheses, orthoses, casts, and specialized shoes. **Table 20.1** provides an example of using this general but systematic approach to identify gait problems commonly experienced by orthotic users and the associated solutions. The table is not intended to be inclusive of all possible gait problems but was developed to illustrate the process. The solutions listed in the table would be implemented differently for different individuals, depending on the specific components and design of their device. **Table 20.2** illustrates an example of the use of this process to identify biomechanical solutions to other functional activities, such as ascending and descending steps. A sound understanding and application of this process will allow practitioners to find effective biomechanical solutions for patient problems, even when new materials and components are developed and used in appliance designs of the future.

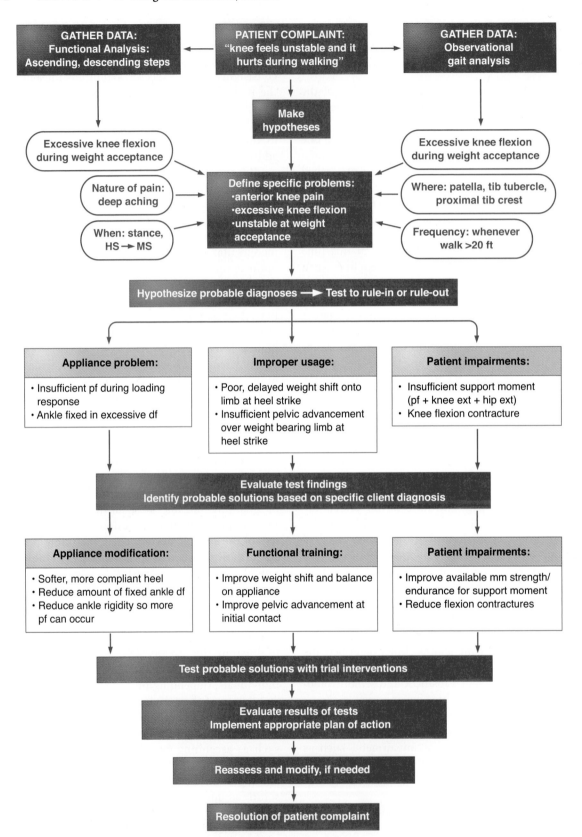

FIGURE 20.2. Application of a clinical decision-making algorithm (see Fig. 20.1) to resolve Ms. Lukas's (case study) complaint of "my knee hurts when I walk." (HS, heel strike; MS, midstance; mm, muscle).

TABLE 20.1	A Systematic Approach to Diagnose Common Orthotic Gait Problems (See Chapter 8 for Prosthetic Problems)			
Problem Functional Activity	**Problem Observed**	**Type of Problem**	**Possible Causes of the Problem (Hypotheses)**	**Corresponding Solutions**
Gait: Stance phase, Weight acceptance to Mid-stance	Excessive knee extension	Appliance problems	• Excessive or too rapid plantarflexion • Ankle fixed in excessive plantarflexion	• Stiffer, less compliant heel • Reduce amount of fixed plantarflexion angle • Use heel lift
		Improper usage, training issues	• Poor weight-shift onto limb • Insufficient pelvic advancement at initial contact	• Weight-shift training • Gait training
		Patient impairments	• Poor hip, trunk control → pelvic retraction • Hip flexion contracture	• Muscle strength, endurance exercise • Stretching exercise
Gait: Mid- to late stance	Excessive knee flexion	Appliance problems	• Ankle fixed in excessive dorsiflexion • "Toe break" occurs too early	• Reduce fixed ankle dorsiflexion angle • Lower heel height • Functionally lengthen foot lever using orthosis with longer footplate)
		Improper usage, training issues	• Insufficient support moment (plantarflexion + knee extension + hip extension)	• Training to improve muscle usage in available components of support moment
		Patient impairments	• Knee flexion contracture • Muscle weakness	• Exercise to increase muscle/capsular length • Muscle strengthening exercise

Continued

TABLE 20.1	A Systematic Approach to Diagnose Common Orthotic Gait Problems (See Chapter 8 for Prosthetic Problems)—cont'd			
Problem Functional Activity	Problem Observed	Type of Problem	Possible Causes of the Problem (Hypotheses)	Corresponding Solutions
Gait: Mid- to late stance (cont'd)	Excessive knee extension	Appliance problems	• Excessive fixed ankle plantarflexion • "Toe break" occurs too late in stance	• Reduce amount of fixed ankle plantarflexion angle • Raise heel height; heel lift • Use orthotic foot plate that is no longer than three-quarter length • Add forefoot rocker to shoe
		Improper usage, training issues	• Insufficient forward rotation of tibia during stance; pelvic retraction	• Gait training for pelvic advance during stance
		Patient impairments	• Insufficient support moment	• Exercise to improve muscle strength, endurance of available components of support moment
Gait: Terminal stance	Insufficient push-off	Appliance problems	• Fixed orthotic ankle joint (no movement)	• Shoe with rocker sole
		Improper usage, training issues	• Short sound-side step length	• Gait training to increase step length, improve pelvic advancement and rollover
		Patient impairments	• Weak plantarflexor muscles	• Dynamic response materials or components in the device

TABLE 20.2	A Systematic Approach to Diagnose Problems During a Functional Activity in Users of Orthotic Devices (See Chapter 8 for Prosthetic Problems)			
Problem Functional Activity	Problem Observed	Type of Problem	Possible Causes of the Problem (Hypotheses)	Corresponding Solutions
Ascending steps: Foot-over-foot method	Difficulty shifting weight onto advancing (higher) limb	Appliance problems	• Insufficient dorsiflexion, knee flexion, or hip flexion passive range of motion (PROM) available from the appliance	• Reduce appliance ankle rigidity to allow more dorsiflexion • Use step-to pattern, leading with limb with greater ankle/ knee ROM
		Improper usage; training issues	• Poor weight-shift	• Functional training
		Patient impairments	• Insufficient dorsiflexion, knee flexion PROM • Insufficient strength to lift body weight	• Stretching exercises • Strengthening exercise • Use step-to pattern, leading with stronger leg • Use railing
Descending steps: Foot-over-foot method	Difficulty shifting weight onto the advancing (lower) limb	Appliance problems	• Insufficient dorsiflexion, knee flexion PROM of limb on higher step	• Reduce appliance ankle rigidity to allow more dorsiflexion
		Improper usage; training issues	• Improper positioning of foot on step	• Position foot with limited dorsiflexion with mid/forefoot extending over edge of step so foot can roll over edge of step without dorsiflexion
		Patient impairments	• Insufficient strength to lower body weight • Insufficient ankle dorsiflexion or knee PROM	• Strengthening exercise • Use railing • Use step-to pattern, leading with weaker leg • Ankle stretching exercise

Box 20.1 illustrates the use of this clinical decision-making process for Janice Simmons. It is important for all clients who use appliances to expect some problems with their devices from time to time. To prevent problems from developing or to minimize their effect, clients should arrange for regular follow-up evaluations by attending prosthetic or orthotic clinics or visiting their prosthetist, orthotist, or physical therapist at appropriate time intervals.

APPLIANCE–ANATOMY INTERACTIONS

As has been indicated throughout the book, there is a dynamic interaction between the client's body and the appliance during functional activities. However, many devices not only affect the parts of the body to which they are directly applied, but also affect other joints and regions of the body. When patients complain of problems in other parts of the body beyond that directly affected by their device, practitioners must consider the device as a possible cause in addition to other hypotheses. Conversely, abnormal movement patterns in parts of the body outside the appliance may also affect how the prosthesis or orthosis functions. The effect of the "limb appliance unit" on the rest of the body is most obvious when the appliance is used in closed-chain conditions. For instance, fixing the ankle in a particular position during weight-bearing activities such as walking and climbing steps affects function not only at the ankle but also at the knee, hip, and trunk. Although most commonly observed in closed-chain conditions, this phenomenon can occur during open-chain activities as well. For example, the use of a wrist splint that holds the wrist in a fixed position also alters the kinematics of the shoulder and elbow.[8] Thus, a client who also has shoulder impairments and is unable to adopt the altered shoulder movements imposed by the wrist splint will most likely abandon use of even a very well-fitted wrist device. Clinicians who prescribe prostheses and orthoses and evaluate appliance problems must be aware of these unintended and possibly deleterious consequences of appliance use. Unexpected undesirable effects of the appliance on parts of the body beyond the device can lead to rejection of the appliance and a lower level of overall function.

Appliances with particular characteristics may be helpful and improve function in certain circumstances, while the same appliance may detract from or make function more difficult during other activities.

BOX 20.1 | The Clinical Decision-Making Process—How It Worked for Patient Janice Simmons

■ **Janice's complaint:** Pain in the left knee and back
■ **Therapist observation:** Left hip drops during stance
■ **Possible hypotheses for problem:**
   ▪ Her residual limb (RL) has shrunk, and she is dropping too far into the socket.
   ▪ The liner has worn and is too thin.
   ▪ She is wearing a shoe with a lower heel/sole than when she was fit for the prosthesis.
   ▪ She has developed hip or knee flexion contractures or lost strength since fitting (eg, she is less physically active as a receptionist than she was as a waitress).
■ **Specific problem (developed after questioning):** The knee and back pain only occur after she walks a while; knee pain is described as pressure at the lower border of the patella.
   ▪ Additional information: No changes were made since final checkout.
      ▫ She has not seen her prosthetist, even though she had an appointment.
      ▫ She still uses the same one-ply sock between liner and socket.
      ▫ She wears the same shoe she did at final checkout.

■ **Tests to rule in or rule out possible hypotheses:**
   ▪ Standing with weight equally on both legs, the left hip is lower than the right (the hips were level on final checkout 6 months ago).
   ▪ The RL is too far down in the socket; the patellar tendon is not at the level of the patellar bar.
   ▪ The shoe (same as at checkout) does not have excessive/abnormal wear.
   ▪ Hip/knee range of motion (ROM) and strength are the same as at final checkout.
■ **Clinical decision (diagnosis):** The most likely cause of her complaint is
   ▪ She has lost RL girth since fitting, causing the limb to slip too far into the socket. This explains the inferior patellar pain. The resultant apparent leg length discrepancy produces the back pain.
■ **Plan of care—interventions to resolve the problem:**
   ▪ Increase ply of sock between socket and liner
   ▪ Encourage patient to schedule follow-up visits with prosthetist or amputee clinic to prevent future problems

For example, an AFO with a rigid ankle fixed in a few degrees of plantarflexion prescribed to enhance stance phase knee extension and prevent knee buckling may improve a patient's ability to walk independently. However, because the rigid ankle restricts ankle dorsiflexion, the patient may have more difficulty with tasks that require dorsiflexion, such as standing up from a seated position or descending steps. In fact, a client may require more assistance to perform these tasks with the orthosis than without it. Clinicians must consider the effects of an appliance on all parts of the body during all the functional activities that are required and important to the client. Prosthetic and orthotic devices must be prescribed and modified to maximize function in all activities that are important for each individual.

Table 20.3 illustrates examples of commonly prescribed prosthetic or orthotic controls and the

TABLE 20.3	Selected Examples of Primary and Secondary Effects of Orthotic/Prosthetic Joint Positioning and Controls		
Joint	**Primary Control Exerted by Appliance**	**Effects on Other Joints or Body Regions (Secondary Effects)**	**Possible Effects on Function**
Ankle	Positioning in plantarflexion with restricted dorsiflexion	• Knee extension position and moment • Hip, trunk flexion • Pelvic retraction	• Enhances knee stability in stance • May produce knee hyperextension • Difficulty rising from chair • Difficulty on steps, foot-over-foot • Difficulty walking up incline
	Positioning in dorsiflexion with restricted plantarflexion	• Knee flexion position and moment • With free knee • Hip flexion • Pelvic retraction in late stance • With locked, extended knee • Hip extension, trunk extension • No push-off	• Prevents knee hyperextension • Difficulty descending incline • May produce midstance knee instability, buckling, drop-off • Shorter contralateral step length
Knee	Locked in extension or delayed, restricted knee flexion	• Shorter contralateral step length • Difficulty producing and clearing foot for swing • Increased hip abduction • Increased lateral trunk movement	• Prevents weight-bearing knee buckling • Reduces gait speed • Increased energy expenditure • On steps, unilateral device requires step-to pattern • On steps, bilateral devices very difficult or impossible • Difficulty sitting down, rising • Difficulty ascending, descending inclines
Hip	Flexed positioning	• Anterior pelvic tilt • Trunk hyperextension • Pelvic retraction	• Short step length • Difficulty initiating normal swing
	Extension lock with restricted hip flexion	• Unable to use reciprocal gait if bilateral • Excessive trunk and pelvic movement	• Prevents unwanted hip flexion • Difficulty sitting down, rising • Difficult or impossible to ascend, descend steps • Difficult, if not impossible, to ascend, descend inclines

secondary effects imposed on other joints or body regions not directly affected by the appliance. Examples of both positive and negative impact on function are also provided. Clinicians and clients must recognize that many components used in prosthetic and orthotic devices produce both positive and negative effects on function. Working together, clients, prosthetists or orthotists, and therapists must use this information to find optimal and individualized solutions to appliance problems that maximize client function and satisfaction.

SUMMARY

Clients who use prosthetic or orthotic devices often develop problems at some point, even when their devices are carefully prescribed and evaluated on delivery and when the wearer receives appropriate training and properly cares for the device after it is received. Therapists, working collaboratively with prosthetists or orthotists and other health-care providers, must employ hypothetico-deductive reasoning in a systematic clinical decision-making process to diagnose the source or sources of the problem and find appropriate solutions. Experienced clinicians may use pattern recognition to diagnose problems; however, care must be taken to avoid cognitive dispositions to respond (biases), such as anchoring and confirmation biases. Patient complaints about their appliances may arise from problems with the device, client physical impairments, such as changes in the client's ROM, strength, or limb volume, or problems in how the client is using the device. Therapists must consider all hypotheses that are consistent with the client's specific presentation of symptoms and test each appropriately to rule it in or out. Accurate diagnosis of the cause of a patient complaint or problem is required to effect an appropriate and efficient plan of care to resolve the problem.

KEYWORDS FOR LITERATURE SEARCH

Clinical Decision Making
  Forward reasoning
  Backward reasoning
  Diagnoses in prosthetics
  Diagnoses in orthotics
  Clinical reasoning

REFERENCES

1. May BJ, Dennis JK: Expert decision making in physical therapy: a survey of. Phys Ther 71:190–206, 1991.
2. Jensen GM, Shepard KF, Hack LM: The novice versus the experienced clinician: insights into the work of the physical therapist. Phys Ther 70:314–323, 1990.
3. Patel VL, Kaufman D, Magder S: The acquisition of medical expertise in complex environments. In Ericsson KA (ed): The road to excellence. Hillsdale, NJ, Lawrence Erlbaum Associates,1996, pp 127–165.
4. Edwards I, Jones M, Carr J, Braunack-Mayer A, Jensen GM: Clinical reasoning strategies in physical therapy. Phys Ther 84:312–330, 2004.
5. Thomas-Edding D: Clinical problem solving in physical therapy and its implication for curriculum development. In Proceedings of the 10th International Congress of the World Confederation for Physical Therapy; May 17–22, 1987; Sydney, Australia. Pages 10G#104.
6. Croskerry P: The importance of cognitive errors in diagnosis and strategies to minimize them. Acad Med 78:775–780, 2003.
7. Croskerry P: The theory and practice of clinical decision-making. Can J Anesth 52:R1, 2005.
8. Chan WYY, Chapparo C: Effect of wrist immobilization on upper limb occupational performance of elderly males. In Chapparo C, Ranka J (eds): Occupational performance model (Australia), Monograph 1, Occupational Performance Network, University of Sydney, Australia, 1997, pp 83–94.

Accommodative foot orthoses Soft or semirigid orthoses designed to have little effect on foot function while providing protection or relief to particular painful or pressure sensitive areas or structures of the foot.

Adjustable positioning orthotic joints Movable single-axis hip joints with additional componentry that allows the orthotist to position the thigh in positions other than frontal and transverse plane neutral.

Alignment stability Stance phase knee extension stability created by aligning the prosthetic or orthotic knee joint posterior to the gravity line or ground reaction force vector.

Amputation The surgical removal of a limb or body part. In this text, the term is used to refer to the removal or absence of a limb.

Anchoring (in clinical reasoning) A cognitive error in the diagnostic process; locking into a particular diagnosis too early and failing to properly consider other plausible alternatives.

Angulation osteotomy A surgical procedure for a medium or long residual humerus where the distal part of the bone is angled and pinned in place to provide an area for socket suspension.

Ankle disarticulation Amputation through the ankle. May also be known as a *Symes amputation*.

Assist An orthotic component or design that produces a force to aid a designated joint motion. For example, a dorsiflexion assist is an orthotic component or design that provides a force to aid dorsiflexion.

Autograft Tissue transplanted from one part of the body to another in the same individual.

Biomechanical analysis The process of methodical observation of a client performing an activity, breaking it into component parts, comparing the movements in each component to typical or effective movement, and identifying the impairments or abnormalities that may limit or restrict the individual's ability to perform the activity.

Bivalved An orthosis or cast that is cut into halves, usually resulting in a front and a back component, with openings on the sides.

Blucher An oxford shoe throat style in which the vamp (the upper) and tongue are made from one piece of material and the quarters lap over the vamp and are free distally. This style is preferred for use with most orthoses because it provides greater adjustability and is generally easier to don and doff.

Body image Each individual's concept of his or her own body as an object in and bound by space independently and apart from all other objects.

Body jacket A total contact molded plastic trunk orthosis, which may be trimmed as a lumbosacral (LSO) or a thoracolumbosacral (TLSO) orthosis.

Body powered A prosthesis in which the force for operating the prosthetic components comes from a motion of the body.

Body sock A garment like a tightly fitting T-shirt that is specially made to fit under spinal orthoses to protect the skin.

Bulbous A term to describe the shape of a residual limb that has a rounded distal end that is larger than the proximal part.

Cauterization Destruction of tissue by burning or freezing; burning was used to close wounds in early days.

Charcot-Marie-Tooth disease A hereditary motor and sensory peripheral neuropathy that primarily affects the lower leg muscles, resulting in gait abnormalities and foot deformities.

Charcot neuroarthropathy A progressive and destructive condition that can occur in individuals with neuropathy. It is characterized by pathological fractures, usually in the foot that produce varying degrees of deformity and functional changes.

Chronic pain Consistent or episodic pain that persists for at least 6 months or more and exceeds the typical amount of time required for healing following an injury or illness.

Compliance A material property that describes a material's ability to yield to pressure or an applied force; following medical orders.

Components The parts of a prosthesis or an orthosis.

Composite plastics Thermoplastics or thermosets that contain glass, carbon (graphite), or other types of fibers, which makes the material stronger than plastic alone.

Confirmation bias (in clinical reasoning) A tendency to look for data that will confirm a particular preliminary hypothesis, while not seeking or ignoring disconfirming evidence.

Conical A residual limb that is smaller circumferentially at the distal end than at the proximal end.

Control strap (varus or valgus) A strap attached to the ankle of an orthosis to restrain unwanted varus or valgus positioning at the ankle. Also called a *T-strap* when used with conventional double upright AFOs.

Conventional orthoses Orthoses constructed from metal componentry with leather or fabric padding and strapping.

Counter A reinforcement of the posterior aspect of a shoe's quarters that cups the heel and stabilizes the hindfoot.

Custom-made orthoses Orthoses individually manufactured and fit for a particular individual by an orthotist or therapist.

Deformational plagiocephaly A condition in which an infant's head is asymmetrically shaped, usually with a flattened surface, caused by mechanical deformation from a sustained posture or position.

Disarticulation Amputation through a joint.

Doff (doffing) To remove or take something off, such as a prosthetic or orthotic appliance or an article of clothing.

Don (donning) To put something on, such as a prosthetic or orthotic appliance or an article of clothing.

Durometer A number (Shore number) that measures the firmness (hardness) of a material. High durometer materials are firm; low durometer materials are softer and more compressible.

Dynamic alignment In a prosthesis, the slight adjustment of foot or knee component in relationship to the socket to provide the client with an optimum gait. Can only be done after the client has learned how to walk with the prosthesis.

Dynamic splint A splint that imparts forces to a target joint to substitute for a weak or paralyzed muscle, to replace muscle contraction to protect a healing tendon, or to apply low load prolonged stresses to increase tissue length.

Dyslipidemia A disturbance of the lipids in the blood, usually too many lipids.

Elastomer A polymer or chemical compound with elastic properties.

Endoprosthetic device Prosthetic device inserted within the body.

Endoskeletal A type of prosthesis that contains a lightweight metal tube that connects the foot to the socket of the prosthesis. The tube may be covered by a soft foam cover that matches the color and configuration of the other leg.

Exoskeletal A type of prosthesis constructed from wood or rigid polyurethane covered with a rigid plastic lamination that connects the foot of the prosthesis to the socket.

External forces Forces that originate from sources outside of the body, such as gravity, the ground reaction force vector, and forces applied by prosthetic and orthotic devices.

External moment The rotation produced when external forces are applied at a distance from the axis of rotation.

Flaps A piece of partially detached tissue, usually including skin and underlying muscles and vessels.

Force A push or a pull exerted by one object on another.

Force couple A pair of parallel forces applied in opposite directions to a rigid segment at different points that produce rotation. Force couples are used in orthoses to control joints or limb segments.

Free motion joint An orthotic joint that does not contain any mechanical stops or restrictions to movement.

Functional analysis The process in which a clinician observes a client performing a functional activity, breaks the activity into component parts, compares the movements in each component to "typical" or effective movement, and identifies impairments that limit or restrict the overall function.

Functional electrical stimulation (FES) orthosis This type of orthosis provides microprocessor controlled trains of electrical stimulation to selected paralyzed muscles or peripheral nerves to produce muscle contractions in a pattern that allows ambulation when applied to the lower extremity or grasp and release when applied to the upper extremity. An FES orthosis is also called a neuroprosthesis.

Functional foot orthosis A rigid or semirigid foot orthosis designed to control the movements of the subtalor joint and support the rear and forefoot during walking or running to minimize the need for compensatory foot movements that may overstress soft tissue structures.

Functional knee orthosis A knee orthosis (KO) used by individuals with ligament instabilities at the knee to provide support and limit motions that may stress the injured ligament.

Functional limitations (also called *activity limitations*) Limitation in the ability of an individual to perform a task or activity, such as basic activities of daily living (eg, walking, climbing steps, or dressing).

Furuncle A boil.

Gait cycle The period between heel contact of one foot and the next heel contact of the same foot. It includes periods of single support stance, double support stance and swing for each leg.

Ground reaction ankle–foot orthosis (GR-AFO) A ground reaction or floor reaction AFO exerts control at the knee without orthotic componentry that crosses (or covers) the knee joint. Positioning the ankle in slight plantarflexion with a dorsiflexion stop produces an extension moment at the knee by positioning the ground reaction force vector (GRFV) anterior to the knee axis. Positioning the ankle in slight dorsiflexion with a plantarflexion stop produces a flexion moment at the knee by positioning the GRFV posterior to the knee axis.

Ground reaction force vector (GRFV) The composite or resultant force vector that represents the magnitude and direction of the force applied to the foot (or feet) by the ground or floor. It is visualized as the line connecting the body's center of mass (CoM) and the point of contact (center of pressure) of the foot with the ground.

Haptic Refers to technology that interfaces to the user via the sense of touch by applying forces, vibrations, and motions to the user. This mechanical stimulation may be used to assist in the creation of virtual objects, for control of such virtual objects, and to enhance the remote control of devices.

Harnessing Refers to the straps of the prosthesis that go around the upper arm and shoulder to provide suspension and power.

Heel lever arm The distance from the end of the prosthetic heel to midpoint of the prosthetic foot.

Hip disarticulation Total removal of the lower extremity by amputation through the hip joint.

Hip spica cast A cast used to immobilize the hip in a particular position. It usually extends from the mid-chest to below the knee. If the problem is with both hips, it extends past both knees; if the problem is on one side, the cast extends below one knee. A hole is left in the groin area to allow for toileting.

Hybrid orthoses Orthoses that are constructed with both molded components and metal or plastic articulated joints.

Hypothetico-deductive system of decision-making An analytical process used to make a diagnosis or decision by generating, testing, and refining possible hypotheses to identify the most likely best diagnosis or decision.

Ilizarov's technique A surgical technique used for limb lengthening based on the principle of distraction osteogenesis (osteo for bone, genesis for formation).

Impairments Problems or abnormalities of body structure (anatomy) or function (physiology), including mental functions.

Internal forces The forces produced by sources within the body, such as muscle contraction, and the viscoelasticity of connective tissues, such as joint capsules and ligaments.

Internal moments The rotation produced when internal forces, such as those produced by muscle contraction and ligaments, are applied at a distance from the axis of rotation. Generally, they offset the effect of *external moments* that are generated by gravity and ground reaction forces.

Kinematics A description of movement in terms of displacement, velocity, and acceleration.

Kinetics The forces, moments, and power produced during movements.

Last A real or virtual model or "statue" of a foot from which a shoe is constructed. The last determines the shoe size, shape, and fit.

Limited motion joint An orthotic or prosthetic joint that has either a flexion or extension stop or both that restricts the joint's motion when the appliance is worn.

Line of gravity The line from an object's center of mass (CoM) to the center of the earth. For the human body, the CoM is just anterior to the second sacral vertebra; also called the gravity line.

Metatarsal ray amputation Removal of one metatarsal and attached digit.

Molded orthoses Orthoses constructed from thermoplastics, thermosetting plastics, or composite materials which are formed by heating the material and molding it over a model of the body part to be braced.

Moment The result of force application at a distance from the rotation center. It is measured as torque or angular motion.

Moment arm The distance between the axis of rotation and the line of action of the force on a body.

Motivation Factors that cause an individual to act toward a particular goal or objective, usually toward a satisfying outcome.

Myodesis The anchoring of muscles to bone when closing an amputation.

Myoelectric prostheses Prostheses operated by electrical impulses generated by muscle actions that are detected by skin electrodes and amplified to power an electric motor.

Myoelectric tester A device used to determine the electric potential generated by various muscles in the residual limb and to assist in selecting sites for myoelectric controls.

Myoplasty Suturing posterior and anterior compartment muscles together over the end of the bone in an amputation.

Negative cast A mold or impression of a limb or body part, usually made by wrapping it in a thin layer of plaster or another type of casting material. A negative cast is used to construct a positive cast of the limb or body part.

Neuroma Any type of tumor composed of nerve cells identified by the specific part of the nerve that is involved. Amputation neuroma is formed by the cut ends of peripheral nerves.

Off-loading Techniques used to reduce plantar pressures to assist in healing plantar foot ulcers.

Orthoses Externally applied devices that apply forces to the body to achieve functional and therapeutic goals, including providing assistance, correction, support, or compensation for impairments related to neuromusculoskeletal disorders or acquired conditions.

Orthotic checkout examination The systematic process of examination of an orthosis both on and off its wearer to ensure proper orthotic fit, function, comfort, and cosmesis. An orthotic checkout examination must be completed on a new orthosis prior to beginning functional training with the orthosis.

Orthotic lock An orthotic component that may be prescribed as part of an orthosis. When engaged, it locks or holds the braced joint in a predetermined position and prevents all movement. When the lock is disengaged, free joint movement is permitted.

Orthotist An individual who makes, adjusts, or fits orthoses. An orthotist who has completed a prescribed course of study and passes a certifying examination uses the initials CO (certified orthotist).

Patellar tendon–bearing ankle–foot orthosis (PTB-AFO) An ankle–foot orthosis that has a molded proximal brim that simulates a patellar tendon–bearing prosthetic socket. This orthosis was originally designed as a fracture brace to partially unload the distal tibia, ankle, and foot.

Patency A state of being open.

Pedorthists Professionals who fit and dispense foot orthoses, shoes, and shoe modifications according to prescription.

Pelvic band An orthotic or prosthetic component that may be prescribed to control the hip joint. It extends between the greater trochanter and the iliac crest, attaches to the orthotic hip joint, and may be unilateral or bilateral. On a prosthesis, it is made of leather and metal, attaches to the lateral proximal border of the prosthetic socket, and fits around the patient's hips. It incorporates a single-axis joint that permits flexion and extension.

Phantom pain Painful sensations related to the part of the body that has been amputated.

Phantom sensation The feeling of a limb or body part that is no longer part of the body.

Pistoning The dropping of the prosthesis away from the residual limb during swing phase of gait. Usually occurs with inadequate suspension.

Plastic A synthetic organic polymer.

Polycentric knee joint In orthotics: An orthotic knee joint designed so its axis of rotation moves during knee flexion and extension to align the orthotic axis with the anatomical axis during swing phase.

In prosthetics: A knee mechanism that provides multiple axes of rotation as the knee flexes and extends during swing phase.

Positive cast A three-dimensional model of the limb or body part on which an orthosis or prosthesis is formed. The positive cast is made by filling the negative mold with plaster of Paris or another material.

Post A wedge of material added to the base of a foot orthosis or a footplate to balance or support a particular region of the foot.

Posterior leaf spring ankle–foot orthosis (PLS-AFO) A type of posterior calf shell molded AFO that is flexible and provides swing phase dorsiflexion assist, but no stance phase control.

Prefabricated orthoses Orthoses that are not manufactured for a particular individual but are usually mass produced for the general population using typical sizing for "average" individuals.

Preorthotic prescription examination Client examination performed to gather the information required to make an orthotic prescription. Examination findings are used to identify the client's functional abilities and limitations as well the impairments that contribute to the client's functional problems.

Pressure The force (F) per surface area (a) of application (P = F/a). Units are pounds per square inch, Pascals or newtons per square meter.

Prosthesis Artificial replacement of a body part.

Prosthetist An individual who makes artificial limbs for the upper or lower extremities. A prosthetist who has completed a prescribed course of study and passed a certifying examination uses the initials CP (certified prosthetist).

Protective sensation The ability to perceive the pressure stimulus of the 5.07 (10 gram) Semmes Weinstein monofilament over the plantar surface of the foot or a vibratory threshold of 30 to 40 volts using a biothesiometer; although impaired, this level of sensory perception is usually sufficient to allow individuals to perceive harmful pressure or loading that may lead to plantar ulceration.

Pylon Metal pipe connecting the prosthetic socket to the foot.

Quarters The part of the upper of a shoe that covers the sides and back of the foot.

Reciprocal orthotic hip joints The type of orthotic hip joints on reciprocal gait orthoses (RGOs). These hip joints are linked by cables or another mechanism to facilitate a reciprocal gait. When the wearer advances one leg, the coupled hip mechanism facilitates concurrent extension of the contralateral hip.

Rehabilitative knee orthosis A knee orthosis (KO) with an adjustable dial lock that is most often used temporarily during the postsurgical period to limit knee range of motion (ROM) to protect healing tissues.

Relief A built-up area (pad or added material) or a concavity (area of reduced material) in an orthosis or prosthesis that offloads a painful or pressure-sensitive area by shifting pressure onto more pressure tolerant structures.

Residual limb The part of the amputated limb remaining after amputation.

Resting splint A static splint that supports the joints within the splint in a nonstressful position.

Revascularization Reestablishing patency of circulation to a part.

Rigid orthoses Orthoses made from molded polyethylene, polypropylene, or other type of rigid plastic or composite material.

Rocker sole A curved external shoe sole modification that allows the foot to roll from heel strike to toe-off without requiring the foot to bend. It is used to relieve pressure from the metatarsal heads or to substitute for ankle or toe motion during gait.

Rotationplasty An operative procedure where a portion of a limb is removed while the remaining limb below the involved portion is rotated and reattached.

Self-concept A person's view of himself or herself.

Serial static splint or cast A type of static splint or cast that provides end-range low-load prolonged stresses to increase range of motion (ROM). Involves making a series of new splints or casts to maintain end-range positioning as ROM increases.

Shank (prosthetic) The part of the prosthesis corresponding to the lower leg of the unamputated limb, or the part that connects the foot to the socket (transtibial) or knee unit (transfemoral). The shank includes the pylon and cosmetic cover of the endoskeletal prosthesis and is the finished part of the exoskeletal prosthesis.

Shank (shoe) A longitudinal reinforcement of the midsole of a nonathletic shoe, typically made of spring steel or carbon fiber that extends from the heel to just proximal of the metatarsal heads and determines where the sole flexes during late stance phase.

Shoe modifications Additional materials added to the inside (internal modifications) or outsole (external modifications) of a shoe to accomplish specific therapeutic goals.

Shrinker A sock-like garment made of elasticized material used to reduce edema in a residual limb.

Single-axis joint A mechanical joint that allows movement only in the sagittal plane.

Socket Prosthetic component into which the residual limb is inserted.

Soft spinal orthoses Orthoses made from fabric, elastic, or synthetic materials that are flexible and exert no forces other than compression. These include corsets, belts, and binders for the trunk and soft foam cervical collars that wrap around the neck.

Solid ankle ankle–foot orthosis (SA-AFO) A type of posterior calf shell molded ankle–foot orthosis that is very rigid and stops all motion in all directions at the ankle.

Splint A term for a device that applies external forces to a body part. The term *splint* is interchangeable with and equivalent to the words *orthosis, brace,* and *support.*

Splint Classification System terminology Function-based terminology used to name upper extremity orthoses.

Stance control orthosis or prosthesis In orthotics: A knee–ankle–foot orthosis (KAFO) with a special knee mechanism that engages its knee lock during stance phase only and disengages it for swing phase.

In prosthetics: a weight activated knee mechanism that remains in extension at the moment of heel contact even if the knee is not fully extended. It usually only activates if the knee mechanism is flexed less that 20 degrees. Some hydraulic and microprocessor-controlled stance control knee mechanisms also provide flexion resistance.

Standing frames Orthotic devices that support static standing which are used with paraplegic individuals to enable weight-bearing through the legs.

Static alignment Placing the prosthetic components in proper relationship to each other in the standing position. The socket, knee component (if used), and foot are placed to duplicate the trochanter, knee, and ankle relationships of the nonamputated leg.

Static progressive A type of static splint that provides end-range low-load prolonged stresses to increase range of motion (ROM). Requires a splint that has the ability to adjust the position of the target joint, so that end range position is maintained as ROM increases.

Static splint A splint that holds a body part in a fixed position.

Stirrup orthosis An ankle orthosis that restricts motion at the subtalar joint but allows plantarflexion and dorsiflexion, which is typically used in the management of lateral ankle sprains

Stop An orthotic component or design that stops joint motion at a predetermined position and prevents joint movement beyond the orthotic stop. Orthotic stops are available for all joints and are named for the movement that is restricted (eg, a plantarflexion stop restricts ankle plantarflexion).

Stump sock A cotton or wool sock designed to fit over the residual limb and worn with the prosthesis or liner.

Subaponeurotic Lying beneath the fibrous membrane or fascia that binds the foot muscles and tendons together.

Support moment The sum of all the sagittal plane internal moments acting at the hip, knee, and ankle during a gait cycle depicted so that extensor moments are positive.

Supracondylar ground reaction ankle–foot orthosis A ground reaction ankle–foot orthosis (GR-AFO) that encases the anterior and supracondylar area of the knee. Because it provides a longer lever arm and a larger contact area, it may be required for larger adults who use GR-AFOs to control knee buckling. This design mimics the shape of the supracondylar suprapatellar transtibial prosthetic socket.

Swivel walker A special type of standing frame with adapted shoe plates which allows the user to ambulate by rocking from side to side and to advance by pivoting.

Terminal device Part of an upper extremity prosthesis that replaces the hand. The terminal device may be an artificial hand or hook.

Therapeutic ambulation Part-time walking for the purpose of exercise and to reduce the health risks of wheelchair sitting. Individuals who perform therapeutic ambulation use a wheelchair for functional mobility.

Thermoplastic A plastic that is solid at room temperature but becomes malleable when heated. These materials can be reheated and reshaped.

Thermosetting plastic A plastic resin that is liquid and hardens or cures when mixed with an appropriate catalyst and promoter. These plastics, once formed, cannot be heated and reshaped.

Three-point bending (counterforce) system A system of three forces that work together to control rotation at an axis. It includes a middle force located close to the axis and two end forces that are opposite in direction to the middle force and are applied at a distance from the axis.

Throat The opening of a shoe, formed by the distal part of the quarters, where the foot enters and where the shoe closures attach.

TKA line A line drawn in the sagittal plane from the greater trochanter, through the knee axis, to the middle of the ankle. Used to align the parts of the prosthesis.

Toe lever arm The distance from the middle of the prosthetic foot to the toe break.

Toe-off ankle–foot orthosis (TO-AFO) A type of anterior ankle–foot orthosis usually constructed from a carbon composite material that functions like a dynamic response prosthetic foot to support the foot for swing phase while it facilitates propulsion during stance phase push-off.

Total contact A term used to describe a prosthesis or orthosis that is in contact with all parts of the enclosed body part and applies appropriate comfortable pressure.

Transfemoral Amputation through the femur.

Transmetatarsal Transverse amputation through the shafts of the metatarsals.

Transpelvic Amputation through the pelvis removing the ischium, pubic ramus, and lower pelvic elements.

Transtibial Amputation through the tibia.

Tricep pad Leather or plastic pad that fits over the tricep and has a housing for the terminal device cable for a body-powered transradial prosthesis.

Trunk orthoses Externally applied orthoses that apply forces to the thoracic and lumbosacral regions, including thoracolumbosacral (TLSOs), lumbosacral (LSOs), and sacroiliac (SI) belts or orthoses.

Voluntary closing (VC) Terminal device of an upper extremity prosthesis that closes by the action of the user and opens with relaxation of the movement. At rest, it is in the open position.

Voluntary knee control Stance phase stability of the transfemoral prosthesis which is controlled by the client's extension of the residual limb against the posterior wall of the socket.

Voluntary opening (VO) Terminal device of an upper extremity prosthesis that is opened by the action of the user and closes with relaxation of the movement. At rest, it is in the closed position.

INDEX

Note: Page numbers followed by "f" denote figures, "b" denote boxes, and "t" denote tables.